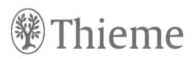

Endovascular Management of Ischemic Stroke

A Case-Based Approach

Vitor Mendes Pereira, MD, MSc
Professor of Radiology and Surgery
Division of Neuroradiology, Department of Medical Imaging
Division of Neurosurgery, Department of Surgery
St. Michael's Hospital, University of Toronto
Toronto, Ontario, Canada

Adam A. Dmytriw, MD, MPH, MSc (Oxon), FRCPC
Neuroradiology & Neurointervention Services
Toronto Western Hospital, University of Toronto
Toronto, Ontario, Canada
Brigham and Women's Hospital, Harvard Medical School
Boston, Massachusetts, USA

Lee-Anne Slater, MBBS(Hons), FRANZCR, MMed, CCINR
Neurointerventional Radiology Monash Health
Monash University, Melbourne, Australia

Sarah Power, PhD, MRCPI, FFR(RCSI)
Consultant Interventional Neuroradiologist
Beaumont Hospital, Dublin, Ireland

Timo Krings, MD, PhD, FRCPC
Professor of Radiology and Surgery
Head, Division of Diagnostic and Interventional Neuroradiology
Joint Department of Medical Imaging of the University Health Network
David Braley and Nancy Gordon Chair of Interventional Neuroradiology
University of Toronto
Chief of Radiology, Toronto Western Hospital
Toronto, Ontario, Canada

239 illustrations

Thieme
New York • Stuttgart • Delhi • Rio de Janeiro

Library of Congress Cataloging-in-Publication Data

Names: Pereira, Vitor Mendes, editor. | Dmytriw, Adam A., editor. | Slater, Lee-Anne, editor. | Power, Sarah, 1976- editor. | Krings, Timo, editor.

Title: Endovascular management of ischemic stroke : a case-based approach / [edited by] Vitor Mendes Pereira, Adam A. Dmytriw, Lee-Anne Slater, Sarah Power, Timo Krings.

Description: New York : Thieme, 2021. | Includes bibliographical references and index. | Summary: "Stroke is the most prevalent cerebrovascular emergency, impacting an estimated 15 million people worldwide every year. Endovascular treatment (EVT) of ischemic stroke has expanded at an unforeseen pace, with EVT the most common neurointerventional procedure performed at most large centers. Endovascular Management of Ischemic Stroke: A Case-Based Approach by renowned stroke pioneer Vitor Mendes Pereira and distinguished co-editors features contributions from a "who's who" of global experts. This practical resource provides straightforward guidance for clinicians who need to learn and master state-of-the-art endovascular interventions reflecting the new, evidence-based treatment paradigm for acute stroke"– Provided by publisher.

Identifiers: LCCN 2021015383 (print) | LCCN 2021015384 (ebook) | ISBN 9781626232754 (paperback) | ISBN 9781626232761 (ebook)

Subjects: MESH: Ischemic Stroke–surgery | Endovascular Procedures–methods | Case Reports

Classification: LCC RC388.5 (print) | LCC RC388.5 (ebook) | NLM WL 356 | DDC 616.8/1–dc23

LC record available at https://lccn.loc.gov/2021015383

LC ebook record available at https://lccn.loc.gov/2021015384

Important note: Medicine is an ever-changing science undergoing continual development. Research and clinical experience are continually expanding our knowledge, in particular our knowledge of proper treatment and drug therapy. Insofar as this book mentions any dosage or application, readers may rest assured that the authors, editors, and publishers have made every effort to ensure that such references are in accordance with **the state of knowledge at the time of production of the book.**

Nevertheless, this does not involve, imply, or express any guarantee or responsibility on the part of the publishers in respect to any dosage instructions and forms of applications stated in the book. **Every user is requested to examine carefully** the manufacturers' leaflets accompanying each drug and to check, if necessary in consultation with a physician or specialist, whether the dosage schedules mentioned therein or the contraindications stated by the manufacturers differ from the statements made in the present book. Such examination is particularly important with drugs that are either rarely used or have been newly released on the market. Every dosage schedule or every form of application used is entirely at the user's own risk and responsibility. The authors and publishers request every user to report to the publishers any discrepancies or inaccuracies noticed. If errors in this work are found after publication, errata will be posted at www.thieme.com on the product description page.

Some of the product names, patents, and registered designs referred to in this book are in fact registered trademarks or proprietary names even though specific reference to this fact is not always made in the text. Therefore, the appearance of a name without designation as proprietary is not to be construed as a representation by the publisher that it is in the public domain.

Thieme Medical Publishers, Inc.
333 Seventh Avenue, 18th Floor
New York, NY 10001, USA
www.thieme.com
+1 800 782 3488, customerservice@thieme.com

Cover design: Thieme Publishing Group
Typesetting by DiTech Process Solutions, India

Printed in the USA by King Printing Company, Inc.   5 4 3 2 1

ISBN 978-1-62623-275-4

Also available as an e-book:
eISBN 978-1-62623-276-1

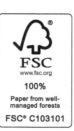

FSC
www.fsc.org
100%
Paper from well-managed forests
FSC® C103101

Dedicated to our patients

Contents

Foreword

There aren't too many times in the history of medicine where five trials in quick succession are published in the *New England Journal of Medicine* and are not only positive but demonstrate the massive treatment effect of endovascular thrombectomy (EVT) with NNTs of 2.5-7. In a subsequent meta-analysis, it is tough to find a sub-group of patients where the treatment is not effective. We, collectively, are at the pinnacle of evidence-based medicine. This is a great achievement for our field. It is also amazing for stroke patients.

However, with that achievement comes responsibility as well. We are now obligated to offer this highly efficacious treatment to all eligible patients at every hour of every day. Additionally, the treatment is a complex neurointerventional procedure. There is a massive amount of data supporting the notion of 'time is brain'. In addition, we know from the HERMES collaboration and other datasets that the quality of reperfusion is directly related to patient outcome.

Herein lies the problem: the field is expanding at an unforeseen pace (for most big centers, EVT is now the commonest neurointervention procedure); there is an expectation to provide the service at all times and additionally, open the vessel fast while keep the complication rate minimal. It is in this context that I admire the work put together by Vitor, Adam, Lee-Anne, Sarah, and Timo. They present an honest, logical approach to EVT. The examples cover the entire breadth of diversity of patient presentations, anatomical variations, intra-procedural problems and their solutions. The authors, of course, based on their previous work, have once again demonstrated exceptional knowledge of neuroanatomy and tools of the trade. The field is changing rapidly. Humans are very good at finding solutions once there is a clear demand, and here the demand is massive. There have been all kinds of innovations that have already happened from the time of the trials, and these are likely to continue for several more years. However, some things are going to remain relatively static: human anatomy, the stress of doing a complex procedure quickly, the artefacts and challenges of doing procedures when the patient is not still, the location of the occlusion, the interpretation of imaging. The principles of thrombectomy might slightly evolve but I suspect will largely be the same. Thus, while many may feel that the time span of such an endeavor as put together by this great team is somewhat limited, I do think that the contents of this book will provide useful information to facilitate continued efforts toward faster and better opening of vessels.

On a personal note, I have the good fortune of knowing the authors well. I do have a special connection to them as I also trained in Toronto, Canada. They are exceptional human beings committed to their patients, practicing medicine at the highest level and creating an environment conducive to innovation in training and education. I can personally vouch for Timo's teaching skills and make it a point to listen to him speak whenever I am presented with the opportunity.

Finally, I would like to congratulate the authors for putting in this immense effort to make this resource available to all of us. I have no doubt that many patients will benefit as we all spend the time to learn from their collective experience and wisdom.

Mayank Goyal, MD, FRCPC, FAHA, FCAR, FCAHS
Professor of Radiology and Clinical Neurosciences,
University of Calgary
Director, Imaging and Endovascular treatment,
Calgary Stroke Program
Calgary, Alberta, Canada

Preface

Four years since the publication of the book *Case-Based Interventional Neuroradiology*, and eight years since *Neurovascular Anatomy in Interventional Neuroradiology: A Case-Based Approach*, it is reasonable to proclaim that the specialty of neurointervention has arrived once again at a new and revolutionary epoch in its growth. While there have undoubtedly been numerous advances across the field such as flow-diversion for aneurysms, novel liquid embolics for shunts and many more innovations, the progress in the endovascular management of stroke will likely stand as a medical miracle of the 21st century.

From head to toe, it is the lot of the interventional community to take on the most challenging and hopeless cases which fail medical or surgical standard of care, and work to build techniques and evidence to prove that the interventionalist has something meaningful to contribute. Just as the management of hemorrhagic lesions became resoundingly endovascular after decades of hard work in research and development, and trials by the stalwart, so too has ischemic stroke followed suit.

In the dark days of numerous failed trials, the faithful remained convinced that the neurointerventional community would come to optimize our tools, patient selection, and workflow. With the invaluable insight of neurologists, who have become an essential part of a wonderful community, yet another standard of care has been placed in the neurointerventional stable.

With this growth comes a notable change in the nomenclature of our texts to *Endovascular Management of Ischemic Stroke* as we cement the series. While simultaneously acknowledging the incredible legacy of teachers, we must also recall that just as interventional radiologists have been responsible for developing cardiovascular (Palmaz, Judkins), cerebrovascular (Lasjaunias, Viñuela) and peripheral (Dotter, Seldinger) intervention, it was paradoxically neurologists (Moniz) and cardiologists (Cournand, Richards) who first sought to obtain diagnostic angiographic images. The common thread between these great individuals was a consuming passion to treat and discover. Pride in provenance and title is misplaced before the welfare of our patients, and our community is at its strongest when a diversity of skills is brought to bear on the devastating specter of ischemic disease.

This book in your hands has been thoughtfully prepared by a global effort of passionate and experienced neurointerventionalists. Herein, the reader will find all manner of scenarios in ischemic stroke, from the rudiments of setup and technique, to a gradual approach to increasingly challenging but realistic scenarios. The text is programmed to ensure the reader receives insight into situations that one is likely to encounter in one's practice. Lastly, we offer important differentials in stroke mimics and explore complications of thrombectomy as well.

We sincerely hope that this book will find a unique place in the educational armamentarium of the neurointerventional community at this critical time as we approach a new learning curve in the wake of a paradigm shift in management of the most prevalent cerebrovascular emergency.

Acknowledgments

We thank all the chapter contributors to this book, and, because the chain of stroke care is only as strong as its weakest link, we specially acknowledge the diagnostic radiologists, intensivists, neurologists, neurosurgeons, paramedics, emergency and primary care physicians, nurses, porters, imaging technologists, physiotherapists and rehabilitation specialists, occupational therapists, speech language pathologists, and dietitians among countless others with whom we have worked.

Contributors

Nimer Adeeb, MD
Department of Neurological Surgery
Ochsner-Louisiana State University Hospital
Shreveport, Louisiana

Farah K. Aleisa, MD
Stroke Neurology
Toronto Western Hospital
University of Toronto
Toronto, Ontario, Canada

Hamed Asadi, MD, PhD, FRANZCR, CCINR, EBIR, FCIRSE
The Florey Institute of Neuroscience and Mental Health
University of Melbourne
School of Medicine, Faculty of Health
Deakin University
Consultant Interventional Neuroradiologist
Austin Health, Monash Health, and St Vincent's Hospital
Melbourne, Australia

Aditya Bharatha, MD, FRCPC
Diagnostic and Interventional Neuroradiology
Deputy Chief of Medical Imaging and Division Head,
    Diagnostic Neuroradiology
St. Michael's Hospital
Associate Professor
Depts. of Medical Imaging and Surgery (Div. of
    Neurosurgery)
University of Toronto
Toronto, Ontario, Canada

Waleed Brinjikji, MD
Associate Professor of Neurosurgery and Radiology
Mayo Clinic
Rochester, Minnesota

Ronil V. Chandra, MBBS, MMed, FRANZCR
Associate Professor of Radiology
Head of Neurointerventional Radiology, Monash Health
School of Clinical Sciences, Monash University
Melbourne, Australia

M. Imran Chaudry, MD
Professor
University of South Carolina School of Medicine
Greenville, South Carolina
Prisma Health - Upstate
Greenville, South Carolina

Albert Ho Yuen Chiu, MBBS (Hons.), FRANZCR, CCINR
Clinical Associate Professor
Division of Internal Medicine/Centre for Medical Research
Faculty of Health and Medical Sciences
University of Western Australia
Consultant Interventional Neuroradiologist
Neurological Intervention & Imaging Service of Western
    Australia (NIISwa)
Sir Charles Gairdner, Royal Perth and Fiona Stanley
    Hospitals
Department of Health
Perth, Western Australia, Australia

Achelle Cortel-LeBlanc, MD, FRCPC
Neurologist, Queensway Carleton Hospital
Lecturer, Faculty of Medicine
University of Ottawa
Ottawa, Ontario, Canada

Jonathan Coutinho, MD, PhD
Stroke Neurologist
Department of Neurology
Amsterdam University Medical Centers
Amsterdam, Netherlands

Hugo Cuellar, MD, PhD, MBA, DABR
Chairman, Department of Radiology
Professor of Radiology, Neurosurgery, and Neurology
Scott and Larene Woodard Professorship in Neurosurgery
Director of Neurointerventional Surgery and
    Neuroradiology
Co-Director, Stroke Center
Louisiana State University Health Sciences Center
Shreveport, Louisiana

Jose Danilo Bengzon Diestro, MD, FPNA
Department of Medical Imaging
Division of Diagnostic and Therapeutic Neuroradiology
St. Michael's Hospital, University of Toronto
Toronto, Ontario, Canada

Adam A. Dmytriw, MD, MPH, MSc (Oxon), FRCPC
Neuroradiology & Neurointervention Services
Toronto Western Hospital, University of Toronto
Toronto, Ontario, Canada
Brigham and Women's Hospital, Harvard Medical School
Boston, Massachusetts

Tadeu A. Fantaneanu, MDCM, CSCN(EEG), FRCPC
Director of the Adult Epilepsy Program and EEG Laboratory
Epilepsy and Neurology, Department of Medicine
The Ottawa Hospital
Assistant Professor, Faculty of Medicine
University of Ottawa
Ottawa, Ontario, Canada

Ana Filipa Geraldo, MD, MSc, PhD candidate
Neuroradiology consultant
Division Chief, Diagnostic Neuroradiology
Centro Hospitalar Vila Nova de Gaia/Espinho (CHVNG/E)
Vila Nova de Gaia, Portugal

Christoph J. Griessenauer, MD, FAANS, FACS
Director of Vascular and Endovascular Neurosurgery
Associate Professor of Neurosurgery
Department of Neurosurgery and Neuroscience Institute
Geisinger Medical Center
Danville, Pennsylvania
Research Institute of Neurointervention
Paracelsus Medical University
Salzburg, Austria

William Guest, MD, PhD, FRCPC
Diagnostic and Interventional Neuroradiology
Department of Medical Imaging
University of Toronto
Toronto, Ontario, Canada

Charles Handley, MBBS(Hons), MMed, FRANZCR
Interventional and Diagnostic Radiology
Monash Imaging, Monash Health
Melbourne, Australia

Manraj Kanwal Singh Heran, MD, FRCPC
Associate Professor of Radiology
Division of Diagnostic & Therapeutic Neuroradiology
Department of Radiology, Vancouver General Hospital
Section of Pediatric Interventional Radiology
Department of Radiology, British Columbia's Children's
    Hospital
University of British Columbia
Vancouver, British Columbia, Canada

Christopher Hilditch, MBBCh, FRCR
Consultant Neuroradiologist
Salford Royal NHS Foundation Trust
Salford, England, United Kingdom

Shivaprakash B. Hiremath, DMRD, DNB, FRCR
Exchange Fellow
Division of Diagnostic and Interventional Neuroradiology
Geneva University Hospitals
Geneva, Switzerland

Peter Howard, MD, FRCPC
Assistant Professor
Division of Neuroradiology
Sunnybrook Health Sciences Centre, University of Toronto
Toronto, Ontario, Canada

Thien J. Huynh, MD, MSc, FRCPC
Diagnostic and Interventional Neuroradiology, Senior
    Associate Consultant
Departments of Radiology and Neurosurgery
Mayo Clinic
Jacksonville, Florida

Anish Kapadia, MD, FRCPC
Diagnostic and Interventional Neuroradiology
Department of Medical Imaging
University of Toronto
Toronto, Ontario, Canada

Christopher Karayiannis, MBChB, PhD, FRACP
General Physician and Geriatrician
Department of Medicine, Peninsula Health
Monash University
Melbourne, Australia

Simon Rupe Khangure, MBBS, BMedSc, FRANZCR
Consultant Radiologist
Fiona Stanley Hospital
Perth, Australia

Timo Krings, MD, PhD, FRCPC
Professor of Radiology and Surgery
Head, Division of Diagnostic and Interventional
    Neuroradiology
Joint Department of Medical Imaging of the University
    Health Network
David Braley and Nancy Gordon Chair of Interventional
    Neuroradiology
University of Toronto
Chief of Radiology, Toronto Western Hospital
Toronto, Ontario, Canada

Hubert Lee, MD, MSc, FRCSC
Diagnostic and Interventional Neuroradiology
Department of Medical Imaging
University of Toronto
Toronto, Ontario, Canada
Department of Neurosurgery
Stanford University School of Medicine
Palo Alto, California

Thabele (Bay) M. Leslie-Mazwi, MD
Director, Endovascular Stroke Services
Neuroendovascular/Neurologic Critical Care
Departments of Neurosurgery and Neurology
Massachusetts General Hospital
Harvard Medical School
Boston, Massachusetts

Nicola Limbucci, MD
Interventional Neuroradiologist
Neurovascular Interventional Unit
Careggi University Hospital
Florence, Italy

Karl-Olof Lövblad, MD
Professor of Radiology
Department of Radiology and Medical Informatics
Geneva University Medical School
Head, Division of Diagnostic and Interventional
  Neuroradiology
Division of Diagnostic and Interventional Neuroradiology
Geneva University Hospitals
Geneva, Switzerland

Emanuele Orrù, MD
Neurointerventional Radiologist
Division of Neurointerventional Radiology
Lahey Hospital and Medical Center
Burlington, Massachusetts
Assistant Professor of Radiology
Tufts University School of Medicine
Boston, Massachusetts

Carmen Parra-Farinas, MD
Department of Medical Imaging
Division of Diagnostic and Therapeutic Neuroradiology
St. Michael's Hospital, University of Toronto
Toronto, Ontario, Canada

Christopher R. Pasarikovski, MD
Department of Surgery
Division of Neurosurgery
University of Toronto
Toronto, Ontario, Canada

Aman B. Patel, MD
Cerebrovascular Neurosurgery
Endovascular Neurosurgery
Massachusetts General Hospital
Harvard Medical School
Boston, Massachusetts

Vitor Mendes Pereira, MD, MSc
Professor of Radiology and Surgery
Division of Neuroradiology, Department of Medical
  Imaging
Division of Neurosurgery, Department of Surgery
St. Michael's Hospital, University of Toronto
Toronto, Ontario, Canada

Kevin Phan, MD, MSc, MPhil
NeuroSpine Surgery Research Group
Prince of Wales Private Hospital
Southwest Sydney Clinical School
Liverpool Hospital, University of New South Wales
Sydney, Australia

Aleksandra Pikula, MD, DABPN, BSc(Hon)
Assistant Professor of Medicine, Division of Neurology
  (Stroke Program)
University of Toronto
Director, Stroke Research Program
University Health Network/Toronto Western Hospital
Toronto, Ontario, Canada

Sarah Power, PhD, MRCPI, FFR(RCSI)
Consultant Interventional Neuroradiologist
Beaumont Hospital
Dublin, Ireland

Stefano Maria Priola, MD
Assistant Professor
Division of Neurosurgery
Northern Ontario School of Medicine
Health Sciences North
Sudbury, Ontario, Canada

Jameel Khalid Rasheedi, MBBS, SB-Neuro, EBN-UEMS
Consultant Stroke Neurologist and Neurointensivist
Division of Neurosciences, Neurology and Neurocritical
  Care Department
King Abdullah Medical City
Mecca, Saudi Arabia
Neurosurgery Department
Sunnybrook Hospital, University of Toronto
Toronto, Ontario, Canada

Robert W. Regenhardt, MD, PhD
Neuroendovascular Service
Departments of Neurosurgery and Neurology
Massachusetts General Hospital
Harvard Medical School
Boston, Massachusetts

Leonardo Renieri, MD
Interventional Neuroradiologist
Neurovascular Interventional Unit
Careggi University Hospital
Florence, Italy

Fateme Salehi, MD, MSc, FRCPC
Assistant Professor of Radiology
Department of Medical Imaging
McMaster University
Juravinski Hospital and Cancer Centre
Hamilton, Ontario, Canada

Amey R. Savardekar, MD
Department of Neurosurgery
Louisiana State University Health Sciences Center
Shreveport, Louisiana

Joanna D. Schaafsma, MD, MSc(hons), PhD
Vascular Neurologist
Department of Medicine, Division of Neurology
University Health Network/University of Toronto
Toronto, Ontario, Canada

Fabio Settecase, MD, MSc, FRCPC
Assistant Professor
Division of Diagnostic and Therapeutic Neuroradiology
Department of Radiology
University of British Columbia
Vancouver General Hospital, UBC Hospital & BC Women's
   Hospital
Vancouver, British Columbia, Canada

Lee-Anne Slater, MBBS, MMed, FRANZCR
Neurointerventional Radiology Monash Health
Monash University
Melbourne, Australia

Cathy Soufan, BBMedSc(Hons), MBBS, DipSurgAnat
Neurointerventional Radiology Monash Health
Monash University
Melbourne, Australia

Alejandro M. Spiotta, MD, FAANS
Professor, Neurosurgery and Neuroendovascular Surgery
Program Director, Neurosurgery Residency
Director, Neuroendovascular Surgery
Medical University of South Carolina
Charleston, South Carolina

Velandai Srikanth, MBBS, FRACP, PhD
Professor of Medicine, Peninsula Health
Peninsula Clinical School, Central Clinical School
Monash University
Melbourne, Australia
Adjunct Professor, Menzies Institute for Medical Research
Hobart, Tasmania, Australia

John Thornton, MB, BCh, BAO, FFR, RCSI, FRCR
Director
National Thrombectomy Service Ireland
Associate Professor
Interventional Neuroradiology
Royal College of Surgeons Ireland
Beaumont Hospital
Dublin, Ireland

Jenny P. Tsai, MDCM, FRCPC
Interventional and Vascular Neurologist
Department of Neurological Surgery
Spectrum Health Medical Group
Assistant Professor of Clinical Neurosciences
Michigan State University College of Human Medicine
East Lansing, Michigan

Anderson Chun On Tsang, MBBS, FRCS(Ed), FCSHK
Clinical Assistant Professor
Division of Neurosurgery
Department of Surgery
The University of Hong Kong
Hong Kong, China

Aquilla S. Turk III, DO
Director, Stroke and Cerebrovascular Program and Professor
   of Surgery
Prisma Health-Upstate
Southeastern Neurosurgical and Spine Institute
Greenville, South Carolina

David Turkel-Parrella, MD
Clinical Assistant Professor of Neurology
Department of Neurology
New York University School of Medicine
Brooklyn, New York

Raymond Turner IV, MD
Stroke and Cerebrovascular Program, Endovascular
   Neurosurgeon
Prisma Health-Upstate
Southeastern Neurosurgical and Spine Institute
Greenville, South Carolina

Vincent M. Tutino, PhD
Research Assistant Professor
Department of Neurosurgery
Department of Pathology and Anatomical Sciences
The State University of New York at Buffalo
Bufffalo, New York

Maria Isabel Vargas, MD
Professor of Radiology and Neuroradiology
Head of Diagnostic Neuroradiology Unit
Division of Diagnostic and Interventional Neuroradiology
Geneva University Hospitals
Faculty of Medicine of Geneva
Geneva, Switzerland

David Volders, MD
Clinical Assistant Professor of Radiology
Division of Diagnostic and Interventional Neuroradiology
QEII Health Sciences Centre, Dalhousie University
Halifax, Nova Scotia, Canada

Ghouth Waggass, MBBS
Department of Medical Imaging
Consultant Diagnostic and Interventional Neuroradiologist
King Faisal Specialist Hospital and Research Centre
Jeddah, Saudi Arabia

Robert A. Willinsky, MD, FRCPC
Professor of Medical Imaging
Division of Neuroradiology, Joint Department of Medical
   Imaging
Toronto Western Hospital, University of Toronto
Toronto, Ontario, Canada

Christoph Wipplinger, MD
Department of Neurological Surgery
Weill Cornell Medicine
New York, New York
Department of Neurosurgery
University of Würzburg
Würzburg, Germany

Victor X. D. Yang, MD, PhD, PEng, FRCSC
Associate Professor of Neurosurgery
Associate Professor of Electrical and Computer Engineering
University of Toronto
Staff Neurosurgeon and Senior Scientist
Sunnybrook Health Science Centre
Toronto, Ontario, Canada

Part I

Evolution of Endovascular Management

1 Intra-arterial Tissue Plasminogen Activator: The First Step

1.1 Case Description

1.1.1 Clinical Presentation

A 64-year-old male presented to the emergency department 100 minutes after acute onset of aphasia, right hemisyndrome, and hemineglect. Clinical examination was suggestive of a partial left middle cerebral artery (MCA) syndrome with National Institutes of Health Stroke Scale (NIHSS) 13.

1.1.2 Imaging Workup and Investigations

- Noncontrast computed tomography (CT) was performed shortly after presentation to the emergency department (135 minutes after symptom onset) revealing early infarction.
- CT angiography revealed occlusion of the distal left M1 segment of the MCA and left MCA bifurcation. There is slow filling of the distal left MCA branches via leptomeningeal collaterals (▶ Fig. 1.1).

1.1.3 Diagnosis

Partial occlusion of the left M1 segment, with early involvement of the MCA territory.

1.1.4 Management

- The patient had no contraindication to intravenous (IV) thrombolysis based on clinical history, clinical assessment, and CT findings.
- He received an initial bolus and infusion of tissue plasminogen activator (tPA) commencing 170 minutes after symptom onset, then subsequently bolus of intra-arterial (IA)-tPA.

1.1.5 Technique

- A 6-Fr guide catheter was placed into the left internal carotid arteries.

- A microcatheter and 014-in wire were placed into the left M1 segment.
- Mechanical clot disruption with a wire and catheter was performed. This was interspersed with IA-tPA. The left M1 segment and upper branch of the left MCA were completely opened after a total of 19 mg of IA-tPA.
- The inferior MCA branch had some residual clot. Supraselective catheterization with mechanical clot disruption was performed with an addition of 5 mg of tPA in this vessel.
- After termination of the procedure, the entire left MCA circulation was open. The patient can now move her right side, whereas she was densely hemiplegic prior to thrombolysis.
- The long, 6-Fr sheath was exchanged with a shorter 6-Fr sheath.
- However, the patient had significant oozing around the second sheath and it was decided to remove the sheath. After compression, the bleeding stopped. No other complications were noted.

1.1.6 Outcome

- Successful complete thrombolysis of left M1 partial thrombus.
- Discharged 4 days after admission to a rehabilitation hospital, with a modified Rankin score of 3.

1.1.7 Discussion

Prior to 1995, no consensus existed on the treatment of acute ischemic stroke. The first treatment to be approved was alteplase, a recombinant human tPA. With the understanding that stroke is caused by arterial occlusion, thrombolysis of thrombus would thus achieve recanalization and salvage ischemic cerebral tissue.

The monumental National Institute of Neurological Disorders and Stroke (NINDS) trial in 1995 randomized patients with acute ischemic stroke to receive either IV alteplase or placebo.[1] This study was divided into two discrete parts. Part 1

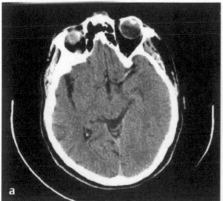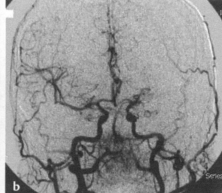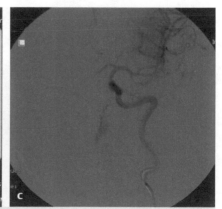

Fig. 1.1 (a) Unenhanced CT demonstrating left M1 occlusion (b) confirmed on digital subtraction angiography. (c) Completion angiography following IA-tPA injection shows recanalization. (Courtesy of Dr. Peter Howard and Vitor Mendes Pereira.)

demonstrated no significant difference between the groups in neurological improvement at 24 hours, but a significant benefit was observed for the treatment group at 3 months in terms of 4-point improvements in the NIHSS. In part 2, patients were assessed for improvements in the Barthel index, modified Rankin scale (mRS), Glasgow outcome scale, and NIHSS at 3 months. It was discovered that patients were at least 30% more likely to have a favorable outcome as measured by these scales (odds ratio [OR] = 1.7; 95% confidence interval [CI]: 1.2–2.6). Thus, NINDS study suggested that the use of IV-tPA within 3 hours of stroke onset has a definite long-term benefit for patients with acute ischemic stroke. However, symptomatic intracerebral hemorrhage (SICH) within 36 hours of symptom onset occurred more frequently in treated patients (6.4 vs. 0.6, $p < 0.001$), suggesting that the use of tPA was not without its risks.[1] Thus, the risks and benefits of this approach must be balanced for optimal treatment. Nevertheless, based on the conclusive results of this trial, the Food and Drug Administration (FDA) approved the use of IV-tPA for the treatment of acute ischemic strokes in 1996.

Elsewhere around the world, similar investigations were underway. The European Cooperative Acute Stroke Study (ECASS) I, II, and III also investigated the use of alteplase for the treatment of acute ischemic stroke.[2,3,4] ECASS I was a double-blind randomized controlled trial (RCT) that randomized 620 patients to receive alteplase or placebo within 6 hours of stroke onset. The trial used both intention-to-treat (ITT) and explanatory analyses for the study's target population (TP). The TP was defined as patients 18 to 80 years old with stable moderate-to-severe hemispheric stroke and few early infarct signs on CT. There was no difference discovered in the primary endpoint after ITT analysis. However, there was a significant difference in the mRS after post-hoc TP analysis. Moreover, Barthel Index and mRS were in favor of treated patient. No mortality differences were detected, but there was a significant increase in the occurrence of large parenchymal hemorrhages in treated patients.[2] The results of this trial served as a reminder that treatment with tPA is associated with hemorrhagic complications, and careful patient selection must be done to exclude those who are unlikely to benefit from treatment.

ECASS II was another RCT that tested the efficacy and safety of a decreased dose of alteplase (0.9 mg/kg body weight from 1.1 mg/kg body weight in ECASS I) in the hope of lowering rates of intracranial hemorrhage. There was still more frequent symptomatic intracranial hemorrhage in the alteplase group, though mortality was not significantly different. The primary endpoint of mRS (0–1) was not significant between the groups, but a post-hoc analysis found less death or dependence (mRS: 3–6) in the treatment group, leaving the benefit of alteplase within 6 hours of stroke onset rather inconclusive.[3]

The more conclusive result came from ECASS III, which specifically examined the administration of alteplase between 3 and 4.5 hours after stroke onset. The trial randomized 821 patients to receive either alteplase or placebo. More patients were found to have a favorable clinical outcome of mRS (0–1) with alteplase (52.4 vs. 42.2%, OR: 1.34, 95% CI: 1.02–1.76). The secondary endpoint of global OR was also in favor of the treatment group. Moreover, similar to the NINDS and ECASS I and II, treatment was associated with higher intracranial hemorrhage but not higher mortality rates. The ECASS III trial demonstrated the

safety and efficacy of alteplase use within the window of 3 to 4.5 hours after stroke onset, extending the effective usage time of 3 hours from NINDS.[4]

Since the approval of tPA, treatment data revealed that alteplase is able to achieve better recanalization rates and long-term clinical benefit (mRS ≤ 1) with distal occlusions rather than proximal ones.[5,6] In fact, only half of the number of patients with proximal MCA occlusion achieved a good clinical outcome (mRS ≤ 1) as compared to those with distal occlusions.[5] Moreover, recanalization rate in proximal MCA was 26.1% as compared with 38.1% distally.[6] The next decade of research in acute ischemic stroke treatment tackled the possibility of delivering thrombolytic drugs intra-arterially to the site of vessel occlusion, in the hopes of achieving better results in proximal occlusions as well as distal ones.

The first RCT exploring the efficacy and safety of IA delivery method was PROACT I, a phase II study conducted between 1994 and 1995 that tested the use of recombinant pro-urokinase (rpro-UK) against placebo within 6 hours of stroke onset in patients with MCA occlusions. The study had a relatively smaller sample size, with 26 in the rpro-UK group and 14 in the placebo group. There was a significantly higher recanalization rate achieved with IA delivery of rpro-UK as compared to placebo (57.7 vs. 14.3%, $p = 0.017$). Moreover, there was a 10 to 20% absolute increase observed in neurological outcomes at 90 days as measured by the Barthel index, mRS, and NIHSS. Yet, perhaps owing to the small sample size, this difference was not statistically significant. As for safety measures, though there was a higher frequency of SICH observed in the treatment group versus placebo (15.4 vs. 7.1%), this difference was also not statistically significant.[7] The higher recanalization rate achieved in patients treated with rpro-UK, along with early indications of safety, prompted further exploration of the usage of IA delivery methods.

The PROACT II study was conducted in 1996, and in 1998 the phase III follow-up to PROACT I took place. In this study, 180 patients with acute ischemic stroke with angiographically proven occlusion of MCA were randomized to receive IA rpro-UK or placebo within 6 hours of stroke onset. The primary outcome was mRS of 2 or less, and this was achieved in 40% of rpro-UK patients as compared to 25% of control patients ($p = 0.04$). The recanalization rate was also higher for the treatment group, at 66% versus only 18% in the control group ($p < 0.001$). This trial was the first to demonstrate a clinical efficacy of IA thrombolysis in treating patients with acute ischemic stroke within 6 hours of symptom onset. Similar to PROACT I, the rate of SICH was higher in the intervention group within 24 hours (10% in intervention vs. 2% in controls). However, this result was still statistically insignificant ($p = 0.06$).[8]

Another trial performed later in Japan also studied the efficacy of IA thrombolysis against placebo, but the results were more equivocal. The MELT trial conducted between 2002 and 2005 randomized 114 patients with MCA occlusions to either receive IA infusion of urokinase (UK) or no therapy, with the exception of osmotic diuretics only if indicated by high intracranial pressure. The trial was stopped early as the primary endpoint failed to achieve significance, and IV-rtPA was approved in Japan for the treatment of acute ischemic stroke in 2005. As of the study's termination, the primary end point of the rate of achieving a good functional outcome (mRS ≤ 2) at

90 days was not significant ($p = 0.345$). Similarly, the difference in proportion of patients with a Barthel Index ≥ 95 was also not significant ($p = 0.128$). However, there was a higher proportion of patients who achieved an excellent functional outcome at day 90 in the treatment group than in the control (42.1 vs. 22.8%, $p = 0.045$). This trial suggested that the clinical benefits of IA thrombolysis with UK were still not clear at the time, and further research was required to elucidate the benefits of IA thrombolysis.[9]

Several trials also looked at a combined IV and IA approach. One such trial was the EMS trial in 1999. This pilot double-blinded RCT randomized patients receiving IA-tPA to either receive IV-tPA or IV placebo within 3 hours of stroke onset. Though recanalization rates were significantly better ($p = 0.03$), the combined approach was not associated with a better clinical outcome. Although no clinical benefits were observed and trial size was relatively small ($n = 35$), the EMS trial demonstrated the feasibility of the combined approach.[10]

The combined approach was explored further in the IMS I and II trials.[11,12] IMS I compared a single arm of 80 patients who received both IV and IA-rtPA with historical controls of IV-tPA and placebo subjects from the 1995 NINDS trial. As compared to the placebo historical controls, all measures of clinical outcome at 3 months were better in the combined intervention group, including the primary endpoint of mRS of 0 to 1. However, the combined intervention group had a similar 3-month outcome in comparison with IV-tPA historical controls. Mortality rates were comparable in both placebo and tPA NINDS subjects, and SICH was higher than placebo controls but similar to NINDS tPA subjects. The IMS I trial demonstrated the safety and efficacy of combined IA/IV-tPA approach and better clinical outcomes in comparison to placebo.[11] However, there was still no evidence that this is a superior approach than IV-tPA alone. IMS II was similar in design to IMS I, as it compared another 80 patients treated with combined IA and IV-tPA to NINDS controls. Yet, this time around, the researchers employed the use of an EKOS microinfusion system to deliver the IA bolus. This system uses low-energy ultrasound to alter the structure of clots, allowing for easier access. Perhaps owing to the advance in delivery method, there was a benefit detected in Barthel Index and Global Test Statistic scores at 90 days for patients treated with the combined approach as compared to NINDS tPA patients. The IMS II was the first study to demonstrate better clinical outcomes of the combined IA and IV approach over IV-tPA alone.[12]

The efficacy of the combined approach was yet again investigated in the RECANALISE study in 2009. This prospective study treated patients in two phases within 3 hours of stroke onset. In phase I, 56 patients were treated with IV-tPA only. In phase II, 107 patients received a combined approach of IV/IA-tPA. In addition, if recanalization was not achieved with IA thrombolysis, patients were eligible to receive further mechanical thrombectomy including the 4-mm snare or balloon angioplasty. The efficacy of the combined approach was clearly evident as recanalization rates were significantly higher in the group receiving the combined approach (87 vs. 52%, RR = 1.49, $p = 0.0002$). Safety was also demonstrated since mortality and SICH rates were similar between the two groups. However, though neurological improvement (mRS: 0–2) at 90 days was achieved by more patients in the combined approach group (60 vs. 39%), the difference was not significant ($p = 0.07$). In RECANALISE, though the combined IV/IA approach resulted in greater recanalization rates, the clinical outcomes did not reveal a clear benefit.[13]

Overall, the combined approach was shown to have better recanalization rates than IV-tPA alone.[13] Yet the clinical benefit of the combined approach was still not clear, with IMS II demonstrating better outcomes on some measures, and IMS I and RECANALISE finding no significant differences.[11,12,13]

From no standard treatment to the combined IV/IA approach, the management of acute ischemic stroke has come a long way. Moreover, around the same time, more exciting techniques were being developed in the treatment of acute ischemic stroke in the field of mechanical thrombectomy.

References

[1] Tissue plasminogen activator for acute ischemic stroke. N Engl J Med. 1996; 334(21):1405–1406

[2] Hacke W, Kaste M, Fieschi C, et al. The European Cooperative Acute Stroke Study (ECASS). Intravenous thrombolysis with recombinant tissue plasminogen activator for acute hemispheric stroke. JAMA. 1995; 274 (13):1017–1025

[3] Hacke W, Kaste M, Fieschi C, et al. Second European-Australasian Acute Stroke Study Investigators. Randomised double-blind placebo-controlled trial of thrombolytic therapy with intravenous alteplase in acute ischaemic stroke (ECASS II). Lancet. 1998; 352(9136):1245–1251

[4] Hacke W, Kaste M, Bluhmki E, et al. ECASS Investigators. Thrombolysis with alteplase 3 to 4.5 hours after acute ischemic stroke. N Engl J Med. 2008; 359 (13):1317–1329

[5] Saqqur M, Uchino K, Demchuk AM, et al. CLOTBUST Investigators. Site of arterial occlusion identified by transcranial Doppler predicts the response to intravenous thrombolysis for stroke. Stroke. 2007; 38(3):948–954

[6] del Zoppo GJ, Poeck K, Pessin MS, et al. Recombinant tissue plasminogen activator in acute thrombotic and embolic stroke. Ann Neurol. 1992; 32 (1):78–86

[7] del Zoppo GJ, Higashida RT, Furlan AJ, Pessin MS, Rowley HA, Gent M. PROACT: a phase II randomized trial of recombinant pro-urokinase by direct arterial delivery in acute middle cerebral artery stroke. PROACT Investigators. Prolyse in Acute Cerebral Thromboembolism. Stroke. 1998; 29(1):4–11

[8] Furlan A, Higashida R, Wechsler L, et al. Intra-arterial prourokinase for acute ischemic stroke. The PROACT II study: a randomized controlled trial. Prolyse in Acute Cerebral Thromboembolism. JAMA. 1999; 282(21):2003–2011

[9] Ogawa A, Mori E, Minematsu K, et al. MELT Japan Study Group. Randomized trial of intraarterial infusion of urokinase within 6 hours of middle cerebral artery stroke: the middle cerebral artery embolism local fibrinolytic intervention trial (MELT) Japan. Stroke. 2007; 38(10):2633–2639

[10] Lewandowski CA, Frankel M, Tomsick TA, et al. Combined intravenous and intra-arterial r-TPA versus intra-arterial therapy of acute ischemic stroke: Emergency Management of Stroke (EMS) Bridging Trial. Stroke. 1999; 30 (12):2598–2605

[11] IMS Study Investigators. Combined intravenous and intra-arterial recanalization for acute ischemic stroke: the Interventional Management of Stroke Study. Stroke. 2004; 35(4):904–911

[12] IMS II Trial Investigators. The Interventional Management of Stroke (IMS) II study. Stroke. 2007; 38(7):2127–2135

[13] Mazighi M, Serfaty JM, Labreuche J, et al. RECANALISE Investigators. Comparison of intravenous alteplase with a combined intravenous-endovascular approach in patients with stroke and confirmed arterial occlusion (RECANALISE study): a prospective cohort study. Lancet Neurol. 2009; 8(9):802–809

2 Transcatheter MERCI Clot Retrieval: The Early Generation

2.1 Case Description

2.1.1 Clinical Presentation

A 67-year-old female with known atrial fibrillation (AF) presented with acute onset of speech disturbance and right-sided weakness. On admission, her clinical examination revealed global aphasia, right hemiplegia, right hemianopia, and eye deviation to the left, suggestive of left middle cerebral artery (MCA) syndrome. Her initial National Institutes of Health Stroke Scale (NIHSS) score fluctuated between 14 and 18.

2.1.2 Imaging Workup and Investigations

- Noncontrast computed tomography (CT) was performed.
- CT perfusion demonstrated distal M1 occlusion. Occluded right internal carotid artery (ICA) and anterior circulation supply predominantly via the left ICA/ACOM. Small posterior communicating arteries (PComms) bilaterally. CTP revealed mismatch with a small insular region of infarct.
- CT angiography revealed occlusion of distal M1 segment of the left MCA (▸ Fig. 2.1).

2.1.3 Diagnosis

Distal M1 occlusion in the context of a patient with AF. Mechanism of embolus was thought to be cardioembolic based on warfarin being stopped and the presence of known AF.

2.1.4 Management

Mechanical thrombectomy of distal M1 segment with MERCI clot retrieval device.

2.1.5 Technique

- The patient was prepped and draped in the usual sterile fashion.
- The right common femoral artery was localized by palpation. A right common femoral artery puncture was performed.
- A 6-Fr shuttle and 125-cm H1 H were used to access the left ICA.
- A mid position was adopted because of an ICA loop.
- A combination of MERCI microcatheter and Xpedion wire was used to gain access beyond the clot.
- Two attempts at clot withdrawal were attempted. Resistance was encountered at the ICA terminus such that the shuttle was being pulled forward on sustained backward tension.
- The clot was shown to be at the ICA terminus on a run performed in this position.
- Vasospasm and vessel distortion of ICA were seen.
- With continued sustained tension, the MERCI device straightened and the clot returned to its distal location.
- A 3 mg of intra-arterial (IA) tPa was administered during the procedure at various times both in and beyond the clot.

- A final attempt at 6 hours post onset to deploy a hyperform balloon was unsuccessful due to looping in the cavernous segment of the ICA. A final cerebral angiography revealed no significant change in clot position. The puncture site was closed with Angio-Seal.

2.1.6 Outcome

- Patient made significant recovery, with NIHSS score decreased to 2 following the procedure. Her NIHSS score at 30 days was 1.

2.1.7 Discussion

Around the same time, IA tissue plasminogen activator (tPA) was being tested for its efficacy in the treatment of acute ischemic stroke, and mechanical thrombectomy was being developed as an adjunctive or alternative measure. Mechanical thrombectomy involves entering the vessel directly to the position of the clot and then removing it by either retrieving the clot distally or proximal aspiration.

The first mechanical thrombectomy system to be approved by the Food and Drug Administration (FDA) is the MERCI Retriever System.[1] This system consists of a nitinol wire that is passed through a catheter distal to the thrombus. When the catheter is removed, the wire assumes a corkscrew shape at its tip. Thereafter, withdrawal of the wire allows the clot to become free. Its safety and efficacy were examined by the MERCI trial. This was a prospective study with patients with contraindication to tPA, or had stroke duration longer than the 3-hour window of intravenous (IV) tPA. Out of the 151 patients who received the MERCI retriever, 69 achieved recanalization in the intention to treat analysis, giving a recanalization rate of 46%. This can be compared to the placebo arm of PROACT-II trial that had a recanalization rate of 18%. However, the rate of MCA recanalization was 45%, less than the 66% reported in PROACT-II using IA prourokinase. The SICH rate was estimated to be 5%, which is higher than that of the placebo arm of NINDS and PROACT-II, but comparable to IV-tPA in the NINDS trial, IA/IV-tPA in the IMS trial and IA prourokinase in PROACT-II. Clinical significant complication rate was 7.1%, again comparable to these historic trials. The overall mortality was high at 44%, due to the patient selection for those with severe strokes and large vessel occlusions.[1] Overall, the results of the MERCI trial suggest that the MERCI retriever is a safe and efficacious alternative for patients with contraindications to tPA or stroke duration outside of the tPA treatment window.[2] While the MERCI trial was underway, advancements were made to the retriever system, and the newer generation of L5 MERCI retriever was tested in the Multi-MERCI trial. Successful recanalization rate was higher with this new version of MERCI retriever (57.3%). Favorable outcomes, defined as modified Rankin scale (mRS) ≤ 2 at 90 days, were achieved in 36% of the patients. The SICH (9.8%) and procedure-related complication rate (5.5%) were again comparable with other stroke trials.[3] The MERCI device was proven to be safe and efficacious by the MERCI and the Multi-MERCI trials, starting a new exciting era of mechanical thrombectomy.

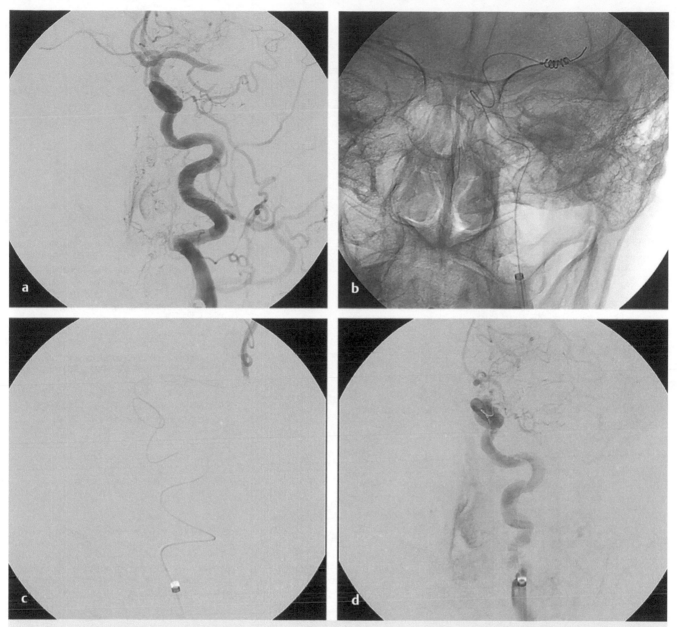

Fig. 2.1 (a) Digital subtraction angiography demonstrating left M1 occlusion; (b) unsubtracted view of MERCI device in situ with (c) subsequent transient bypass effect; (d) unsuccessful clot withdrawal with retraction to the ICA terminus. (Courtesy of Dr. Peter Howard and Victor Yang.)

Another mechanical thrombectomy device similar to the MERCI retriever was the CATCH device, a nitinol wire construct that assumes the shape of a basket when pulled out of the catheter. A retrospective case series examined the use of CATCH in 40 patients, most of who received IV-tPA. The recanalization rate was 65% and favorable clinical outcome of mRS ≤2 was 39%. Additionally, the SICH rate was 18% and procedural complication rate was 15%. These outcomes were all comparable to the MERCI and the PROACT-II trials.[4]

Then in 2010, the new generation of stent retrievers came into existence, the first of which was named Solitaire. The device contains a stent that is deployed within the thrombus. This allows the stent to expand into the thrombus, thus entrapping it within. The clot is removed when the stent is withdrawn from the vessel. The SWIFT trial compared patient outcomes with the MERCI device. The results vastly favored the new stent retrievers, with recanalization rate of 64% in comparison to the 24% recanalization rate achieved using MERCI. Good 90-day neurological outcomes were also achieved more frequently in the Solitaire group than in the MERCI group (58 vs. 33%). Similarly, the use of Solitaire also resulted in less mortality (29 vs. 69%). The SWIFT trial highlighted the vast improvement of the Solitaire stent retriever device over MERCI.[5] The technique and devices of mechanical thrombectomy were ever improving.

Other stent retrievers came into existence around the same time. The Trevo and Revive devices are similar to the Solitaire device, with the exception that Revive employs a closed basket at the end for better clot removal.[6,7,8] Their safety and efficacy were tested in prospective studies and randomized controlled trials (RCTs). The TREVO study was a single-center prospective trial with 60 patients receiving the Trevo device within 8 hours of stroke onset in the anterior circulation and within 12 hours of onset in the posterior circulation. The recanalization rate was 73.3% with Trevo alone, and went up to 86.7% when IA-tPA or other devices were used additionally. Good outcome as defined by mRS ≤ 2 was 45% at 90 days. Mortality was 28.3% and SICH was 11.7%. The Trevo device was further compared to the MERCI device in TREVO 2, an RCT with 88 patients receiving treatment with Trevo and 90 patients receiving MERCI. Recanalization was achieved in a greater number of patients treated with Trevo than with MERCI (86 vs. 60%). In addition, more patients achieved a good functional outcome (mRS ≤ 2) in the Trevo group when compared to the MERCI group (40 vs. 22%).[7] The Revive device was examined in the small scale REVIVE study. Vessel recanalization was successful in all patients who received Revive and 60% of patients achieved a clinical improvement of greater than 8 points on the NIHSS or a NIHSS score of 0 to 1.[8] The results of SWIFT, TREVO, TREVO 2, and REVIVE provided evidence for the safety and efficacy of this new generation of mechanical thrombolytic devices. All stent retrievers achieved better recanalization rates and clinical outcomes than the older MERCI-type devices, and were shown to be equally safe.

As early as 2008, the FDA gave approval to Penumbra, a mechanical thrombolytic device that works by aspirating the clot proximally. This device first breaks up the clot into smaller pieces, then uses both aspiration and direct extraction to remove it from the vessel.[9] The safety and efficacy of the device were assessed in three single-arm studies: SPEED, Pivotal, and POST.[9,10,11] In these studies, revascularization rate ranged from 81.6 to 91%, and good clinical outcome of mRS ≥ 2 at 90 days ranged from 25 to 40%. The rate of SICH was 11.2 and 14% in the Pivotal and SPEED studies, respectively, and the rate of serious procedure-related adverse events was 5.7% in the POST study. All-cause mortality ranged from 20 to 32.8%. The Pivotal, SPEED, and POST studies proved that Penumbra is both an efficacious and safe device, but these were single-arm studies without comparison to other devices or treatment options.[9,10,11]

Throughout the years, there has been a wide range of mechanical thrombectomy devices developed, including the distal clot removal devices (MERCI and Catch), the stent retrievers (Solitaire, Trevo, and Revive), and the aspiration device (Penumbra). Each of these were examined in studies and proven to be efficacious and safe. These mechanical thrombectomy devices along with IA-tPA had shifted the focus of acute ischemic stroke management from bedside infusion of IV-tPA to the neuroangiography suite. However, the clinical effectiveness and safety of these endovascular treatments still needed to be compared with the effectiveness of IV-tPA in RCTs.

References

[1] Smith WS, Sung G, Starkman S, et al. MERCI Trial Investigators. Safety and efficacy of mechanical embolectomy in acute ischemic stroke: results of the MERCI trial. Stroke. 2005; 36(7):1432–1438

[2] Becker KJ, Brott TG. Approval of the MERCI clot retriever: a critical view. Stroke. 2005; 36(2):400–403

[3] Smith WS, Sung G, Saver J, et al. Multi MERCI Investigators. Mechanical thrombectomy for acute ischemic stroke: final results of the Multi MERCI trial. Stroke. 2008; 39(4):1205–1212

[4] Mourand I, Brunel H, Costalat V, et al. Mechanical thrombectomy in acute ischemic stroke: catch device. AJNR Am J Neuroradiol. 2011; 32(8):1381–1385

[5] Saver JL, Jahan R, Levy EI, et al. SWIFT Trialists. Solitaire flow restoration device versus the MERCI Retriever in patients with acute ischaemic stroke (SWIFT): a randomised, parallel-group, non-inferiority trial. Lancet. 2012; 380(9849):1241–1249

[6] San Román L, Obach V, Blasco J, et al. Single-center experience of cerebral artery thrombectomy using the TREVO device in 60 patients with acute ischemic stroke. Stroke. 2012; 43(6):1657–1659

[7] Nogueira RG, Lutsep HL, Gupta R, et al. TREVO 2 Trialists. Trevo versus MERCI retrievers for thrombectomy revascularisation of large vessel occlusions in acute ischaemic stroke (TREVO 2): a randomised trial. Lancet. 2012; 380(9849):1231–1240

[8] Rohde S, Haehnel S, Herweh C, et al. Mechanical thrombectomy in acute embolic stroke: preliminary results with the revive device. Stroke. 2011; 42(10):2954–2956

[9] Frei D, Gerber J, Turk A, et al. The SPEED study: initial clinical evaluation of the Penumbra novel 054 Reperfusion Catheter. J Neurointerv Surg. 2013; 5(May) Suppl 1:i74–i76

[10] Penumbra Pivotal Stroke Trial Investigators. The penumbra pivotal stroke trial: safety and effectiveness of a new generation of mechanical devices for clot removal in intracranial large vessel occlusive disease. Stroke. 2009; 40(8):2761–2768

[11] Tarr R, Hsu D, Kulcsar Z, et al. The POST trial: initial post-market experience of the Penumbra system: revascularization of large vessel occlusion in acute ischemic stroke in the United States and Europe. J Neurointerv Surg. 2010; 2(4):341–344

3 Penumbra Clot Aspiration Technique: The Dark Days

3.1 Case Description

3.1.1 Clinical Presentation

- A 78-year-old female presented to the emergency department 4 hours after acute onset of left arm and left leg weakness with vertigo symptoms. Clinical examination was suggestive of proximal M1 occlusion and revealed National Institutes of Health Stroke Scale (NIHSS) score of 14.

3.1.2 Imaging Workup and Investigations

- Noncontrast CT demonstrated hyperdense right M1 (▶ Fig. 3.1).
- CT angiography demonstrated corresponding occlusion.

3.1.3 Diagnosis

- Right M1 occlusion.

3.1.4 Management

- IV-tPA and suction thrombectomy.

3.1.5 Technique

- The patient was prepped and draped in the usual sterile fashion.
- The right common femoral artery was localized by palpation. 1 mL L/A was utilized for anesthesia.
- A right common femoral artery puncture was performed.
- A 6-Fr shuttle sheath was placed and attached to a continuous heparinized flush.
- A 5-Fr, 125-cm H1 H catheter was advanced through the sheath over a guide wire into the left common carotid artery (CCA).
- The H1 H was used as a coaxial technique to gain access to proximal CCA for the shuttle given the marked proximal tortuosity of the arch.
- A 6-Fr neuron was placed into the left ICA. Combination of 0.54 penumbra and prowler superselect was navigated into M1 and was able to traverse the occlusion.
- Suction was applied with dissipation of clot and restoration of TICI 3 recanalization (▶ Fig. 3.2).

3.1.6 Outcome

- The catheters were removed. The sheath was removed and Angio-Seal applied. There was good hemostasis. There were no complications.
- The patient had a normal recovery and uneventful postprocedural course.
- The NIHSS score was 1 at 24 hours and 0 at 30-day follow-up.
- On 6-month follow-up, he remained at his functional baseline.

3.1.7 Discussion

The early results of randomized controlled trials (RCTs) comparing conventional intravenous tissue plasminogen activator (IV-tPA) to endovascular methods, including intra-arterial (IA) tPA and mechanical thrombectomy, were anything but promising. In 2013, the publications of the three negative trials (IMS III, SYNTHESIS, and MR RESCUE) cast a shadow over the future of endovascular thrombectomy.

The IMS III was an international phase III RCT comparing endovascular therapy plus IV-tPA to IV-tPA alone in patients who have received tPA within 3 hours of stroke onset and with an NIHSS score ≥ 10. The trial was conducted in the United States, Canada, Australia, and Europe. The study randomized in a 2:1 fashion with 434 patients receiving the endovascular therapy and 222 patients receiving only IV-tPA, but was stopped early due to futility. At its termination, there were no significant differences observed in overall good clinical outcome (as defined by modified Rankin scale [mRS] ≤ 2), good clinical outcome in subgroup analyses of NIHSS score above 20, good clinical outcome in subgroup analysis of NIHSS score below 19, and mortality at 90 days or symptomatic hemorrhage rates.[1] While the result of the trial was negative, the investigators as well as critics recognized the limitations of IMS III.

A number of factors could have contributed to the negative outcome, one of which is long mean time from symptom onset to reperfusion. In an analysis of the data from IMS III, clinical outcomes were correlated with perfusion times. In particular, every 30-minute delay was correlated with a 12% reduction in the relative likelihood of good clinical outcome.[2] Conversely, with a decrease in reperfusion time, there would be greater chance of having a good clinical outcome. Another factor that provoked criticism was the use of outdated mechanical thrombectomy devices. The trial included the use of many endovascular treatment methods such as MERCI, Penumbra, or IA-tPA with EKOS or the standard catheter, with only a small proportion of Solitaire before study termination.[1] While the first-generation devices were shown to be safe and efficacious, the stent retrievers (i.e., Solitaire and Trevo) consistently proved to achieve greater recanalization rates and have better clinical outcomes. The predominant use of first generation devices did not reflect the full potential of endovascular therapy at the time. Finally, over the course of the study, a baseline computed tomography angiography (CTA) became the standard of care for patients with acute stroke. Thus, over half of the patients enrolled in the study did not have a confirmed diagnosis of a large artery occlusion on CTA.[1] Thus, the study included many patients who were unlikely to benefit from endovascular therapy. Taken together, the delay in reperfusion time, use of older generation devices, and lack of CTA at baseline contributed to the negative outcome of the IMS III trial.

The SYNTHESIS trial took a different approach and compared endovascular therapy alone with IV-tPA alone. The study was a multicenter trial conducted in Italy. In this trial, 362 patients within 4.5 hours of stroke onset were randomized to either endovascular therapy or IV-tPA in a 1:1 ratio. Endovascular therapy involved IA-tPA or mechanical thrombectomy

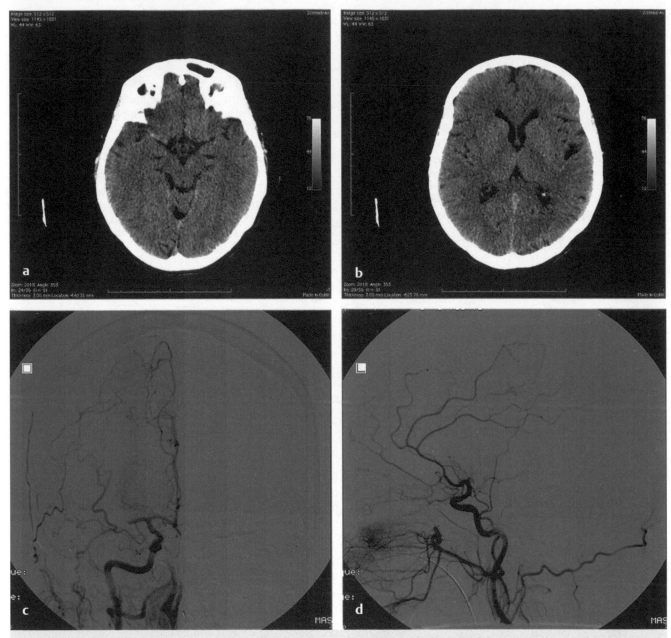

Fig. 3.1 **(a)** Noncontrast CT demonstrating hyperdense right M1 with **(b)** no early signs of ischemia; **(c)** frontal and **(d)** lateral confirmed M1 occlusion.

(Solitaire, Trevo, MERCI, and Penumbra), but no IV-tPA was administered to this group. The primary end point of an excellent clinical outcome (mRS ≤ 1) was not significantly different (30.4% for endovascular group and 34.8% for IV-tPA group). There were no significant differences in symptomatic hemorrhage occurrences, other serious adverse events, or the case fatality rate between the two arms.[3]

The limitations of SYNTHESIS were similar to those of IMS III. There was a 1-hour delay between treatment with endovascular therapy and IV-tPA (3.75 vs. 2.75 hours, respectively). As mentioned earlier, symptomatic stroke to therapy time is critically important to ensure good clinical outcome, and the delay in therapy time likely minimized the effects of endovascular therapy. The newer generation of stent retrievers was again underutilized in this study. Out of those who ultimately

received endovascular therapy, the majority of patients (66%) were treated with IA-tPA, and only 14% were treated with the stent retrievers. Lastly, CTA or magnetic resonance (MR) angiography was not an inclusion criterion for endovascular therapy, due to the lack of availability of these image modalities at the start of the trial. Thus, patients who underwent endovascular treatments did not have a confirmed large artery occlusion. All of these limitations undermined the effectiveness of endovascular therapy, contributing to the trial's negative result.[3]

3.1.8 Further Attempts and Critiques

A third negative trial published around the same time was MR RESCUE, an RCT conducted in North America comparing mechanical embolectomy (MERCI or Penumbra) and standard

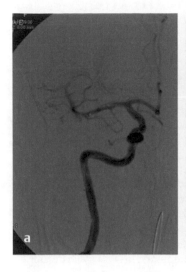
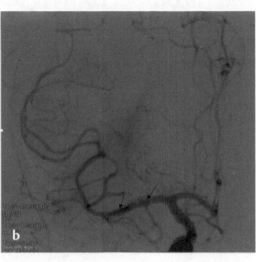

Fig. 3.2 (a) Post–suction thrombectomy DSA showing recanalization and clearance of the (b) site of occlusion. (Courtesy of Dr. Peter Howard and Victor Yang.)

medical care (IV-tPA). This was the first trial to employ CT or MRI at baseline for patient selection regarding treatment decisions. After undergoing imaging, patients were stratified to either a favorable or a nonfavorable penumbral pattern, to examine whether a favorable penumbra predicted benefit from endovascular therapy. The trial included 118 patients randomized to four groups with a sample size of 20 to 34 each. The results showed no significant differences in mean mRS achieved between embolectomy and thrombectomy and the standard therapy groups, or in the stratified subgroups based on the penumbra pattern. There was no interaction between imaging pattern and treatment. Across the four groups, there were no differences achieved in 90-day mortality or symptomatic hemorrhage rates. The trial result suggested that mechanical embolectomy was not significantly different from the effect of IV-tPA, and a favorable penumbral pattern did not identify patients who would benefit from embolectomy.[4]

Similar to IMS III and SYNTHESIS, MR RESCUE was also limited by the lack of usage of the stent retrievers. Unfortunately, the stent retrievers were not introduced prior to the end of the trial enrolment. In addition, the use of imaging in this study significantly delayed the time from stroke onset to embolectomy. The mean time from onset to embolectomy was 6 hours, significantly longer than that in other previous trials. Perhaps the largest limitation of this trial was the relatively smaller sample size in each group. The small sample size may not have had enough power to detect a difference, particularly when there were also crossovers present between the groups. Lastly, there was heterogeneity in the core volumes predicted using CT and MRI. CT tended to give a higher predicted core volume than MRI, impacting the accuracy of the penumbral pattern stratification. The MR RESCUE had similar limitations to IMS III and SYNTHESIS, but also had many limitations of its own.[4]

In summary, the three RCTs published in 2013 all showed a negative result when comparing the effectiveness of endovascular approaches to IV-tPA. However, in one form or another, these RCTs did not accurately represent modern endovascular management of acute ischemic stroke at the time. Some common shared issues were the delay in treatment time, the lack of baseline imaging, and the lack of usage of the newer generation stent retrievers. Further investigations were required to compare the clinical effectiveness of the more efficacious stent retrievers against medical standard care, using modern management of baseline CTA with an emphasis on shortening treatment delays.

References

[1] Broderick JP, Palesch YY, Demchuk AM, et al. Interventional Management of Stroke (IMS) III Investigators. Endovascular therapy after intravenous t-PA versus t-PA alone for stroke. N Engl J Med. 2013; 368(10):893–903

[2] Khatri P, Yeatts SD, Mazighi M, et al. IMS III Trialists. Time to angiographic reperfusion and clinical outcome after acute ischaemic stroke: an analysis of data from the Interventional Management of Stroke (IMS III) phase 3 trial. Lancet Neurol. 2014; 13(6):567–574

[3] Ciccone A, Valvassori L, Nichelatti M, et al. SYNTHESIS Expansion Investigators. Endovascular treatment for acute ischemic stroke. N Engl J Med. 2013; 368(10):904–913

[4] Kidwell CS, Jahan R, Gornbein J, et al. MR RESCUE Investigators. A trial of imaging selection and endovascular treatment for ischemic stroke. N Engl J Med. 2013; 368(10):914–923

4 Trevo Stent-Retriever Thrombectomy: Light on the Horizon

4.1 Case Description

4.1.1 Clinical Presentation

A 79-year-old female, previously well, was undergoing rehabilitation on the ward post elective right knee replacement. She developed sudden left hemiparesis and aphasia. A stroke code was called; the patient was not a candidate for tissue plasminogen activator (tPA).

4.1.2 Imaging and Workup

- Noncontrast CT head was performed, which demonstrated hyperdense right M1 sign.
- CT angiography demonstrated proximal vessel occlusion, with mismatch on CT perfusion.
- Decision was made to take the patient urgently to the angio suite for mechanical thrombectomy. Risks include death, hemorrhage, reperfusion injury, pseudoaneurysm, hematoma, and vascular injury, and informed consent was obtained.

4.1.3 Diagnosis

- Right middle cerebral artery (MCA) M1 segment occlusion.

4.1.4 Technique

- Right femoral single-wall puncture after standard prep and drape.
- Under ultrasound guidance, 5 to 7 Fr dilators were used with 8-Fr sheath. 2,000 units of heparin was infused.
- Considering the tortuous anatomy off the aortic arch and great vessel origins, Mani catheter with a Terumo advantage exchange wire was used to gain access to the right external carotid artery.

- Concentric balloon catheter of 8 Fr was then exchanged up, and positioned into the proximal right internal carotid artery (ICA).
- Initial anteroposterior (AP), lateral angiograms demonstrated a proximal right M1 occlusion, with cross-filling into the left anterior cerebral artery territory, and cortical collateral filling at a very delayed stage.
- Trevo 18 microcatheter was then prepared, using a transcend soft tip microguidewire, and gained access into right M2 segment, with microcatheter injection demonstrating intraluminal position (▸ Fig. 4.1).
- Trevo ProView mechanical thrombectomy stent was then deployed, with single shot angiogram demonstrating appropriate expansion of the stent. This was incubated for 5 minutes.
- With the stent in situ, transient bypass effect with observed on AP and lateral angiograms.
- The stent was pulled back with inflation of the concentric balloon guide catheter, and simultaneous suction to obtain flow arrest.
- Repeat angiogram demonstrated recanalization of the M1, and the superior M2 branch, with occlusion of the inferior M2 branch persisting.
- Recanalization of the inferior branch was not pursued. The sheath was sewn in.

4.1.5 Outcome

- Immediate neurological assessment was performed, which showed motor improvement.
- The patient was discharged home on postoperative day 3 with an NIHSS score of 0.
- At 6-month follow-up in the neurointerventional clinic, her NIHSS and modified Rankin scale scores were 0.

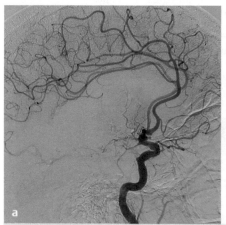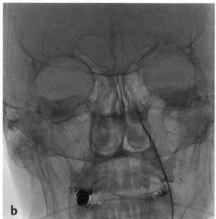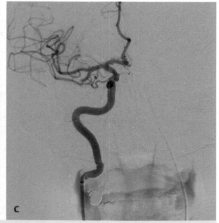

Fig. 4.1 (a) Lateral digital subtraction angiography demonstrating right M1 occlusion and (b) unsubtracted view of the Trevo device in situ. (c) Complete MCA recanalization. Courtesy of Dr. Victor Yang.

4.1.6 Discussion

The next-generation RCTs were conducted with lessons from IMS III, SYNTHESIS, and MR RESCUE. Since the publication of these negative studies, a couple of new trials were designed to primarily test the new stent retrievers, utilize baseline imaging as an inclusion criteria, and aim for a faster stroke onset to procedure time. These trials included MR CLEAN, ESCAPE, EXTEND IA, SWIFT PRIME and REVASCAT, THRACE, and THERAPY. With the exception of THERAPY, which was underpowered at the time of its termination, all of these trials yielded conclusive positive results that favored mechanical thrombectomy.

The MR CLEAN was a Dutch trial wherein 233 patients were randomized to intra-arterial (endovascular) treatments with usual care and 267 were randomized to usual standard of care alone. Out of those in the endovascular arm, 196 underwent endovascular treatment, of which 190 were treated with modern stent retrievers. Patient inclusion criteria involved a large vessel occlusion in the anterior circulation as confirmed via CTA, feasibility of endovascular treatment within 6 hours of stroke onset, and NIHSS of ≥ 2. There were significant differences observed among the patients who achieved a good functional outcome (modified Rankin scale [mRS] ≤ 2): 32.6% in the endovascular arm vs. 19.1% in usual care. The adjusted odds ratio was 1.67 (95% confidence interval [CI]: 1.21–2.30). There were no significant differences in mortality, rate of symptomatic intracerebral hemorrhage (SICH), or other serious adverse events.[1] The positive result of MR CLEAN owes itself to the use of stent retrievers and baseline imaging. Other factors were contributory as well; for instance, most patients in the trial were included after they have failed to respond within 1 hour of IV-tPA. It was then not surprising that usual care would be less effective than expected. Moreover, the Dutch health system allowed only endovascular therapy for acute ischemic stroke to be performed within the trial. This avoided the biased selection of patients who were easy to treat, making it more congruent with the reality of stroke care. Lastly, the safety result of the trial demonstrated that all the intervention procedures were performed in a safe manner.[2] Though the MR CLEAN results were positive, it should be mentioned that they are not as frankly so as the other four positive trials discussed, perhaps owing to the long stroke onset to groin puncture time of 260 minutes.[2,3] Regardless of its limitations, the MR CLEAN demonstrated the safety and effectiveness of endovascular therapy in acute ischemic stroke involving a large artery occlusion of the anterior circulation within 6 hours of stroke onset.

Similar to MR CLEAN, ESCAPE is a trial that compared endovascular treatment plus standard care with standard care alone. This international trial randomized 165 patients to the endovascular plus standard care arm and 150 patients to the standard care arm. Also akin to MR CLEAN, patients were enrolled with proximal intracranial occlusions in the anterior circulation, but the timeline was extended to within 12 hours of symptom onset. The inclusion criteria specified patients with small infarct cores, occlusion in proximal anterior circulation artery, and moderate-to-good collateral circulation as identified via noncontrast CT and CTA. The trial was stopped early due to demonstrable efficacy. Significantly more proportion of patients in the endovascular group achieved functional independence (mRS ≤ 2) at 90 days (53.0 vs. 29.3%). The common OR

was 2.6, favoring the intervention. The number needed to treat (NNT) to achieve one more independent functional outcome was only 4. Moreover, there was also significantly reduced mortality (10.4 vs. 19%) associated with intervention, while the SICH rate was not significantly different between the groups. Better results were gained from ESCAPE than from MR CLEAN. ESCAPE also used baseline imaging and the majority of patients were treated with stent retrievers. However, a few key differences were notable. The investigators of the ESCAPE trial emphasized efficient workflow, setting time targets for CT to groin puncture and reperfusion times. The mean time from symptom onset to groin puncture was 185 minutes, which is significantly shorter than the 260 minutes of MR CLEAN.[2,3] Moreover, imaging was used to exclude patients with large infarcts and poor collateral circulation. This selection process allowed patients who would most likely to benefit from endovascular therapy. There was also an emphasis on decreasing the use of general anesthesia. As such, complications due to general anesthesia were less likely to occur. With an emphasis on efficient workflow, innovative patient selection, a decreased use of general anesthesia, and the use of stent retrievers, the ESCAPE trial was able to demonstrate both an increase in functional outcome and a decrease in mortality favoring endovascular therapy.[3]

EXTEND IA, SWIFTPRIME, and REVASCAT were trials that compared the effectiveness of Solitaire plus IV-tPA and IV-tPA alone. EXTEND IA was conducted in Australia and New Zealand that randomized patients already receiving IV-tPA within 4.5 hours of stroke onset to receive endovascular therapy using Solitaire or continued medical care. The plan was to enroll 100 patients with occlusions of the internal carotid or MCA and evidence of salvageable brain tissue on CT. One of the major innovations in this study is the use of RAPID software to automatically identify salvageable brain tissue, decreasing the delay to endovascular therapy. However, the trial was stopped early with 35 patients randomized to each arm due to efficacy. The co-primary outcomes of 24-hour MRI reperfusion and 3-day NIHSS both vastly favored endovascular intervention. At 24 hours, there was 100% reperfusion of the ischemic territory with Solitaire, as compared to only 37% with IV-tPA. Early neurological improvement at 3 days, defined as ≥ 8-point reduction on the NIHSS, or a score of 0 or 1, was achieved in 80% of Solitaire patients and 37% of IV-tPA patients. More patients in the Solitaire group also achieved a good functional outcome at 90 days than IV-tPA patients (71 vs. 40%). There were no significant differences in SICH rate or mortality. Similar to ESCAPE, this trial was also vastly more positive than the results of MR CLEAN. EXTEND IA employed CT perfusion imaging as an inclusion criteria, selecting for patients who were more likely to benefit from therapy. The time from stroke onset to groin puncture was yet again shorter than the time in MR CLEAN (210 minutes in EXTEND IA vs. 260 minutes in MR CLEAN). Another contributor to the positive result was the higher rate of revascularization (86%) achieved with Solitaire as compared with previous trials.[4]

SWIFT PRIME was a trial conducted in the United States, Canada, and Europe that planned to randomize 477 patients who were receiving IV-tPA to either treatment with Solitaire or continued treatment with IV-tPA. Patients were included only if it was possible to perform endovascular therapy within 6 hours of stroke onset. The selection criteria included confirmed occlusions in the proximal arteries in the anterior circulation (intracranial ICA, M1, or carotid terminus) and absence of large ischemic core lesions on CTA or MRA. This trial was again stopped early due to efficacy after enrolling 196 patients with 98 in each group. The primary outcome of disability at 90 days as assessed by the mean of mRS demonstrated a favorable shift in the endovascular arm. The NNT for a less-disabled outcome was 2.6. The rate of functional independence (mRS ≤ 2) was achieved in 60% of the intervention group and 35% of the control, and the NNT for functional independence was 4.0. There were no differences in mortality and SICH rates. This trial had a stroke onset to groin puncture time of 224 minutes, yet again highlighting the importance of decreased time to better result. The percentage of functional independence achieved was higher than that of MR Clean and comparable to other previous trials (MR CLEAN: 33%, ESCAPE: 53%, EXTEND IA: 71%, and SWIFT PRIME: 60%). The SWIFT PRIME trial provided even more solid evidence for the use of stent retriever in treating acute ischemic stroke due to occlusions in the proximal arteries of the anterior circulation within 6 hours of onset.[5]

The REVASCAT was a trial conducted in Spain. Its study population was those who were refractory or contraindicated to IV-tPA. In addition, patients had confirmed proximal anterior circulation occlusion. Patients were excluded if they had a large ischemic core, as identified by the Alberta Stroke Program Early Computer Tomography Score (ASPECTS) on noncontrast CT or diffusion-weighted MRI. They were randomized to receive treatment with Solitaire or medical therapy. The trial was stopped early after enrolling 206 patients due to efficacy concern, with 103 in each group. The primary outcome was reduction in severity of disability over the range of mRS. The odds ratio for 1 point improvement on the mRS scale was 1.7 (95% CI: 1.05–2.8), slightly favoring the intervention. Higher rate of functional independence (mRS ≤ 2) at 90 days was achieved in the intervention group (43.7%) than in the control group (28.2%). The NNT to prevent functional dependence was 6.5. Neither the rate of symptomatic hemorrhage nor death was clinically significant. This trial was similar to MR CLEAN but different from ESCAPE, EXTEND IA, and SWIFT PRIME in that it excluded patients with an early response to IV-tPA. This criteria resulted in longer times from hospital arrival to reperfusion, and thus lower rates of reperfusion in comparison to ESCAPE, EXTEND IA, and SWIFT PRIME. Moreover, patient selection in this trial was done with the ASPECTS scoring alone, which allowed the inclusion of patients with larger infarct sizes. Hence, results were positive but not as drastically positive as that of ESCAPE, EXTEND IA, and SWIFT PRIME.[6]

While MR CLEAN, ESCAPE, SWIFTPRIME, EXTEND IA, and REVASCAT were published in 2015, the results of THRACE and THERAPY were published a year later. THRACE was a trial conducted in France. Similar to MR CLEAN and ESCAPE, this study compared IV-tPA alone with IV-tPA plus mechanical thrombectomy. The mechanical thrombectomy procedures used were primarily stent retrievers, as well as some aspiration devices. Patients were enrolled based on a confirmed occlusion in a large vessel of the anterior circulation or superior basilar artery as evident on CTA or MRA. Unfortunately only two patients were enrolled with occlusions of the superior basilar artery; thus, the results of the trial reflect strokes only in the anterior

circulation. IV-tPA had to be initiated within 4 hours of stroke onset and thrombectomy within 5 hours of onset. An unplanned interim analysis was done after the results from MR CLEAN were released. This analysis showed superiority of the mechanical thrombectomy and the trial was thus stopped early. At the termination of the trial, 208 patients were randomized to receive tPA alone and 204 patients were to receive tPA plus mechanical thrombectomy. The primary endpoint of functional independence (mRS ≤ 2) at 90 days was achieved in more proportion of the patients in the intervention group (53%) compared to the control group (42%) (OR: 1.55, 95% CI: 1.05–2.30). There were no differences in mortality or SICH rates.

While the THRACE trial affirms the results of the trials published in 2015, there were some differences in its methodology. One major difference is that patient selection was not performed based on the size of the ischemic core. In THRACE, 30% of patients who scored 0 to 4 on ASPECTS achieved functional independence at 90 days. Thus, the potential benefit of treatment in this group of patients should not be overlooked. Another difference in methodology is the short delay from IV-tPA to randomization compared to other studies, and thus patients were not excluded based on their response to IV-tPA. Moreover, this resulted in a large proportion (30%) of crossover from the mechanical thrombectomy group to the control group, because many patients did not receive mechanical thrombectomy. The time from randomization to groin puncture was also longer than that of other studies. All of these factors contributed to the decreased absolute difference in functional independence as compared with other trials. Nevertheless, THRACE demonstrated the efficacy of mechanical thrombectomy without exclusion of patients with large ischemic cores and an initial response to IV-tPA.

Around the same time as THRACE, results from THERAPY were also published. This was a trial conducted in the United States and Germany with a planned enrolment of 692 patients. However, enrolment was stopped early at 108 patients after results from MR CLEAN were made available and it was subsequently considered unethical to treat patients with tPA alone. The major difference between THERAPY and other trials is that it investigated only the efficacy of the Penumbra aspiration device. It compared treatment with IV-tPA plus penumbra with IV-tPA alone. The key inclusion criterion was patients with large vessel occlusions of thrombus length ≥ 8 mm. The primary efficacy endpoint of functional independence at 90 days failed to reach significance, as the study was underpowered at the time of termination. However, the data favored intervention over control (OR: 1.76, 95% CI: 0.86–3.59). Moreover, per-protocol analyses of primary and secondary endpoints consistently favored the intervention, with some secondary endpoints reaching statistical significance. There were no differences in mortality or SICH rates. THERAPY was the first study to examine the effect of aspiration devices alone. While it was stopped early and underpowered, the results suggested a potential benefit of aspiration devices over standard medical management. What must be noted is that this trial did not answer the question of whether aspiration or stent retrievers were more efficacious, and further RCTs comparing these two currently favored procedures will be required to provide a definitive answer.

With the publication of MR CLEAN, ESCAPE, EXTEND IA, SWIFT PRIME, THRACE, and THERAPY, the case for endovascular therapy had become stronger. These trials learned from the earlier lessons of IMS III, SYNTHESIS, and MR RESCUE. Using mainly stent retrievers, stream-lining workflow to reduce door to treatment times, and employing innovating imaging techniques for optimal patient selection, these new trials had discovered a significant benefit in the functional outcomes, neurological improvement, reperfusion rates, and even mortality. The NNT to prevent one functional disability is staggeringly low, ranging from 4 to 6.5.[6] Moreover, endovascular therapy has consistently been proven to be just as safe as medical treatment. These results provide a strong case for using endovascular therapy as standard care for acute ischemic stroke patients.

References

[1] Berkhemer OA, Fransen PSS, Beumer D, et al. MR CLEAN Investigators. A randomized trial of intraarterial treatment for acute ischemic stroke. N Engl J Med. 2015; 372(1):11–20

[2] Pierot L, Pereira VM, Cognard C, von Kummer R. Teaching lessons by MR CLEAN. AJNR Am J Neuroradiol. 2015; 36(5):819–821

[3] Goyal M, Demchuk AM, Menon BK, et al. ESCAPE Trial Investigators. Randomized assessment of rapid endovascular treatment of ischemic stroke. N Engl J Med. 2015; 372(11):1019–1030

[4] Campbell BCV, Mitchell PJ, Kleinig TJ, et al. EXTEND-IA Investigators. Endovascular therapy for ischemic stroke with perfusion-imaging selection. N Engl J Med. 2015; 372(11):1009–1018

[5] Saver JL, Goyal M, Bonafe A, et al. SWIFT PRIME Investigators. Stent-retriever thrombectomy after intravenous t-PA vs. t-PA alone in stroke. N Engl J Med. 2015; 372(24):2285–2295

[6] Jovin TG, Chamorro A, Cobo E, et al. REVASCAT Trial Investigators. Thrombectomy within 8 hours after symptom onset in ischemic stroke. N Engl J Med. 2015; 372(24):2296–2306

5 Solitaire Stent-Retriever Thrombectomy: Building the Evidence

5.1 Case Description

5.1.1 Clinical Presentation

- A 37-year-old female presented to the emergency department approximately 30 minutes after acute onset of left-sided hemiplegia.
- Clinical examination revealed severe dysarthria, hemiplegia of the left side, and neglect to the left side (National Institutes of Health Stroke Scale [NIHSS] score of 18).

5.1.2 Imaging and Workup

- Noncontrast CT demonstrated dense middle cerebral artery (MCA) sign on the right side.
- CT angiography showed right internal carotid artery (ICA) occlusion consistent with dissection and right MCA occlusion.
- MRI confirmed the ICA dissection and demonstrated restricted diffusion limited to the lenticulostriate distribution of the MCA.

5.1.3 Diagnosis

- Right ICA occlusion consistent with dissection and right MCA occlusion.
- She was given intravenous tissue plasminogen activator IV-tPA 1 hour 10 minutes after symptom onset; however, the patient continued to display persistent left hemiplegia with no clinical improvement.
- After interdisciplinary discussion, the decision was made for mechanical thrombectomy of the occluded M1 segment.

5.1.4 Technique

- The procedure was performed under conscious sedation. The patient was prepped and draped in the usual sterile fashion. The right common femoral artery was localized by ultrasound and palpation. A right common femoral artery

puncture was performed. An 8-Fr short arterial sheath was placed.

- An 8-Fr MERCI Balloon guide catheter was then prepared. Using a coaxial technique with a 5-Fr, 125-cm HH1 catheter and a Terumo glide wire, the 8-Fr balloon guide catheter was advanced into the right common carotid artery. Injection of the right common carotid artery confirmed occlusion of the right ICA just above the bifurcation, with flame-shaped tapering in keeping with an internal carotid dissection.
- Using road map technique, the Terumo glide wire was carefully advanced beyond the occlusion, taking care to remain within the true lumen of the vessel. The HH1 and 8-Fr Balloon guide catheters were then advanced into the right ICA, to about the C2–C3 level.
- Angiography performed through the guide now showed the intracranial ICA. The carotid termination and the right A1 segment were patent. The right M1 segment was occluded proximally. There were some late leptomeningeal collaterals (poor). Following injection, there was stasis of contrast in the ICA, in keeping with the proximal ICA occlusion.
- A Rebar 18 microcatheter was prepared, and attached to a flush system. Using roadmap technique, the microcatheter was navigated along with the Transend Soft Tip Guidewire into the upper M2 trunk of the right MCA.
- A Solitaire 5 mm × 40 cm stent retriever device was placed across the MCA clot, from the M2 upper trunk to the supraclinoid ICA, and it was unsheathed to deploy. With stent deployment, antegrade flow was seen in the right MCA. The stent was left in position for 5 minutes, and then retrieved. The balloon was not inflated on the guide, as the dissection of the ICA was already occluding the ICA. Continuous suction was applied to the balloon guide during stent retrieval. Thrombus was observed on the retrieved stent. The guiding catheter and hub were meticulously aspirated and flushed. Postretrieval hand and pump injections showed good patency of the M1 segment of the MCA and most M2 branches. The ACA remained patent, with flash filling. There was still ICA stasis in keeping with the proximal occlusion (▶ Fig. 5.1).

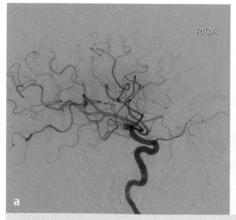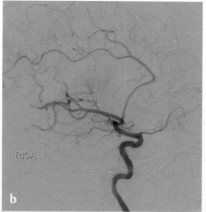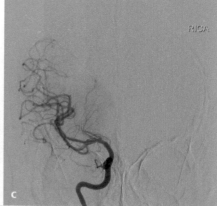

Fig. 5.1 (a) Digital subtraction angiography showing right M1 occlusion in the context of ICA dissection (not shown) with (b) Solitaire device in situ permitting transient bypass. (c) Postthrombectomy bypass demonstrating recanalization. (Courtesy of Dr. Peter Howard.)

- Attention was then turned to the proximal ICA dissection. The guide catheter was carefully withdrawn into the common carotid artery. A hand injection of contrast showed irregularity of the ICA at the site of prior dissection, with less than 50% luminal narrowing and no evidence of hemodynamic compromise. The possibility of stenting to preserve the proximal ICA patency was discussed with neurology. It was agreed not to stent to avoid use of aspirin and Plavix.
- A repeat common carotid angiogram was performed after a 15-minute delay. The MCA remained patent. The ICA had improved in appearance, with less narrowing than on the previous angiogram.
- At this point, it was decided to terminate the procedure. The guiding catheter was removed. The 8-Fr groin sheath was sewn in place. On the day following the procedure, the groin sheath was removed and manual compression for about 30 to 40 minutes gave good hemostasis. The patient had a dramatic improvement in right arm and leg motor function following the procedure.

5.1.5 Outcome

- Recanalization of right MCA occlusion using Solitaire stent retriever device was technically successful.
- Patient also had an occlusive dissection of the proximal right ICA as seen on the CTA prior to procedure. Following placement of the large guide catheter across the dissection into the distal true lumen, and subsequent retrieval of the catheter into the CCA, the proximal ICA was recanalized and remained patent without evidence of hemodynamic compromise.
- Early neurological improvement was noted after the procedure. At discharge 7 days later, the NIHSS score was 2, and she made an excellent functional recovery.

5.1.6 Discussion

After publication of the positive trials in 2015, many systematic reviews and meta-analyses sought to pool together the data from these trials to make a more robust claim for mechanical thrombectomy. Four meta-analyses were published in 2016 that used a variety of methods to pool together patient data and perform further analyses across the RCTs.

The first of these meta-analyses was published in November 2015 in *JAMA*. This meta-analysis included eight RCTs with published results at the time: IMS III, SYNTHESIS, MR RESCUE, MR CLEAN, ESCAPE, EXTEND-IA, SWIFT-PRIME, and REVASCAT. A total of 2,423 patients were included, with 1,313 who received endovascular therapy and 1,110 who received standard medical treatment. The study discovered that endovascular therapy was associated with an improvement of modified Rankin scale (mRS) scores (odds ratio [OR]: 1.56, 95% confidence interval [CI]: 1.14–2.13). Moreover, 12% more patients in the endovascular group achieved functional independence (mRS ≤ 2) at 90 days (OR: 1.71, 95% CI: 1.18–2.49). There were also significantly higher rates of revascularization achieved with endovascular thrombectomy (75.8%) than tPA alone (34.1%; OR: 6.49, 95% CI: 4.79–8.79). There were no differences in symptomatic intracerebral hemorrhage (SICH) or all-cause mortality at 90 days.

However, the heterogeneity between the studies was high for the mRS. Thus, subgroup and sensitivity analyses were performed. In particular, functional outcomes were significantly better in patients with confirmed proximal artery occlusions on imaging, those who received a combination therapy of both endovascular and tPA, and those who received the stent retrievers. In addition, there was interaction between the study year and functional outcomes in that, unsurprisingly, the older trials revealed less effect sizes. This meta-analysis synthesized the results from multiple RCTs, and despite the presence of heterogeneity among the trials, endovascular therapy was still shown to result in better functional outcomes and better revascularization rates when compared with standard medical management.[1]

Another meta-analysis was published in *Stroke* in March 2016, and it included patient-level data from ESCAPE, SWIFT PRIME, EXTEND-IA, and REVASCAT, RCTs that primarily used the Solitaire device. The primary analysis included 787 patients from all four trials, of which 401 were randomized to endovascular group and 386 to the standard medical therapy. The primary outcome was functional score at 90 days as defined by the mRS. Secondary outcomes were functional independence (mRS ≤ 2), mortality, and SICH rates. In the primary analysis, the common odds ratio (cOR) for mRS improvement was 2.7 (95% CI: 2.0–3.5). The number needed to treat (NNT) to reduce disability was 2.5 and the NNT for a better independent functional outcome was 4.25. Mortality and SICH rates were not significant. Two sensitivity analyses were performed as well, excluding patients in whom Solitaire was not the first device used and excluding ESCAPE where other devices were allowed. The results of these sensitivity analyses were similar to the primary analysis. The benefit of thrombectomy was consistently observed in all predefined subgroups, regardless of age, sex, NIHSS score, the site of lesion, presence of tandem cervical carotid occlusions, ASPECTS score, and administration of IV-tPA. Furthermore, though older age is frequently an exclusion criterion for thrombectomy, the result from this meta-analysis suggests that there is no evidence of reduced benefit in the elderly patient (≥ 80 years of age). In fact, there was an observed clinically significant 20% absolute reduction in mortality rates. Moreover, in IMS III and MR CLEAN, NIHSS was a selection criterion for patients. This meta-analysis found no significant difference in benefit in patients with NIHSS ≤ 15 in comparison to patients with NIHSS > 20. Lastly, the pool data affirmed that better functional outcome is achieved with decreased time from onset to intervention. The result from this meta-analysis suggests that the Solitaire device is safe and effective in treating large vessel occlusions, leading to improvement in functional outcome and reduced disability in all patient subgroups.[2]

A systematic review published in the *BMJ* was conducted by researchers in Portugal. This study included all RCTs comparing medical care with endovascular therapy. All of the 2,925 patients from 10 studies were included, those from IMS III, SYNTHESIS, MR RESCUE, MR CLEAN, ESCAPE, EXTEND-IA, SWIFT-PRIME, REVASCAT, THERAPY, and THRACE. With the pool analysis, endovascular treatment had higher proportion of patients with good or excellent functional outcomes (mRS ≤ 2 or 1). The risk ratio of a good functional outcome was 1.37 (95% CI: 1.14–1.64). Mortality and SICH rates were not significant. However, heterogeneity of the studies was high. After excluding the 2013 trials, MR RESCUE, SYNTHESIS, and IMS III, there were no longer heterogeneity among the trial results, and the risk ratio of a good functional increased to 1.56 (95% CI: 1.38–1.75). Due to methodological issues with MR RESCUE, SYNTHESIS, and IMS III, the OR of 1.56 was deemed to be a more accurate reflection of endovascular therapy's true effect. This systematic review provided moderate- to high-quality evidence that endovascular therapy 6 to 8 hours after acute ischemic stroke onset provides benefit in functional outcomes.[3]

The final meta-analysis included data only from the five RCTs published in 2015: MR CLEAN, ESCAPE, EXTEND-IA, SWIFT-PRIME, and REVASCAT. This meta-analysis was published in the *Lancet*, and included data from 1,287 patients with 634 randomized to endovascular thrombectomy and 653 to medical therapy. The pooled results indicate that endovascular treatment was associated with significant reduction of disability, as measured by mRS, at 90 days (adjusted cOR: 2.49, 95% CI: 1.76–3.53). Moreover, the NNT to reduce at least one score of mRS was 2.6. Mortality and SICH rates did not differ between the intervention and control groups. There were many subgroups of clinical interest associated with a significant effect favoring endovascular thrombectomy. In particular, patients older than 80 years achieved a cOR of 3.68 (95% CI: 1.95–6.92) favoring the intervention. Patients who were randomized 300 minutes after onset of symptoms achieved cOR of 1.79 (95% CI: 1.05–2.97). Patients who were not eligible for IV-tPA had cOR of 2.43 (95% CI: 1.30–4.55). This result shows benefit for patients who are older, those who underwent randomization later, and those in which IV-tPA was contraindicated.[4,5,6]

With these systematic reviews and meta-analysis, it is more evident than ever that endovascular thrombectomy is more effective than tPA alone in treating patients with acute ischemic strokes. The functional outcome was better with intervention even with patient data included from the negative 2013 trials. When results from only the newer trials were analyzed, the effect size was considerably larger. There was also new evidence that the intervention is effective regardless of patient age, NIHSS score, ASPECTS score, site of lesion, presence of tandem cervical carotid occlusions, whether concomitant tPA was administered, and whether randomization was delayed.[2,3,4] Essentially, endovascular therapy is safe and effective in almost all patient groups. With the current solid evidence, endovascular therapy should be the standard of care for large artery occlusions in the anterior circulation. Policy makers around the world have since been urged by investigators to put a greater emphasis on building health care systems that increase the accessibility of advanced stroke services to the population.

References

[1] Bracard S, Ducrocq X, Mas JL, et al. THRACE Investigators. Mechanical thrombectomy after intravenous alteplase versus alteplase alone after stroke (THRACE): a randomised controlled trial. Lancet Neurol. 2016; 15(11):1138–1147

[2] Mocco J, Zaidat OO, von Kummer R, et al. THERAPY Trial Investigators. Aspiration thrombectomy after intravenous alteplase versus intravenous alteplase alone. Stroke. 2016; 47(9):2331–2338

[3] Badhiwala JH, Nassiri F, Alhazzani W, et al. Endovascular thrombectomy for acute ischemic stroke: a meta-analysis. JAMA. 2015; 314(17):1832–1843

[4] Campbell BCV, Hill MD, Rubiera M, et al. Safety and efficacy of solitaire stent thrombectomy: individual patient data meta-analysis of randomized trials. Stroke. 2016; 47(3):798–806

[5] Rodrigues FB, Neves JB, Caldeira D, Ferro JM, Ferreira JJ, Costa J. Endovascular treatment versus medical care alone for ischaemic stroke: systematic review and meta-analysis. BMJ. 2016; 353(January):i1754

[6] Goyal M, Menon BK, van Zwam WH, et al. HERMES collaborators. Endovascular thrombectomy after large-vessel ischaemic stroke: a meta-analysis of individual patient data from five randomised trials. Lancet. 2016; 387(10029):1723–1731

Part II

Case Selection

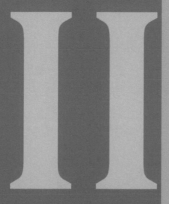

6 Timing in Stroke and the Tissue Clock

6.1 Case Description

Completed stroke in a young patient within 1 hour of ictus.

6.1.1 Clinical Presentation

A 39-year-old woman developed left hemiparesis while driving. Her father noted she was also confused. The patient was transferred to the emergency department via ambulance, presenting 50 minutes following symptom onset.

Examination revealed expressive dysphasia, dense left hemiparesis, and severe neglect. She was noted to be ambidextrous. The patient had no significant past medical history and was on no medication.

6.1.2 Imaging Workup and Investigations

- Noncontrast computed tomography (NCCT) was performed at 1 hour. This demonstrated hypodensity involving grey and white matter in the right lenticulostriate territories and temporal lobe, ASPECTS score 6. Right M1 linear density was suggestive of acute thrombus (▶ Fig. 6.1).
- Perfusion maps showed increased mean transit time (MTT) throughout the entire right middle cerebral artery (MCA) territory, with decreased cerebral blood volume (CBV), consistent with core infarction in the right lateral lenticulostriate territories, right temporal lobe, and paracentral gyri (▶ Fig. 6.2).
- CT angiography revealed a right internal carotid artery dissection causing total occlusion from the level of the axis to the petrous portion of the intracranial carotid artery. Right M1 segment occlusion was confirmed.
- MRI demonstrated a large area of diffusion restriction (approximately 180 cc) involving the right MCA territory (▶ Fig. 6.3).

6.1.3 Diagnosis

M1 segment occlusion and right internal carotid artery dissection (▶ Fig. 6.3).

6.1.4 Treatment

- Given the large volume core infarct, the patient was treated medically with aspirin and statin alone. She also received intensive physical, occupational, and speech therapy.

6.1.5 Outcome

- She made moderate improvements in dysphasia and mild in weakness. Rankin disability score was 4 on discharge.
- Following discharge, the patient had a residual left-sided dyspraxia, weakness, and mild cognitive impairment. Her recovery was complicated by the development of secondary generalized tonic/clonic seizures.

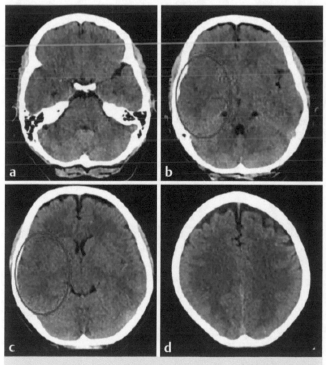

Fig. 6.1 (a, top left) Right M1 linear density was suggestive of acute thrombus; (b–d) NCCT demonstrating hypodensity involving the right lenticulostriate territories and temporal lobe.

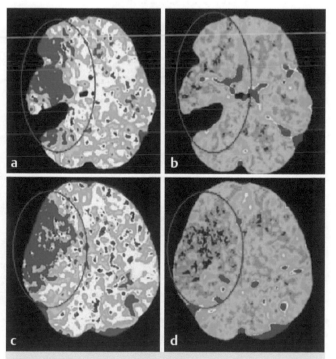

Fig. 6.2 (a, top left) MTT at level of basal ganglia; (b, top right) CBV at level of basal ganglia; (c, bottom left) MTT cortical slice; (d, bottom right) CBV cortical slice.

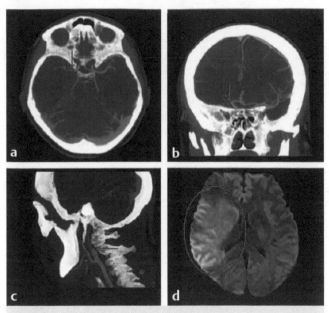

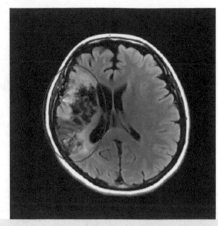

Fig. 6.4 Follow-up FLAIR image showing established right MCA infarct with extensive encephalomalacia and cavitation.

Fig. 6.3 (a, top left) axial CT angiogram maximum intensity projection (MIP); (b, top right) coronal CT angiogram MIP; (c, bottom left) sagittal CT angiogram neck MIP; (d, bottom right) axial diffusion-weighted MR image.

- Follow-up MRI revealed established right MCA infarct with extensive encephalomalacia and cavitation (▶ Fig. 6.4). New infarction was also noted in the posterior limb of the right internal capsule.

6.2 Companion Case

Elderly patient with only a small core and large penumbra 5 hours and 50 minutes after ictus.

6.2.1 Clinical Presentation

A 73-year-old man developed sudden-onset expressive dysphasia and right hemiparesis following admission the previous night with new-onset atrial fibrillation. He had been last seen well 3 hours 30 minutes prior.

His past history included ischemic heart disease, treated with a cardiac stent, dyslipidemia, hypertension, and chronic airways disease.

6.2.2 Imaging Workup and Investigations

- NCCT performed 2 hours 20 minutes following presentation (5 hours 50 minutes following last known well time) showed no established infarct, ASPECTS score 10 (▶ Fig. 6.5a).
- CTA demonstrated left M1 segment occlusion (▶ Fig. 6.5b).
- Perfusion imaging revealed a large region of left MCA territory ischemia, highlighted with increased MTT. CBV maps indicated only a small region of core infarction (▶ Fig. 6.5c, d).

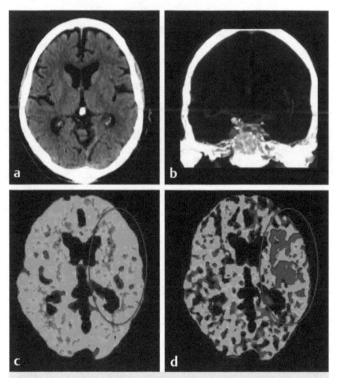

Fig. 6.5 (a, top left) NCCT at the level of the basal ganglia; (b, top right) coronal CT angiogram maximum intensity projection (MIP); (c, bottom left) CBV map at the level of the basal ganglia; (d, bottom right) MTT map at the level of the basal ganglia.

- MRI imaging was performed to confirm a small infarct core prior to determining the treatment course. MRI demonstrated restricted diffusion, consistent with core infarct of less than 10 cc involving the left corona radiata, left caudate body, and possibly the posterior limb of the internal capsule (▶ Fig. 6.6).

6.2.3 Diagnosis

Left M1 occlusion.

6.2.4 Treatment

- With new-onset atrial fibrillation, the patient had received therapeutic Clexane, and as such was not a candidate for conventional tissue plasminogen activator.

6.2.5 Endovascular

- Clot retrieval was performed 4 hours after symptoms were discovered, 7.5 hours after the last known well time, with a 5MAX penumbra aspiration catheter.
- Left M1 clot was withdrawn with aspiration on the 5MAX and 7-Fr shuttle catheters (▶ Fig. 6.7).
- TICI 2B reperfusion left MCA territory was demonstrated.

6.2.6 Outcome

- Some neurological improvement was noted immediately, with an improvement in the right upper limb power. NIHSS was 9 in the afternoon following retrieval. Ultimately, the patient made a good recovery with an NIHSS score of 3.
- Repeat MRI showed minimal growth of the preexisting diffusion-weighted imaging infarct core, confirming lenticulostriate perforator territory of the left MCA.
- On outpatient review, there was minimal residual dysphasia and hemiparesis. The patient was independent with all activities of daily living, with a Rankin score of 1.

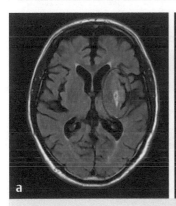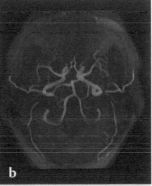

Fig. 6.6 FLAIR image showing a small infarct core less than 10 cc with persistent occlusion.

6.2.7 Discussion

Achieving good outcome in acute ischemic stroke is dependent on multiple factors not the least of which include successful revascularization and duration of symptoms. Much of the benefits seen in the recently published stroke trials is attributed to both superior device selection allowing for improved revascularization as well as organized systems of care which allowed for rapid triage of patients and decreased time to revascularization.[1,2,3,4,5] However, we have grown to understand that achieving excellent revascularization (i.e., mTICI of 2c or 3) in a timely manner does not guarantee an excellent functional outcome.[1,2,3,4,5] Likewise, there are many cases in which patients are revascularized outside a given time window, yet still achieve an excellent neurological outcome (**Case 2**). This can be explained by other factors at play including the "tissue clock." This concept is important as it demonstrates that patients should not be triaged for mechanical thrombectomy based on time from symptom onset alone (**Case 1**).

Large vessel occlusions result in a rapid decrease in cerebral blood flow (CBF). Normally, CBF is about 50 mL/100 g/min. However, if CBF decreases to 23 mL/100 g/min clinical signs of ischemia begin to occur. When CBF decreases to below 15 mL/100 g/min, cortical evoked potentials precipitously decrease. The cessation of cortical evoked potentials (CEPs) is secondary to neurons conserving energy by decreasing cell metabolism to the minimal possible level and represents one of the final stages prior to infarction.[6,7]

The depth of cerebral ischemia is basically a function of CBF. As the depth of cerebral ischemia decreases, the amount of time available to salvage brain tissue decreases as well. Thus, the time available to salvage brain tissue in acute ischemic stroke is not only dependent on factors within our control (i.e., achieving a timely complete revascularization) but is also dependent on the depth of ischemia (i.e., reduction in CBF) that is causing the patient's clinical symptoms.[6,7] For example, a patient with a left MCA occlusion with a CBF of 20 mL/100 g/min may have the exact same symptoms as one with a CBF of 11 mL/100 g/min due to the fact that the CBF in both cases is well below the threshold that results in signs of cerebral ischemia. However, the amount of time which the patient with the CBF reduction of 11/mL/100 mg/min can sustain the ischemic insult without suffering irreversible injury is much less than that of the patient

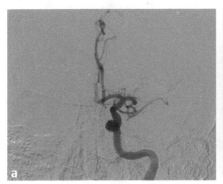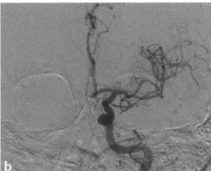

Fig. 6.7 (a) Cerebral angiogram demonstrating left M1 occlusion; (b) reperfusion following clot retrieval.

with a CBF of 20 mL/100 g/min.[7] This explains the concept of the tissue clock as "every person has his or her own time."[6]

The tissue clock is dependent on multiple factors, the most important of which is collateral blood flow. The greater the extent of collaterals, the greater the CBF in the ischemic territory and the "slower" the tissue clock. It is for this reason that some recently published trials such as ESCAPE put such a large emphasis on the imaging of collaterals to determine patient selection.[5,8] The role of collaterals in patient selection and outcome of acute ischemic stroke is described in Chapter 7 of this book. Other factors which affect the tissue clock include temperature, blood glucose, and neuronal metabolism. Over the past two decades, extensive research has been performed to address these aspects of the tissue clock.[9] The goal of this approach is to somehow impede the ischemic cascade through the introduction of neuroprotective agents. However, despite significant success of this strategy in preclinical and animal models, no human trials to date have demonstrated efficacy of the neuroprotective strategy.[9] Nonetheless, as we begin to achieve successful revascularization rates in 80 to 90% of patients, it is possible that renewing investigations into slowing down the tissue clock could prove useful.

6.2.8 Pearls and Pitfalls

- The degree of cerebral blood flow reduction determines the length of time one can tolerate cerebral ischemia.
- The tissue clock is a function of multiple patient-specific factors including collateral blood flow, temperature, blood glucose, and neuronal metabolism.

- Selection of patients based on the extent of collaterals is well established.
- Further research is needed to determine if other neuroprotective strategies aimed at slowing down the tissue clock will be useful.

References

[1] Berkhemer OA, Fransen PS, Beumer D, et al. MR CLEAN Investigators. A randomized trial of intraarterial treatment for acute ischemic stroke. N Engl J Med. 2015; 372(1):11–20

[2] Boers AM, Marquering HA, Jochem JJ, et al. MR CLEAN Investigators. Automated cerebral infarct volume measurement in follow-up noncontrast CT scans of patients with acute ischemic stroke. AJNR Am J Neuroradiol. 2013; 34(8):1522–1527

[3] Campbell BC, Mitchell PJ, Kleinig TJ, et al. EXTEND-IA Investigators. Endovascular therapy for ischemic stroke with perfusion-imaging selection. N Engl J Med. 2015; 372(11):1009–1018

[4] Demchuk AM, Goyal M, Menon BK, et al. Endovascular treatment for Small Core and Anterior circulation Proximal occlusion with Emphasis on minimizing CT to recanalization times (ESCAPE) trial: methodology. Int J Stroke. 2015; 10(3):429–438

[5] Goyal M, Demchuk AM, Menon BK, et al. ESCAPE Trial Investigators. Randomized assessment of rapid endovascular treatment of ischemic stroke. N Engl J Med. 2015; 372(11):1019–1030

[6] Al-Ali F, Elias JJ, Filipkowski DE, Faber JE. Acute ischemic stroke treatment, part 1: patient selection "the 50% barrier and the capillary index score". Front Neurol. 2015; 6:83

[7] Jones TH, Morawetz RB, Crowell RM, et al. Thresholds of focal cerebral ischemia in awake monkeys. J Neurosurg. 1981; 54(6):773–782

[8] Menon BK, d'Esterre CD, Qazi EM, et al. Multiphase CT angiography: a new tool for the imaging triage of patients with acute ischemic stroke. Radiology. 2015; 275(2):510–520

[9] Fisher M. New approaches to neuroprotective drug development. Stroke. 2011; 42(1) Suppl:S24–S27

7 Role of Leptomeningeal Collaterals

7.1 Case Description

7.1.1 Clinical Presentation

A 72-year-old female presented to the emergency department with a 90-minute history of sudden-onset right hemiparesis, global aphasia, and neglect. Initial National Institutes of Health Stroke Scale (NIHSS) score was 25. Past medical history was significant for hypertension, dyslipidemia, and atrial fibrillation. Medications at the time of presentation included aspirin 81 mg daily and multiple antihypertensive agents. She had previously been anticoagulated with warfarin; however, this had been discontinued 2 years previously due to episodes of significant epistaxis.

7.1.2 Imaging Workup and Investigations

- Noncontrast computed tomography (NCCT) and CT angiography (CTA) were completed within 2 hours from the onset of symptoms showing left M1 occlusion (▶ Fig. 7.1).

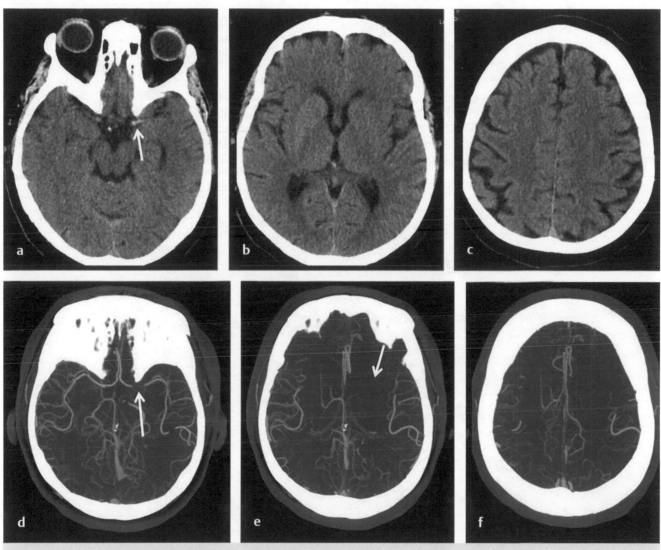

Fig. 7.1 Non–contrast-enhanced CT brain (**a–c**) demonstrated a hyperdense vessel sign in the region of carotid termination and proximal M1 segment on the left (**7.1a**, *arrow*). There was loss of gray-white matter differentiation in the region of the caudate nucleus and insular ribbon on left (ASPECTS score of 8). No other early or established ischemic change was seen. There was no evidence of hemorrhage. Single-phase CT angiogram performed from the level of the aortic arch demonstrated occlusion of the left carotid terminus and proximal M1 segment of left MCA. There was, however, good leptomeningeal collateralization of the occluded left MCA territory, with filling of left MCA branches back to the M1 segment and distal face of the thrombus (**d–f**). The thrombus could be seen as a relatively short length filling defect in the vessel (**d**, *arrow*). Note was made of relative paucity of vessels in the region of the left lenticulostriate territory compared to the contralateral side (**e**, *arrow*) with absent opacification of the left internal cerebral vein. The left ACA was patent, filling through a patent anterior communicating artery.

7.1.3 Diagnosis

Left carotid terminus occlusion with good leptomeningeal collateralization to left middle cerebral artery (MCA) territory.

7.1.4 Treatment

Full-dose intravenous tissue plasminogen activator (IV-tPA) was administered which was initially used as a bridge to mechanical thrombectomy.

Material Used

An 8-Fr short angiographic sheath; 8-Fr MERCI balloon guide catheter; 5-Fr VTK slip catheter; 0.035 Terumo Advantage guidewire wire; Synchro 14 microguidewire; Trevo 18 microcatheter; Trevo Pro 4×20 mm stent retriever; 8-Fr Angio-Seal closure device.

Technique

- Intervention was performed with conscious sedation, and local anesthetic. A single-wall right common femoral artery puncture was performed, and the 8-Fr short vascular access sheath inserted. Following puncture, 2,000 international units of heparin was administered intravenously.

- The 8-Fr balloon guide catheter was advanced to the left internal carotid artery (ICA) over a 5-Fr VTK slip catheter with the aid of an advantage guidewire. Left internal carotid angiogram demonstrated persistent occlusion of the left carotid terminus (▶ Fig. 7.2), with abrupt cut-off of contrast in the supraclinoid ICA at the level of the anterior choroidal artery origin.

- A Trevo 18 microcatheter was navigated through the occluded left carotid terminus and M1 segment and into the left proximal inferior division of left MCA. Control injection through the microcatheter (not shown) confirmed position distal to thrombus in a patent good caliber M2 branch. A 4×20 mm Trevo Pro stent retriever was then deployed from the proximal M2 to the level of the supraclinoid ICA. The tip of the stent retriever is depicted by arrow in ▶ Fig. 7.2a.

- After leaving the stent in situ for 5 minutes to allow incorporation of thrombus, retrieval was performed with flow arrest and continuous aspiration through the balloon guide catheter. Thrombus fragments were retrieved from the stent and aspiration tubing and further thrombus was obtained from aspiration of the guide catheter. The guide catheter balloon was deflated.

- Control angiogram showed complete recanalization of the index lesion, and complete reperfusion of the distal MCA territory with no evidence of thromboembolic complication. The left ACA territory was patent and was now seen filling

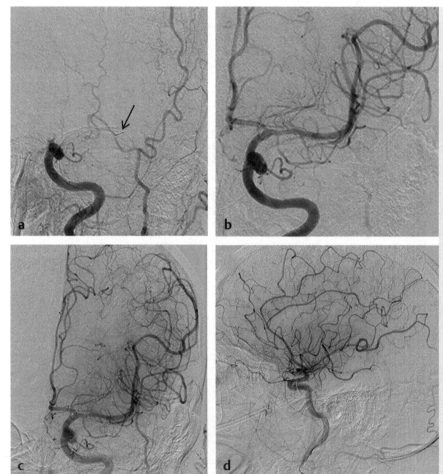

Fig. 7.2 Left internal carotid angiogram showing persistent occlusion of the left carotid terminus (**a**), with abrupt cut off of contrast in the supraclinoid ICA at the level of the anterior choroidal artery origin and tip of the stent retriever (*arrow*). Control angiogram showed complete recanalization (**b**) after stent retriever and adjunctive suction, and distal reperfusion (**c,d**).

from the left ICA injection. The procedure was completed within 4 hours of symptom onset.

- All devices were removed. An 8-Fr Angio-Seal closure device was placed for hemostasis.

7.2 Postprocedure Care/Outcome

The patient demonstrated on table improvement to NIHSS score of 7, with mild right sided weakness and dysphasia remaining. Postprocedure the patient was transferred to high-dependency stroke unit for further care.

Repeat NCCT of the brain was performed at 24 hours postprocedure (▶ Fig. 7.3). This demonstrated low attenuation change consistent with small volume infarction in the left caudate and lentiform nucleus, as well as insular and frontal opercular region. Gray-white matter differentiation was otherwise preserved in the left hemisphere with no evidence of more widespread infarction. Following CT, the patient was commenced on 81 mg aspirin daily. In view of the atrial fibrillation and prior history of significant epistaxis, the patient was assessed by the ENT service, and subsequently recommended on anticoagulation at 10 days poststroke. Blood pressure control was optimized and lipid lowering medication was commenced. The patient continued to improve throughout her inpatient stay with almost complete resolution of symptoms, and she was discharged 5 days following presentation to rehabilitation.

7.3 Companion Case

7.3.1 Clinical Presentation

A 75-year-old male presented to the emergency department with a 90-minute history of sudden onset right facial droop, hemiparesis, global aphasia, and neglect. NIHSS score was 28. Past medical history was significant for hypertension, dyslipidemia, and atrial fibrillation. Medications at the time of presentation included warfarin, with INR of 2.7 on testing.

7.3.2 Imaging Workup and Investigations

- NCCT of the brain and CT angiogram were completed within 2 hours of symptom onset. CT of the brain (▶ Fig. 7.4) demonstrated loss of gray-white matter differentiation in the left insula, and cortical zones M5 and M6. CT ASPECTS score 7. Hyperdense vessel sign was noted in the region of the left carotid terminus and proximal M1 segment.
- Single-phase arch-to-vertex CT angiography was performed. This demonstrated occlusion of the left supraclinoid ICA to carotid terminus as well as nonfilling of left A1 segment of ACA and left MCA. There was filling of the more distal left ACA territory presumably through the A Comm from the contralateral side. Axial reconstructed MIP images demonstrated overall poor collateralization to the majority of the left MCA territory. There was some filling of leptomeningeal collaterals in the left posterior temporal and inferior parietal region but relative paucity of collaterals elsewhere in the left MCA territory, particularly in the left frontal and anterior parietal region.

7.3.3 Diagnosis

Left carotid terminus occlusion with poor leptomeningeal collateralization to left MCA territory.

7.3.4 Treatment

As the patient was on warfarin with INR of 2.7, IV-tPA was contraindicated and so not administered. The patient was therefore brought directly to the interventional suite for endovascular treatment. Vitamin K was administered prior to intervention.

Material Used

- 8 Fr short angiographic sheath.
- 8-Fr MERCI balloon guide catheter.
- 5-Fr H1 slip catheter.

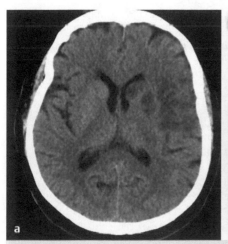
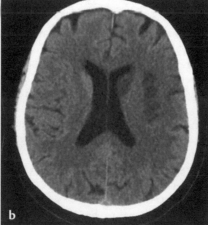
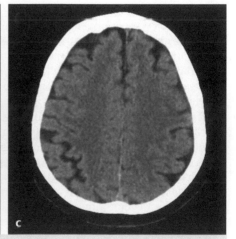

Fig. 7.3 A 24-hour follow-up NCCT (**a–c**) showing low attenuation change consistent with small-volume infarction in the left caudate and lentiform nucleus, as well as insular and frontal opercular region.

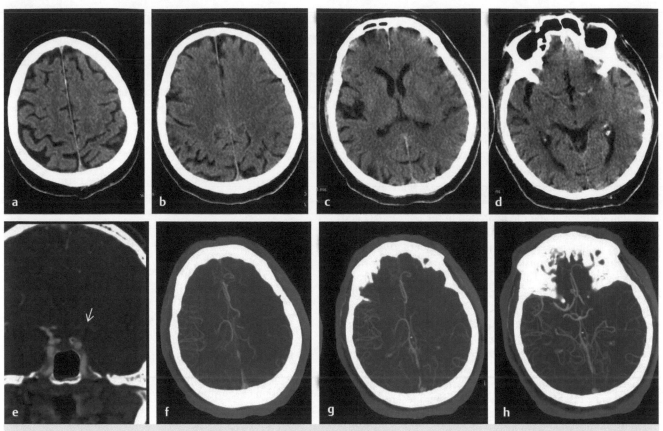

Fig. 7.4 NCCT within 2 hours of symptom onset showing (**a–c**) loss of gray-white matter differentiation in the left insula, and cortical zones M5 and M6, (ASPECTS score of 7) and hyperdense vessel (**d**). Single-phase CTA, showing occlusion of the left supraclinoid ICA to carotid terminus as well as non-filling of left A1 and M1 segments (**e**). Axial reconstructed MIP images demonstrated overall poor collateralization to the majority of the left MCA territory (**f–h**).

- 0.035 angled Terumo guidewire wire.
- Synchro 14 microguidewire.
- Rebar 18 microcatheter.
- Solitaire AB 6 × 30 mm.
- Trevo Pro 4 × 20 mm stent retriever.

Technique

- Intervention was performed with conscious sedation and local anesthetic. A single-wall right common femoral artery puncture was performed, and the 8-Fr short vascular access sheath was inserted. The 8-Fr balloon guide catheter was advanced to the left ICA over a 5-Fr H1 slip catheter with the aid of a Terumo guidewire.
- Left internal carotid angiogram demonstrated persistent occlusion of the left carotid terminus, with abrupt cutoff of contrast in the supraclinoid ICA. There was no filling of left ACA or MCA territory from the carotid injection.
- A Rebar 18 microcatheter was navigated through the occluded left carotid terminus and M1 segment with the aid of a Synchro 14 guidewire. A 6 × 30 mm Solitaire AB stent was deployed from the M1 segment of MCA to the left supraclinoid ICA (▶ Fig. 7.5a). There was no evidence of antegrade flow through the deployed stent on left ICA control injection.

- The stent was left in situ for 5 minutes and then retrieved with flow arrest and continuous aspiration. A large volume of thrombus was retrieved in the stent. Control angiography demonstrated recanalization of the carotid terminus, left A1, and proximal left MCA to the level of the distal M1 segment with some distal filling of temporal and anterior division of MCA branches (▶ Fig. 7.5b, c).
- Two further passes were performed in a similar fashion, from the M2 to M1 segment of MCA, first with the Solitaire 6 × 30 mm and secondly with a 4 × 20 mm Trevo Pro stent retriever. This resulted in complete recanalization of the left M1 segment of MCA and reperfusion of the distal MCA territory (▶ Fig. 7.5d–f).
- There was spasm in both the M1 segment and ICA. A total of 5 mg of intra-arterial (IA) verapamil was administered through the guide catheter with good effect. The patient was recanalized within 5 hours of symptom onset.

There was great difficulty in attempting to place closure device at the puncture site in view of extreme tortuosity of the iliac vessels and due to the patient's body habitus, as there was a large amount of soft tissue between the skin surface and the sheath entry site into the femoral artery. A groin hematoma was also present. Hemostasis was achieved by manual compression.

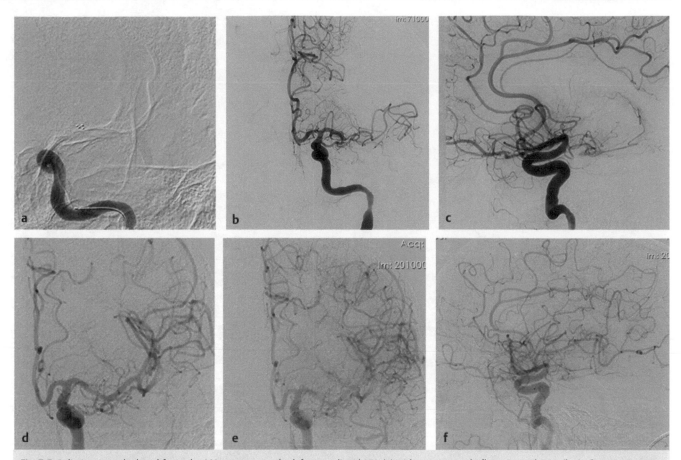

Fig. 7.5 Solitaire stent deployed from the M1 segment to the left supraclinoid ICA (**a**) with no antegrade flow. Control DSA (**b,c**) after continuous aspiration and stent retrieval shows recanalization of the carotid terminus, left A1, and proximal left MCA to the level of the distal M1 segment with some distal filling of temporal and anterior division of MCA branches. DSA (**d–f**) after two further passes from the M2 to M1 segment with the Solitaire 6 × 30 mm and secondly with a 4 × 20 mm Trevo Pro stent retriever showing complete recanalization of the left M1 segment of MCA and reperfusion of the distal MCA territory.

7.4 Postprocedure Care/Outcome

The patient's clinical condition was not significantly changed postprocedure. The following morning, NIHSS score was 26, which was a slight improvement from 28 on admission. CT at 24 hours postthrombectomy (▶ Fig. 7.6a–d), however, demonstrated large left MCA infarct, with relative sparing of the left posterior temporal lobe (a site where there were collaterals present on initial CTA). There was hemorrhagic transformation of the infarct in the region of the left basal ganglia with associated mass effect, midline shift, effacement of the left lateral ventricle, and also intraventricular extension of blood. Neurosurgery was consulted; however, it was felt that prognosis even with decompressive craniectomy would be poor; therefore, further intervention was not performed. The poor prognosis was discussed with the patients' family and palliative care service was consulted. The patient died on the eighth day of hospital admission.

7.4.1 Discussion

The greatest differentiating factor between these two similar cases with very different outcomes was most likely the degree of collateralization to the occluded left MCA territory. In the first case, there was excellent leptomeningeal collateralization with retrograde filling of MCA branches back to the M1 segment on CTA at presentation. In the second patient, who went on to infarct almost the entire territory, CTA performed at the same time from symptom onset showed poor collateralization particularly in the left frontal and parietal region, and there was already some loss of frontal gray-white matter differentiation at 2 hours from symptom onset.

Leptomeningeal collaterals, also referred to as leptomeningeal anastomoses or pial collaterals, are direct arteriole–arteriole connections, approximately 50 to 400 μm in caliber, joining terminal cortical branches of major cerebral arteries (i.e., anterior, middle, and posterior cerebrals) along the brain surface. Dormant under normal conditions (i.e., when blood flow from the major cerebral arteries is not impeded), they provide a route for retrograde filling of the territory distal to an occluded artery.

Carotid terminus occlusion has been shown to be an independent predictor for poor outcome in stroke, most likely because the occlusion of the carotid terminus cuts off the most important channel for collateral blood supply, the circle of Willis. Provided the patient has a patent anterior communicating artery, the ACA ipsilateral to the occlusion will fill antegradely from the contralateral side. There is, however, no

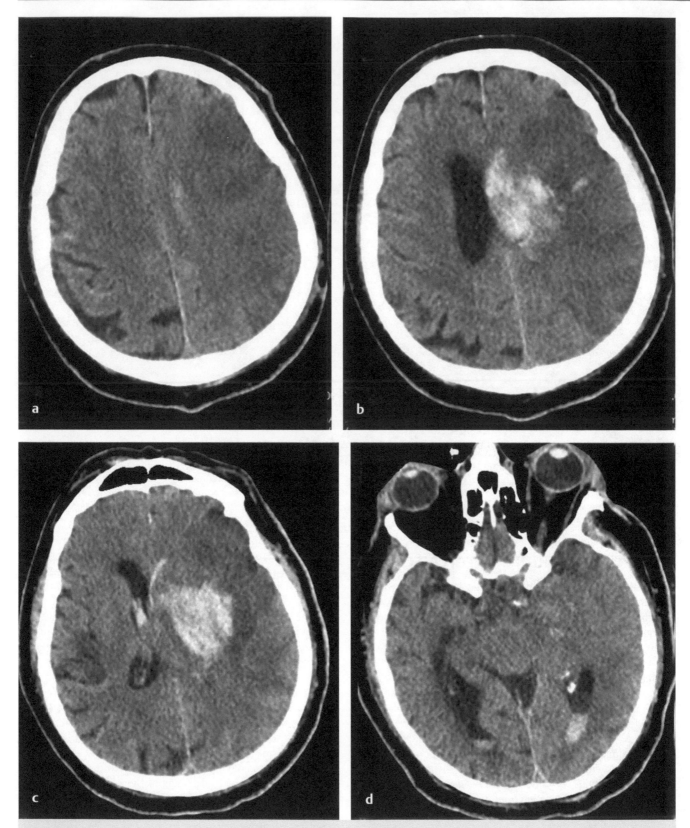

Fig. 7.6 NCCT at 24 hours postthrombectomy (**a–d**) demonstrated large left MCA infarct, with relative sparing of the left posterior temporal and hemorrhagic transformation in the region of the left basal ganglia with associated mass effect, midline shift, effacement of the left lateral ventricle, and intraventricular blood.

possibility of antegrade supply to the MCA territory, and collateral supply, if it exists, must therefore be retrograde due to filling of leptomeningeal collaterals from the ipsilateral ACA or PCA territory.

Numerous studies, using several imaging modalities and grading methods, suggest that good leptomeningeal collaterals confer a benefit in stroke. Relationship has been shown between collateral flow and the "known" predictors of good outcome in stroke. For example, good leptomeningeal collateral supply has been shown to be associated with lower NIHSS score at presentation, higher baseline ASPECTS score, lower admission diffusion-weighted imaging (DWI) lesion volume, less infarct growth, smaller final infarct size, and higher follow-up CT ASPECTS score. Poor collateralization has been associated with higher incidence and larger size of hemorrhage following IA thrombolytic therapy.

7.4.2 Workup and Diagnosis

Patient History

Targeted patient history should be obtained with a view to determining time interval from onset of symptoms, and contraindications to IV thrombolysis.

Examination and Investigations

Findings on physical examination in patients presenting with acute stroke will depend on the territory involved, and collateral supply to the occluded territory. Stroke severity should be assessed with the NIHSS. Patients with good leptomeningeal collateral supply have been shown to have lower NIHSS score at presentation. For example, Miteff et al[0] demonstrated significant difference in median acute NIHSS between good and reduced collateral groups in patients presenting with carotid T and M1 occlusion (NIHSS: 16 vs. 18; $p = 0.012$). Left and right hemisphere strokes were equally distributed between the groups. Menon et al[0] demonstrated that in multivariable analysis a poor collateral score was associated with higher baseline NIHSS score (odds ratio [OR]: 1.1 per 1 point increase in NIHSS; $p = 0.04$).

In determining eligibility for IV thrombolysis in a patient on warfarin, point-of-care INR testing in the emergency department will allow rapid determination of INR. IV-tPA administration can be considered in patients on warfarin with INR below 1.7.

NCCT will rule out hemorrhage as a cause for presentation and should be scrutinized for evidence of early ischemic changes such as loss of gray-white matter differentiation and early sulcal effacement. This is particularly important in patients with poor leptomeningeal collateral status as infarction may already be present even at short intervals from symptom onset as highlighted in section "Companion Case." Lima et al[0] demonstrated that patients with "equal" or "greater" collaterals had significantly higher baseline CT ASPECTS score than those with "less" collaterals ($p = 0.02$).

CTA is an important tool in the workup of the acute stroke patient. It is widely available, is easily accessible, and serves as a quick and highly accurate method for detecting occlusive thrombus in proximal cerebral arteries, and if performed from the level of the aortic arch it allows assessment of the extracranial vasculature. CTA has the added benefit of giving additional information regarding collateralization to the occluded vascular territory, and allows assessment of leptomeningeal collaterals. There are numerous proposed grading systems for leptomeningeal collaterals in the literature, as discussed in greater detail later in the "Imaging" section. Throughout numerous studies in both medically managed and endovascular cohorts, good collateral status has been shown in multivariate analysis to be an independent predictor for good functional outcome. Patients with poor collateral status are more likely to have a poor outcome following large artery occlusive stroke, despite treatment. Collateral status therefore does have a role to play in patient selection.

CT perfusion can be used as an adjunctive technique in patients presenting with acute stroke. Territory distal to the occlusion will typically show reduced time to peak (TTP), prolonged mean transit time (MTT), reduced relative cerebral blood flow (rCBF), and preserved or reduced relative cerebral blood volume (rCBV). A region of rCBV is taken to represent already infarcted tissue (i.e., "core infarct"). Regions of tissue with reduced TTP, rCBF, and prolonged MTT that do not have reduced rCBV are taken to represent tissue that is hypoperfused, and therefore at risk, but not yet infarcted, referred to as ischemic "penumbra." There are, however, downsides to CT perfusion. In addition to the extra radiation, CT perfusion requires postprocessing which takes time, there is a lack of standardization of postprocessing tools across vendors, and there is a lack of robust evidence validating its use in reliably identifying penumbra. There remains disagreement in the literature about its utility in routine clinical practice to guide early treatment decisions.

As a modality, CT is usually more accessible than MRI in the acute setting, it is also a quicker study to perform, and it does not require the extensive patient safety screening of MRI. MRI, however, remains the initial hyperacute stroke imaging investigation of choice in some centers. The basic MRI stroke protocol can be relatively fast and usually includes an axial DWI, axial T2*/susceptibility-weighted imaging, and axial fluid-attenuated inversion recovery, as well as intracranial time-of-flight or gadolinium-enhanced MRA to demonstrate site of occlusion. While MRA may provide information about the status of circle of Willis collaterals, it does not possess enough spatial resolution to evaluate the more distal leptomeningeal bed. CTA is superior to MRA for depicting and evaluating leptomeningeal collaterals.[0] Significant negative correlation has been demonstrated between CTA collateral score and baseline DWI lesion volume[0]; patients with higher and therefore better collateral scores have been shown to have lower lesion volume on DWI at baseline ($p < 0.001$).

7.4.3 Imaging Findings

There are numerous proposed grading systems for leptomeningeal collaterals in the literature using a variety of imaging techniques. Already in 2012, a systematic review published by McVerry et al in *AJNR* found 81 publications describing 63 different methods for grading leptomeningeal collateral supply on the basis of conventional angiography (digital subtraction angiography [DSA]), CTA, MRA, and transcranial Doppler (TCD).[0]

Conventional angiography can reveal retrograde collateral flow in a dynamic fashion; published methods for the assessment of flow are, however, heterogeneous. The most frequently used scale was proposed by the American Society of Interventional and Therapeutic Neuroradiology and Society of Interventional Radiology in an effort to homogenize grading with angiography. Extent of collateral flow to the territory of the occluded artery is assessed based on extent and speed of retrograde filling of the territory. This is a 5-point scale, where a score of 0 reflects no filling of collaterals and a score of 4 reflects complete and rapid collateral blood flow to the vascular bed in the entire territory by retrograde perfusion. Angiographic assessment of collaterals gives temporal resolution. Angiographic assessment is, however, invasive, and even when used in an interventional population complete assessment of collateral circulation on DSA would require injection of multiple vascular territories which can introduce an unacceptable time delay to reperfusion. It is therefore preferable that cross-sectional imaging techniques are used to assess collateral flow in stroke patients. Techniques such as CTA will confirm the presence of a large vessel occlusion, and allow assessment of collateral flow. While TCD and MRA may provide some information about collateral status, they do not possess enough spatial resolution to evaluate the more distal leptomeningeal bed. CTA has a higher degree of anatomic resolution and can more accurately depict the leptomeningeal collaterals.

Diverse CTA collateral scoring methods have been proposed using CTA source images and axial CTA maximum intensity projection (MIP) images. Although there is no standard scoring system, CTA allows prediction of clinical outcome with moderate to excellent interobserver agreement. On conventional single-phase CTA, published grading systems vary from simple 2-point scales where collateral score is dichotomized as "poor" or "good" to more complex 5-point scoring systems where collaterals are graded as absent, less, equal to, greater than, and exuberant compared to the contralateral hemisphere. The more complicated the grading system, the more predictive it will be in terms of outcome; however, the less easy it is to apply in day-to-day clinical use. Outside of a research situation, ease of use trumps predictive value, and a scoring system that is easy to apply with good interobserver variation would be favorable. One of the clinical randomized controlled trials published in 2015 which proved benefit for endovascular management of patients with large artery occlusive stroke was the ESCAPE study.[0] This trial used collateral vessel imaging on CTA as one of the approaches to improve the accuracy of assessing early ischemic change on unenhanced CT images and exclude patients with moderate to large core where recanalization/reperfusion was more likely to be futile. Patients were excluded from entry to the trial if there was no or minimal collateral filling in a region greater than 50% of the MCA territory when compared with pial filling on the contralateral side. Based on this, one could consider a dichotomized scale of "poor" versus "good" collaterals as determined by filling of less than or greater than 50% of the occluded arterial territory using the contralateral normal side as a comparison. The leptomeningeal collaterals on CTA depicted in ▶ Fig. 7.1d–f would therefore represent a good collateral grade, while those collaterals

depicted in ▶ Fig. 7.4f–h would therefore depict poor grade. As shown, collaterals are best assessed on reconstructed axial MIP images (24-mm thickness recommended). This has the added benefit of minimizing artifacts from patient motion.

While leptomeningeal collaterals have been shown as an important prognostic factor in large artery occlusive stroke, small numbers of patients with poor collaterals on standard single-phase CTA have been shown in studies to still have good clinical outcome. This may well relate to the static nature of conventional single-phase CTA, which provides a single snap shot in time of intracranial arterial contrast opacification. If images are acquired in the early arterial phase, it is possible that a patient with good collateral supply could be misclassified as having poor collateralization as acquisition may be too early to display collaterals with delayed filling.

Various imaging strategies have been proposed to counteract this potential pitfall of single-phase CTA. The static nature of conventional CTA can be overcome with time resolved, dynamic, the so-called 4D, techniques which are now possible on the newer CT systems which allow volumetric perfusion CT (VPCT) of the whole brain. This allows more detailed analysis of collateral flow in a time-resolved fashion which is less dependent on contrast bolus timing. The necessary image data can be reconstructed from the VPCT acquisition without additional contrast administration or radiation exposure. Frölich et al[0] have shown excellent interobserver reliability for scoring collaterals using this technique. In their study, the total extent of collateral flow was best visualized on temporally fused MIP (tMIP). Collateral grade was associated with favorable functional outcome and the strength of this relationship increased from earlier to later phases of dynamic CTA with collaterals on tMIP showing the strongest correlation with outcome. Smit et al[0] compared conventional single-phase CTA with timing invariant CTA (TI-CTA) derived from CT perfusion data in patients presenting with large artery occlusive stroke. Patients with poor collateral circulation on conventional CTA were still found to have good clinical outcome in 31% of cases; however, on TI-CTA, this subgroup of patients was found to actually have good collaterals. Conversely, all patients with poor collateral status on TI-CTA were found to have poor outcome. These studies support the fact that, if acquired too early, CTA will underestimate collateral flow.

The ESCAPE trial introduced another imaging innovation, multiphase CTA. This technique generates time-resolved cerebral angiograms of the intracranial vasculature from skull base to vertex in three phases following contrast administration using a multidetector CT scanner.[0] The first phase is an aortic arch to vertex acquisition, timed to be in peak arterial phase of normal brain using bolus tracking technique. The remaining two phases are from skull base to vertex in mid- and late-venous phase without addition of any extra contrast material. Images are then presented for assessment as reconstructed 24-mm axial MIP images. For multiphase CTA, a 6-point collateral score grading system has been detailed[0] which scores collaterals by looking at delay through phases, prominence, and extent of collaterals in the occluded territory compared to the contralateral hemisphere. A score of 0 reflects that compared to the asymptomatic contralateral side, there are no vessels visible in any phase within the occluded vascular territory. In contrast, for the highest score of 5, compared to the asymptomatic contralateral hemisphere, there is no delay and normal or increased prominence of peripheral vessels and normal extent within the occluded arteries territory within the symptomatic hemisphere. This 6-point scale can be collapsed to a 3-point scale of good, intermediate, and poor collaterals. Comparative efficacy of multiphase CTA has been compared with other imaging paradigms and its utility in clinical decision making confirmed.

Why some patients have better leptomeningeal collaterals than others remains unclear. There are certain anatomical situations which could contribute to poor collateral score in a patient with carotid terminus occlusion, for example, if the origin of an ipsilateral left fetal type PCA was covered by supraclinoid ICA thrombus, or where there is incomplete circle of Willis and the ipsilateral ACA cannot fill from the contralateral side. Such anatomical caveats would not explain poor collateral status for a solely M1 segment of MCA occlusion, however. Still, variant anatomy can be a contributing factor, and should be sought out on CTA. In the authors' experience, a situation where there is embolic occlusion of the left A2 segment of ACA together with either carotid terminus or M1 segment occlusion will invariably result in a poor collateral score for the MCA territory. A collateral score of 0 therefore should prompt a search for multifocal intracranial arterial occlusion, paying particular attention to ACA, as distal ACA occlusions can be easily missed, and are best identified on coronal and sagittal reconstructions.

7.4.4 Decision-Making Process

Throughout numerous studies in both medically managed and endovascular cohorts, good collateral status has been shown in multivariate analysis to be an independent predictor for good functional outcome. Degree of collateralization to the occluded territory therefore does play a role in patient selection.

A number of large randomized controlled clinical trials published in early 2015 have proven benefit for endovascular treatment with mechanical thrombectomy in patients with large artery occlusive stroke, and mechanical thrombectomy is now the standard of care for patients with proven large artery occlusion. "Correct" patient selection for thrombectomy, however, remains an important issue, and several imaging paradigms have been proposed to aid with patient selection, such as NCCT with CTA, NCCT with CTP, and MRI with DWI. To look at the NCCT and CTA paradigm, with collateral grading for patient selection, there is no doubt now from the literature that patients with good collaterals should be treated. It has not, however, as yet been shown across the literature that patients with poor collateral score have a ubiquitously poor outcome. As outlined in previous sections, this may reflect the fact that there are different collateral scoring systems, and most likely also relates to the assessment of collaterals on a single phase rather than multiphase or dynamic CTA. Therefore at present, while prognosis is guarded in these patients, a poor collateral score alone is not yet considered an absolute contraindication to stroke treatment and intervention. It is likely that further evidence will come in the form of post hoc analyses from the recent randomized controlled trials, but is as yet not available at the time of writing this book. It is important that standardized assessments of collateral score be put in place, and collaterals assessed on multiphase or dynamic CTA.

What may, however, be useful, while uncertainty persists, is considering adjunctive imaging in such patients. A dynamic CTA will also provide CT perfusion data which should give some additional information regarding core infarct volume and may be useful for this group if early change is not already apparent on NCCT. Alternatively, obtaining DWI in this patient group could also be considered with a view to avoiding futile recanalization, although there is recent literature suggesting that early DWI changes may be reversible with reperfusion.

7.4.5 Management

Medication

In the recently published randomized controlled trials (MR CLEAN, ESCAPE, EXTEND-IA, SWIF PRIME, and REVASCAT), patients in the endovascular arm received IV-tPA in addition to mechanical thrombectomy unless contraindicated. Current standard of care for the management of acute stroke with large intracranial arterial occlusion therefore still includes administration of IV-tPA in patients presenting within the 4.5-hour time window unless contraindicated. Those patients with large artery occlusion should, however, proceed to endovascular treatment immediately rather than waiting for an assessment of response to IV thrombolysis, as minimizing time to reperfusion remains the ultimate aim of treatment.

Endovascular

There is now level-1 evidence that endovascular thrombectomy improves patient outcome in large artery occlusive stroke. This is the new standard of care for patients with intracranial large artery occlusion.[0,0] Appropriate imaging investigations must be performed to prove intracranial arterial occlusion and allow exclusion of patients with a large area of irreversibly injured brain tissue.

In the recently published trials which proved benefit for thrombectomy, the number needed to treat to achieve one patient with independent functional outcome was in the range of 3.2 to 7.1. Evidence provided by these trials is largely for stent retriever thrombectomy. In another trial, the THERAPY trial, aspiration thrombectomy was performed using the Penumbra aspiration system. Patients were randomly assigned to IV-tPA alone, or to IV-tPA plus aspiration thrombectomy. The trial was stopped early after only 108 of the planned 692 patients were enrolled due to the favorable data on endovascular treatment from other recently published trials. The trial was therefore underpowered to show significance; however, there was a strong trend toward better outcomes in the endovascular arm compared with controls. It would seem therefore that both stent retriever thrombectomy and aspiration thrombectomy are both valid options for endovascular treatment of large artery occlusive stroke.

7.4.6 Postprocedural Care

If possible, a closure device should be used to achieve hemostasis at the puncture site. If a closure device is not used, then consideration can be given to leaving the sheath in situ until tPA/heparin is no longer in the system, and then obtaining hemostasis with manual pressure. Postprocedure patients should be managed in a dedicated stoke unit, high dependency unit, or intensive care unit depending on clinical condition and level of care required. Follow-up imaging should be obtained at 24 hours postprocedure, or earlier if clinical condition deteriorates, to determine extent of established infarction and assess for any hemorrhagic change.

In the literature, on multivariate analysis, association has been shown between collateral score and final infarct size; patients with better leptomeningeal collaterals have been shown to have significantly smaller final infarct volumes ($p = 0.04$).[0] Similarly, better collateral status has shown strong correlation with higher follow-up CT ASPECTS score (Spearman $r = 0.58$; $p < 0.001$).[0] In patients treated with IA thrombolysis, poor pial collateral formation has been identified on multivariate analysis as a statistically significant predictor for symptomatic hemorrhage (OR: 6.8, $p = 0.0286$).[0]

It seems intuitive that hypotension be avoided in the after care of the incompletely recanalized stroke patient, or in cases of failed recanalization, in an effort to maintain cerebral perfusion through the leptomeningeal collaterals. At present, however, the use of devices to augment cerebral blood flow is not well established, and similarly the usefulness of drug-induced hypertension in stroke patients is not well established.

7.4.7 Literature Synopsis

Numerous studies in the literature have shown association between better leptomeningeal collateral status and improved functional outcome following large artery occlusive stroke. For example, Miteff et al[0] showed that in multivariate analysis good collateral status on CTA was an independent predictor of good outcome (modified Rankin scale [mRS]: 0–2 at 3 months). Menon et al also demonstrated in multivariate analysis that CTA collateral score was an independent predictor of good clinical outcome (mRS: 0–2 at 3 months, OR: 16.7 for good vs. poor collateral score; OR: 9.2 for medium vs. poor collateral score).[0] Lima et al[0] found that pattern of leptomeningeal collaterals on CTA was significantly associated with good outcome (mRS: 0–2 at 6 months, OR: 1.93; $p = 0.03$). These results, however, reflect largely medically managed patients. In *AJNR* in 2012, Souza et al[0] defined a collateral score of 0 (CS = 0) as a malignant collateral profile, associated with a high risk of poor clinical outcome. Subgroup analysis was performed in this study according to the method of treatment (i.e., no treatment, IV treatment only, IA treatment with or without IV). There was significant difference in terms of outcome between patients with CS = 0 compared with collateral score of greater than 0 (CS > 0). Patients with CS = 0 had higher median 3-month mRS than CS > 0 (5 vs. 3, $p = 0.02$) and were more likely than CS > 0 to be dead or dependent on follow-up (96 vs. 64%, $p < 0.01$).

For endovascularly treated patient cohorts, good leptomeningeal collateral supply has also been shown to confer benefit in terms of functional outcome following large artery occlusive stroke. Nambiar et al[0] assessed the relationship between CTA collateral status, recanalization, and clinical outcome in 81 patients with M1 occlusion brought for IA intervention. Treatments took place between 2004 and 2009; therefore, recanalization rates (TICI 2b–3: 38.1%) and outcomes (overall mRS: 0–2: 35.8%) reflect the time period of the study and the techniques used. Patients were trichotomized to three groups based on CTA collateral status: good, intermediate, and poor. Patients with good collaterals had significantly lower NIHSS score at presentation, significantly higher baseline CT ASPECTS score, and significantly smaller baseline infarct volumes. For recanalized patients, infarct growth was significantly lower in the good collateral group compared to intermediate or poor groups ($p = 0.05$). There were also higher rates of good clinical outcome (mRS: 0–2) among patients with good collateral status ($p = 0.04$): 100% of recanalized patients with good collateral status had good outcome, compared with 58.8% of patients with intermediate collateral status and 33.3% of patients with poor collateral status. In contrast, for patients in whom the occluded artery could not be recanalized, there was no significant difference in infarct growth when stratified by collateral status ($p = 0.09$), and no significant difference in good clinical outcome when stratified by collateral status ($p = 0.67$). In a multivariate model, interaction between collateral status and recanalization was relevant ($p = 0.08$). Of patients with good or intermediate collaterals where the artery was recanalized, 70% had good outcome. For patients with good or intermediate collaterals in whom the artery could not be recanalized, only 23.3% had a good outcome; therefore, recanalization is important for patients with good collaterals. However, in patients with poor collaterals, only 33.3% of recanalized patients had good outcome, and only 18.2% of failed recanalization patients had good outcome. Therefore, patients with good and intermediate collaterals who achieve recanalization with endovascular treatment do well when compared to those who do not achieve recanalization. Patients with poor collaterals do not do well even if recanalization is achieved with endovascular therapy. This study therefore provided evidence for the use of a CTA collaterals assessment–based paradigm in selecting patients for IA therapy.

Seeta Ramaiah et al[0] also assessed impact of arterial collateralization on outcome after IA therapy for acute ischemic stroke in patients with intracranial carotid or MCA occlusion treated intra-arterially. Collateral status was measured noninvasively with CTA, and a score of 0 to 3 assigned. There were 87 patients with ICA and/or MCA occlusion brought for IA intervention. Interventional techniques included Solitaire (75%), MERCI (12%), Penumbra (3%), and IA-tPA (15%). Recanalization to TICI 2b–3 was achieved in 69% of patients, and 54% of patients were mRS 0 to 2 at 3 months. On multivariate analysis, patients with collateral score of 3 had higher odds of good functional outcome even after adjustment for age, baseline NIHSS score, IV-tPA, and TICI grade (OR = 2.985, $p = 0.045$). There was also a trend toward higher death rate with collateral score of 0 to 2 (OR = 0.239, $p = 0.07$).

Liebeskind et al[0] performed post hoc assessment of collaterals in the SWIFT trial, to determine impact of collaterals on revascularization outcomes with stent retriever technology. The SWIFT trial randomized patients with large artery occlusive stroke to treatment with either the Solitaire or MERCI device. Collaterals were retrospectively analyzed on conventional angiography in SWIFT subjects. Adequate angiographic views were available in 119 of 144 subjects (83%), and collateral score was assessed using the ASITN/SIR scale. Almost all of the MCA occlusions could be assessed and approximately half of the carotid terminus lesions could be assessed. Collaterals were strongly related to baseline ASPECTS score ($p < 0.001$), collaterals were strongly related to 24-hour ASPECTS score ($p < 0.001$), there was a trend toward partial or worse collaterals with symptomatic hemorrhage ($p = 0.075$), and better collaterals were linked with TICI 2b/3 reperfusion ($p = 0.019$). In multivariate analysis, collateral grade was an independent predictor of good functional outcome (mRS: 0–2) at 90 days (OR: 4.63, $p < 0.001$).

These data were for the whole 119 patients, who were therefore treated with either Solitaire or MERCI device. In the supplementary tables from the study, the data for Solitaire alone are presented. This too, as expected, showed significant difference in patient outcome across different collateral groups. Patients with a score of 0 to 1 (i.e., poor collaterals) had good outcome in only 14.1% of cases, while patients with collateral grades 3 and 4 had good functional outcomes in 59.3 and 50% of cases, respectively.

In summary, collaterals have therefore been shown as a pivotal factor in the clinical outcomes of subjects in interventional cohorts reinforcing the growing literature on collateral perfusion as a key variable in acute ischemic stroke. It should be noted, however, that there is great heterogeneity in the published literature regarding CTA scoring systems for grading degree of leptomeningeal collateralization. Also, as discussed in detail in previous sections, single-phase CTA may give the false impression of poor collaterals as it can miss the delayed filling of what may actually be good collaterals. This may account for the small percentage of patients with poor collaterals in published studies still having a good outcome. Acquisition techniques and grading of leptomeningeal collaterals should be homogenized to allow a standardized system of assessing collateral flow to allow a CTA collaterals assessment–based paradigm in selecting patients for treatment and endovascular therapy.

7.4.8 Pearls and Pitfalls

- Leptomeningeal collaterals provide a route for retrograde filling of the territory distal to an occluded artery, numerous studies, using several imaging modalities and grading methods, suggest that good leptomeningeal collaterals confer a benefit in stroke.
- Good leptomeningeal collateral supply has been shown to be significantly associated with lower NIHSS score at presentation, higher baseline ASPECTS score, lower admission DWI lesion volume, less infarct growth, smaller final infarct size, higher follow-up CT ASPECTS score, and improved functional outcome on follow-up.
- Indirect assessment of leptomeningeal collaterals by noninvasive methods is preferable and will allow a collaterals assessment–based paradigm in selecting patients for treatment and endovascular therapy.
- CTA has a high degree of anatomic resolution and can accurately depict leptomeningeal collaterals. Single-phase CTA, however, lacks temporal resolution, and can potentially mislabel patients as having poor collaterals. Multiphase CTA or dynamic CTA is preferred for collateral assessment.
- Diverse CTA collateral grading methods have been proposed. The more complicated the grading system, the more

predictive it will be in terms of outcome; however, the less easy it is to apply in day-to-day clinical use. Outside of a research situation, ease of use trumps predictive value, and a scoring system that is easy to apply would be favorable. One could consider a dichotomized scale of "poor" versus "good" collaterals as determined by filling of less than or greater than 50% of the occluded arterial territory using the contralateral normal side as a comparison.

- Collaterals are best assessed on reconstructed axial MIP images (24-mm thickness recommended).
- Collaterals have been shown as a pivotal factor in the clinical outcomes of subjects in interventional cohorts reinforcing the growing literature on collateral perfusion as a key variable in acute ischemic stroke.
- Patients with good and intermediate collaterals who achieve recanalization with endovascular treatment do well when compared to those who do not achieve recanalization.
- Patients with poor collaterals overall do not do well even if recanalization is achieved with endovascular therapy. A ubiquitously poor outcome for patients with poor collaterals has not, however, been shown across all studies. This most likely relates to the assessment of collaterals on a single phase rather than multiphase or dynamic CTA. Therefore, at present, while prognosis is guarded in these patients, a poor collateral score alone is not yet considered an absolute contraindication to stroke treatment and intervention. It is likely that further studies may provide this evidence; however, it is as yet not available at the time of writing this book.
- A collateral score of 0 requires careful scrutiny of NCCT for developing infarction, a search for multifocal intracranial arterial occlusion, and consideration of other adjunctive imaging technique to rule out a large area of already infarcted tissue in order to avoid futile recanalization.
- Acquisition techniques and grading of leptomeningeal collaterals should be homogenized to allow a standardized system of assessing collateral flow and allow a CTA collaterals assessment–based paradigm in selecting patients for treatment and endovascular therapy.

Further Reading

Miteff F, Levi CR, Bateman GA, Spratt N, McElduff P, Parsons MW. The independent predictive utility of computed tomography angiographic collateral status in acute ischaemic stroke. Brain. 2009; 132(Pt 8):2231–2238

Menon BK, Smith EE, Modi J, et al. Regional leptomeningeal score on CT angiography predicts clinical and imaging outcomes in patients with acute anterior circulation occlusions. AJNR Am J Neuroradiol. 2011; 32(9):1640–1645

Lima FO, Furie KL, Silva GS, et al. The pattern of leptomeningeal collaterals on CT angiography is a strong predictor of long-term functional outcome in stroke patients with large vessel intracranial occlusion. Stroke. 2010; 41(10):2316–2322

Kinoshita T, Ogawa T, Kado H, Sasaki N, Okudera T. CT angiography in the evaluation of intracranial occlusive disease with collateral circulation: comparison with MR angiography. Clin Imaging. 2005; 29(5):303–306

Souza LCS, Yoo AJ, Chaudhry ZA, et al. Malignant CTA collateral profile is highly specific for large admission DWI infarct core and poor outcome in acute stroke. AJNR Am J Neuroradiol. 2012; 33(7):1331–1336

McVerry F, Liebeskind DS, Muir KW. Systematic review of methods for assessing leptomeningeal collateral flow. AJNR Am J Neuroradiol. 2012; 33(3):576–582

Goyal M, Demchuk AM, Menon BK, et al. ESCAPE Trial Investigators. Randomized assessment of rapid endovascular treatment of ischemic stroke. N Engl J Med. 2015; 372(11):1019–1030

Frölich AMJ, Wolff SL, Psychogios MN, et al. Time-resolved assessment of collateral flow using 4D CT angiography in large-vessel occlusion stroke. Eur Radiol. 2014; 24(2):390–396

Smit EJ, Vonken EJ, van Seeters T, et al. Timing-invariant imaging of collateral vessels in acute ischemic stroke. Stroke. 2013; 44(8):2194–2199

Menon BK, d'Esterre CD, Qazi EM, et al. Multiphase CT angiography: a new tool for the imaging triage of patients with acute ischemic stroke. Radiology. 2015; 275 (2):510–520

Menon BK, Goyal M. Imaging paradigms in acute ischemic stroke: a pragmatic evidence-based approach. Radiology. 2015; 277(1):7–12

Campbell BCV, Donnan GA, Lees KR, et al. Endovascular stent thrombectomy: the new standard of care for large vessel ischaemic stroke. Lancet Neurol. 2015; 14 (8):846–854

Powers WJ, Derdeyn CP, Biller J, et al. 2015 American Heart Association/American Stroke Association focused update of the 2013 guidelines for the early management of patients with acute ischemic stroke regarding endovascular treatment: a guideline for healthcare professionals from the American Heart Association/American Stroke Association. Stroke. 2015; 46(10):3020–3035

Tan IYL, Demchuk AM, Hopyan J, et al. CT angiography clot burden score and collateral score: correlation with clinical and radiologic outcomes in acute middle cerebral artery infarct. AJNR Am J Neuroradiol. 2009; 30(3):525–531

Christoforidis GA, Karakasis C, Mohammad Y, Caragine LP, Yang M, Slivka AP. Predictors of hemorrhage following intra-arterial thrombolysis for acute ischemic stroke: the role of pial collateral formation. AJNR Am J Neuroradiol. 2009; 30 (1):165–170

Nambiar V, Sohn SI, Almekhlafi MA, et al. CTA collateral status and response to recanalization in patients with acute ischemic stroke. AJNR Am J Neuroradiol. 2014; 35(5):884–890

Seeta Ramaiah S, Churilov L, Mitchell P, Dowling R, Yan B. The impact of arterial collateralization on outcome after intra-arterial therapy for acute ischemic stroke. AJNR Am J Neuroradiol. 2014; 35(4):667–672

Liebeskind DS, Jahan R, Nogueira RG, Zaidat OO, Saver JL, SWIFT Investigators. Impact of collaterals on successful revascularization in Solitaire FR with the intention for thrombectomy. Stroke. 2014; 45(7):2036–2040

8 Importance of Clot Burden and Clot Location

8.1 Case Description

8.1.1 Clinical Presentation

A 64-year-old male patient presented to an outside institution with a 2-hour history of dense right hemiplegia, neglect, and slurred speech. He did not have any significant background medical condition except for a recent right foot fracture. National Institutes of Health Stroke Scale (NIHSS) was assessed to be 17.

8.1.2 Imaging Workup and Investigations

A noncontrast computed tomography (NCCT) of the brain and CT angiography (CTA) at the referring institution was performed approximately 10 minutes after patient's arrival (▶ Fig. 8.1). NCCT demonstrated long-segment hyperdensity of the left supraclinoid internal carotid artery (ICA), carotid terminus, and M1 segment of the left middle cerebral artery (MCA). There was loss of definition of head of caudate, lentiform nucleus, and insular gray-white matter differentiation, as well as loss of gray-white matter differentiation in M3 region of the left MCA territory, consistent with an ASPECTS score of 6. There was no evidence of hemorrhage.

Cerebral CTA performed as a single-phase study from the level of the aortic arch showed patent left common carotid artery, with the absence of contrast opacification of the left ICA from the level of the carotid bulb through to carotid terminus, as well as absence of contrast opacification of the left M1 segment of MCA (▶ Fig. 8.2). There was no evidence of significant calcific atherosclerotic plaque in the region of the carotid bifurcation.

The extent of the collaterals was poor on the single-phase CTA study, with less than 50% of left MCA territory filling (▶ Fig. 8.3); however, this could be an inaccurate reflection of the collaterals as no additional phases were performed. CT perfusion was not performed.

8.1.3 Diagnosis

Occlusion of the left MCA, as well as the left ICA involving at least carotid terminus, with possible occlusion of more proximal ICA, and high clot burden score on CTA.

8.1.4 Treatment

Initial Management

After the initial CT investigation, intravenous tissue plasminogen activator (IV-tPA) was commenced at 2.5 hours after symptom onset. Following discussion between stroke physician in

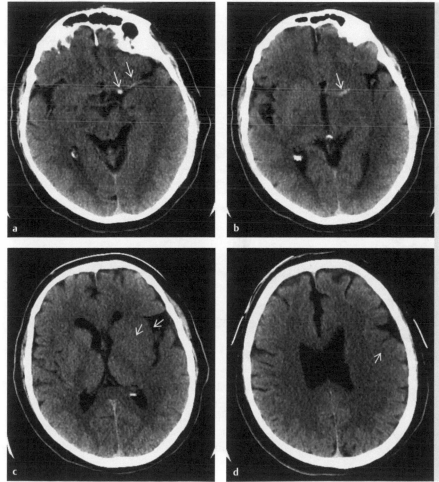

Fig. 8.1 Noncontrast CT of the brain demonstrated hyperdense left carotid terminus and M1 segment of MCA (**a,b**). There was loss of insular ribbon, and gray-white matter differentiation of basal nuclei, (**c,d**) as well as slight blurring of gray-white matter differentiation in the left superior temporal region.

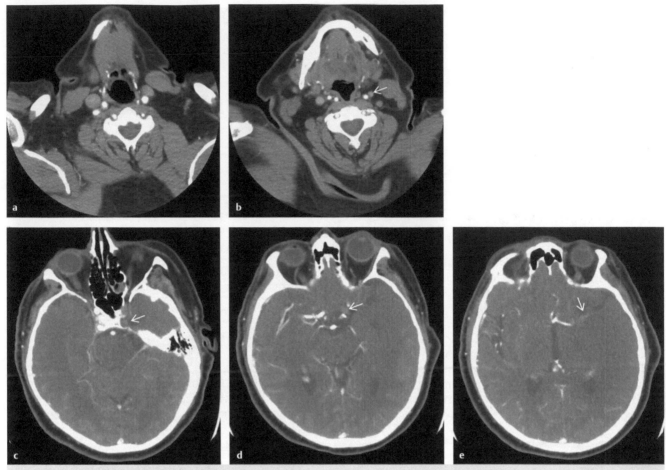

Fig. 8.2 Single-phase CT angiography performed from aortic arch to vertex showed patent left common carotid artery (a), with absent contrast opacification of the ICA from the level of the carotid bulb through to carotid terminus (b–d), as well as in the left proximal MCA. (e) There was filling of the left ACA via the anterior communicating artery.

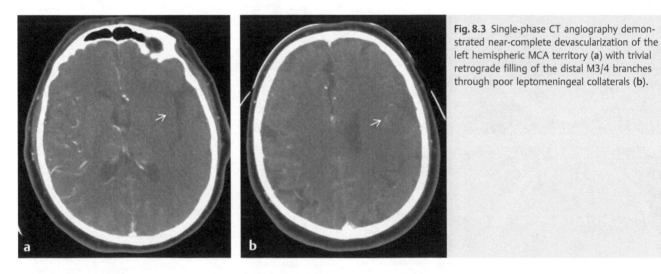

Fig. 8.3 Single-phase CT angiography demonstrated near-complete devascularization of the left hemispheric MCA territory (a) with trivial retrograde filling of the distal M3/4 branches through poor leptomeningeal collaterals (b).

admitting center and interventional neuroradiology, the patient was transferred to the regional endovascular stroke center for further management. The admitting hospital was located approximately 55 km from the regional endovascular stroke center, and the patient was transferred by ambulance.

The patient arrived in the regional endovascular stroke center at approximately 4 hours from symptom onset. At that time, tPA infusion was completed, with no improvement in patient symptoms and stable NIHSS score of 17; the patient was therefore immediately transferred to the angiosuite.

Endovascular Treatment

Material Used

The procedure was performed in a biplane angiographic suit with usual angiographic prep and drape equipment:

- Angiographic pack including suction syringes.
- Arterial access needle.
- 8-Fr arterial access sheath.
- 0.38-in hydrophilic guidewire.
- 0.35-in metal guidewire.
- 6-Fr Weinberg diagnostic catheter.
- 8-Fr Mach guide catheter.
- 5-Fr intermediate catheter (5MAX-ACE).
- 3-Fr intermediate catheter (3MAX)
- Rebar-27 microcatheter.
- 0.14-in Transend-EX microwire.
- 3- to 6-mm stent retrievers (6 × 30 mm Solitaire, 5 × 21 mm EmboTrap stent retriever).
- 8-Fr Angio-Seal closure device.

Procedure and Technique

Ten minutes after arrival, while patient was awake, after infiltration of soft tissues at the puncture site with local anesthetic, a single wall right CFA puncture was performed and an 8-Fr short Cordis arterial sheath placed for vascular access. A preassembled coaxial 6-Fr Weinberg through an 8-Fr Mach guide catheter was used to gain access to the left common carotid artery over a 0.035-in wire. Left common carotid angiography demonstrated patent proximal ICA with no significant atherosclerotic disease or stenosis and an unopacified column of blood distally (▶ Fig. 8.4a, b). At this point, it was still difficult to be certain of the exact site of the occlusion. Therefore, the coaxial system was advanced into the proximal internal carotid and the 8-Fr guide catheter was positioned just above the carotid bulb by sliding it over the 6-Fr inner catheter guidewire. The system was already connected to a pressurized heparin saline flush bag via a large bore rotating hemostatic valve. Subsequently, a 5MAX-ACE intermediate catheter was placed through the guide catheter and advanced over a 0.38-in Terumo-Glide guidewire until its tip was positioned in the mid-cervical ICA. Angiographic runs via the intermediate 5MAX-ACE catheter demonstrated patency of mid to distal cervical ICA with distal cutoff of contrast filling at the level of the cavernous ICA (▶ Fig. 8.4c, d).

A Rebar-27 microcatheter with inner Transend-EX microguidewire was introduced into the 5MAX-ACE intermediate catheter and initially positioned within the distal cavernous ICA. The microwire and subsequently microcatheter were advanced through the occluded segment and navigated to the level of the left M1 bifurcation. Microcatheter injection confirmed intraluminal position of microcatheter. Filling defect consistent with thrombus was seen distal to the microcatheter tip in the region of the left M1 segment bifurcation and involving proximal divisions of the left MCA (▶ Fig. 8.5).

A 6 × 30 mm Solitaire stent retriever was deployed. Angiographic runs demonstrated minimal reconstitution through the stent with no convincing flow distally (▶ Fig. 8.6a, b). The stent retriever was withdrawn after 2 minutes with a small volume of thrombus extracted in the stent (▶ Fig. 8.6c); retrieval was performed with suction through the 5MAX-ACE catheter.

Postretrieval angiography showed minimal improvement of flow. A second pass of Solitaire was performed; the carotid terminus was partially recanalized, with contrast opacification seen in relation to the very proximal portion of left A1 and M1, as well as filling of the left posterior communicating artery (▶ Fig. 8.6d, e). This was followed by deployment of an EmboTrap stent retriever across the MCA bifurcation (▶ Fig. 8.7) with further smaller clot fragments removed, and further recanalization of the carotid terminus noted on the follow-up runs.

There was, however, persistent occlusion of the left M1 segment of MCA. The 5MAX-ACE was advanced into the left M1 segment. A 3MAX reperfusion catheter was then advanced through the 5MAX-ACE to abut the proximal face of the left MCA thrombus and aspiration thrombectomy was attempted four times with a moderate amount of thrombus extracted using a 50-mL VacLok syringe. On each occasion, the 3MAX was advanced further into the superior division of the left MCA as clot removal was achieved gradually in an incremental way (▶ Fig. 8.8). The final point of deployment of the 3MAX was to the level of the M2/M3 segment junction. This was followed by two further Solitaire passes through the other M2 branches of the superior division, with more thrombus retrieved.

At this stage, the left M1 was cleared and antegrade flow was established into the superior division; however, the inferior division and temporal branch of MCA remained occluded, and there was visible thrombus within the left A2 segment of ACA with near-complete occlusion. Therefore, a single EmboTrap retrieval was performed through the left A2 segment (▶ Fig. 8.9) with moderate amount of thrombus removed and the artery was completely recanalized (▶ Fig. 8.10).

Three more retrievals were performed through the left MCA superior and inferior divisions and temporal branch with more thrombus extracted; however, eventually only the superior division of MCA and the proximal segment of the anterior temporal branch were reopened. Total number of stent retriever passes was 9 with the resultant thrombolysis in cerebral infarction (TICI) 2a recanalization of the arteries. Angiographic runs from the cervical carotid showed no residual thrombus, with patent bifurcation, and no significant stenosis; therefore, no carotid intervention was needed (▶ Fig. 8.10). The procedure took 109 minutes from the first to the last run.

Postprocedural Care/Outcome

Patient was cooperative during the procedure and his clinical condition remained relatively stable with no significant neurological change during the procedure. At the end of the procedure, groin hemostasis was achieved using an 8-Fr Angio-Seal. Postprocedure, the patient was stable, and transferred by ambulance back to the referring hospital escorted by a stroke physician and a nurse.

Blood pressure control was instigated with a target mean arterial pressure of less than 120 mm Hg to prevent reperfusion injury. However, the patient gradually deteriorated overnight with drop in Glasgow Coma Scale (GCS). A repeat NCCT of the brain was performed 24 hours postthrombectomy demonstrating a large left MCA territory infarct with multiple regions of hemorrhagic transformation (▶ Fig. 8.11a).

Following further discussion and consultation with neurosurgeon, the patient was transferred back to the regional

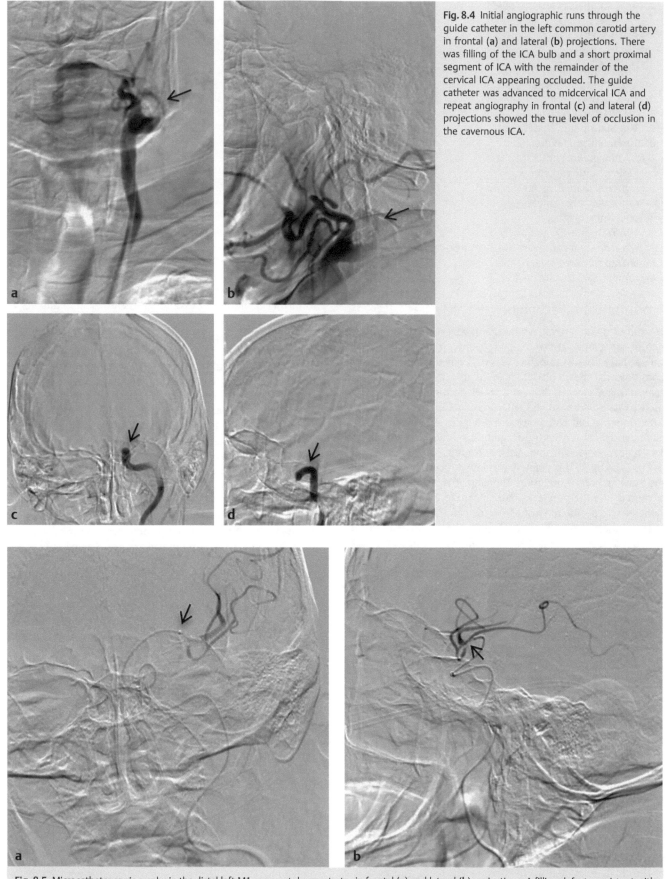

Fig. 8.4 Initial angiographic runs through the guide catheter in the left common carotid artery in frontal (a) and lateral (b) projections. There was filling of the ICA bulb and a short proximal segment of ICA with the remainder of the cervical ICA appearing occluded. The guide catheter was advanced to midcervical ICA and repeat angiography in frontal (c) and lateral (d) projections showed the true level of occlusion in the cavernous ICA.

Fig. 8.5 Microcatheter angiography in the distal left M1 segment demonstrates in frontal (a) and lateral (b) projections. A filling defect consistent with thrombus was seen distal to the microcatheter tip in the region of the left M1 segment bifurcation and involving proximal divisions of left MCA.

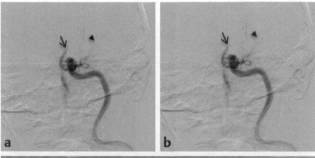
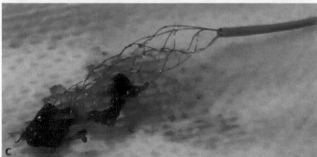
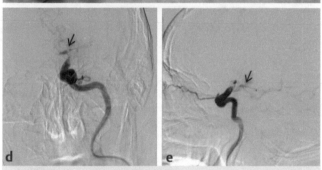

Fig. 8.6 *Arrowheads* indicate the distal strut markers on the initial angiographic run following Solitaire stent retriever deployment in frontal (a) and lateral (b) projections. There was partial flow reconstitution, with improved filling of the para and supraclinoid ICA, and ophthalmic artery opacification (*arrow*). The retrieved Solitaire is shown within the microcatheter with extracted thrombus in the stent (c). Following second pass with the Solitaire, the carotid terminus was partially recanalized, with contrast opacification seen in relation to the very proximal portion of left A1 and M1, as well as filling of the left posterior communicating artery (d,e).

endovascular stroke center for further management. An external ventricular drain was inserted and the patient underwent left hemispheric decompressive craniectomy and duraplasty the same day (▶ Fig. 8.11b, c) with gradual resolution of the resultant mass effect, and moderate improvement in GCS. Subsequently a ventriculoperitoneal shunt was inserted.

The patient remained hemiplegic with no further significant change in the clinical status and was transferred to a rehabilitation facility with moderate but consistently improving functional capabilities, and plan for later cranioplasty and replacement of the bone flap (▶ Fig. 8.12).

8.1.5 Discussion

Background

Despite the relative success of intravenous thrombolysis, limitations in recanalization of proximal intracranial arterial occlusion of less than 50% have spurred development of various endovascular techniques.[1,2] The introduction of stent retrievers was a major advancement; however, despite their high recanalization rate, up to approximately 90%,[3] they are not perfect and interventionalists sometimes encounter thrombus which is not retrievable by applying conventional techniques.[4]

Nevertheless, this is of great importance, considering the overwhelming result of recent randomized controlled trials which undeniably confirmed superiority of endovascular intervention in terms of final clinical outcome.[5,6] In fact metaanalyses of the randomized controlled trials comparing adjunct endovascular therapy versus medical management alone in acute ischemic stroke have shown superior functional outcomes in subjects receiving endovascular therapy, with noninferiority to medical management in terms of important clinical end points of mortality and symptomatic intracerebral hemorrhage.[7] This supports recommendations for including earlier endovascular therapy in patients with imaging-demonstrated large-vessel occlusions.

It is important to remember that recanalization is likely the strongest predictor of at-risk-tissue rescue and patient outcome in acute large artery occlusive stroke. A meta-analysis showed an odds ratio of approximately 5 for having a good functional

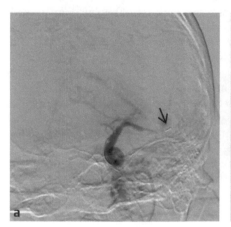
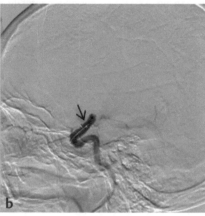

Fig. 8.7 EmboTrap positioned through the occluded MCA segment, distal leading short wire at the tip of the stent is depicted by *arrow* in (a) (frontal projection). The proximal stent marker is depicted by *arrow* in (b) (lateral projection).

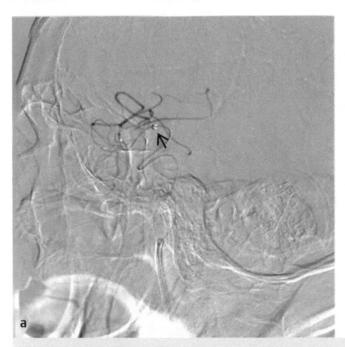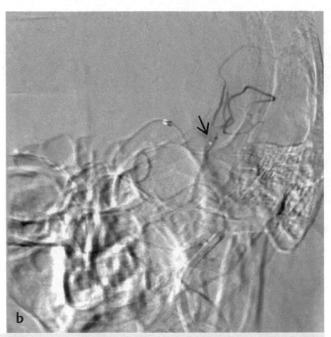

Fig. 8.8 5MAX-ACE catheter within mid M1 segment of left MCA (**a**, lateral projection, *arrow*) with the tip of the 3MAX catheter abutting the proximal end of the thrombus beyond the MCA bifurcation (**b**, frontal projection, *arrow*).

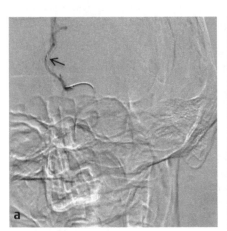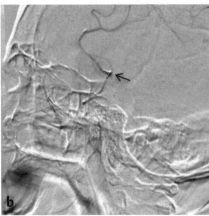

Fig. 8.9 EmboTrap in the left A2 segment of ACA, with the leading tip proximal to origin of callosomarginal branch (**a**, frontal projection, *arrow*). Proximal end of the stent is in the distal left A1 segment (**b**, lateral projection, *arrow*).

outcome at 3 months poststroke for those patients with near-complete recanalization, TICI 2b/3, compared with poor or no recanalization after intervention.[8] Recanalization of the occluded artery depends on multiple different factors including thrombus type, location, and the extent of the occlusion.[9] It is well known that when using IV thrombolysis, recanalization rates are lower in proximal versus distal arteries[2,8,10,11,12]; hence, the best IV-tPA outcome in patients with anterior circulation stroke is usually seen in those with distal MCA occlusion compared to occlusion of the carotid terminus[13] who are likely the group with poor prognosis if not fully recanalized.

It has been well established that the clot length is also an independent predictor of the outcome in IV thrombolysis.[14] There is now emerging evidence that clot burden can be also considered a predictor for outcome in those who received endovascular treatment.[10] There have been attempts in proposing standard methods in quantifying thrombus burden in patients, assisting prognostication based on site and extent of the intracranial occlusion.[10,15]

Clinical trials have also shown that the likelihood of recanalization negatively correlates with the thrombus burden, with those having a clot less than 8 mm in length having a much better chance to achieve recanalization.[9,16]

Clot composition may also determine effectiveness of thrombolysis. A study found that fibrin-rich cardioembolic thrombus achieved faster and more frequent recanalization with tPA compared to large-vessel atherosclerotic lesions.[17] In a case series with complete or partial MCA recanalization after IV-tPA, 20% of patients had early reocclusion, and risk factors for this include NIHSS score more than 16 at baseline and severe ipsilateral carotid artery disease, which was defined as more than 70% stenosis in this study.[18]

8.1.6 Workup and Diagnosis

Like all other emergencies, it is usually difficult to gather relevant information, and although in the setting of an acute ischemic stroke, it is possible to relatively accurately localize

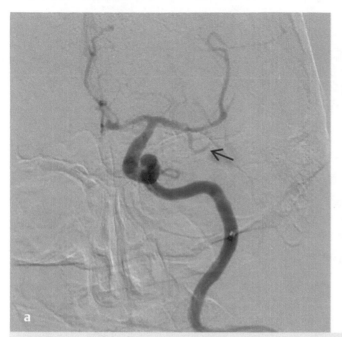
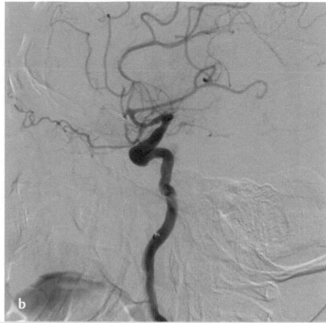

Fig. 8.10 Final angiographic run in frontal (a) and lateral (b) projections demonstrating recanalized left M1 segment and superior division of MCA as well as ACA, with opacification of an occluded temporal branch stump (a, *arrow*).

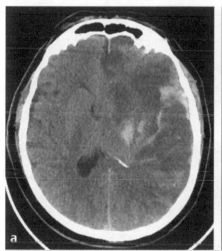
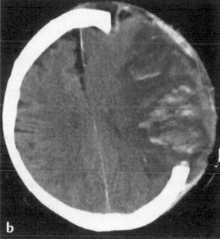
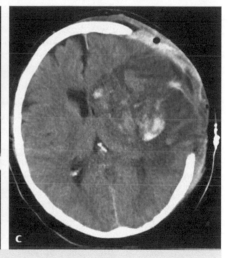

Fig. 8.11 Non–contrast-enhanced CT of the brain shows large area of infarction in the left MCA territory, and left inferior frontal region, with hemorrhagic transformation in the left MCA territory. Evidence of associated mass effect with sulcal effacement and subfalcine herniation (a). Subsequent decompressive craniectomy and duraplasty (b) with further evolution of hemorrhagic transformation (c).

the ischemic territory involved based on the clinical findings; it is usually not possible to estimate the extent and severity of the underlying arterial occlusion. Information regarding previous transient ischemic attacks (TIAs) may increase the possibility of an underlying carotid stenosis and potential tandem occlusion. The presence of other known risk factors will clearly increase risk of atherosclerosis in the patient.

Standard imaging, in addition to the NCCT of the brain, now includes a CTA from the aortic arch to the vertex, which not only identifies the intracranial occlusion but also helps clarify potential cervical ICA or vertebral thrombosis and tandem occlusions. CTA gives excellent demonstration of the relevant anatomy aiding in procedural planning. It is also important to evaluate the remainder of the cerebral vasculature, assess collateral circulation, and look for associated abnormalities such as atrial/aortic arch thrombus or contralateral stenosis. MRA may also be useful in the diagnosis of cervical arterial thrombosis, but is normally less accessible and usually more time consuming, and may overestimate a severe arterial stenosis as occlusion due to the slow flow, in particular on time-of-flight imaging. Ultrasound is of minimal use in an acute setting and should be solely preserved for the workup in those presented with TIAs.

All preprocedural assessment aside, catheter angiography remains the gold standard and most of the information is in fact gathered when the first angiographic run is performed during the endovascular intervention.

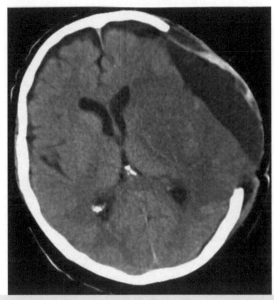

Fig. 8.12 Follow-up noncontrast CT of the brain showed decreased mass effect and expected evolution of the left MCA territory infarct.

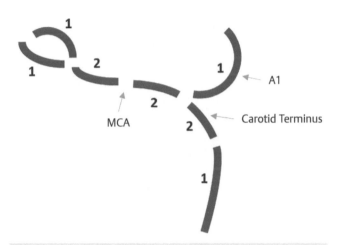

Fig. 8.13 Schematic diagram of ICA, MCA, and ACA segments for clot burden scoring.

8.1.7 Imaging Findings

Although the length of arterial hyperdensity on NCCT of the brains is generally thought to correspond with the length of thrombus,[14,19] it is frequently found to be an inaccurate estimate of thrombus length and at best to be proportional with the clot burden rather than a true measurement of its length. It is likely because in addition to the technical differences related to the acquisition parameters which could influence the measurement of the hyperdense segment, there are potential interoperator variabilities. The exact source of increased density following intracranial arterial occlusion is somewhat unclear and it has been shown that CT appearance of clot very much depends on thrombus composition.[20,21] This means that the low-attenuating parts of clot could be less well discernible.[20]

Susceptibility vessel sign on MRI, which is related to the presence of deoxyhemoglobin causing inhomogeneities in local magnetic field and signal loss on T2* sequences, has also been associated with the length of thrombus; however, it is probably an inaccurate measure of the true clot burden and its correlation with the recanalization success and the final outcome is debated.[22] Therefore, CTA has been proposed as a better investigative method for clot burden scoring as it is widely available and can be performed rapidly and safely.[10,23]

CTA-based clot burden assessment, as a semiquantitative score, has also been shown to be a predictor of recanalization and also to correlate with the final clinical outcome.[10,22] In this scoring system, 10 points are allocated to the normal anterior circulation tree from ICA to M2 branches which decreases with the number of segments exhibiting a visible clot[22,24] (▶ Fig. 8.13). A score of 10 is normal, implying absence of thrombus, but 2 points are subtracted from 10 for thrombi found in the supraclinoid ICA and each of the proximal and distal halves of the MCA trunk. In addition, one point is subtracted for thrombi found in the infraclinoid ICA and A1 segment and for each affected M2 branch.

CTA is very useful to assess potential calcific atherosclerotic plaques over the ICA bifurcations, indicating possible underlying stenosis. However, one of the most important pitfalls is its inability to differentiate complete ICA occlusion either chronic or acute from a stagnant nonopacified column of blood (i.e., pseudo-occlusion). Such a situation arises when there is a complete occlusion distally with unopacified blood within the ICA proximally, delaying the passage of the contrast, and giving the false impression of an occluded artery, as in our case with potentially falsely overcalculated clot burden score of 1.

A similar problem can also occur when there is severe proximal ICA stenosis or even when there is a short segment ICA occlusion at the origin, which could potentially be confused with an extensive arterial thrombosis on the CTA. This pseudo-occlusion is a very important consideration as occlusion length and hence clot burden has been shown to be an important determinant of the efficacy and complication rates of mechanical thrombectomy.

Such a dilemma can be resolved by performing either multiphase CTA or by acquiring a delayed CT following the initial CTA which can distinguish a true ICA occlusion from a severe ICA stenosis. In multiphase CTA, the second and third phases of the CTA are usually just of the intracranial circulation; however, the ICA at the level of the skull base would be visible. MRI/MRA has also been proposed as a potential solution to this problem, but it is worth mentioning that it also can be susceptible to slow flow, in particular if time-of-fight technique is used, and contrast-enhanced MRA will suffer the same problems as contrast-enhanced CTA unless a multiphase study is obtained. Overall, although intuitively these multiphase angiographic studies are most likely of benefit in assessing and estimating the clot burden in victims of acute ischemic stroke and are certainly recommended; strictly speaking, they still lack level-I evidence in their effectiveness in the final outcome.

Perfusion studies are usually severely abnormal in those with large clot burden, with increased time to peak, mean transit time, decreased relative cerebral blood flow, and preserved or reduced relative cerebral blood volume. This pattern is also usually noted in MR perfusion either acquired by dynamic contrast enhancement or arterial spin labeling. Although the extent of abnormality on perfusion studies can be suggestive of a heavy clot burden, it is very much dependent on the status of the collaterals and the underlying anatomy of the circle of Willis, and is therefore an unreliable measure. The cost–benefit (time value) of the perfusion studies is still a matter of debate and the exact role that they can play in stratifying the patients regarding endovascular management is still controversial.

Catheter angiography remains gold standard for the exact assessment of the extent of the arterial occlusion and clot burden. However, it is also important to consider that early angiographic runs from carotid by proximal injection into CCA may suffer from the same pitfall as CTA due to the presence of column of unopacified blood within ICA, as shown on initial angiographic runs in the case presented here. The exact extent of clot can only be determined after selective cannulation in a distally occluded but not stenosed ICA or proximally stenosed/occluded ICA without distal thrombus.

8.1.8 Decision-Making Process

Heavy clot burden poses a challenge in the management of acute ischemic stroke. It is now well accepted that these patients are unlikely to recanalize with IV-tPA alone and benefit from endovascular intervention; however, intra-arterial treatment of this condition is often not easy either.

Depending on the other underlying conditions (e.g., severely stenosed or occluded ICA or vertebral origin, or extensive thrombosis alone), different strategies should be considered and appropriate course of action determined, which may include angioplasty and stenting or extensive thrombectomy with aspiration, stent retriever thrombectomy, or both.

If the underlying problem is due to severe stenosis from atherosclerotic disease, careful catheterization of the arterial ostium is required, occasionally with the need for balloon angioplasty prior to introduction of the guide catheter for thrombectomy. Depending on the arterial status postangioplasty, insertion of a stent may also be deemed necessary. If a stent is placed before thrombectomy, one must advance the guide catheter through the stent for thrombectomy in order to avoid catching the stent retriever on the stent. If the guide catheter can be advanced without the need for angioplasty or stenting, it allows for more rapid distal recanalization and the proximal stenosis can be considered after this is achieved. However, in case of a dissection as the underlying cause for compromised flow and thrombosis, the challenge is to stay in the true lumen and angiography must be used to confirm this before stenting or thrombectomy.

One of the most difficult decisions to make while endovascularly treating a stroke patient with heavy clot burden is when to stop. Although after the introduction of the stent retrievers recanalization rate has significantly increased with statistics up to 95% reported in the literature, there is no doubt that there are patients in whom successful recanalization is not achievable despite multiple attempts. It is well shown that in these patients, who usually present with high NIHSS score, failure of endovascular intervention is likely associated with very poor outcomes. Therefore, the authors are of the opinion that repeat attempts should continue as long as reasonably possible in these patients, and multiple different techniques in combination should be used with different instruments utilized to optimize the chance for a successful recanalization. In the authors' experience, it is not uncommon that an initial failure in recanalization is overcome on subsequent attempts, in particular when switching between different stent retrievers or alternating with suction thrombectomy.

Each one of the instruments available in the market has specified recommendations regarding the number of safe attempts; however, this need not be considered as a limiting factor in recanalization attempts with further devices. It is also intuitively expected that persistence and repeat attempts will increased the cumulative risk for potential complications; however, at least anecdotally, this increase does not appear significant compared with the potential benefit to the patient if successful recanalization is achieved.

In addition to the conventional methods of thrombectomy, other more innovative techniques such as combining stent retrievers with suction thrombectomy should not be forgotten. In the authors' experience, the use of distal access intermediate catheters such as the 5MAX-ACE, combined with 3 or 4 Fr inner catheters such as the 4MAX or 3MAX, can be very useful for a successful aspiration thrombectomy from intracranial arteries or even the ICA. Aspiration can be performed manually, or with an aspiration thrombectomy pump such as the Penumbra pump.

There have been recent case reports of using two stent retrievers at the same time in tandem or even Y configuration for recanalization of long thrombi extending into the larger parent vessels or saddle emboli, in particular at the MCA bifurcation, which are not extracted despite multiple single stent retrievers attempted through different divisions individually (► Fig. 8.14).[25] This technique has also been previously discussed for concurrent A1–M1 thrombi.[26] However, even this technique is not always successful. Particular attention should be given to the potential risks associated with some of these maneuvers and should only be performed with due diligence in specific cases, where conventional techniques have been unsuccessful.

8.1.9 Postprocedural Care

Unfortunately intravenous thrombolysis has low rate of successfully recanalizing the occluded arteries in those patients with heavy clot burden, but based on the current evidence endovascular intervention combined with IV-tPA is superior over IV-tPA alone; therefore, IV-tPA infusion is recommended if there is no contraindication for all patients regardless of the exact extent and severity of the arterial occlusion.

However, necessity of IV-tPA for those undergoing quick mechanical thrombectomy is currently being questioned, particularly given the cost associated with it and potential critical time which can be wasted. But the jury is still out and if subgroup analyses of the recent studies cannot definitely answer this question, a comparative randomized controlled study may be required; until then, IV-tPA will likely stay as a standard part of the current pharmacomechanical treatment.[27]

In view of the higher potential risk of failure to completely recanalize, as well as ischemic and hemorrhagic complications,

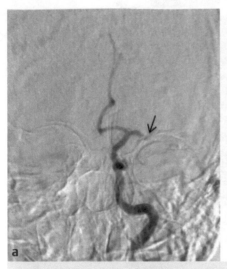
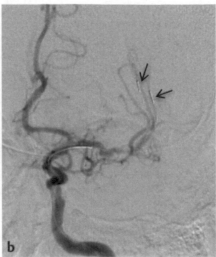
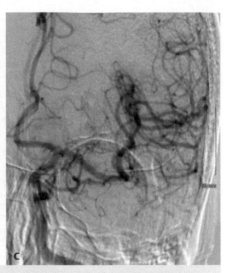

Fig. 8.14 (b) Catheter angiography confirming mid-MCA occlusion in a 76-year-old male patient presented 2 hours post onset of dense right hemiplegia with NIHSS of 16 (a). Following five unsuccessful recanalization attempts made from superior and inferior divisions, double-stent technique with stents deployed into superior and inferior MCA divisions concurrently was tried (b). Single-pass successful stent retrieval with complete MCA recanalization (c).

patients with heavy clot burden probably need more stringent monitoring and assessment which is normally available only in the setting of intensive care unit or high dependency units. In such a setting, stringent control over the blood pressure and monitoring for the signs of increased intracranial pressure are also possible. Urgent intervention may be required more frequently in this patient group. In our case, early deterioration required emergent craniectomy.

8.1.10 Pearls and Pitfalls

- Clinical trials have also shown that the likelihood of recanalization negatively correlates with the thrombus burden, with clot lengths less than 8 mm having greater likelihood of recanalization.
- CTA-based clot burden scoring has been shown to be a predictor of recanalization and also to correlate with the final clinical outcome.
- The static nature of conventional CTA does not allow assessment of flow. The main potential pitfall is in the assessment of the ICA in either a significant proximal stenosis or distal occlusion, where a slow flow situation arises, giving a "false occlusion/pseudoocclusion sign." Pseudo-occlusion may lead to erroneous overestimation of thrombus length. On CTA, delayed imaging or a multiphase study can be performed to overcome this dilemma.
- Acute stroke patients with intracranial arterial occlusion and heavy clot burden may have a challenging management with difficult recanalization. On the other hand, they are unlikely to benefit IV-tPA alone, making endovascular intervention and thrombectomy almost always necessary.
- Failure in recanalization and hence unsuccessful reperfusion in patient with heavy clot burden carry significant risk of a large infarction with likely catastrophic outcome. Therefore, extensive attempt to recanalize occluded arteries is recommended in these patients using different endovascular techniques, with stent retrievers and suction thrombectomy as needed.

- Collaborative meta-analyses of the pooled patient-level data from multiple randomized controlled trials (HERMES) demonstrated benefit from endovascular thrombectomy for patients with large clot burden as well. A total of 122 out of 1,132 stroke patients were included in these studies with concomitant tandem occlusions of the extracranial ICA.[28]

References

[1] Ferrell AS, Britz GW. Developments on the horizon in the treatment of neurovascular problems. Surg Neurol Int. 2013; 4 Suppl 1:S31–S37

[2] Saqqur M, Uchino K, Demchuk AM, et al. CLOTBUST Investigators. Site of arterial occlusion identified by transcranial Doppler predicts the response to intravenous thrombolysis for stroke. Stroke. 2007; 38(3):948–954

[3] Saver JL, Jahan R, Levy EI, et al. SWIFT Trialists. Solitaire flow restoration device versus the MERCI Retriever in patients with acute ischaemic stroke (SWIFT): a randomised, parallel-group, non-inferiority trial. Lancet. 2012; 380(9849):1241–1249

[4] Nogueira RG, Lutsep HL, Gupta R, et al. TREVO 2 Trialists. Trevo versus MERCI retrievers for thrombectomy revascularisation of large vessel occlusions in acute ischaemic stroke (TREVO 2): a randomised trial. Lancet. 2012; 380 (9849):1231–1240

[5] Fransen PS, Beumer D, Berkhemer OA, et al. MR CLEAN Investigators. MR CLEAN, a multicenter randomized clinical trial of endovascular treatment for acute ischemic stroke in the Netherlands: study protocol for a randomized controlled trial. Trials. 2014; 15:343

[6] McDowell MM, Ducruet AF. Time is brain: a critical analysis of the EXTEND-IA and ESCAPE trials. World Neurosurg. 2015; 83(6):949–951

[7] Bush CK, Kurimella D, Cross LJ, et al. Endovascular treatment with stent-retriever devices for acute ischemic stroke: a meta-analysis of randomized controlled trials. PLoS One. 2016; 11(1):e0147287

[8] Rha J-H, Saver JL. The impact of recanalization on ischemic stroke outcome: a meta-analysis. Stroke. 2007; 38(3):967–973

[9] Blackham KA, Meyers PM, Abruzzo TA, et al. Society for NeuroInterventional Surgery. Endovascular therapy of acute ischemic stroke: report of the Standards of Practice Committee of the Society of NeuroInterventional Surgery. J Neurointerv Surg. 2012; 4(2):87–93

[10] Puetz V, Dzialowski I, Hill MD, et al. Calgary CTA Study Group. Intracranial thrombus extent predicts clinical outcome, final infarct size and hemorrhagic transformation in ischemic stroke: the clot burden score. Int J Stroke. 2008; 3(4):230–236

[11] Wunderlich MT, Goertler M, Postert T, et al. Duplex Sonography in Acute Stroke (DIAS) Study Group, Competence Network Stroke. Recanalization after

intravenous thrombolysis: does a recanalization time window exist? Neurology. 2007; 68(17):1364–1368

[12] Lee K-Y, Han SW, Kim SH, et al. Early recanalization after intravenous administration of recombinant tissue plasminogen activator as assessed by pre- and post-thrombolytic angiography in acute ischemic stroke patients. Stroke. 2007; 38(1):192–193

[13] Linfante I, Llinas RH, Selim M, et al. Clinical and vascular outcome in internal carotid artery versus middle cerebral artery occlusions after intravenous tissue plasminogen activator. Stroke. 2002; 33(8):2066–2071

[14] Kamalian S, Morais LT, Pomerantz SR, et al. Clot length distribution and predictors in anterior circulation stroke: implications for intra-arterial therapy. Stroke. 2013; 44(12):3553–3556

[15] Sims JR, Rordorf G, Smith EE, et al. Arterial occlusion revealed by CT angiography predicts NIH stroke score and acute outcomes after IV tPA treatment. AJNR Am J Neuroradiol. 2005; 26(2):246–251

[16] Riedel CH, Zimmermann P, Jensen-Kondering U, Stingele R, Deuschl G, Jansen O. The importance of size: successful recanalization by intravenous thrombolysis in acute anterior stroke depends on thrombus length. Stroke. 2011; 42(6):1775–1777

[17] Molina CA, Montaner J, Arenillas JF, Ribo M, Rubiera M, Alvarez-Sabín J. Differential pattern of tissue plasminogen activator-induced proximal middle cerebral artery recanalization among stroke subtypes. Stroke. 2004; 35 (2):486–490

[18] Rubiera M, Alvarez-Sabín J, Ribo M, et al. Predictors of early arterial reocclusion after tissue plasminogen activator-induced recanalization in acute ischemic stroke. Stroke. 2005; 36(7):1452–1456

[19] Riedel CH, Jensen U, Rohr A, et al. Assessment of thrombus in acute middle cerebral artery occlusion using thin-slice nonenhanced Computed Tomography reconstructions. Stroke. 2010; 41(8):1659–1664

[20] Frölich AM, Schrader D, Klotz E, et al. 4D CT angiography more closely defines intracranial thrombus burden than single-phase CT angiography. AJNR Am J Neuroradiol. 2013; 34(10):1908–1913

[21] Puig J, Pedraza S, Demchuk A, et al. Quantification of thrombus Hounsfield units on noncontrast CT predicts stroke subtype and early recanalization after intravenous recombinant tissue plasminogen activator. AJNR Am J Neuroradiol. 2012; 33(1):90–96

[22] Legrand L, Naggara O, Turc G, et al. Clot burden score on admission T2*-MRI predicts recanalization in acute stroke. Stroke. 2013; 44(7):1878–1884

[23] Lev MH, Farkas J, Rodriguez VR, et al. CT angiography in the rapid triage of patients with hyperacute stroke to intraarterial thrombolysis: accuracy in the detection of large vessel thrombus. J Comput Assist Tomogr. 2001; 25(4):520–528

[24] Tan IY, Demchuk AM, Hopyan J, et al. CT angiography clot burden score and collateral score: correlation with clinical and radiologic outcomes in acute middle cerebral artery infarct. AJNR Am J Neuroradiol. 2009; 30(3):525–531

[25] Asadi H, Brennan P, Martin A, et al. Double stent-retriever technique in endovascular treatment of middle cerebral artery saddle embolus. J Stroke Cerebrovasc Dis. 2016; 25(2):e9–e11

[26] Hsieh K, Verma RK, Schroth G, et al. Multimodal 3 Tesla MRI confirms intact arterial wall in acute stroke patients after stent-retriever thrombectomy. Stroke. 2014; 45(11):3430–3432

[27] Chandra RV, Leslie-Mazwi TM, Mehta BP, et al. Does the use of IV tPA in the current era of rapid and predictable recanalization by mechanical embolectomy represent good value? J Neurointerv Surg. 2016; 8(5):443–446

[28] Goyal M, Menon BK, van Zwam WH, et al. HERMES Collaborators. Endovascular thrombectomy after large-vessel ischaemic stroke: a meta-analysis of individual patient data from five randomised trials. Lancet. 2016; 387(10029):1723–1731

9 ASPECTS: When Not to Treat

9.1 Case Description

9.1.1 Clinical Presentation

A 76-year-old female patient presented to the emergency department 130 minutes after sudden onset of left arm and leg weakness with facial droop. Clinical examination confirmed a right middle cerebral artery (MCA) syndrome, National Institutes of Health Stroke Scale (NIHSS) 12.

9.1.2 Imaging Workup and Investigations

- Noncontrast computed tomography (NCCT) performed shortly after presentation to the emergency department (145 minutes after symptom onset) reveals early infarction in the right insular, frontal, and temporal lobes, ASPECTS 6 (▶ Fig. 9.1).
- CT angiography (CTA) reveals occlusion of the right MCA-dominant M2 superior division (▶ Fig. 9.1), and moderate collateral circulation.
- CT perfusion (CTP) reveals increased mean transit time in the MCA cortical branch territories, with reduced cerebral blood volume (CBV) and cerebral blood flow (CBF) corresponding to the areas of early infarction on NCCT, but surrounding areas of normal CBV with mildly reduced CBF indicating tissue at risk of infarction, but potentially salvageable with reperfusion.

9.1.3 Diagnosis

Right M2 superior division occlusion with early infarction in the MCA territory. Abnormally perfused tissue surrounding the infarct (mismatch on CTP) indicating tissue at risk of infarction, but potentially salvageable with reperfusion.

9.1.4 Management

- The patient had no contraindication to intravenous (IV) thrombolysis based on clinical history, clinical assessment, and CT findings.
- She received an initial bolus and infusion of tissue plasminogen activator (tPA) commencing 190 minutes after the symptom onset. Endovascular therapy was considered appropriate based on time from onset of symptoms, location of the arterial occlusion, and CT findings suggesting potentially salvageable tissue. The time from symptom onset to groin puncture was 235 minutes.

9.1.5 Endovascular Treatment

Materials

- 8-Fr short vascular access sheath.
- Cello balloon guide catheter.
- 5-Fr Slip-Cath.
- Terumo guidewire.
- 5-Fr Navien guiding catheter.
- Rebar 18 microcatheter.
- Synchro 14 guidewire.
- Solitaire 4 mm × 20 mm stent retriever.

Technique

- Right common femoral artery puncture with placement of an 8-Fr short vascular access sheath into the common femoral artery.
- Cello balloon guide catheter placed in the right common carotid artery after advancing it coaxially over a slip-cath and terumo guidewire.
- Control anteroposterior and lateral angiographic runs confirmed persistent M2 superior division occlusion.
- A 5-Fr Navien guiding catheter was advanced into the distal right internal carotid artery.
- A Rebar 18 microcatheter was navigated distally over a Synchro 14 guidewire into the occluded M2 segment.
- A 4 mm × 20 mm solitaire AB stent retriever was placed along the occluded segment proximally extending into the M1 segment.
- After 5 minutes, the stent was retrieved with simultaneous continuous aspiration. Small clots recovered. Repeat angiographic runs did not demonstrate satisfactory recanalization. A second pass was made with the same technique.
- Final angiographic runs demonstrated satisfactory distal perfusion (TICI2b), with distal occlusion of an angular branch.

9.1.6 Postprocedural Care

- Transferred to the neurology high dependency unit for monitoring.
- Six hours after the thrombectomy procedure, an emergent NCCT was performed due to a change in neurological status, revealing a small parenchymal hematoma within the infarcted territory and a moderate volume of subarachnoid hemorrhage/contrast staining (▶ Fig. 9.2). A small area of new infarct was now discernible in periventricular white matter.
- The patient was closely monitored with subsequent improvement in neurological status over 24 hours. Repeat NCCT 24 hours later showed no change in size of the hematoma, partial resolution of subarachnoid hemorrhage, and no further infarct extension.

9.1.7 Outcome

- Right MCA infarct with hemorrhagic transformation.
- Reperfusion therapy with IV-tPA and mechanical thrombectomy. Final infarct volume based on day 5 NCCT (▶ Fig. 9.3) remained largely similar to the initial NCCT, and significantly smaller than the predicted infarct on CTP.
- Discharged 5 days after admission to a rehabilitation hospital, with a modified Rankin score of 3.

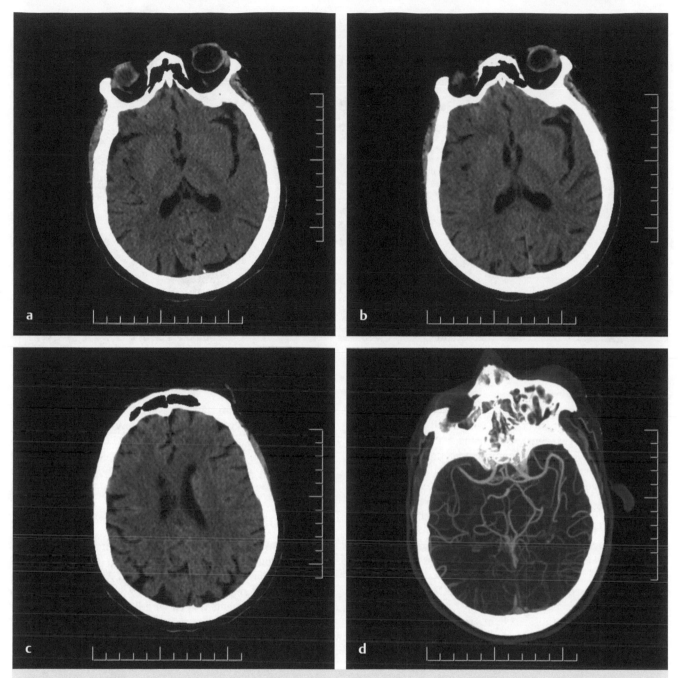

Fig. 9.1 NCCT and CTA in a 79-year-old female patient performed 145 minutes after onset of a right MCA syndrome. There is early infarction in the right MCA territory, affecting the insular cortex, M1, M2, and M4 cortex—ASPECTS 6. Right M2 (dominant branch) occlusion on CTA.

9.1.8 Background

The Alberta Stroke Program Early CT Score (ASPECTS) is a standardized, quantitative, topographical scoring system for assessment of early ischemic changes in the MCA territory on CT. The early European Cooperative Acute Stroke Studies (ECASS) excluded patients with early ischemic changes on CT in greater than one-third of the MCA territory.[1,2] The rationale for the exclusion was that early ischemic change in greater than one-third of the MCA territory was associated with severe stroke, poor outcome, higher frequency of spontaneous hemorrhagic transformation, and suggested proximal occlusion with poor collateral circulation, thus less likely to respond to thrombolytic therapy.[1] This led to the "1/3 MCA rule"; early ischemic changes on CT in greater than one-third of the MCA territory is a recommended contraindication for IV-tPA therapy. However, assessing volume of infarcted territory on axial CT sections is difficult, and utilizing this technique to determine the presence of infarction in greater than one-third of the MCA territory is considered unreliable with poor interobserver variability.[3,4,5] To attempt to address these problems of the 1/3 MCA rule, the ASPECTS study group developed the ASPECTS scoring system to allow a simplified, standardized, alternative method of quantifying early ischemic changes on CT.[6] The initial ASPECTS study

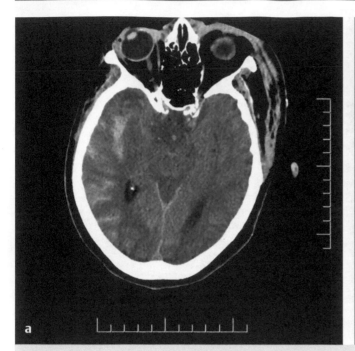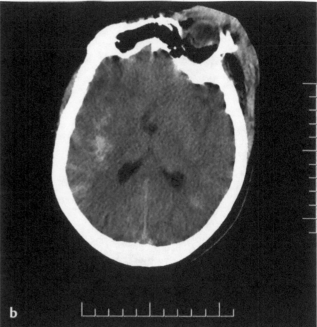

Fig. 9.2 NCCT performed 6 hours after thrombectomy reveals a small parenchymal hematoma within the part of the infarcted territory, and surrounding subarachnoid blood/contrast staining.

retrospectively reviewed imaging, clinical data, and outcomes of 203 consecutive patients treated with tPA at two stroke centers. Initial CT images were graded using ASPECTS and according to the 1/3 MCA rule. They found that for stroke neurologists, radiology trainees, and experienced neuroradiologists, the use of dichotomized ASPECTS (≤ 7 vs. > 7) had better interobserver agreement than the 1/3 MCA rule. In addition, the dichotomized ASPECTS had better sensitivity and specificity than the 1/3 MCA rule for functional outcome. Baseline ASPECTS had an inverse correlation with NIHSS score and was a significant predictor of both functional outcome and symptomatic hemorrhage.[6]

The ASPECTS scoring system divides the MCA territory into 10 discrete regions. Regions are weighed on a functional rather than a volume basis; thus, eloquent areas such as the internal capsule have the same weighing as larger volumes of MCA cortex. The MCA territory is divided into three subcortical and seven cortical regions. The subcortical regions are the caudate nucleus (C), lentiform nucleus (L), and internal capsule (IC). The cortical regions are the insular cortex (I); anterior, middle, and posterior MCA cortex at the level of the basal ganglia (M1–3); and anterior, middle, and posterior MCA cortex rostral to the basal ganglia (M4–6)[6] (▶ Fig. 9.4). An ASPECTS is calculated by assessing each of the 10 regions, awarding 1 point for each normal region, and no point for a region that has early ischemic change, giving a total score out of 10. A score of 10 indicates a normal scan with no feature of early ischemia, and a score of 0 indicates ischemia throughout the MCA territory. Changes of early ischemia may be parenchymal hypoattenuation (abnormally reduced attenuation of a brain structure relative to other parts of the same structure or the contralateral hemisphere), loss of differentiation between gray and white matters, or focal swelling (sulcal or ventricular effacement due to compression by adjacent brain). At its inception, ASPECTS were calculated by

assessing two 10-mm NCCT axial sections, one at and one just rostral to the level of the basal ganglia.[6] With increase in use of thinner sections on CT imaging, the ASPECTS scoring system has been modified to include all axial sections that include basal ganglia or supraganglionic structures, the boundary between these regions at the level of the caudate head.

9.1.9 Discussion

ASPECTS has value in prognosticating, and may assist with patient selection for acute stroke treatment. In the initial ASPECTS study, a baseline, pretreatment ASPECTS of 7 or less was strongly associated with an increase in the rates of death and functional dependency in patients treated with IV-tPA.[6] Subsequent larger studies confirm the strong correlation between pretreatment ASPECTS and probability of excellent functional outcome (modified Rankin score of 0–1) after treatment with IV-tPA, the Canadian Alteplase for Stroke Effectiveness Study demonstrating this effect in a relatively linear fashion.[7] Post hoc analysis of the pivotal National Institute of Neurological Disorders and Stroke (NINDS) tPA study found that higher ASPECTS (scores of 8–10) were associated with a greater extent of benefit from IV thrombolysis, a trend toward reduced mortality and smaller final infarct volumes.[8] Post hoc analysis of the ECASS-2 trial found an increased rate of thrombolysis-related parenchymal hematoma in patients with a pretreatment ASPECTS of ≤ 7.[9] Post hoc analysis of the Prourokinase Acute Cerebral Infarct Trial (PROACT-II), and review of the Interventional Management of Stroke (IMS-1) trial scans using ASPECTS, identified a clear treatment interaction when ASPECTS was used in a dichotomized fashion. In PROACT-II, patients with a pretreatment ASPECTS of > 7 treated with intra-arterial (IA) prourokinase did better than controls, in contrast to those with a pretreatment ASPECTS of ≤ 7 who had no benefit.[10] In a review of IMS-1, patients treated with

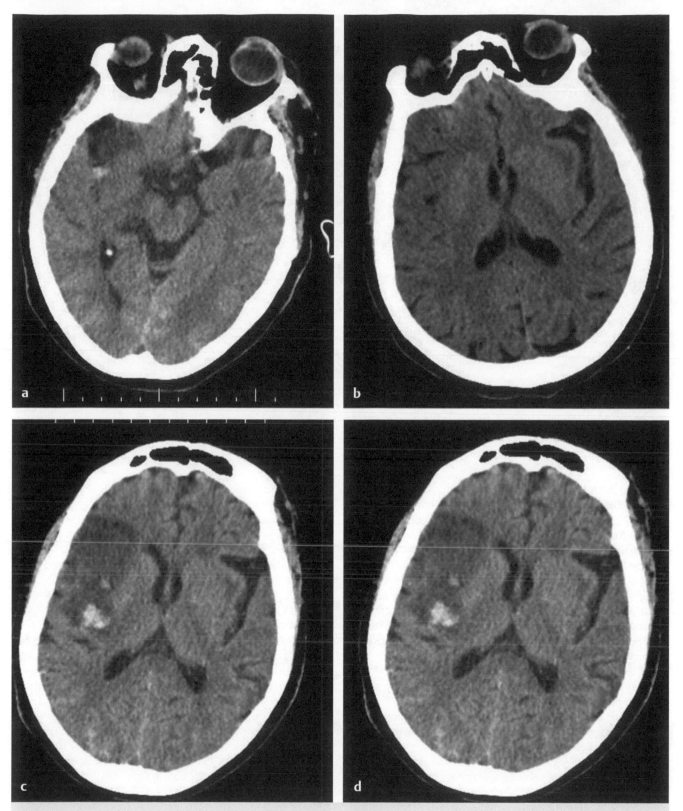

Fig. 9.3 NCCT performed on day 5 after admission reveals the final infarct volume, similar to areas of early infarction on the initial NCCT. Note the small area of infarction in right periventricular white matter that first became apparent on the NCCT performed 6 hours after thrombectomy. The final infarct is significantly smaller than the predicated infarct on CT perfusion. The parenchymal hematoma has reduced in size when compared with the postthrombectomy NCCT (see ▶ Fig. 9.2).

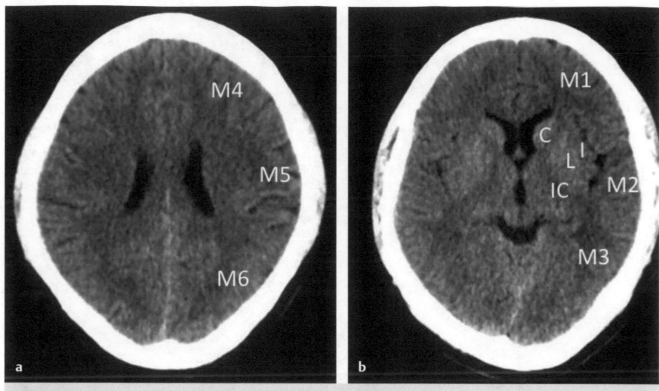

Fig. 9.4 ASPECTS map. Scores are calculated rostral to (**a**) and at (**b**) the level of the basal ganglia, the boundary between these regions at the level of the caudate head. Subcortical regions: caudate nucleus (**c**), lentiform nucleus (**l**), and internal capsule (**ic**). Cortical regions: insular cortex (**i**); anterior, middle, and posterior MCA cortex at the level of the basal ganglia (M1–3); and anterior, middle, and posterior MCA cortex rostral to the basal ganglia (M4–6).

combined IV-IA therapy were compared with matched subjects from the NINDS ASPECTS analysis. Patients with a pretreatment ASPECTS of >7 were more likely to benefit from combined IV-IA therapy than from IV therapy alone. Patients with a pretreatment ASPECTS ≤7 were less likely to benefit from combined therapy and more likely to be harmed.[11] The IMS-3 trial compared outcomes from acute stroke patients treated with IV-tPA therapy plus endovascular therapy with IV-tPA therapy alone. The trial failed to show benefit of endovascular therapy and was terminated early due to futility.[12] One criticism of the trial and possible contributing factor for the lack of an outcome difference between therapies was recruitment of patients with low ASPECTS. Imaging criteria for exclusion in the trial included infarction in greater than one-third of the MCA territory on baseline CT. Supplementary methods state that "an ASPECTS of less than 4 could be used as a guideline when evaluating more than one-third region of territory involvement but was not considered a specific exclusion."[12] Post hoc analysis of IMS-3[13] revealed that 92 patients had an ASPECTS of 0 to 4, and 186 patients had an ASPECTS of 5 to 7. After analysis, pretreatment ASPECTS was found to be a strong predictor of outcome—subjects with an ASPECTS of 8 to 10 were almost twice as likely to achieve a favorable outcome as those ≤7. Pretreatment ASPECTS was also a predictor of reperfusion with combined IV-IA therapy. However, the authors of the post hoc analysis concluded that there was insufficient evidence of a treatment by ASPECTS interaction.[13]

In the case highlighted in this chapter, ASPECTS was only one of many clinical and imaging factors influencing the decision to treat and the chosen treatment methods. The patient had excellent baseline functional status, no significant medical comorbidities, evidence of potentially salvageable tissue on CTP, and a desire to undergo the available treatments. A baseline ASPECTS of 7 or less is not a contraindication for IV-tPA, and ASPECTS should not be used in isolation to prognosticate or select treatment. Notwithstanding, the potential for poorer outcome with lower ASPECTS may be useful to assist with patient selection for therapy.

A very low ASPECTS (0–3) implies a large area of early ischemic change in the MCA territory, and may be a predictor of malignant MCA infarction (▶ Fig. 9.5, ▶ Fig. 9.6).[14] Patients with very low ASPECTS on presentation should undergo early repeat imaging to assess for potentially malignant MCA swelling, and aid in identifying patients who may benefit from surgical decompression. Determining infarct core size prior to acute reperfusion therapy is of increasing interest, as core size is a predictor of clinical outcome and response to therapy. In particular, patients with core volumes of more than 70 to 100 cc are more likely to have poor functional outcome regardless of reperfusion.[15,16,17] NCCT ASPECTS has a reasonable correlation with DWI MRI ASPECTS and thus for core infarct size,[18,19] but remains inferior to CTP.[20] The application of ASPECTS to CTA source data and perfusion maps has been investigated[20,21,22,23,24,25]; however, such applications are not widely utilized in a clinical setting.

There are limitations to the ASPECTS scoring system. ASPECTS can only attempt to quantify early ischemic change in the MCA territory, and thus has no value in infarction of other vascular territories. For example, a patient may have a disabling or potentially fatal stroke in the posterior circulation territory but will have a normal ASPECTS. Interobserver reliability of

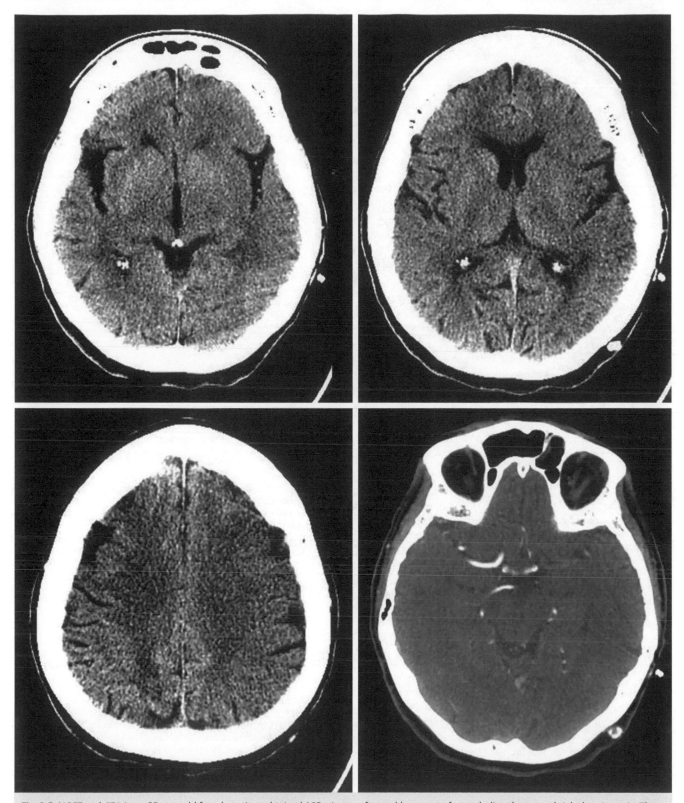

Fig. 9.5 NCCT and CTA in an 85-year-old female patient obtained 165 minutes after sudden onset of speech disturbance and right hemiparesis. There is occlusion of the carotid terminus and left MCA. Early infarction is evident throughout nearly the entire left MCA territory (ASPECTS 1). Only the M3 cortex is spared.

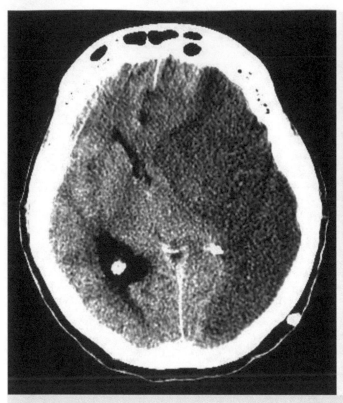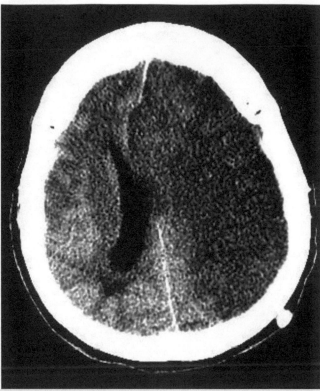

Fig. 9.6 A 24-hour follow-up NCCT of a patient presenting with a complete left MCA territory infarct (see ▶ Fig. 9.5). Evolution of the left MCA infarct with low attenuation throughout the MCA territory with swelling and mass effect including midline shift. Infarction of the left ACA territory is now evident. Due to comorbid conditions and poor clinical status, craniotomy was not performed. Palliative care measures were instituted and the patient died 24 hours later.

total ASPECTS is good but not excellent, although it is superior to that of the "1/3 MCA rule."[6,26,27,28] This is most likely secondary to the standardized and structured technique of ASPECTS. Given the potential for ASPECTS to prognosticate and modify patient selection for acute stroke therapy as discussed previously, the reliability of the score has been evaluated when used in a dichotomized fashion. The interobserver reliability falls to only moderate when ASPECTS is dichotomized at 7 (≤ 7 vs. > 7), which may impact on its utility.[29]

9.1.10 Pearls and Pitfalls

- All CT axial sections that include basal ganglia or supraganglionic structures must be assessed when assessing for early ischemic change to calculate ASPECTS.
- Pretreatment ASPECTS is a predictor of prognosis.
- When used in a dichotomized fashion, pretreatment ASPECTS of ≤ 7 is associated with an increase in the rates of hemorrhage, death, and functional dependency.
- ASPECTS should not be used in isolation to prognosticate or select treatment.

References

[1] Hacke W, Kaste M, Fieschi C, et al. The European Cooperative Acute Stroke Study (ECASS). Intravenous thrombolysis with recombinant tissue plasminogen activator for acute hemispheric stroke. JAMA. 1995; 274 (13):1017–1025

[2] Hacke W, Kaste M, Fieschi C, et al. Second European-Australasian Acute Stroke Study Investigators. Randomised double-blind placebo-controlled trial of thrombolytic therapy with intravenous alteplase in acute ischaemic stroke (ECASS II). Lancet. 1998; 352(9136):1245–1251

[3] Schriger DL, Kalafut M, Starkman S, Krueger M, Saver JL. Cranial computed tomography interpretation in acute stroke: physician accuracy in determining eligibility for thrombolytic therapy. JAMA. 1998; 279(16):1293–1297

[4] Grotta JC, Chiu D, Lu M, et al. Agreement and variability in the interpretation of early CT changes in stroke patients qualifying for intravenous rtPA therapy. Stroke. 1999; 30(8):1528–1533

[5] Wardlaw JM, Dorman PJ, Lewis SC, Sandercock PA. Can stroke physicians and neuroradiologists identify signs of early cerebral infarction on CT? J Neurol Neurosurg Psychiatry. 1999; 67(5):651–653

[6] Barber PA, Demchuk AM, Zhang J, Buchan AM. Validity and reliability of a quantitative computed tomography score in predicting outcome of hyperacute stroke before thrombolytic therapy. ASPECTS Study Group. Alberta Stroke Programme Early CT Score. Lancet. 2000; 355(9216):1670–1674

[7] Hill MD, Buchan AM, Canadian Alteplase for Stroke Effectiveness Study (CASES) Investigators. Thrombolysis for acute ischemic stroke: results of the Canadian Alteplase for Stroke Effectiveness Study. CMAJ. 2005; 172 (10):1307–1312

[8] Demchuk AM, Hill MD, Barber PA, Silver B, Patel SC, Levine SR, NINDS rtPA Stroke Study Group, NIH. Importance of early ischemic computed tomography changes using ASPECTS in NINDS rtPA Stroke Study. Stroke. 2005; 36(10):2110–2115

[9] Dzialowski I, Hill MD, Coutts SB, et al. Extent of early ischemic changes on computed tomography (CT) before thrombolysis: prognostic value of the Alberta Stroke Program Early CT Score in ECASS II. Stroke. 2006; 37(4):973–978

[10] Hill MD, Rowley HA, Adler F, et al. PROACT-II Investigators. Selection of acute ischemic stroke patients for intra-arterial thrombolysis with pro-urokinase by using ASPECTS. Stroke. 2003; 34(8):1925–1931

[11] Hill MD, Demchuk AM, Tomsick TA, Palesch YY, Broderick JP. Using the baseline CT scan to select acute stroke patients for IV-IA therapy. AJNR Am J Neuroradiol. 2006; 27(8):1612–1616

[12] Broderick JP, Palesch YY, Demchuk AM, et al. Interventional Management of Stroke (IMS) III Investigators. Endovascular therapy after intravenous t-PA versus t-PA alone for stroke. N Engl J Med. 2013; 368(10):893–903

[13] Hill MD, Demchuk AM, Goyal M, et al. IMS3 Investigators. Alberta Stroke Program early computed tomography score to select patients for endovascular treatment: Interventional Management of Stroke (IMS)-III Trial. Stroke. 2014; 45(2):444–449

[14] Krieger DW, Demchuk AM, Kasner SE, Jauss M, Hantson L. Early clinical and radiological predictors of fatal brain swelling in ischemic stroke. Stroke. 1999; 30(2):287–292

[15] Singer OC, Kurre W, Humpich MC, et al. MR Stroke Study Group Investigators. Risk assessment of symptomatic intracerebral hemorrhage after thrombolysis using DWI-ASPECTS. Stroke. 2009; 40(8):2743–2748

[16] Albers GW, Thijs VN, Wechsler L, et al. DEFUSE Investigators. Magnetic resonance imaging profiles predict clinical response to early reperfusion: the diffusion and perfusion imaging evaluation for understanding stroke evolution (DEFUSE) study. Ann Neurol. 2006; 60(5):508–517

[17] Yoo AJ, Verduzco LA, Schaefer PW, Hirsch JA, Rabinov JD, González RG. MRI-based selection for intra-arterial stroke therapy: value of pretreatment diffusion-weighted imaging lesion volume in selecting patients with acute stroke who will benefit from early recanalization. Stroke. 2009; 40(6):2046–2054

[18] Barber PA, Hill MD, Eliasziw M, et al. ASPECTS Study Group. Imaging of the brain in acute ischaemic stroke: comparison of computed tomography and magnetic resonance diffusion-weighted imaging. J Neurol Neurosurg Psychiatry. 2005; 76(11):1528–1533

[19] Nezu T, Koga M, Nakagawara J, et al. Early ischemic change on CT versus diffusion-weighted imaging for patients with stroke receiving intravenous recombinant tissue-type plasminogen activator therapy: stroke acute management with urgent risk-factor assessment and improvement (SAMURAI) rt-PA registry. Stroke. 2011; 42(8):2196–2200

[20] Lin K, Rapalino O, Law M, Babb JS, Siller KA, Pramanik BK. Accuracy of the Alberta Stroke Program Early CT Score during the first 3 hours of middle cerebral artery stroke: comparison of noncontrast CT, CT angiography source images, and CT perfusion. AJNR Am J Neuroradiol. 2008; 29(5):931–936

[21] Coutts SB, Lev MH, Eliasziw M, et al. ASPECTS on CTA source images versus unenhanced CT: added value in predicting final infarct extent and clinical outcome. Stroke. 2004; 35(11):2472–2476

[22] Aviv RI, Shelef I, Malam S, et al. Early stroke detection and extent: impact of experience and the role of computed tomography angiography source images. Clin Radiol. 2007; 62(5):447–452

[23] Aviv RI, Mandelcorn J, Chakraborty S, et al. Alberta Stroke Program Early CT Scoring of CT perfusion in early stroke visualization and assessment. AJNR Am J Neuroradiol. 2007; 28(10):1975–1980

[24] Parsons MW, Pepper EM, Chan V, et al. Perfusion computed tomography: prediction of final infarct extent and stroke outcome. Ann Neurol. 2005; 58 (5):672–679

[25] Kloska SP, Dittrich R, Fischer T, et al. Perfusion CT in acute stroke: prediction of vessel recanalization and clinical outcome in intravenous thrombolytic therapy. Eur Radiol. 2007; 17(10):2491–2498

[26] Pexman JH, Barber PA, Hill MD, et al. Use of the Alberta Stroke Program Early CT Score (ASPECTS) for assessing CT scans in patients with acute stroke. AJNR Am J Neuroradiol. 2001; 22(8):1534–1542

[27] Coutts SB, Demchuk AM, Barber PA, et al. VISION Study Group. Interobserver variation of ASPECTS in real time. Stroke. 2004; 35(5):e103–e105

[28] Finlayson O, John V, Yeung R, et al. Interobserver agreement of ASPECT score distribution for noncontrast CT, CT angiography, and CT perfusion in acute stroke. Stroke. 2013; 44(1):234–236

[29] Gupta AC, Schaefer PW, Chaudhry ZA, et al. Interobserver reliability of baseline noncontrast CT Alberta Stroke Program Early CT Score for intra-arterial stroke treatment selection. AJNR Am J Neuroradiol. 2012; 33 (6):1046–1049

10 Microbleeds Are Not a Contraindication to Thrombolysis in Acute Stroke

10.1 Case Description

10.1.1 Clinical Presentation

A 68-year-old man presented with a reduced conscious state associated with focal neurology on examination. His wife reported acute onset of left facial droop and altered conscious state at home. An ambulance was called and he was intubated in the community. He arrived at the emergency department 1 hour after onset of symptoms.

The patient had a known history of chronic atrial fibrillation (AF), and was on aspirin due to nonadherence with recommended warfarin therapy. He also had a history of congestive cardiac failure, and essential hypertension. Prior to intubation, the Glasgow Coma Score (GCS) was 4; the patient had no verbal response or eye opening, and had an extensor response to pain. Examination revealed left facial droop, extensor posturing, and positive left Babinski reflex.

10.1.2 Imaging Workup and Investigations

- Noncontrast computed tomography (NCCT) performed 2 hours after symptom onset demonstrates no acute ischemic changes (▶ Fig. 10.1).
- Subsequent CT angiography (CTA) demonstrated a filling defect in the tip of the basilar artery extending into the left and right P1 segments.

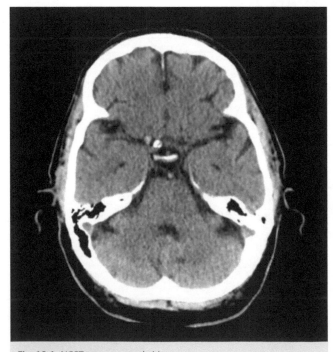

Fig. 10.1 NCCT was unremarkable.

10.2 Diagnosis

Occlusive basilar artery thrombosis.

10.3 Treatment

10.3.1 Initial Management

- Patient received intravenous thrombolysis 4.5 hours after the onset of symptoms.

10.3.2 Endovascular Management

- Endovascular clot retrieval was conducted at 5.5 hours with Trevo device.
- 1-cm clot was removed from basilar artery with Trevo device. Some residual clot was seen in the right superior cerebellar artery (SCA) (▶ Fig. 10.2).

10.3.3 Outcome

- The patient had an excellent response to therapy. He was able to follow commands after sedation was weaned on the same day.
- He was extubated on day 2 of admission, and discharged from intensive care on day 3.
- He was discharged from the hospital 2 weeks later; on discharge he was able to ambulate independently, with some residual deficits in dynamic balance.
- MRI performed 3 months later showed a large infarct involving the pons, as well as multiple small cerebellar infarcts (▶ Fig. 10.3). Multiple cerebral microbleeds (CMBs) were also identified in a lobar distribution (▶ Fig. 10.4).

10.4 Discussion

10.4.1 Background

Thrombolysis and mechanical thrombectomy are therapies proven to improve clinical outcomes following acute ischemic stroke.[1,2,3,4,5,6] However, tissue plasminogen activator (tPA) increases the risk of intracerebral hemorrhage (ICH).[7] The risk of ICH may also be increased in people with multiple lobar CMBs.[8] Identification of CMBs on MRI therefore invites the question, is thrombolysis indicated in patients with CMBs who present with acute ischemic stroke?

CMBs are small hypointense lesions, visible on susceptibility weight imaging and gradient echo (GRE) MRI sequences that represent hemosiderin-laden macrophage deposits in areas of angiopathy.[9] Risk of CMBs increases with age, with prevalence of CMBs reported to be around 25% in a general older population of mean age 68 years.[10,11] They are a marker of frailty, have been shown to correlate with severity of white matter lesions

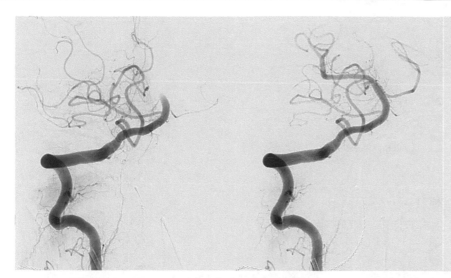

Fig. 10.2 Basilar artery thrombosis before (left) and after (right) successful mechanical thrombectomy.

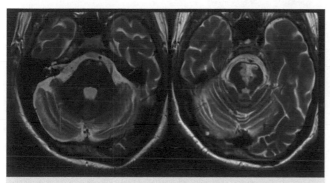

Fig. 10.3 Red oval—MRI T2 sequence showing pontine infarcts; red arrows—small cerebellar infarct.

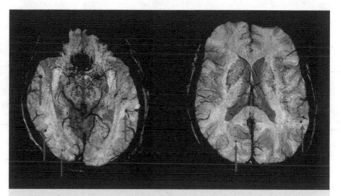

Fig. 10.4 Red arrows—multiple cerebral microbleeds in a lobar distribution.

(WML), and found to be an independent predictor of cognitive dysfunction.[12,13]

CMBs that occur in the lobar regions have been associated with cerebral amyloid angiopathy, carriage of the apolipoprotein e4 allele, and raised diastolic blood pressure (BP), while those that are infratentorial or deep are associated with cardiovascular risk factors such as hypertension, as well as subcortical infarcts, and WML on MRI.[11,14,15]

In observational studies, CMBs have been associated with an increased risk of ICH, and an increased risk of hematoma expansion in patients with ICH.[8,16,17,18] CMBs may also increase the risk of ICH in patients taking antiplatelet drugs.[18,19]

In a recent meta-analysis of five observational studies by Shoamanesh et al, there was a nonsignificant trend toward an increased risk of symptomatic and asymptomatic ICH after thrombolysis, in patients with CMBs compared to those without.[20] These studies were limited by small sample size and inconsistent methodology; thus, further studies are required.

10.4.2 Workup and Diagnosis

History

The patient's history of AF, congestive cardiac failure, hypertension, and age put him at high risk for cardioembolic stroke. Risk stratification using the CHA$_2$DS$_2$VASc criteria gives him a score of 3, which is associated with an annual risk of AF-related thromboembolism of around 5%.[21]

Examination and Investigations

On presentation, there were clear focal neurological symptoms, associated with a reduced conscious state. The patient's thrombolysis was delayed to confirm the stroke team clinical suspicion of basilar thrombosis by obtaining CTA. Obtaining further imaging after NCCT should not delay intravenous thrombolysis where it is indicated.

MRI performed subacutely showed a large pontine infarct accounting for the patient's altered consciousness and other symptoms, as well as multiple cerebellar infarcts that resulted in the residual deficits in dynamic balance.

10.4.3 Decision-Making Process

The decision to perform thrombolysis requires a diagnosis of ischemic stroke causing a measurable neurological deficit, with onset of symptoms no longer than 4.5 hours prior to beginning treatment in patients 18 years or older.[1] See ▶ Table 10.1 for a list of absolute and relative exclusion criteria. Endovascular clot retrieval has been shown to be superior to thrombolysis alone.[2]

Table 10.1 Exclusion criteria for thrombolysis for acute ischemic stroke[1]

Absolute exclusion criteria
Patient may not receive thrombolysis if any of the below criteria are met

- Significant head trauma or prior stroke in previous 3 mo
- Symptoms suggest subarachnoid hemorrhage
- History of previous intracranial hemorrhage
- Intracranial neoplasm, arteriovenous malformation
- Elevated blood pressure (systolic > 185 mm Hg or diastolic > 110 mm Hg)
- Arterial puncture at noncompressible site in previous 7 d
- CT demonstrates multilobar infarction (hypodensity > 1/3 cerebral hemisphere)
- Recent intracranial or intraspinal surgery
- Active internal bleeding
- Platelet count < 100,000/mm³
- Heparin received within 48 h, resulting in elevated aPTT
- Current use of anticoagulant with INR > 1.7
- Current use of direct thrombin inhibitors or direct factor Xa inhibitors with elevated sensitive laboratory tests
- Blood glucose concentration < 50 mg/dL (2.7 mmol/L)
- Acute bleeding diathesis

Relative exclusion criteria
Patient may receive thrombolysis after consideration of risk versus benefit, if one or more of the below criteria are met

- Only minor or rapidly improving stroke symptoms
- Pregnancy
- Seizure at onset with postictal residual neurological impairments
- Acute myocardial infarction in last 3 mo
- Major surgery or serious trauma within previous 14 d
- Recent gastrointestinal or urinary tract hemorrhage (within previous 21 d)

10.5 Literature Synopsis

Although multiple CMBs may increase the risk of ICH in some patients, the presence of CMBs is not a contraindication to thrombolysis in ischemic stroke.[1] Had this patient had an MRI performed at the time of, or before, the event, the presence of microbleeds should not have affected the decision to perform thrombolysis.

10.6 Pearls and Pitfalls

- The presence of cerebral microbleeds is not a contraindication to thrombolysis for acute ischemic stroke.
- Check for absolute and relative contraindications to thrombolysis.
- The presence of multiple cerebral microbleeds may increase the risk of bleeding after thrombolysis, but the magnitude and associated predictors are not clear.

10.7 References

[1] Jauch EC, Saver JL, Adams HP, Jr, et al. American Heart Association Stroke Council, Council on Cardiovascular Nursing, Council on Peripheral Vascular Disease, Council on Clinical Cardiology. Guidelines for the early management of patients with acute ischemic stroke: a guideline for healthcare professionals from the American Heart Association/American Stroke Association. Stroke. 2013; 44(3):870–947

[2] Campbell BC, Mitchell PJ, Kleinig TJ, et al. EXTEND-IA Investigators. Endovascular therapy for ischemic stroke with perfusion-imaging selection. N Engl J Med. 2015; 372(11):1009–1018

[3] Jovin TG, Chamorro A, Cobo E, et al. REVASCAT Trial Investigators. Thrombectomy within 8 hours after symptom onset in ischemic stroke. N Engl J Med. 2015; 372(24):2296–2306

[4] Goyal M, Demchuk AM, Menon BK, et al. ESCAPE Trial Investigators. Randomized assessment of rapid endovascular treatment of ischemic stroke. N Engl J Med. 2015; 372(11):1019–1030

[5] Berkhemer OA, Fransen PS, Beumer D, et al. A randomized trial of intraarterial treatment for acute ischemic stroke. N Engl J Med. 2015; 372 (1):1–20

[6] Saver JL, Goyal M, Bonafe A, et al. SWIFT PRIME Investigators. Solitaire™ with the Intention for Thrombectomy as Primary Endovascular Treatment for Acute Ischemic Stroke (SWIFT PRIME) trial: protocol for a randomized, controlled, multicenter study comparing the Solitaire revascularization device with IV tPA with IV tPA alone in acute ischemic stroke. Int J Stroke. 2015; 10(3):439–448

[7] Hacke W, Kaste M, Bluhmki E, et al. ECASS Investigators. Thrombolysis with alteplase 3 to 4.5 hours after acute ischemic stroke. N Engl J Med. 2008; 359 (13):1317–1329

[8] Stemer A, Ouyang B, Lee VH, Prabhakaran S. Prevalence and risk factors for multiple simultaneous intracerebral hemorrhages. Cerebrovasc Dis. 2010; 30 (3):302–307

[9] Charidimou A, Gang Q, Werring DJ. Sporadic cerebral amyloid angiopathy revisited: recent insights into pathophysiology and clinical spectrum. J Neurol Neurosurg Psychiatry. 2012; 83(2):124–137

[10] Poels MM, Ikram MA, van der Lugt A, et al. Incidence of cerebral microbleeds in the general population: the Rotterdam Scan Study. Stroke. 2011; 42 (3):656–661

[11] Poels MM, Vernooij MW, Ikram MA, et al. Prevalence and risk factors of cerebral microbleeds: an update of the Rotterdam scan study. Stroke. 2010; 41(10) Suppl:S103–S106

[12] Akoudad S, de Groot M, Koudstaal PJ, et al. Cerebral microbleeds are related to loss of white matter structural integrity. Neurology. 2013; 81(22):1930–1937

[13] Poels MM, Ikram MA, van der Lugt A, et al. Cerebral microbleeds are associated with worse cognitive function: the Rotterdam Scan Study. Neurology. 2012; 78(5):326–333

[14] Yates PA, Sirisriro R, Villemagne VL, Farquharson S, Masters CL, Rowe CC, AIBL Research Group. Cerebral microhemorrhage and brain β-amyloid in aging and Alzheimer disease. Neurology. 2011; 77(1):48–54

[15] Jia Z, Mohammed W, Qiu Y, Hong X, Shi H. Hypertension increases the risk of cerebral microbleed in the territory of posterior cerebral artery: a study of the association of microbleeds categorized on a basis of vascular territories and cardiovascular risk factors. J Stroke Cerebrovasc Dis. 2014; 23(1):e5–e11

[16] Martí-Fàbregas J, Delgado-Mederos R, Granell E, et al. RENEVAS Group (Stroke Research Network, RETICS, Instituto de Salud Carlos III). Microbleed burden and hematoma expansion in acute intracerebral hemorrhage. Eur Neurol. 2013; 70(3–4):175–178

[17] Fluri F, Jax F, Amort M, et al. Significance of microbleeds in patients with transient ischaemic attack. Eur J Neurol. 2012; 19(3):522–524

[18] Gregoire SM, Jäger HR, Yousry TA, Kallis C, Brown MM, Werring DJ. Brain microbleeds as a potential risk factor for antiplatelet-related intracerebral haemorrhage: hospital-based, case-control study. J Neurol Neurosurg Psychiatry. 2010; 81(6):679–684

[19] Vernooij MW, Haag MDM, van der Lugt A, et al. Use of antithrombotic drugs and the presence of cerebral microbleeds: the Rotterdam Scan Study. Arch Neurol. 2009; 66(6):714–720

[20] Shoamanesh A, Kwok CS, Lim PA, Benavente OR. Postthrombolysis intracranial hemorrhage risk of cerebral microbleeds in acute stroke patients: a systematic review and meta-analysis. Int J Stroke. 2013; 8(5):348–356

[21] Olesen JB, Lip GY, Hansen ML, et al. Validation of risk stratification schemes for predicting stroke and thromboembolism in patients with atrial fibrillation: nationwide cohort study. BMJ. 2011; 342:d124

Further Reading

Charidimou A, Werring DJ. Cerebral microbleeds as a predictor of macrobleeds: what is the evidence? Int J Stroke. 2014; 9(4):457–459

Jauch EC, Saver JL, Adams HP, et al. Guidelines for the early management of patients with acute ischemic stroke: a guideline for healthcare professionals from the American Heart Association/American Stroke Association. Stroke. 2013; 44 (3):870–947

11 Stroke Etiologies: Hemodynamic, Embolic, and Perforator Stroke

11.1 Case Description

11.1.1 Clinical Presentation

A previously healthy 69-year-old, right hand–dominant woman was brought to the emergency department (ED) with sudden-onset right middle cerebral artery (MCA) syndrome while driving. She was last seen well 45 minutes prior to arrival in the ED. Initial vital signs show a blood pressure of 168/72 mm Hg and a regular heart rate of 86 beats per minute, and were otherwise normal. Neurological examination was notable for right gaze preference, left homonymous hemianopsia, dysarthria, left hemiparesis, hemibody sensory loss affecting the face, upper and lower extremities, and left hemineglect with somatagnosia. Total National Institutes of Health Stroke Scale (NIHSS) score was 10.

On further history, she denied headache, nausea, or vomiting. A detailed review of systems was negative. She had no known past medical history and did not take regular medications. She was a lifelong nonsmoker, rarely drank alcohol, and there was no recreational drug use history.

11.1.2 Imaging Workup and Investigations

- Noncontrast computed tomography (NCCT) of the head showed absence of hemorrhage. The ASPECTS score was 9, with 1 point deducted for loss of gray-white matter differentiation in the right insular ribbon. CT angiography (CTA) of the head and neck was significant for an abrupt cutoff of the right MCA in the distal M1 segment (▶ Fig. 11.1a, b).

- CT perfusion (▶ Fig. 11.1c–f) demonstrated a small area of severely decreased relative cerebral blood volume (rCBV) and relative cerebral blood flow (rCBF) in the right parietal lobe. There was, however, a large area of increased mean transit time (MTT) and time to maximal residue (Tmax) noted in the right lateral frontal, temporal, and parietal lobes, with sparing of the right lentiform nucleus. Appearances therefore indicated a large area of perfusion mismatch in the right MCA territory.

- Laboratory investigations were normal, including complete blood count, creatinine, and coagulation profile. Electrocardiography demonstrated no evidence of cardiac ischemia.

11.1.3 Diagnosis

Right MCA territory ischemic stroke secondary to acute right M1 occlusion.

11.1.4 Treatment

- In the absence of contraindications, intravenous (IV) thrombolysis was initiated in the ED and the patient was promptly transported to the angiography suite for intra-arterial thrombectomy.

Equipment

- Standard 8-Fr femoral access.
- 6-Fr, 90 cm AXS Infinity guide catheter (Stryker, Kalamazoo, MI).
- 5-Fr, 120 cm Berenstein-tip Select catheter (Penumbra, Alameda, CA).

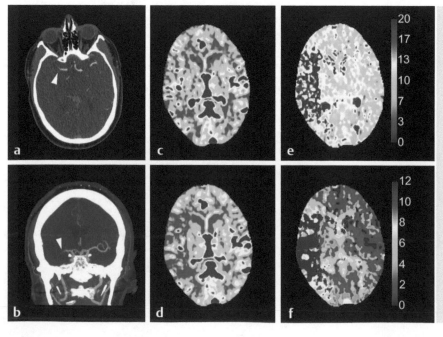

Fig. 11.1 Case 1: Initial CT angiography (**a**, axial source image; **b**, coronal maximal intensity projection) demonstrates cutoff (*white arrows*) in the distal M1 segment of the right MCA. CT perfusion (**c**, rCBV; **d**, rCBF; **e**, MTT; **f**, Tmax) reveals corresponding perfusion mismatch with sparing of the basal ganglia, indicating an occlusion distal to the origin of the lateral lenticulostriate artery.

- Intermediate aspiration catheter (6 Fr Sofia Plus; MicroVention Terumo, Aliso Viejo, CA).
- 0.027" microcatheter (Marksman 150 cm; Medtronic, Minneapolis, MN).
- 0.016" microwire (Fathom; Medtronic, Minneapolis, MN).
- 4 × 20 mm mechanical thrombectomy device and microcatheter (Solitaire X, Medtronic, Minneapolis, MN).
- Aspiration pump and tubing (Penumbra, Alameda, CA).

Technique

- An 8-Fr vascular sheath was placed following groin access, and a 6-Fr Shuttle sheath was advanced over a 5-Fr diagnostic catheter. The 5-Fr catheter was used to select the right internal carotid artery, and a diagnostic injection demonstrated filling defect consistent with thrombus in the distal right M1 segment (▶ Fig. 11.2a).
- The 6-Fr shuttle sheath was positioned in the distal cervical internal carotid artery. The angiographic catheter was removed and the intermediate aspiration catheter was advanced over a coaxial system of the 0.027" Marksman microcatheter over a 0.016" Fathom microwire.
- The right MCA was selected using the microwire and the microcatheter tip was positioned distal to the thrombus in the inferior M2 segment. The guidewire was removed and a 4 × 20 mm stent retriever was introduced. The device was deployed across the thrombus (▶ Fig. 11.2b) and the microcatheter was removed. The aspiration catheter was

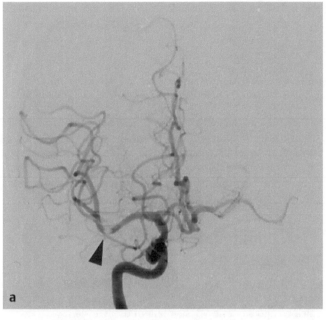
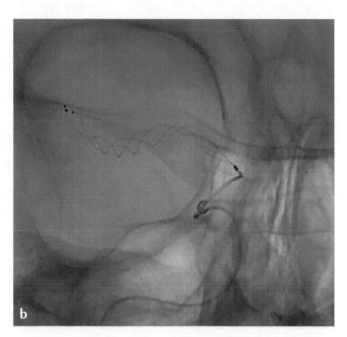
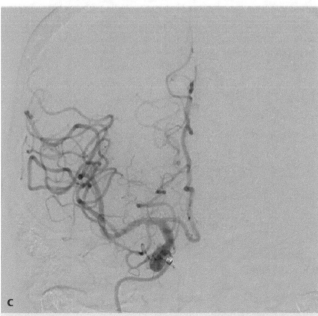
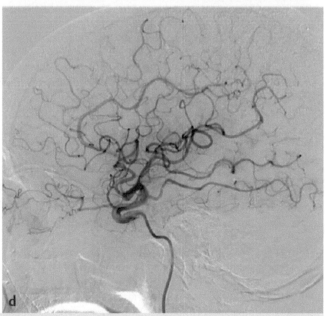

Fig. 11.2 Case 1: Initial diagnostic injection demonstrates a filling defect (**a**, *black arrow*) in the distal right MCA corresponding to the thrombus. Flow is visible across the lesion, though with incomplete filling of distal branches. A stent retriever is placed across the lesion (**b**). Following thrombectomy, normal anterograde flow is reestablished, with opacification of all distal vessels (**c**), with a final mTICI score of III (**d**).

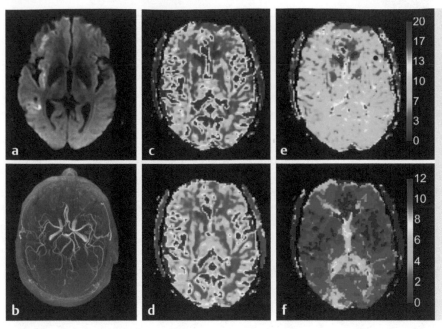

Fig. 11.3 Case 1: Diffusion-weighted images on postoperative day 1 MRI demonstrates a moderate-sized infarct involving isolated cortical areas (a). Collapsed view of MR angiography shows persistent patency of the right MCA (b). Perfusion-weighted images on MRI show normalization of perfusion deficit. Right hemispheric relative CBV (c) and CBF (d) is slightly increased in the recently reperfused right hemisphere, while mean transit time (e) and time to maximal residue function (Tmax, f) have largely normalized.

advanced to the face of the thrombus and connected to the aspiration system.

- The stent retriever was then partially withdrawn into the aspiration catheter until flow arrest, signaling capturing of the thrombus between the stent retriever and the aspiration catheter. The stent retriever and aspiration catheter were then removed as a unit. The guide catheter was allowed to back-bleed, and when no thrombus was seen, it was flushed forward. Follow-up angiography of the right anterior circulation demonstrated complete recanalization and reperfusion (► Fig. 11.2c, d).

Follow-up

Follow-up MRI on postoperative day 1 demonstrated limited infarct burden, with patency of the right MCA. Perfusion-weighted imaging shows normalization of the previously seen perfusion mismatch (► Fig. 11.3).

Paroxysmal atrial fibrillation was diagnosed on extended cardiac monitoring following discharge, and was felt to be the most likely stroke etiology in this patient.

11.2 Companion Case

11.2.1 Clinical Presentation

A 77-year-old, right hand–dominant woman was brought to the emergency department with moderate aphasia, right facial droop, and right upper extremity paresis and numbness. She was last seen well 5 hours prior. Initial blood pressure was 93/65 mm Hg, with a regular heart rate of 116 beats per minute. Neurological exam, with head-of-bed at 60 degrees, was remarkable for decreased verbal expression and intermittent ability to follow single-step commands, inability to move right arm against gravity, a prominent right lower facial droop, and right arm numbness. Total NIHSS score was 8. Repeat examination after IV fluid administration, at a systolic blood pressure of

150 mm Hg, with head-of-bed at 5 degrees, showed improved fluency and comprehension of speech as well as right arm pronator drift and improvement in facial droop, with persistent arm numbness. Repeat NIHSS was 4. Past medical history was notable for medically controlled hypertension and dyslipidemia. The patient has no prior history of stroke.

11.2.2 Imaging Workup and Investigations

NCCT of the head showed a focus of calcification in vicinity of proximal left MCA. CTA of the head and neck demonstrated a calcified and stenotic M1 segment of the left MCA, with no significant extracranial carotid disease (► Fig. 11.4a, b). Left MCA territory distal to the stenosis demonstrated CT perfusion abnormality, with increased Tmax and MTT, reduced rCBF, and relatively normal rCBV (► Fig. 11.4c–e).

11.2.3 Diagnosis

Hemodynamically significant proximal M1 segment of MCA stenosis due to intracranial atherosclerotic disease.

11.2.4 Treatment

- The patient was placed on bedrest and initiated on antiplatelet and statin therapy. She was admitted to the neurocritical care unit for neuromonitoring and hypertensive therapy. Transthoracic echocardiogram confirmed normal cardiac function.
- IV fluids and vasopressors were administered, with close volume status and blood pressure monitoring. Postural and activity tolerance gradually improved over subsequent days under careful medical supervision.
- Systolic blood pressure target to > 160 mm Hg was maintained for more than 3 months as the patient had

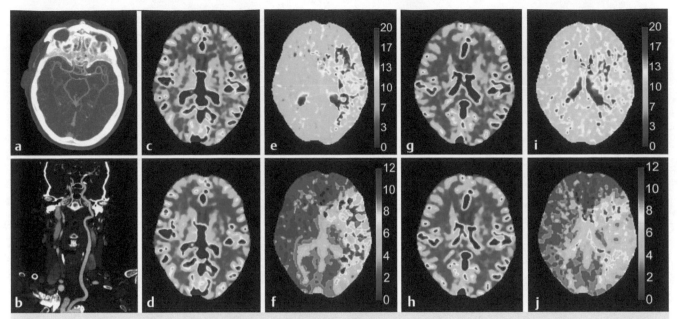

Fig. 11.4 Companion Case 1: Initial CT angiogram (**a**, axial maximal intensity projection; **b**, left ICA reconstruction) reveals a short calcified plaque in the proximal left MCA with complete and symmetric filling of distal vessels. CT perfusion (**c**, rCBV; **d**, rCBF; **e**, MTT; **f**, Tmax) demonstrates non-matched perfusion defect affecting the entire left MCA territory, with reduced rCBF, prolonged MTT, prolonged Tmax, without reduced rCBV. Follow-up CT perfusion on day 4 of admission shows improvement of perfusion defect following augmentation of systolic blood pressure (**g–j**).

recurrent intermittent and transient right upper limb numbness lasting several minutes at a time.

- Blood pressure target was subsequently gradually normalized. The patient was asymptomatic at 9-month follow-up.

11.3 Additional Companion Case

11.3.1 Clinical Presentation

A 57-year-old, right hand–dominant woman with poorly controlled vascular risk factors presented with a history of slurred speech and mild right hemiparesis on awakening. She was last seen well 9 hours previously. Neurological examination showed mild dysarthria, right facial droop, and right pronator drift, for a total NIHSS score of 4.

Past medical history was significant for long-standing, uncontrolled systolic hypertension, insulin-dependent type 2 diabetes mellitus, obstructive sleep apnea, and obesity. She was a current smoker, with a 20-pack-year history of tobacco use. She did not consume alcohol or take recreational drugs.

11.3.2 Imaging Findings

MRI demonstrated a small diffusion-restricting lesion involving the posterior limb of the internal capsule on the left (▶ Fig. 11.5a). MR angiogram showed no evidence of intracranial large artery occlusion or atherosclerotic disease (▶ Fig. 11.5b).

11.3.3 Diagnosis

Lacunar infarct involving the posterior limb of the left internal capsule.

11.3.4 Treatment

- After confirming safety to swallow, aspirin (ASA) 325 mg was administered orally in the ED, followed by ASA 81 mg daily.
- Three antihypertensive agents were then sequentially initiated, titrated over days to achieve a blood pressure target of 110 to 140/60 to 90 mm Hg. High-dose statin was initiated, with target low-density lipoprotein (LDL) level of < 80 mg/dL (2 mmol/L).

11.4 Discussion

11.4.1 Background

The three cases discussed earlier illustrate the common presentation of an MCA syndrome due to three different etiologies: M1 occlusion such as from an embolic source, hemodynamic stroke with M1 stenosis, and perforator stroke. However, only the patient with acute MCA occlusion is a candidate for acute endovascular therapy. Consideration of the physiology and pathophysiology associated with cerebral ischemia is important to understand these differential diagnoses.

Impaired regional perfusion is at the basis of symptoms and signs associated with cerebral ischemia. Normal physiology ensures cerebrovascular autoregulation over a large range of mean arterial pressure, to ensure maintenance of blood flow (CBF) above ischemic threshold. In general, normal cerebral function is maintained at a mean CBF of approximately 50 mL/min/ 100 g of brain tissue. Below this threshold, transient loss of function of the affected cerebral region may become clinically apparent, with chance of normalization with early reestablishment of normal CBF. However, if CBF falls and remains under 10 to 12 mL/min/100 g of brain tissue at any time, infarction occurs.

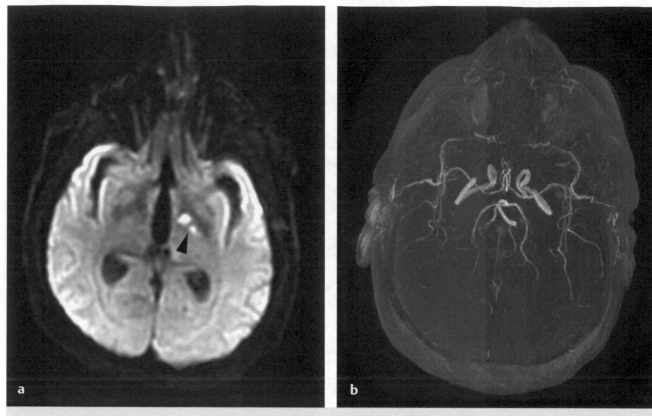

Fig. 11.5 Companion Case 2: Diffusion-weighted imaging on presentation demonstrates a small infarct affecting the posterior limb of the left internal capsule (**a**, *black arrow*). Collapsed view of the MR angiography shows no large-artery occlusive lesion (**b**).

The threshold for irreversible infarction increases over time, and stabilizes at 17 to 18 mL/min/100 g of the brain tissue by 3 hours.

This physiological basis of regional cerebral ischemia implies that clinical presentations are almost exclusively reflective of hypoperfused parenchymal neuroanatomical structures, but may not directly relate to stroke etiology. Therefore, an MCA syndrome may result from loss of anterograde blood flow in an acute M1 segment occlusion, from relative hypoperfusion distal to a high-grade MCA stenosis, or from a perforator vessel occlusion resulting in a lacunar stroke. In other words, any ischemic insult to the frontoparietal motor and sensory cortices or tracts may result in a clinical syndrome of hemiparesis, numbness, and dysarthria. Therefore, appropriate triage and emergent neuroimaging is essential in differentiating between stroke etiologies, and allowing appropriate case selection for emergency endovascular treatment through early identification of large-vessel occlusions. A similar situation exists in the posterior circulation, where, for example, differentiation between a basilar artery occlusion, basilar stenosis with hypoperfusion, and perforator infarction is essential in order to instigate appropriate management.

11.4.2 Workup and Diagnosis

History and Examination

History and clinical examination can help with differentiation of stroke etiologies. Two features are particularly helpful in their distinction:

- The absence of cortical symptoms suggests likely subcortical or perforator infarction. Several common signs and symptoms of hemispheric strokes, including gaze deviation, aphasia, and cortical sensory loss (such as inattention or extinction), localize to cortical areas and are often spared in perforator strokes.
- Hemodynamic fluctuation in symptom severity. While fluctuations in collateral flow with intravascular volume status, blood pressure, and head-of-bed elevation can result in changes in symptom severity in patients with large-vessel occlusion, complete resolution of presenting symptoms with improved flow is rare in these patients. On the contrary, profound fluctuations in symptom severity inversely correlated with increased cerebral perfusion can be observed with patients with symptomatic high-grade stenoses. This feature defines "hemodynamically significant" lesions.

11.4.3 Imaging Findings

Noncontrast Enhanced CT

The conventional initial NCCT of the head rules out intracerebral hemorrhage and demonstrates any early ischemic changes, if present. In the absence of bleeding, large area of infarction, or other clinical contraindications, the patient may benefit from IV thrombolytic therapy if presenting within 4.5 hours.

Angiographic Imaging

Angiography is necessary to confirm location of the arterial occlusive lesion, and can be performed through different imaging modalities, most commonly CT or MR angiography. CTA is associated with short scan time, and affords high luminal definition. It can also be rapidly acquired for both the head and neck following NCCT of the head, as a part of the same examination. Accessibility makes CTA a powerful early-assessment tool to rule in (or out) patient candidacy for endovascular therapy in an emergency situation. In addition, a multiphasic CTA protocol would permit evaluation of the collateral circulation, a vascular surrogate measure that can be used to estimate infarct growth rate. The downside of CTA is its obligatory contrast and ionizing radiation exposure, limiting its use in patients with severe nephropathy or iodine contrast allergy.

For centers with ready access to MRI and in patients without contraindications, MR angiography (MRA) may similarly demonstrate the presence or absence of intracranial occlusive or stenotic lesion with or without contrast. The time-of-flight technique allows image acquisition in as little as 2 to 2.5 minutes without use of contrast agent. Concomitant acquisition of diffusion-weighted imaging (DWI), which provides the highest diagnostic sensitivity for infarct core identification in hyperacute stroke, is another frequent reason for using MRI. MRA, however, may not always reliably differentiate slow flow or critical stenosis from a complete occlusion. It should be noted that flow-related artifacts are less common with contrast-enhanced than time-of-flight MRA. Other notable limitations of MRI include longer study time, susceptibility to motion artifacts, and contraindication in the presence of some implanted or external devices.

Perfusion Imaging

Routine use of perfusion imaging in all hyperacute strokes remains center-specific. Perfusion imaging can be performed by MRI (perfusion-weighted imaging, or PWI) or CT (CTP), and allows for direct measure of averaged tissue perfusion over time within each voxel. By MRI, a mismatch between DWI and PWI identifies patients with over five times greater odds of favorable response to reperfusion. CT perfusion has the benefit of wider accessibility and shorter acquisition time, though at the expense of ionizing radiation exposure. CT perfusion predicts probable infarcts in absence of reperfusion, and optimal core and penumbra parameters remain objects of debate, though rCBF and Tmax are commonly used in conjunction with automated segmentation softwares.

11.4.4 Decision-Making Process

A rapid-sequence decision-making process is crucial when evaluating a patient with acute ischemic stroke.
1. Ensure patient stability from an airway–breathing–circulation perspective.
2. Ensure cerebral perfusion. In instances of hypotension without clinical evidence of increased intracranial pressure, immediate steps, including fluid resuscitation and lowering head of bed while maintaining a safe airway, may be associated with improved cerebral blood flow in ischemic territory.
3. Establish basic patient characteristics: age, symptoms, and the time the patient was last known at neurological baseline. The acuity of symptom *onset* should be verified. A complete medical history, including current use of any anticoagulant, antiplatelet, or antihypertensive agents, has potential impact on immediate management.
4. Obtain neuroimaging to rule out hemorrhage and large or completed infarcts, and to identify arterial occlusive lesion amenable to thrombectomy. Preference for first imaging modality is given to CT for its wide availability and rapid acquisition in eligible patients, and angiography should be part of the study. Perfusion imaging, if available, provides visualization of the ischemic penumbra, and allows for evaluation and selection of patients suitable for mechanical thrombectomy. In patients without a large-vessel occlusion, it provides a radiological correlate to guide blood pressure management and further optimization of cerebral perfusion.
5. Where clinical suspicion for stroke is high, and intracranial large artery occlusion has not been found, MRI allows confirmation of ischemic stroke using DWI with high diagnostic sensitivity and specificity. Diffusion restriction within an infarct can be seen as early as within 30 minutes, peaks within 3 to 5 days, offers the highest sensitivity within the first 2 weeks, and normalizes within 1 to 4 weeks. DWI can clearly outline the ischemic lesions, and allows for further distinction of various stroke etiologies (e.g., lacunar infarct or large vessel occlusion) and will also help distinguish true stroke from stroke mimics.

Management

Currently, the standard of care is that all patients with acute ischemic stroke, presenting within 3 to 4.5 hours and without contraindications for IV thrombolysis, should be given IV tissue plasminogen activator (tPA) without delay, whether they are considered for mechanical thrombectomy or not. This approach is recommended by the 2019 American Heart Association/American Stroke Association Guidelines for the Early Management of Patients with Acute Ischemic Stroke; the *2018 Canadian Stroke Best Practices Recommendations* by the Heart and Stroke Foundation of Canada; and the 2018 *Guidelines on Mechanical Thrombectomy in Acute Ischemic Stroke* by the European Stroke Organisation (ESO), and the European Stroke and Minimal Invasive Neurological Therapy.

Meanwhile, endovascular therapy is the key focus prompting updated guidelines and recommendations since 2015. In addition to IV-tPA, patients with embolic intracranial large-artery occlusion should be treated with endovascular intervention without delay if presenting within 24 hours of last-known-well time. The results of several randomized controlled trials published since 2015 have provided the highest level of evidence for endovascular therapy in these patients.

In patients with a hemodynamically significant stenosis, augmentation of cerebral perfusion is the first-line treatment option. This can be achieved by lowering head of bed, increasing intravascular volume, or using vasopressors. Permissive hypertension reinforces anterograde blood flow across a hemodynamically significant stenosis and collateral flow to the ischemic region. In the instance of severe stenosis of an extracranial vessel, flow may also cross over from the circle of Willis. Intracranial stenting may be considered in patients with refractory hypoperfusion secondary to a flow-limiting stenosis.

Although an etiology-based treatment is the ideal, it is important to bear in mind that revascularization therapy is time sensitive: "Time is brain." Not all evidence pointing to a clear stroke pathophysiology or etiology is necessarily available when considering possible thrombolytic therapy and mechanical thrombectomy early in patient assessment. Observational studies provide evidence suggesting that patients in whom contraindications for IV-tPA are carefully ruled out have low risk of complications. Therefore, when in doubt in assessing a patient eligible for IV thrombolysis and without clinical or radiographic (early signs of infarction on CT or large infarct), it is reasonable to err on the side of treating the patient as soon as possible, with further investigations to follow. Of note, severe hypertension is associated with worse outcome after thrombolysis, and judicious blood pressure monitoring and control is indicated to achieve safe optimization of cerebral perfusion in all patients. Higher level of care in an intensive care unit setting is often required.

This approach to initial treatment equally applies for lacunar, or perforator-associated, strokes. Though the pathophysiology of lacunar infarcts is often thought to be related to lipohyalinosis or thickening of small arterial and arteriolar walls from long-standing cardiovascular risk factors, especially hypertension, acute stroke treatment for patients eligible for IV-tPA is the same. Aggressive optimization of secondary stroke prevention therapy should ensue.

11.4.5 Literature Synopsis

In 2015, a number of large, international, randomized controlled trials were published, which proved benefit for endovascular therapy for acute large-vessel occlusion involving the internal carotid artery and the MCA in the M1 segment (ESCAPE, MR CLEAN, REVASCAT, EXTEND-IA, and SWIFT PRIME). The number needed to treat (NNT) across these studies averaged to approximately four patients to achieve one patient with functional independence at 90 days (NNT = 4). Contrasting with a prior generation of large randomized controlled trials, these recent studies highlighted the importance of a target occlusion that is accessible for current devices for endovascular therapy. Other important conclusions include identifying a small core and a large penumbra, and shortening time to therapy. The result is the need for a rapid diagnosis and understanding of the etiology for the patient's acute deterioration. In 2018, two more randomized controlled studies (DAWN and DEFUSE 3) demonstrated the efficacy of mechanical thrombectomy up to 24 hours, in select patients with large vessel occlusion and clinical or radiographic mismatch, resulting from a small infarct core and a large penumbra.

While mechanical thrombectomy has become standard of care for acute large-vessel occlusions presenting within 24 hours of stroke onset, evidence supports maximal medical management as best first-line therapy for critical intracranial stenosis. The Stenting and Aggressive Medical Management for the Prevention of Recurrent Stroke in Intracranial Stenosis (SAMMPRIS) trial demonstrated the combination of daily aspirin 325 mg, clopidogrel 75 mg, and rosuvastatin, to be superior to intracranial angioplasty and stenting as first-line therapy.

SAMMPRIS is an important study in addressing the management of intracranial stenosis versus a strictly optimized medical treatment. However, SAMMPRIS had significant limitations, including insufficiently stringent patient selection criteria. Retrospectively, the majority of SAMMPRIS patients treated did not meet clinical criteria supporting benefit for intracranial stenting per pre-existing clinical evidence. Meanwhile, SAMMPRIS optimized the medical arm of the study with closer monitoring and intervention than feasible in most clinical contexts, therefore heightening the benefits of strictly optimized medical therapy. SAMMPRIS suggested that intracranial angioplasty and stenting are most likely to benefit carefully selected patients with recurrent strokes despite best medical therapy, and those with hemodynamically symptomatic high-grade intracranial stenosis.

The Wingspan Stent System Post Market Surveillance (WEAVE) trial ensued. With strict inclusion of patients with recurrent stroke in the territory of the high-grade (70-99%) target stenotic segment, and timing limited to over 8 days after the most recent event, the study demonstrated a dramatic drop in the rate of adverse events. While SAMMPRIS demonstrated a 14.7% composite serious adverse events rate, WEAVE had a composite complication rate of 2.6%. The study was stopped early in October 2017, having met its safety endpoint of less than 4% complication rate.

Current first-line treatment for high-grade intracranial stenosis is medical therapy. For patients with recurrent strokes attributable to a high-grade intracranial stenosis, and despite maximal medical therapy, intracranial stenting and angioplasty is a reasonable therapeutic option. More data are needed to support long-term efficacy of intracranial stenting.

Moderate systolic hypertension at approximately 170 to 190 mm Hg may be associated with better outcome in hyperacute stroke, though systolic pressures exceeding this level may increase the risk of hemorrhage. Some evidence supports the safe use of phenylephrine to achieve hypertension in acute stroke, but data are limited.

11.4.6 Pearls and Pitfalls

- Similar stroke symptoms may result from a proximal vessel occlusion, a hemodynamic stenosis, or a lacunar infarct.
- Identification of an arterial occlusive lesion amenable to thrombectomy is necessary for acute endovascular therapy.
- Guidelines and recommendations in the United States, Canada, and Europe suggest that all patients meeting eligibility criteria for IV thrombolysis should be given IV-tPA.
- Medical management should be considered as first-line therapy in critical intracranial stenosis. It includes the use of antiplatelet(s), a statin, and permissive hypertension as safely as possible to support collateral perfusion.
- Intracranial angioplasty and stenting play a role in patients with critical intracranial stenosis with failure of first-line maximal medical therapy.

Further Reading

Mui K, Yoo AJ, Verduzco L, et al. Cerebral blood flow thresholds for tissue infarction in patients with acute ischemic stroke treated with intra-arterial revascularization therapy depend on timing of reperfusion. AJNR Am J Neuroradiol. 2011; 32 (5):846–851

Albers GW, Thijs VN, Wechsler L, et al. DEFUSE Investigators. Magnetic resonance imaging profiles predict clinical response to early reperfusion: the diffusion and perfusion imaging evaluation for understanding stroke evolution (DEFUSE) study. Ann Neurol. 2006; 60(5):508–517

Campbell BCV, Donnan GA, Lees KR, et al. Endovascular stent thrombectomy: the new standard of care for large vessel ischaemic stroke. Lancet Neurol. 2015; 14 (8):846–854

Campbell BC, Mitchell PJ, Kleinig TJ, et al. EXTEND-IA Investigators. Endovascular therapy for ischemic stroke with perfusion-imaging selection. N Engl J Med. 2015; 372(11):1009–1018

Saver JL, Goyal M, Bonafe A, et al. SWIFT PRIME Investigators. Stent-retriever thrombectomy after intravenous t-PA vs. t-PA alone in stroke. N Engl J Med. 2015; 372(24):2285–2295

Jovin TG, Chamorro A, Cobo E, et al. REVASCAT Trial Investigators. Thrombectomy within 8 hours after symptom onset in ischemic stroke. N Engl J Med. 2015; 372 (24):2296–2306

Berkhemer OA, Fransen PS, Beumer D, et al. MR CLEAN Investigators. A randomized trial of intraarterial treatment for acute ischemic stroke. N Engl J Med. 2015; 372 (1):11–20

Goyal M, Demchuk AM, Menon BK, et al. ESCAPE Trial Investigators. Randomized assessment of rapid endovascular treatment of ischemic stroke. N Engl J Med. 2015; 372(11):1019–1030

Rusanen H, Saarinen JT, Sillanpää N. The association of blood pressure and collateral circulation in hyperacute ischemic stroke patients treated with intravenous thrombolysis. Cerebrovasc Dis. 2015; 39(2):130–137

Olavarría VV, Arima H, Anderson CS, et al. Head position and cerebral blood flow velocity in acute ischemic stroke: a systematic review and meta-analysis. Cerebrovasc Dis. 2014; 37(6):401–408

Derdeyn CP, Chimowitz MI, Lynn MJ, et al. Stenting and Aggressive Medical Management for Preventing Recurrent Stroke in Intracranial Stenosis Trial Investigators. Aggressive medical treatment with or without stenting in high-risk patients with intracranial artery stenosis (SAMMPRIS): the final results of a randomised trial. Lancet. 2014; 383(9914):333–341

Zaidat OO, Fitzsimmons B-F, Woodward BK, et al. VISSIT Trial Investigators. Effect of a balloon-expandable intracranial stent vs medical therapy on risk of stroke in patients with symptomatic intracranial stenosis: the VISSIT randomized clinical trial. JAMA. 2015; 313(12):1240–1248

Albers GW, Marks MP, Kemp S, et al. Thrombectomy for stroke at 6 to 16 hours with selection by perfusion imaging. N Engl J Med. 2018; 78(8):708–718

ALexander MJ, Zauner A, Chaloupka JC, et al. WEAVE trial: final results in 152 on-label patients. Stroke. 2019; 50(4):889–894

Nogueira RG, Jadhav AP, Haussen DC, et al. Thrombectomy 6 to 24 hours after stroke with a mismatch between deficit and infarct. N Engl J Med. 2018; 378(1):11–21

12 Endovascular Therapy in a Patient with a Proximal MCA Occlusion and No Neurological Deficits

12.1 Case Description

12.1.1 Clinical Presentation

An 84-year-old woman developed acute-onset left-sided weakness and dysarthria. She had a medical history of hypertension, dyslipidemia, and diabetes, and had suffered a TIA 3 months ago with similar clinical manifestations as the current event. She arrived at the hospital approximately 2 hours after symptom onset, at which time she had completely recovered from her deficits (National Institutes of Health Stroke Scale [NIHSS] 0).

12.1.2 Imaging Workup and Investigations

- Noncontrast computed tomography (NCCT) done 150 minutes after onset of symptoms revealed a hyperdense artery sign in the right MCA (▶ Fig. 12.1). There were no early ischemic changes (ASPECTS score 10).
- CTA showed an occlusion of the right M1 segment with an intraluminal clot at the carotid terminus (▶ Fig. 12.2). The patient had excellent collaterals filling the right MCA territory and retrograde filling of the distal part of the MCA.

- On CTP, there was a large perfusion abnormality visible in the territory of the right MCA with increased mean transit time and time to peak, and normal to increased cerebral blood volume (▶ Fig. 12.3).

12.1.3 Diagnosis

Transient episode of neurological dysfunction of the right hemisphere with an occlusion of the right MCA and a large area of perfusion mismatch without signs of acute infarction.

12.1.4 Treatment

- Because of the proximal M1 occlusion in combination with a large area of perfusion mismatch, it was feared that the patient had a high risk of developing an infarct due to failure of collateral circulation, despite the fact that she had no neurological deficits at this time.
- After a discussion with the patient and her family, the decision was made to treat the patient with endovascular reperfusion therapy. She was not given intravenous (IV) thrombolysis.
- Occlusion of the M1 segment was confirmed on catheter angiography. The vessel was opened with a 4 × 20 mm stent

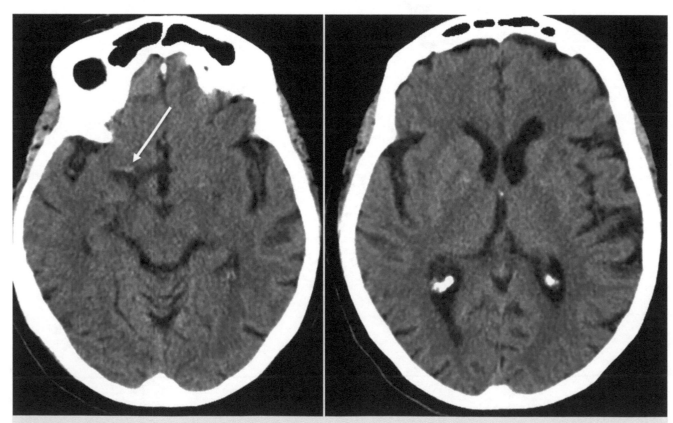

Fig. 12.1 Axial NCCT of the brain, performed 150 minutes after symptom onset. There is a hyperdense artery sign of the right MCA (*arrow*). No early ischemic changes are visible (ASPECTS 10).

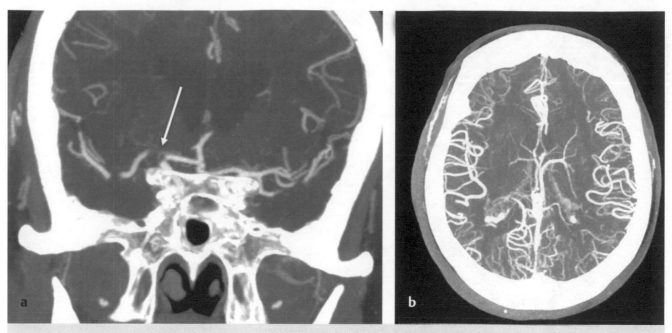

Fig. 12.2 Coronal CT angiography (**a**) performed directly after the NCCT shows an occlusion of the M1 segment of the right MCA (*arrow*). There are excellent collaterals filling the MCA territory (**b**) and retrograde filling of the distal MCA.

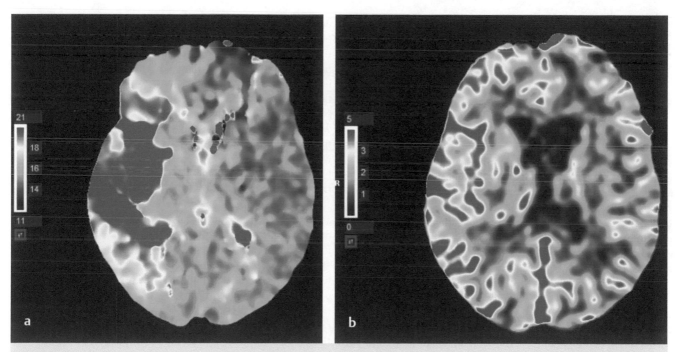

Fig. 12.3 CT perfusion showing increased mean transit time (**a**) and normal to increased cerebral blood volume (**b**) of the right MCA territory.

retriever (Trevo). After a single pass, TICI 3 reperfusion was achieved.

- There was some irregularity of the proximal M1 segment due to vasospasm (▶ Fig. 12.4). Treatment with 5-mg intra-arterial verapamil resulted in resolution of the irregularity.

12.1.5 Outcome

- There were no complications during the procedure and the patient had no neurological deficits afterward.
- MRI was performed 2 days after endovascular treatment, which showed small infarctions in the right basal ganglia, due

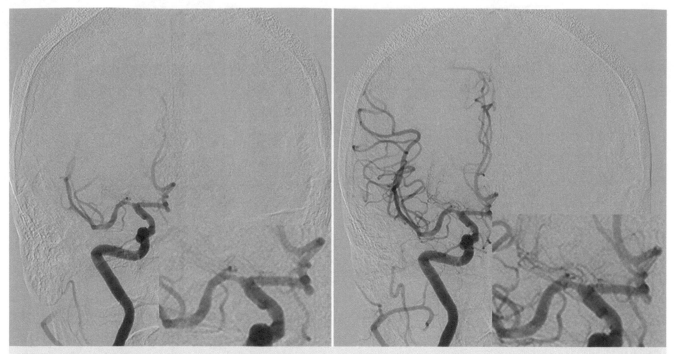

Fig. 12.4 Catheter angiography of the right ICA after the first pass with a stent retriever shows TICI 3 reperfusion. There is an irregularity visible in the proximal M1 segment, which resolved after treatment with verapamil.

to prolonged occlusion of the lenticulostriate arteries (▶ Fig. 12.5).

- The patient was discharged home on the third day after admission with an NIHSS score of 0.

12.2 Discussion

12.2.1 Background

There is almost no evidence from randomized trials on the use of endovascular therapy in patients with mild or no neurological deficit. Most of the recent thrombectomy studies excluded this patient population.[1,2,3,4,5] The protocols of the EXTEND-IA and Mr Clean trial did allow randomization of patients with mild deficits. In the case of Mr Clean, a minimum baseline NIHSS score of 2 was required for randomization.[4] The EXTEND-IA protocol did not specify a minimal NIHSS score, but stated that the patient had to be eligible for IV thrombolysis treatment.[6] However, despite the fact that these studies allowed recruitment of patients with mild deficits, hardly any of these patients were actually included. In EXTEND-IA and Mr Clean, the median NIHSS scores of the patients randomized to intervention were 17 (IQR: 13–20) and 17 (IQR: 14–21), respectively.[4,5]

Even before the widespread introduction of endovascular therapy, there was already uncertainty about the optimal strategy to manage patients with acute ischemic stroke and rapidly improving or mild symptoms (RIMS). Cohort studies have shown that RIMS is one of the most common reasons to withhold IV thrombolysis, despite the fact that the outcome in about a third of these patients is unfavorable.[7,8] In a retrospective single-center study, Rajajee et al examined risk factors for poor outcome in patients with RIMS.[9] Among 39 patients with RIMS who did not receive reperfusion therapy, 8 (21%) were dead or

dependent at the time of discharge. The strongest predictor of a poor outcome was the presence of a large vessel occlusion in the territory of the stroke, which was present in 8 of 39 patients. Of these, four patients (50%) had a poor outcome and infarct expansion was found on MRI in three patients. In contrast, of the patients without a large-vessel occlusion, only 13% (4/31) had a poor outcome. Thus, the odds of a poor outcome were seven times higher in patients with an occlusion, compared to those without an occlusion. The 95% confidence interval of this risk estimate, however, is wide (1.2–38), due to the low sample size of the study. Alexandrov et al used transcranial Doppler and they also found that large vessel occlusion was the strongest predictor of poor outcome in patients with RIMS.[10] Secondary deterioration occurred in 62% of patients with an occlusion, compared to only 4% of patients with a normal flow in the intracranial arteries. Finally, results from a prospective study from Canada in which patients with TIA or minor stroke were evaluated with MRI and MRA confirmed that a proximal occlusion is an important predictor of recurrent stroke.[11]

Based on the presence of a proximal occlusion and the CT perfusion abnormalities, our patient was feared to have a high risk of developing an infarct. Although the pathophysiology of infarct expansion in patients with a proximal occlusion and RIMS is incompletely understood, the most plausible mechanism is failure of collateral flow. Patients with RIMS and an occlusion of a major supplying artery probably initially have sufficient perfusion from collateral circulation, similar to our patient. This is the likely reason for the mild neurological deficits. If no recanalization of the proximal occlusion has occurred by this time, either spontaneously or after therapy, this process can result in expansion of the infarct.

Because of the high risk of poor outcome in patients with RIMS and a proximal occlusion, reperfusion therapy should be

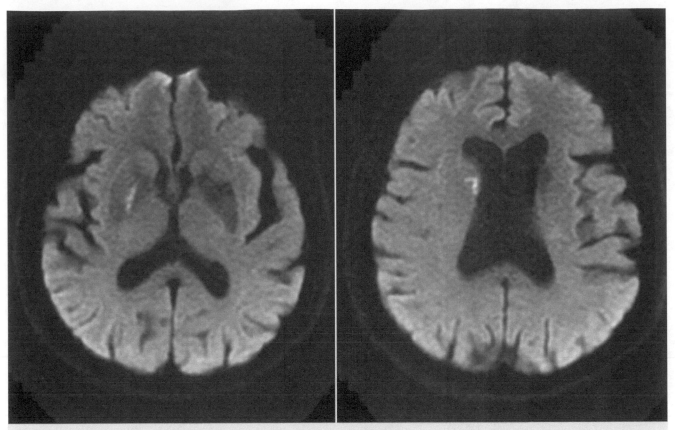

Fig. 12.5 MRI (axial DWI sequence) performed 2 days after the endovascular procedure shows small infarcts in the area of the right basal ganglia.

considered in these patients. In a recent phase 1 study in which the safety of IV tenecteplase for patients with RIMS and a proximal occlusion was examined, patients in whom recanalization occurred had a higher chance of a good clinical outcome at follow-up compared to those with persistent occlusion (relative risk: 1.65).[12] Despite the fact that our patient arrived at the hospital within the timeframe for IV treatment, we decided not to use IV thrombolysis. In the guideline of the American Heart Association, RIMS is listed as a relative (but not an absolute) contraindication for IV thrombolysis.[13] However, it also states that for the use of IV thrombolysis, a patient should have a "measurable neurological deficit," which was not the case in our patient. In fact, according to the most recent AHA definition, our patient had a TIA at the time of admission, not an ischemic stroke.[14] Other arguments against the use of IV thrombolysis were the risk of symptomatic hemorrhage,[15] and the fact that proximal M1 occlusions generally respond poorly to IV therapy.[16] Based on these considerations, we decided to treat the patient directly with mechanical thrombectomy, instead of bridging with IV thrombolysis.

12.3 Pearls and Pitfalls

- Ischemic stroke patients with mild neurological deficits and a proximal occlusion can have a high risk of poor clinical outcome.
- Infarct expansion, probably due to failure of collateral circulation, is the most plausible cause of secondary neurological deterioration in these patients.

- Recanalization of the occluded vessel is associated with a higher chance of good outcome and endovascular reperfusion therapy should therefore be considered in patients with mild deficits and a proximal occlusion.

References

[1] Saver JL, Goyal M, Bonafe A, et al. SWIFT PRIME Investigators. Stent-retriever thrombectomy after intravenous t-PA vs. t-PA alone in stroke. N Engl J Med. 2015; 372(24):2285–2295

[2] Jovin TG, Chamorro A, Cobo E, et al. REVASCAT Trial Investigators. Thrombectomy within 8 hours after symptom onset in ischemic stroke. N Engl J Med. 2015; 372(24):2296–2306

[3] Goyal M, Demchuk AM, Menon BK, et al. ESCAPE Trial Investigators. Randomized assessment of rapid endovascular treatment of ischemic stroke. N Engl J Med. 2015; 372(11):1019–1030

[4] Berkhemer OA, Fransen PS, Beumer D, et al. MR CLEAN Investigators. A randomized trial of intraarterial treatment for acute ischemic stroke. N Engl J Med. 2015; 372(1):11–20

[5] Campbell BC, Mitchell PJ, Kleinig TJ, et al. EXTEND-IA Investigators. Endovascular therapy for ischemic stroke with perfusion-imaging selection. N Engl J Med. 2015; 372(11):1009–1018

[6] Campbell BC, Mitchell PJ, Yan B, et al. EXTEND-IA Investigators. A multicenter, randomized, controlled study to investigate EXtending the time for Thrombolysis in Emergency Neurological Deficits with Intra-Arterial therapy (EXTEND-IA). Int J Stroke. 2014; 9(1):126–132

[7] Smith EE, Abdullah AR, Petkovska I, Rosenthal E, Koroshetz WJ, Schwamm LH. Poor outcomes in patients who do not receive intravenous tissue plasminogen activator because of mild or improving ischemic stroke. Stroke. 2005; 36(11):2497–2499

[8] Barber PA, Zhang J, Demchuk AM, Hill MD, Buchan AM. Why are stroke patients excluded from TPA therapy? An analysis of patient eligibility. Neurology. 2001; 56(8):1015–1020

[9] Rajajee V, Kidwell C, Starkman S, et al. Early MRI and outcomes of untreated patients with mild or improving ischemic stroke. Neurology. 2006; 67 (6):980–984

[10] Alexandrov AV, Felberg RA, Demchuk AM, et al. Deterioration following spontaneous improvement: sonographic findings in patients with acutely resolving symptoms of cerebral ischemia. Stroke. 2000; 31(4):915–919

[11] Coutts SB, Simon JE, Eliasziw M, et al. Triaging transient ischemic attack and minor stroke patients using acute magnetic resonance imaging. Ann Neurol. 2005; 57(6):848–854

[12] Coutts SB, Dubuc V, Mandzia J, et al. TEMPO-1 Investigators. Tenecteplase-tissue-type plasminogen activator evaluation for minor ischemic stroke with proven occlusion. Stroke. 2015; 46(3):769–774

[13] Jauch EC, Saver JL, Adams HP, Jr, et al. American Heart Association Stroke Council, Council on Cardiovascular Nursing, Council on Peripheral Vascular Disease, Council on Clinical Cardiology. Guidelines for the early management of patients with acute ischemic stroke: a guideline for healthcare professionals from the American Heart Association/American Stroke Association. Stroke. 2013; 44(3):870–947

[14] Easton JD, Saver JL, Albers GW, et al. American Heart Association, American Stroke Association Stroke Council, Council on Cardiovascular Surgery and Anesthesia, Council on Cardiovascular Radiology and Intervention, Council on Cardiovascular Nursing, Interdisciplinary Council on Peripheral Vascular Disease. Definition and evaluation of transient ischemic attack: a scientific statement for healthcare professionals from the American Heart Association/American Stroke Association Stroke Council; Council on Cardiovascular Surgery and Anesthesia; Council on Cardiovascular Radiology and Intervention; Council on Cardiovascular Nursing; and the Interdisciplinary Council on Peripheral Vascular Disease. The American Academy of Neurology affirms the value of this statement as an educational tool for neurologists. Stroke. 2009; 40(6):2276–2293

[15] Wardlaw JM, Murray V, Berge E, del Zoppo GJ. Thrombolysis for acute ischaemic stroke. Cochrane Database Syst Rev. 2014; 7(7):CD000213

[16] del Zoppo GJ, Poeck K, Pessin MS, et al. Recombinant tissue plasminogen activator in acute thrombotic and embolic stroke. Ann Neurol. 1992; 32 (1):78–86

13 MRI in Stroke (Core Size, Mismatch, and New Advances)

13.1 Case Description

13.1.1 Clinical Presentation

A 61-year-old male patient presented with a headache and visual disturbance for 3 days. On arrival to the emergency department (ED), the patient had an episode of seizures with tongue bite. Associated comorbidities include hypertension and moderate valvular aortic stenosis.

13.1.2 Imaging Workup and Investigations

The patient underwent CT angiography and perfusion. CT images were unremarkable with no evidence of loss of gray-white differentiation or hypodensity in the posterior fossa (▶ Fig. 13.1). Postcontrast CT images showed atheromatous plaque causing near-total stenosis of the V4 segment of the left vertebral artery.

MR imaging performed later showed infarction involving left cerebellar hemisphere confirming to superior cerebellar artery territory (▶ Fig. 13.2), multiple punctate infarcts involving thalami, and bilateral parieto-occipital region (▶ Fig. 13.3). Susceptibility-weighted imaging (SWI) showed the absence of hemorrhagic transformation. Diffusion-weighted imaging–fluid-attenuated inversion recovery (DWI–FLAIR) mismatch suggestive of hyperacute nature of infarction was present.

3D time of flight (TOF) MR angiography revealed significant stenosis involving V4 segment of the left vertebral artery with significant stenosis involving proximal basilar artery (i.e., exaggerated stenosis due to flow-dependent nature of TOF

angiography). Postcontrast MR angiography revealed similar findings as in TOF angiography.

Conventional angiography confirmed stenosis involving the V4 segment of the left vertebral artery with mild stenosis of the proximal basilar artery. The stenosed segment of the vertebral artery was treated with thromboaspiration and stent placement.

13.1.3 Diagnosis

Severe stenosis involving left vertebral artery with mild stenosis involving proximal basilar artery.

13.1.4 Treatment

Mechanical thrombectomy by thromboaspiration and stenting.

13.1.5 Outcome

The patient showed significant improvement of motor weakness, cerebellar ataxia, and left superior quadrantanopia.

13.2 Companion Case

Middle Cerebral Artery Thrombosis.

13.2.1 Clinical Presentation

A 77-year-old female patient presented with right faciobrachiocrural hemiplegia and motor aphasia. Clinical examination

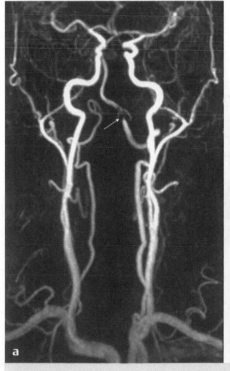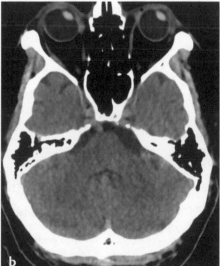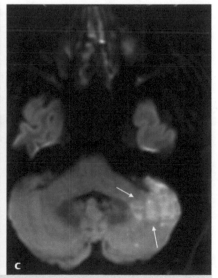

Fig. 13.1 MR angiography image (**a**) shows near-total stenosis of V4 segment of left vertebral artery (*arrow*). Axial CT section (**b**) at the level of pons fails to demonstrate ischemic changes involving cerebellum well visualized on trace image (**c**) of DWI (*arrow*).

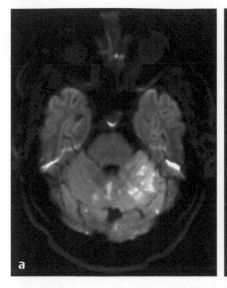

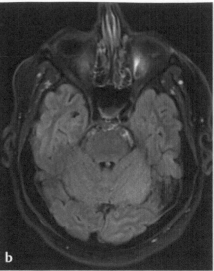

Fig. 13.2 Axial trace image of DWI (**a**) shows multiple foci of restricted diffusion involving superior aspect of cerebellar hemisphere and nodulus of vermis predominantly on left side. Axial FLAIR image (**b**) shows no evidence of altered signal intensity in areas with restricted diffusion suggestive of DWI–FLAIR mismatch.

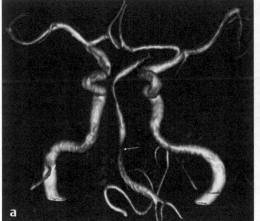

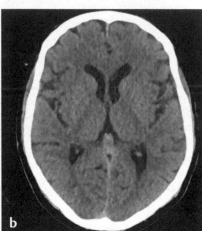

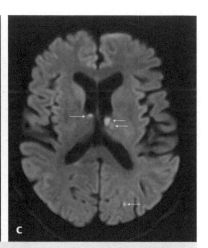

Fig. 13.3 3D TOF MR angiography (**a**) shows significant stenosis (*arrow*) involving proximal basilar artery with small ischemic foci involving bilateral thalami and left parietal region not seen on axial CT (**b**). However, axial trace image (**c**) of DWI at the same level shows restricted diffusion involving bilateral thalami and left occipital region (*arrow*).

revealed an NIHSS score of 20. The patient was a case of paroxysmal atrial tachycardia and dyslipidemia. The patient was not a candidate for thrombolysis due to the recent history of surgery and established stroke.

13.2.2 Imaging Workup and Investigations

MR imaging performed at the peripheral hospital showed ischemic changes involving the left parietal region, insular cortex, head of the caudate nucleus, and posterior aspect of the lentiform nucleus. Axial FLAIR showed hyperintense vessel sign involving cortical branches of the left MCA suggestive of slow arterial flow along with multiple foci of encephalomalacic changes involving right parietotemporal and left frontal region. 3D TOF MR angiography showed abrupt cutoff involving M1 segment of the left MCA with gradient images showing susceptibility vessel sign. No evidence of hemorrhagic transformation on gradient recalled echo images. CT angiography showed occlusion at the level of M1 MCA on the left side along with

significant mismatch on perfusion imaging. The patient underwent mechanical thrombectomy with complete recanalization of MCA (TICI 3).

13.2.3 Diagnosis

Left middle cerebral artery thrombosis.

13.2.4 Treatment

Mechanical thrombectomy with complete recanalization (TICI 3).

13.2.5 Outcome

MR imaging performed postthrombectomy showed no increase in the size or extent of ischemic changes (▶ Fig. 13.4).

The patient was treated with speech, physio, and ergotherapy. The patient showed partial improvement of motor weakness with an NIHSS score of 7 and modified Rankin scale of 4 at the time of discharge.

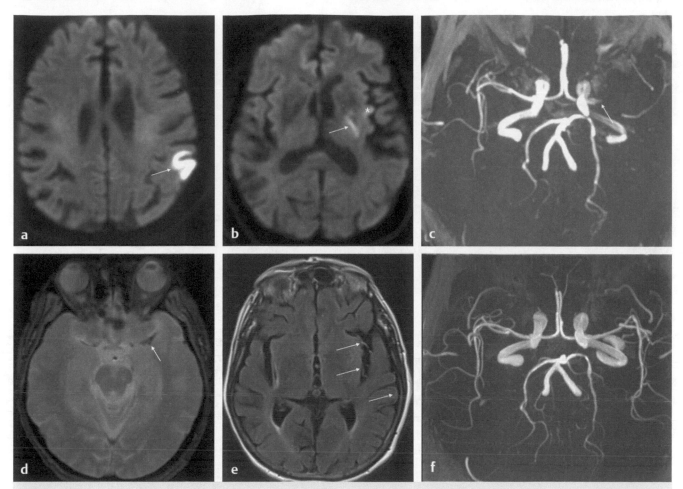

Fig. 13.4 Axial trace image (**a**) of DWI shows infarct involving the left parietal region. Axial trace image (**b**) of DWI shows ischemic changes involving the posterior aspect of the left lentiform nucleus and in the insular cortex. 3D TOF angiography (**c**) shows total occlusion of M1 segment of left MCA with susceptibility vessel sign on gradient recalled echo (**d**). Axial FLAIR image (**e**) shows hyperintense vessel sign involving cortical branches of left MCA. 3D TOF angiography (**f**) post mechanical thrombectomy shows complete recanalization of left MCA.

13.3 Discussion

13.3.1 Background

The radiologists in training are the ones to perform an initial evaluation of stroke imaging in emergencies usually. Hence, the awareness of early signs of ischemia becomes necessary for accurate and reliable diagnosis especially in challenging situations such as imaging on low strength magnets (≤ 1.5 T) using fast imaging sequences (time is brain).

13.3.2 Early Signs

The early and useful signs of hyperacute stroke to be recognized on MR imaging include the presence of hyperintensity on trace images with low apparent diffusion coefficient (ADC) values (i.e., restricted diffusion); FLAIR hyperintense vessel (FHV; ► Fig. 13.5) sign in involved vascular territory (i.e., ACA, MCA, and PCA territories); susceptibility vessel sign suggestive of thrombosis with prominence of deep medullary veins on T2*GRE or SWI; vascular stenosis or occlusion on 3D TOF angiography; and the presence of intramural T1 hyperintensity on 3D VISTA suggestive of dissection; abnormalities including

decreased cerebral blood volume (CBV), cerebral blood flow (CBF), and increased mean transit time (MTT) and time to peak (TTP) on perfusion-weighted imaging (PWI).[1,2,3,4,5,6,7]

13.4 Imaging Sequences

13.4.1 Diffusion-Weighted Imaging

DWI is a technique based on spin echo echoplanar imaging which utilizes different gradient strengths and magnitude (*b*-value) to look for tissue differences in the rate of diffusion. It comprises imaging at different *b*-values (i.e., 0 and 1,000 for routine clinical imaging). Although the *b*-values can be varied from 1,000 to 3,000, high *b*-value DWI only accentuates the hyperintense signal on trace images without any significant change in sensitivity to diagnose an infarction.[8,9] The DWI comprises of *b* = 0, trace, and ADC images for each slice position. Calculation of the ADC values helps in the quantification of the degree of restriction of water motion. The presence of restricted diffusion is suggested by hyperintensity on trace images with the corresponding hypointensity on ADC images (i.e., low ADC values). The presence of significantly low ADC values is usually associated with the irreversible nature of

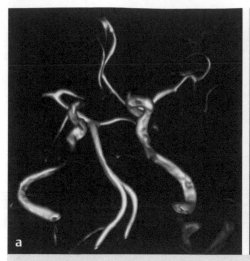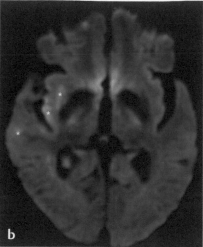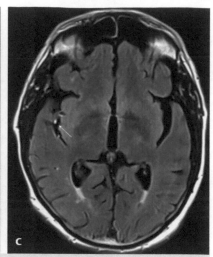

Fig. 13.5 Images from another patient with right MCA stroke. 3D TOF angiography (**a**) shows abrupt cutoff involving right M1 MCA. Axial trace image of DWI (**b**) shows subtle hyperintensity involving right insular cortex (*asterisk*). Axial FLAIR image (**c**) shows hyperintense vessel sign involving cortical branches of MCA (*arrow*) in right sylvian cistern.

infarct, tissue necrosis, and increased risk of hemorrhagic transformation post intravenous or endovascular management.[10]

DWI shows a sensitivity of 75 to 95% in the detection of lacunar stroke. However, DWI can be negative in large arterial stroke and lacunar infarction due to imaging performed either before the appearance of changes on DWI or because of hypoperfusion severe enough to cause symptoms in lacunar strokes but not enough to cause restricted diffusion or due to its size smaller than the slice thickness and interval.[11,12] In cases with suspected stroke showing the absence of restricted diffusion, the lack of flow-related enhancement on TOF involving cerebral vasculature; the presence of thrombus along with prominent deep medullary veins on T2*GRE/SWI involving M1–M4 segments of MCA, A1 and A2 segments of ACA, P1 and P2 segments of PCA; and the presence of FHV sign on 2D FLAIR along with perfusion abnormalities should highlight the presence of ischemia. In addition, the presence of FHV sign on FLAIR, visualization of deep medullary and cortical veins on gradient, and SWI with perfusion abnormalities also indicate the presence of salvageable cerebral parenchyma (i.e., penumbra).

Along with depicting early signs of ischemia, DWI also throws some light on the likely etiology of stroke depending on the distribution of the vascular lesions. Involvement of multiple vascular territories and diffuse nature suggests embolic origin; involvement pertaining to a vascular territory suggests thrombotic etiology; unilateral involvement and infarcts in border zone territory suggests hypoperfusion as in ICA stenosis and bilateral diffuse watershed infarcts with involvement of basal ganglia and hippocampus with or without cerebral cortical involvement; and predominantly perirolandic involvement is suggestive of hypoxia–hypoperfusion complex.

The radiologist needs to be aware of imaging findings in hyperacute stroke as they are subtle and can be missed easily. Stroke onset shows a diurnal variation with the majority of them presenting early in the morning.[13] In cases with wakeup stroke, the presence of DWI–FLAIR mismatch serves as a reliable marker in the identification of hyperacute stroke less than 4.5 hours which aids in the selection of patients for reperfusion

therapy since the hyperintense signal on FLAIR is visualized in all patients after 7 hours.[14]

The presence of susceptibility artifacts in the basifrontal and temporal region can mimic areas of restricted diffusion in some cases. The knowledge of the occurrence of such artefacts and comparison with available previous imaging helps us avoid the misdiagnosis.

13.4.2 Fluid-Attenuated Inversion Recovery

FLAIR is an inversion recovery-based sequence which suppresses the signal from cerebrospinal fluid and accentuates visualization of signal intensity changes involving cerebral parenchyma.

The predominant role of FLAIR imaging in stroke is in the identification of DWI–FLAIR mismatch, the presence of FHV sign, to differentiate between coexisting hyperacute and subacute infarct and depict parenchymal changes of differential etiology. However, early visualization of altered signal intensity (<6 hours) involving cerebral parenchyma is associated with increased risk of hemorrhagic transformation of infarct due to posttherapeutic intervention.[15]

The presence of FHV sign is attributed to large vessels occlusion and retrograde leptomeningeal collaterals. It serves as an indirect marker of the penumbra, associated with smaller lesions, decreased rate of infarct progression, and better prognosis, and disappears spontaneously about 10 days after reperfusion.[16,17,18]

13.4.3 Susceptibility-Weighted Imaging

SWI is a gradient-based sequence which uses magnetic susceptibility differences in the tissues and has increased sensitivity in the detection of paramagnetic substances.[19]

SWI is useful in the detection of thrombosis (susceptibility vessel sign, sensitivity ≈ 90%), prominence deep medullary veins, hemorrhagic transformation of infarct, and preexisting microbleeds.[4,20] The susceptibility vessel sign helps in the identification of thrombosis, accentuated hypointensity (due to the presence of deoxyhemoglobin) larger than the caliber of the vessel. As the degree of blooming is related to the number of RBCs in the thrombus, the intense blooming of thrombus on SWI suggests cardiac etiology.[21]

The accentuated hypointensity in the cortical vessels is of possible venous origin as confirmed by angiography studies. The dilated deep medullary veins, an indirect indicator of the presence of penumbra, and their extent correlates with the volume of the salvageable tissue.[22]

SWI is most sensitive compared to T2*GRE and CT in the detection of microbleeds or preexisting hemorrhagic areas. Mechanical thrombectomy could be preferred over intravascular thrombolysis in patients with preexisting hemorrhagic sequelae (microbleeds, superficial siderosis, and hemorrhage), and the presence of microbleeds should not exclude the possible mechanical thrombectomy in an indicated patient.[10,23]

The drawbacks of SWI include nonvisualization of classically described susceptibility vessel sign in the vicinity of skull base involving carotid siphon, A1 segment of ACA, basilar trunk, and V4 segment of the vertebral artery due to bone–air interface causing susceptibility artefact. It can also be absent in cases with an old clot or with a white clot (i.e., platelet-rich thrombus).[21]

13.4.4 Time of Flight Angiography

TOF angiography is a gradient-based 2D or 3D sequence which shows flow-related enhancement, used to evaluate the status of the intracranial vasculature. The increased magnetic field strength at 3 T allows an excellent display of the cortical branches of MCA.

TOF angiography shows abrupt cutoff or stenosis of the vessel supplying the ischemic territory. It also aids in the detection of vascular dissection with T1-hyperintense crescent sign.[5] However, caution has to be exerted in interpreting the TOF images in cases with MCA occlusion as the proximal patent stump of M1 MCA can mimic an aneurysm and in those with dissection, the vessel can appear patent due to T1 effect of the hematoma.

The pitfalls of TOF angiography include suboptimal evaluation of the anterior aspect of the carotid siphon and extracranial vessels. The laminar flow in the center of the blood vessel with TOF effect leads to blood flow artefact which mimics a dissection on 3D TOF angiography. This artefact can be overcome by changing the orientation of the phase encoding gradient and by application of spatial presaturation pulses.[24] Postcontrast CT and MR angiography are superior to TOF, as the signal intensity on TOF is flow dependent leading to diminished signal in vessels distal to the stenosis. They also enable visualization of the extracranial vasculature with short acquisition times.

13.4.5 MR Perfusion-Weighted Imaging

MR perfusion imaging is widely used in clinical practice, although a few study groups have used perfusion imaging in their trials. The MR perfusion techniques can be broadly classified into noncontrast techniques (i.e., arterial spin labeling [ASL]) and postcontrast perfusion imaging including dynamic T1-weighted perfusion and dynamic susceptibility contrast perfusion techniques. The common sequence used in ischemic stroke is dynamic susceptibility contrast perfusion which is based on T2* effect leading to signal drop post–gadolinium injection.

The primary aim of this sequence is in identifying the penumbra (i.e., the tissue at risk of ischemia). The postprocessing of perfusion imaging needs reformation techniques available within the scanner or online free vendor software. The maps used in the analysis include CBF, CBV, MTT, and TTP. The transit through the collateral circulation explains the delay in the arrival of the contrast in the area of the penumbra. The transit of contrast is reflected on imaging as an increase in MTT and TTP with a decrease in CBF in penumbra, with a significant reduction in CBV generally in infarct core.[6,25]

The DWI–PWI mismatch allows differentiation of tissue at risk of ischemia (altered perfusion on PWI) from the infarct core (restricted diffusion on DWI) and the presence of penumbra, a criterion for selection of patients for thrombolysis. The raw data of the PWI can be automatically sent from the scanner to the modern softwares which perform the analysis, and the results are sent to the interventional radiologist, which decreases the time needed to select and perform mechanical thrombectomy.

ASL is a noncontrast perfusion technique which involves tagging of moving blood and scanning the area of interest after a postlabeling delay (inversion delay). ASL is not commonly used in emergencies due to decreased signal-to-noise ratio, spatial resolution, and long acquisition times. The other disadvantages include overestimation of infarct size on ASL in comparison to DSC perfusion.[26]

13.4.6 Evolution of Stroke on MR Imaging

Hyperacute stroke and its imaging features are elaborated in the previous sections of the discussion. Acute stroke shows accentuation of the hyperintensity on trace images with a reduction in ADC values, the appearance of hyperintensity on T2-weighted images, and FLAIR. The occluded vessel could show recanalization posttherapeutic intervention or rarely spontaneous recanalization. Subacute infarct shows pseudonormalization of diffusion and hyperintensity on T2 and FLAIR images with enhancement on postcontrast T1-weighted images. The susceptibility images could show punctate foci of blooming in the event of hemorrhagic transformation of the infarct. Chronic infarcts appear as areas of encephalomalacia (i.e., T1 hypointensity, hyperintense on T2 with suppression on FLAIR, and lack of postcontrast enhancement).

13.4.7 CT versus MRI in Stroke

In comparison, CT allows shorter imaging times, which is particularly useful in unstable patients. CT angiography and perfusion are commonly used as an initial imaging modality as they enable analysis of cerebral parenchyma, perfusion, and the status of intracranial and extracranial vasculature. It also serves as a roadmap for endovascular management with shorter imaging time. However, it needs adequate technical expertise to perform and training to interpret the advanced imaging protocols. MRI is superior to CT in accurate identification of ischemic changes in hyperacute and lacunar stroke.

References

[1] Lövblad KO, Wetzel SG, Somon T, et al. Diffusion-weighted MRI in cortical ischaemia. Neuroradiology. 2004; 46(3):175–182

[2] González RG, Schaefer PW, Buonanno FS, et al. Diffusion-weighted MR imaging: diagnostic accuracy in patients imaged within 6 hours of stroke symptom onset. Radiology. 1999; 210(1):155–162

[3] Lee KY, Latour LL, Luby M, Hsia AW, Merino JG, Warach S. Distal hyperintense vessels on FLAIR: an MRI marker for collateral circulation in acute stroke? Neurology. 2009; 72(13):1134–1139

[4] Cho KH, Kim JS, Kwon SU, Cho AH, Kang DW. Significance of susceptibility vessel sign on T2*-weighted gradient echo imaging for identification of stroke subtypes. Stroke. 2005; 36(11):2379–2383

[5] Schievink WI. Spontaneous dissection of the carotid and vertebral arteries. N Engl J Med. 2001; 344(12):898–906

[6] Copen WA, Schaefer PW, Wu O. MR perfusion imaging in acute ischemic stroke. Neuroimaging Clin N Am. 2011; 21(2):259–283, x

[7] Lövblad KO, Altrichter S, Viallon M, et al. Neuro-imaging of cerebral ischemic stroke. J Neuroradiol. 2008; 35(4):197–209

[8] Kim HJ, Choi CG, Lee DH, Lee JH, Kim SJ, Suh DC. High-b-value diffusion-weighted MR imaging of hyperacute ischemic stroke at 1.5 T. AJNR Am J Neuroradiol. 2005; 26(2):208–215

[9] Purroy F, Begue R, Quílez A, Sanahuja J, Gil MI. Contribution of high-b-value diffusion-weighted imaging in determination of brain ischemia in transient ischemic attack patients. J Neuroimaging. 2013; 23(1):33–38

[10] Dietemann, J-L. Imagerie des Accidents Vasculaires Cérébraux et Médullaires [Internet]. [cited 2018 Dec 28]. Available at: https://www.livres-medicaux.com/imagerie-des-accidents-vasculaires-cerebraux-et-medullaires-9791030301762.html. Accessed September 20, 2019

[11] Makin SD, Doubal FN, Dennis MS, Wardlaw JM. Clinically confirmed stroke with negative diffusion-weighted imaging magnetic resonance imaging: longitudinal study of clinical outcomes, stroke recurrence, and systematic review. Stroke. 2015; 46(11):3142–3148

[12] Gass A, Ay H, Szabo K, Koroshetz WJ. Diffusion-weighted MRI for the "small stuff": the details of acute cerebral ischaemia. Lancet Neurol. 2004; 3(1):39–45

[13] Wouters A, Lemmens R, Dupont P, Thijs V. Wake-up stroke and stroke of unknown onset: a critical review. Front Neurol. 2014; 5:153

[14] Thomalla G, Cheng B, Ebinger M, et al. STIR and VISTA Imaging Investigators. DWI-FLAIR mismatch for the identification of patients with acute ischaemic stroke within 4·5 h of symptom onset (PRE-FLAIR): a multicentre observational study. Lancet Neurol. 2011; 10(11):978–986

[15] Kufner A, Galinovic I, Brunecker P, et al. Early infarct FLAIR hyperintensity is associated with increased hemorrhagic transformation after thrombolysis. Eur J Neurol. 2013; 20(2):281–285

[16] Huang X, Liu W, Zhu W, et al. Distal hyperintense vessels on FLAIR: a prognostic indicator of acute ischemic stroke. Eur Neurol. 2012; 68(4):214–220

[17] Liu W, Xu G, Yue X, et al. Hyperintense vessels on FLAIR: a useful non-invasive method for assessing intracerebral collaterals. Eur J Radiol. 2011; 80(3):786–791

[18] Pérez de la Ossa N, Hernández-Pérez M, Domènech S, et al. Hyperintensity of distal vessels on FLAIR is associated with slow progression of the infarction in acute ischemic stroke. Cerebrovasc Dis. 2012; 34(5–6):376–384

[19] Haacke EM, Mittal S, Wu Z, Neelavalli J, Cheng YC. Susceptibility-weighted imaging: technical aspects and clinical applications, part 1. AJNR Am J Neuroradiol. 2009; 30(1):19–30

[20] Mittal S, Wu Z, Neelavalli J, Haacke EM. Susceptibility-weighted imaging: technical aspects and clinical applications, part 2. AJNR Am J Neuroradiol. 2009; 30(2):232–252

[21] Liebeskind DS, Sanossian N, Yong WH, et al. CT and MRI early vessel signs reflect clot composition in acute stroke. Stroke. 2011; 42(5):1237–1243

[22] Huang P, Chen C-H, Lin W-C, Lin RT, Khor GT, Liu CK. Clinical applications of susceptibility weighted imaging in patients with major stroke. J Neurol. 2012; 259(7):1426–1432

[23] Shi Z-S, Duckwiler GR, Jahan R, et al. Mechanical thrombectomy for acute ischemic stroke with cerebral microbleeds. J Neurointerv Surg. 2016; 8(6):563–567

[24] Vargas MI, Delavelle J, Kohler R, Becker CD, Lovblad K. Brain and spine MRI artifacts at 3Tesla. J Neuroradiol. 2009; 36(2):74–81

[25] Lövblad K-O, El-Koussy M, Oswald H, Baird AE, Schroth G, Mattle H. Magnetic resonance imaging of the ischaemic penumbra. Swiss Med Wkly. 2003; 133(41–42):551–559

[26] Huang Y-C, Liu H-L, Lee J-D, et al. Comparison of arterial spin labeling and dynamic susceptibility contrast perfusion MRI in patients with acute stroke. PLoS One. 2013; 8(7):e69085

Part III

Fundamentals and Standard Approaches

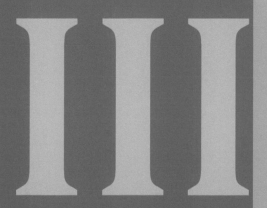

14 The Classical Setup: Carotid-T with Balloon

14.1 Case Description

14.1.1 Clinical Presentation

A 62-year-old female presented 4 hours 30 minutes after sudden-onset facial asymmetry, dysarthria, and left-sided weakness and numbness. She had a National Institutes of Health Stroke Scale (NIHSS) score of 18.

14.1.2 Imaging Workup and Investigations

- Noncontrast CT of the brain demonstrated no early ischemic changes (▶ Fig. 14.1). There is evidence of a hyperdense vessel sign seen in the region of the right internal carotid artery (ICA) terminus.
- CT perfusion demonstrated a large perfusion mismatch involving the right middle cerebral artery (MCA) and ACA territory (▶ Fig. 14.2).

14.1.3 Diagnosis

- Right anterior circulation stroke secondary to an ICA T occlusion.

14.1.4 Treatment

- Given the patient had no contraindications for intravenous (IV) recombinant tissue plasminogen activator, IV thrombolysis was commenced. The patient demonstrated no clinical improvement and findings were compatible with a large vessel occlusion; so, the patient was taken to the angiography suite for endovascular treatment.

Endovascular Therapy

Equipment

- 8-Fr short vascular access sheath.
- 8-Fr balloon-guiding catheter.
- 6-Fr diagnostic catheter.
- 4 × 40 mm Solitaire platinum stent retriever device.
- 2.95-Fr microcatheter.

The procedure was performed with local anesthesia only. Puncture of the right CFA was performed and an 8-Fr short vascular access sheath was inserted over a slip catheter (see upcoming cases for the different types of slip catheters best suited to accessing the right and left carotid arteries for different arch anatomy).

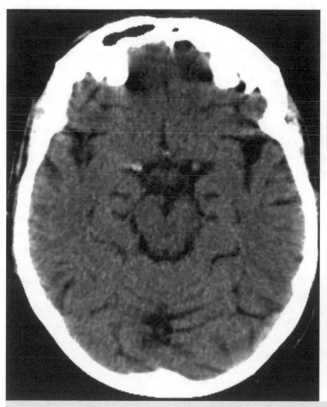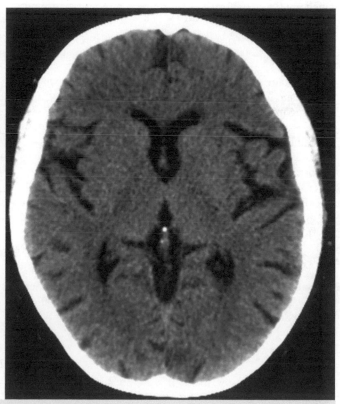

Fig. 14.1 Noncontrast CT of the brain demonstrated no early ischemic changes. There is evidence of a hyperdense vessel sign seen in the region of the right ICA terminus.

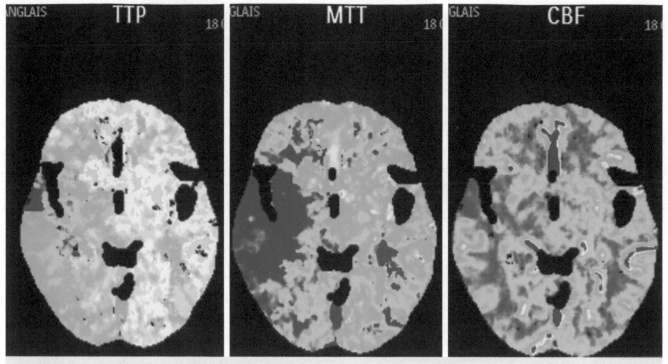

Fig. 14.2 CT perfusion demonstrates a large perfusion mismatch involving the right MCA and ACA territory.

Once the balloon guide catheter (BGC) was in place, right ICA angiography was performed confirming the right ICA terminus occlusion (▶ Fig. 14.3).

The microcatheter was then advanced intracranially into the ICA and then the tip was left in the proximal M2 (▶ Fig. 14.4).

The Solitaire stent retriever was then delivered via the microcatheter and unsheathed in the right M1 (▶ Fig. 14.5).

After 5 minutes, the balloon on the BGC was inflated (▶ Fig. 14.6) and the Solitaire device slowly withdrawn while maintaining constant aspiration on the BGC.

Once the Solitaire device was within the microcatheter outside of the body, the rotating hemostatic device was removed so as to not pull the solitaire device through the valve and strip the clot or damage the device. The balloon was deflated and the BGC allowed to back bleed. The clot was successfully extracted and TICI 3 reperfusion achieved with a single pass (▶ Fig. 14.7).

Outcome

Follow-up CT of the brain demonstrated no infarct. The patient was discharged on day 2 with an NIHSS score of 1 and 90-day modified Rankin scale (mRS) of 0.

14.2 Discussion

The case demonstrates the typical setup and technique for mechanical thrombectomy. Prior to starting the procedure, the operator should know the details of the patient's history, neuroimaging, and neurological status. After establishing access and navigating into the affected ICA, a diagnostic angiogram is performed to confirm the presence of a large vessel occlusion.

Depending on the IV thrombolysis agent used, 10 to 22% of large vessel occlusions may recanalize by the time the initial angiogram is performed.[1] However, observation for clinical response after IV thrombolysis before activating institutional protocols for endovascular therapy is not recommended, as it leads to longer times from symptom onset to reperfusion, which in turn results in inferior clinical outcomes.[2,3]

Once the proximal end of the occlusion is identified, a microcatheter is tracked through a guidewire across the identified thrombus and placed in a position distal to the occlusion (proximal M2 in this case). This placement allows for the mesh of the stent retriever to be embedded across the entire clot later on. In ideal situations, stent retrievers work initially by establishing reperfusion after deployment followed by eventual retrieval of the entire clot.[4] After allowing for some time for device to sit inside the clot following device deployment, the stent retriever is carefully pulled into a more proximally located catheter. Especially true for long segment thrombi (> 8 mm),[5] clot fragmentation that leads to distal emboli may occur during clot retrieval. The case employed the use of constant aspiration through a BGC during this retrieval period. This method has been shown to result in less distal embolization by inducing flow arrest.[6] Furthermore, mechanical thrombectomy with the use of a BGC has been demonstrated to decrease the total time to reperfusion and increase the rate of first pass recanalization, angiographic success (mTICI: 2b–3), and favorable 90-day clinical outcomes.[7,8] Similar to BGC use, employing a 5-minute "wait time" after initial stent deployment has also been reported to improve first pass recanalization and angiographic success.[9]

After the first pass, the stent retriever must be carefully cleaned and resheathed because only 46.8% of patients will have recanalization after the first retrieval attempt. After three

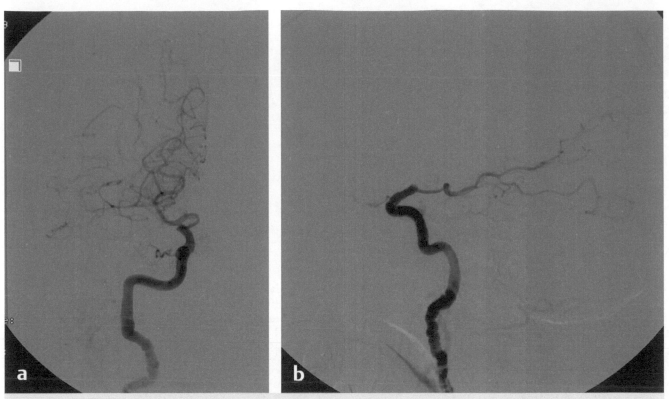

Fig. 14.3 (a) AP and (b) lateral right ICA angiograms demonstrate no opacification of the ICA above the level of the posterior communicating artery in keeping with occlusion of the terminal ICA.

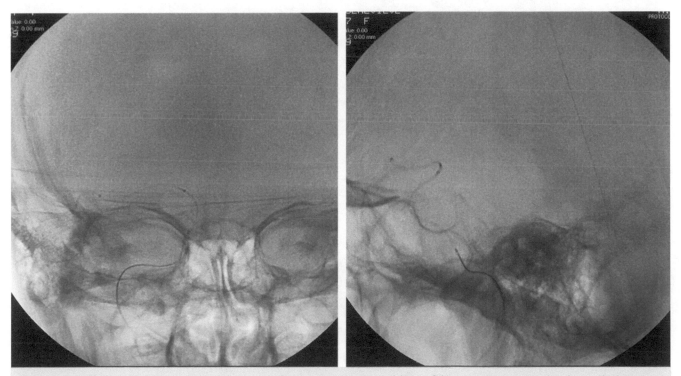

Fig. 14.4 AP and lateral native images demonstrate microcatheter positioning prior to delivery of the stent retriever. Note that the standard ICA views are used so that the microwire and microcatheter can be navigated safely along the expected course of the MCA despite no roadmap being available due to the occlusion.

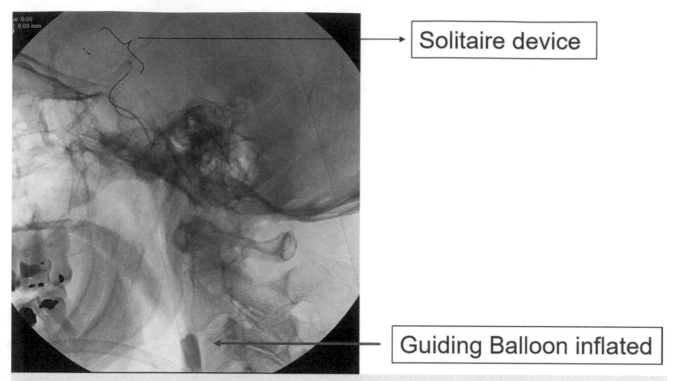

Fig. 14.5 AP and lateral native angiographic images demonstrate the Solitaire stent partially unsheathed in the M1.

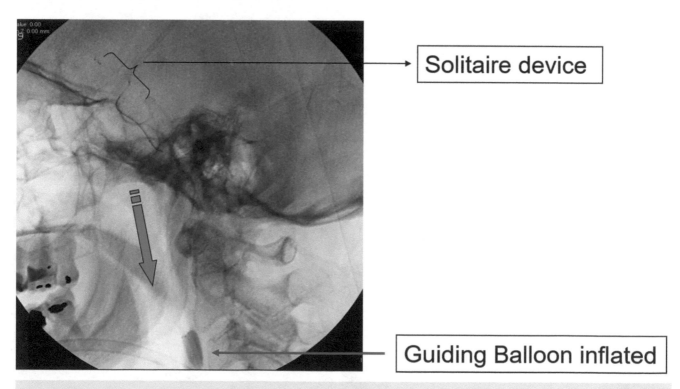

Fig. 14.6 Image demonstrates contrast in the inflated balloon and the Solitaire device as it is being withdrawn. The *blue and green arrows* mark the markers at the proximal and distal ends of the device and the *black arrow* denotes the tip of the microcatheter.

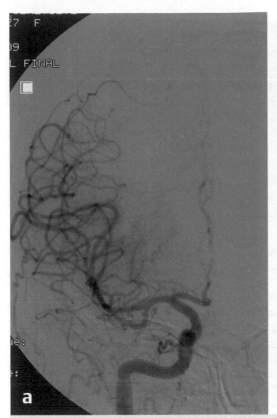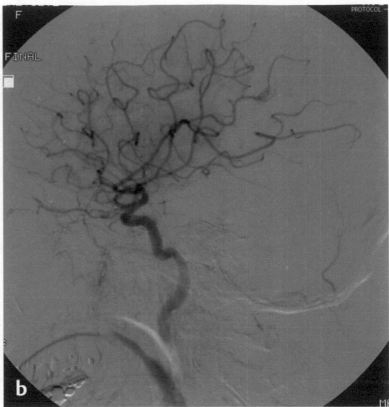

Fig. 14.7 (a) AP and (b) lateral control angiography following mechanical thrombectomy demonstrates TICI 3 reperfusion.

passes, about 67.9% of patients will attain recanalization.[10] Following reestablishing flow but prior to securing the access site, the operator should ascertain that the patient's neurologic status has not significantly deteriorated. Complications brought about by the procedure such as nontarget embolization can result in new or worsening neurologic deficits that may need immediate intervention.

The classical setup outlined here for internal carotid terminus occlusions may not work as well in other clinical scenarios. Other neurointerventional techniques and devices may be utilized to address clots that do not yield to mechanical thrombectomy with BGC use. In approaching ischemic strokes from large vessel occlusions, many factors such as tortuosity in the proximal vasculature, anatomical location of target location, length of the thrombus, and the presence of tandem lesions need to be kept in mind in selecting materials and planning maneuvers for reperfusion.[5] All these considerations will be discussed at length in the subsequent chapters.

14.2.1 Pearls and Pitfalls

- The operator should be aware of the patient's neurological status throughout the perioperative period.
- The use of a BGC can improve radiologic and clinical outcomes in mechanical thrombectomy for large vessel occlusion.
- The setup presented in this chapter applies to straightforward carotid terminus occlusions but may need to be modified for more complex cases.

References

[1] Campbell BCV, Mitchell PJ, Churilov L, et al. EXTEND-IA TNK Investigators. Tenecteplase versus alteplase before thrombectomy for ischemic stroke. N Engl J Med. 2018; 378(17):1573–1582

[2] Powers WJ, Rabinstein AA, Ackerson T, et al. American Heart Association Stroke Council. 2018 guidelines for the early management of patients with acute ischemic stroke: a guideline for healthcare professionals from the American Heart Association/American Stroke Association. Stroke. 2018; 49 (3):e46–e110

[3] Saver JL, Goyal M, van der Lugt A, et al. HERMES Collaborators. Time to treatment with endovascular thrombectomy and outcomes from ischemic stroke: a meta-analysis. JAMA. 2016; 316(12):1279–1288

[4] Pierot L, Soize S, Benaissa A, Wakhloo AK. Techniques for endovascular treatment of acute ischemic stroke: from intra-arterial fibrinolytics to stent-retrievers. Stroke. 2015; 46(3):909–914

[5] Leung V, Sastry A, Srivastava S, Wilcock D, Parrott A, Nayak S. Mechanical thrombectomy in acute ischaemic stroke: a review of the different techniques. Clin Radiol. 2018; 73(5):428–438

[6] Lee DH, Sung JH, Kim SU, Yi HJ, Hong JT, Lee SW. Effective use of balloon guide catheters in reducing incidence of mechanical thrombectomy related distal embolization. Acta Neurochir (Wien). 2017; 159(9):1671–1677

[7] Brinjikji W, Starke RM, Murad MH, et al. Impact of balloon guide catheter on technical and clinical outcomes: a systematic review and meta-analysis. J Neurointerv Surg. 2018; 10(4):335–339

[8] Zaidat OO, Mueller-Kronast NH, Hassan AE, et al. STRATIS Investigators. Impact of balloon guide catheter use on clinical and angiographic outcomes in the STRATIS Stroke Thrombectomy Registry. Stroke. 2019; 50(3):697–704

[9] Yi HJ, Lee DH, Sung JH. Clinical usefulness of waiting after stent deployment in mechanical thrombectomy: effect of the clot integration. World Neurosurg. 2018; 119:e87–e93

[10] Flottmann F, Leischner H, Broocks G, et al. Recanalization rate per retrieval attempt in mechanical thrombectomy for acute ischemic stroke. Stroke. 2018; 49(10):2523–2525

15 M1 Anatomy and Role of Perforators in Outcome

15.1 Case Description

15.1.1 Clinical Presentation

A 76-year-old female presented with a 90-minute history of severe left-sided weakness, involving upper and lower limb, left facial droop, dysarthria, and gaze deviation. National Institutes of Health Stroke Scale (NIHSS) score was 18. Comorbidities included a previous history of unprovoked pulmonary embolus, hypercholesterolemia, and bipolar disorder. Although the patient denied a previous history of stroke, subsequent imaging showed an old lacunar infarct involving the right head of caudate nucleus. There were no other relevant comorbidities and no other cardiovascular risk factors.

15.1.2 Imaging Workup and Investigations

Noncontrast enhanced CT of the brain (▶ Fig. 15.1a, b) demonstrated old lacunar infarct right basal ganglia, but no evidence of early infarction. There was no evidence of hemorrhage. CT angiography (CTA) demonstrated occlusion of the mid and distal M1 segment of the right middle cerebral artery (MCA), involving the very proximal M2 segments. There was, however, excellent collateralization to the MCA territory, with filling of MCA branches back to the level of the proximal M2 segments, showing the relatively short length of thrombus (▶ Fig. 15.1c).

CT perfusion demonstrated significant mismatch with prolonged time to peak (TTP) within the right MCA territory (▶ Fig. 15.2a), and preservation of relative cerebral blood volume (▶ Fig. 15.2b).

15.1.3 Diagnosis

Right M1 segment of MCA occlusion.

15.1.4 Treatment

In view of the high NIHSS score, presentation clearly within the time window, lack of early change on CT, presence of large artery occlusion on CTA, and the excellent collateral supply to the occluded territory, decision was made to proceed with treatment and intervention.

Initial Management

- Full-dose intravenous tissue plasminogen activator (tPA) was administered.

Endovascular Treatment

Material

- 8-Fr short angiographic sheath.
- 8-Fr MERCI balloon guide catheter.
- 5-Fr H1 slip catheter.
- 0.035 angled hydrophilic wire.
- Trevo 18 microcatheter.
- Synchro 14 microguidewire.
- Trevo 4 × 20 mm stent retriever.
- 8-Fr Angio-Seal closure device.

Technique

Intervention was performed with conscious sedation and local anesthetic. A single-wall right common femoral artery puncture was performed, and the 8-Fr short vascular access sheath inserted. The 8-Fr balloon guide catheter was advanced to the right internal carotid artery (ICA) over a 5-Fr H1 slip catheter with the aid of an angled Terumo guidewire using roadmap guidance. Right ICA angiography confirmed the presence of occlusive thrombus in the M1 segment of the right MCA (▶ Fig. 15.3a). There was good leptomeningeal collateralization

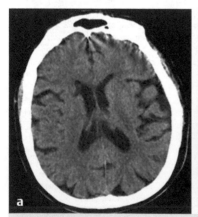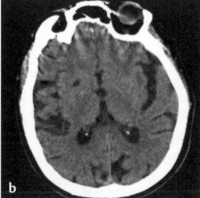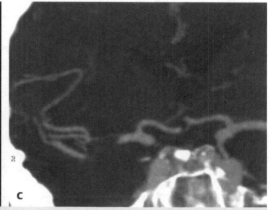

Fig. 15.1 Noncontrast enhanced CT of the brain, axial images (**a,b**) shows an old lacunar infarct right basal ganglia, but no evidence of early infarction, and no hemorrhage. CT angiography coronal reconstruction (**c**) shows occlusion of the mid to distal M1 segment of right MCA and proximal M2 segments; distal MCA branches fill through collaterals back to the level of the proximal M2 segments demonstrating the relatively short length of thrombus (**Fig. 15.1c**).

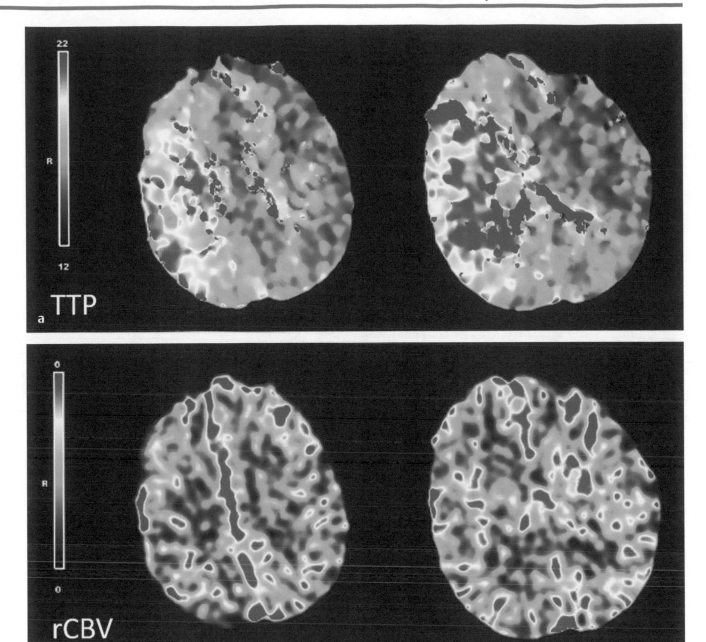

Fig. 15.2 CT perfusion shows significant mismatch with prolonged time to peak within the right MCA territory (▶ Fig. 15.2a), and preservation of relative cerebral blood volume (▶ Fig. 15.2b).

to the right MCA territory from anterior cerebral artery (ACA; ▶ Fig. 15.3b) with retrograde filling of MCA to the M2 level in arterial phase of angiography. The presence of occlusive M1 thrombus resulted in occlusion of lenticulostriate perforators. There was some filling of the medial lenticulostriate territory through perforators arising from the very proximal patent right M1 segment and A1 segment.

A Trevo 18 microcatheter was navigated to the right MCA over Synchro 14 microwire. The M1 occlusion was traversed and the microcatheter placed in the proximal superior division of the right MCA. Microcatheter injection confirmed position

distal to thrombus. A Trevo 4 × 20 mm stent retriever was then deployed from the M2 division of MCA, across the M1 thrombus to the level of supraclinoid ICA. The stent was left in situ for 5 minutes to allow incorporation of thrombus. Control angiography with the stent retriever deployed demonstrated some antegrade flow in the right MCA with filling defects consistent with thrombus in the stent (▶ Fig. 15.3c, *arrow* depicts stent retriever distal tip). After 5 minutes, the guide catheter balloon was inflated in the proximal right ICA, and stent retrieval performed with flow arrest and continuous manual aspiration. Despite this, clot was not retrieved in the stent retriever, and control

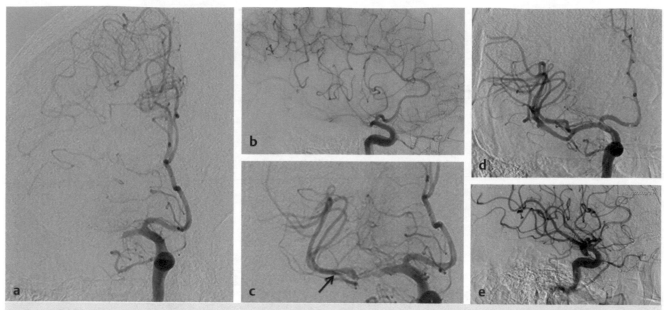

Fig. 15.3 Frontal view of right ICA angiography shows occlusive thrombus in the M1 segment of right MCA (**a**) with occlusion of lenticulostriate perforators. There was some filling of the medial lenticulostriate territory through perforators arising from the very proximal patent right M1 segment and A1 segment. Lateral view of right ICA angiography shows good leptomeningeal collateralization to the right MCA territory from ACA (**b**) with retrograde filling of MCA to the M2 level in arterial phase of angiography. Control angiography with a Trevo 4 × 20 mm stent retriever deployed across the thrombus shows some antegrade flow in the right MCA with filling defects consistent with thrombus in the stent (**c**, *arrow* depicts stent retriever distal tip). Final angiography following four stent retriever passes shows complete restoration of flow through the right M1 segment (**d**, frontal; **e**, lateral projection) with normal filling of the territory beyond the occlusion, and filling now of the lenticulostriate perforators (**d**).

angiography showed unchanged appearance of the right M1 occlusion. In total, four passes of stent retriever were required to fully recanalize the right M1 occlusion, with thrombus retrieved in the stent on the third and fourth passes. Final angiography demonstrated complete restoration of flow through the right M1 segment, with normal filling of the territory beyond the occlusion (▶ Fig. 15.3d, e). There was filling of the lenticulostriate perforators (▶ Fig. 15.3d). No evidence of arterial narrowing or spasm was seen at the site of thrombectomy.

All devices were removed. Hemostasis of the femoral artery puncture site was achieved by insertion of an 8-Fr Angio-Seal.

Postprocedure Care/Outcome

The patient demonstrated on-table improvement following recanalization of the occluded artery, with improved power on the left side. She was transferred to the neuro high dependency unit in stable condition for further monitoring and care. Her subsequent course in hospital was uneventful. Noncontrast CT performed at 24 hours postprocedure (▶ Fig. 15.4) showed infarction in the right putamen and in the posterior limb of internal capsule superiorly. There was no hemorrhagic transformation. Aspirin 81 mg once daily was commenced following the CT. She remained normotensive throughout her hospital stay. On day 5 postprocedure, the patient was discharged to rehabilitation center; her symptoms had almost completely resolved with just mild left-sided weakness remaining. On 3-month follow-up, she had further improved with complete resolution of the left-sided weakness.

15.2 Companion Case

15.2.1 Clinical Presentation

A 56-year-old woman presented with a 1-hour history of left facial droop, mild left upper limb weakness with pronator drift on examination, and left arm numbness with profound sensory deficit in the left arm. Examination also revealed mild dysarthria and left-sided neglect. NIHSS score was 7. Past medical history was significant for rheumatic heart disease with mitral stenosis and hypertension. There were no other cardiovascular risk factors, and family history was noncontributory.

15.2.2 Imaging Workup and Investigations

Noncontrast enhanced CT of the brain was performed at 70 minutes from symptom onset, with no evidence of early or established ischemic change and no hemorrhage (▶ Fig. 15.5a–c). ASPECTS score was 10. Hyperdensity consistent with thrombus in an M2 branch was identified in the right sylvian fissure (▶ Fig. 15.5b, c, *arrow*). CTA confirmed occlusion of a large caliber M2 branch of the right MCA (▶ Fig. 15.5d, sagittal oblique reconstruction, *arrow*). The right M1 segment of MCA and lenticulostriate perforators from the M1 segment were patent.

CT perfusion demonstrated significant mismatch with a wedge-shaped area of prolonged TTP and mean transit time within the right MCA territory (▶ Fig. 15.6a, b), as well as reduction in relative cerebral blood flow with preservation of relative cerebral blood volume (▶ Fig. 15.6c, d).

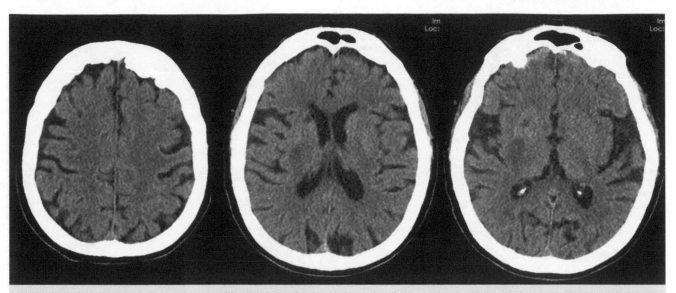

Fig. 15.4 Noncontrast CT, axial images, performed at 24 hours postprocedure shows infarction in the right putamen and posterior limb of right internal capsule superiorly, with sparing of remainder of the right MCA territory.

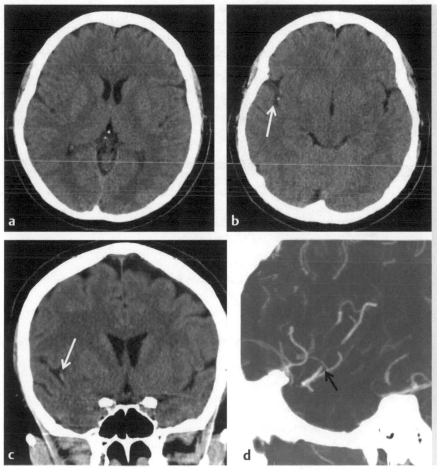

Fig. 15.5 Noncontrast enhanced CT of the brain, axial images (**a,b**), and coronal reconstruction (**c**) show no evidence of early or established ischemic change and no hemorrhage. Hyperdensity consistent with thrombus in an M2 branch is seen in the right sylvian fissure (**b, c**, *arrow*). CTA, sagittal reconstruction, shows occlusion of a large caliber M2 branch of the right MCA (**d**, *arrow*).

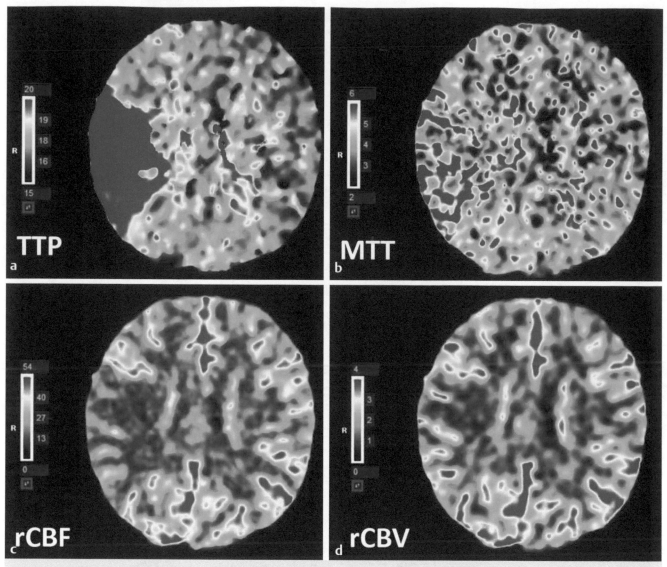

Fig. 15.6 CT perfusion shows mismatch with wedge-shaped area of prolonged time to peak (**a**) and mean transit time (**b**) within the right MCA territory, as well as reduction in relative cerebral blood flow (**c**) with preservation of relative cerebral blood volume (**d**).

15.2.3 Diagnosis

Right M2 branch occlusion.

15.2.4 Treatment

In view of the NIHSS score of 7, presentation clearly within the time window, lack of early change on CT, and the presence of large artery occlusion on CTA with mismatch on CT perfusion, decision was made to proceed with treatment and intervention.

Initial Management

Full-dose intravenous tPA was administered.

Endovascular Treatment

Material

• 8-Fr short angiographic sheath.

• 5-Fr Berenstein diagnostic catheter.
• 0.035 Angled hydrophilic wire.
• 0.035 Advantage exchange length guidewire.
• 8-Fr MERCI balloon guide catheter.
• Rebar 18 microcatheter.
• Synchro 14 microguidewire.
• Solitaire AB 3 × 20 mm stent retriever.
• 8-Fr Angio-Seal closure device.

Technique

Intervention was performed with conscious sedation and local anesthetic. A single-wall right common femoral artery puncture was performed, and the 8-Fr short vascular access sheath inserted. A 5-Fr Berenstein diagnostic catheter was advanced to the right proximal ICA over a 0.035 angled Terumo glide wire. Angiography confirmed persistent right M2 branch occlusion (▶ Fig. 15.7a, b, *arrows*). There was normal variant anatomy with right M1 segment trifurcation. The occluded branch gave supply

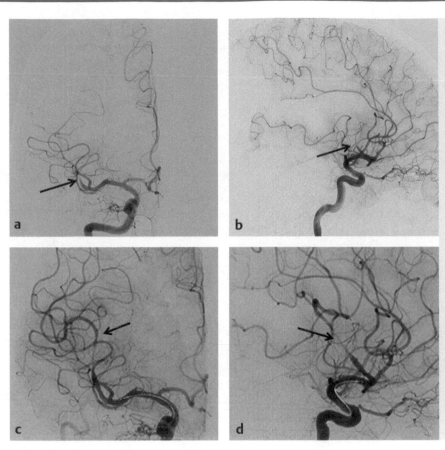

Fig. 15.7 Frontal (**a**) and lateral (**b**) projections of right ICA angiography, showing right M2 branch occlusion (*arrow*). Normal variant anatomy with right M1 segment trifurcation (**a**). Lateral view shows absent filling of central group, parietal, and angular branches of MCA (**b**). The right M1 segment and lenticulostriate perforators are patent (**a**). Control angiography in frontal (**c**) and lateral (**d**) projections with a 3 × 20 mm Solitaire deployed across the thrombus shows partial reopening of the occluded branch (*arrows*).

to the central group, parietal and angular branches of MCA, with collateralization from ACA evident on late arterial to venous phase of angiography (not shown). The right M1 segment and lenticulostriate perforators were patent. A standard exchange maneuver was performed in the right ECA, with the Advantage exchange length guidewire, and the 8-Fr MERCI balloon occlusion guide catheter advanced to the right cervical ICA. Through this, a Rebar 18 microcatheter was navigated through the M1 segment, and across the M2 occlusion with the aid of a Synchro 14 guidewire. Microcatheter injection confirmed position distal to the thrombus. A 3 × 20 mm Solitaire was then deployed across the thrombus. Control angiography with the stent retriever in situ showed partial reopening of the occluded branch (▶ Fig. 15.7 c, d, *arrows*), with filling of the central group but no filling of posterior parietal or angular arteries. It was presumed that the lesion constituted a "Y"-shaped thrombus, or else covered the origin of these branches. The stent was left in situ for 5 minutes to allow incorporation of thrombus, after which retrieval was performed with flow arrest and suction. Three large clot fragments were obtained from the stent and suction syringe. Control angiography showed complete recanalization of the occluded branch and reperfusion of the entire distal territory, including the posterior parietal and angular branches (▶ Fig. 15.8a, b). There was mild spasm seen in the M2 branch at the site where stent retriever had been deployed (▶ Fig. 15.8a, b, *arrows*).

The guide catheter was removed. The 8-Fr Angio-Seal device was placed at the puncture site for hemostasis.

Postprocedure Care/Outcome

The patient demonstrated on-table improvement, with improvement of the facial droop, left upper limb weakness, dysarthria, and neglect. Some residual sensory disturbance remained, which resolved over her hospital stay. Postprocedure she was transferred to the neuro high dependency unit in stable condition for further monitoring and care. Her subsequent course in hospital was uneventful. MRI was performed at 24 hours postprocedure (▶ Fig. 15.8c) and demonstrated a small region of restricted diffusion involving the posterior third of the right insular cortex, extending slightly into the lateral-most aspect of the right precentral gyrus, with no evidence of diffusion restriction elsewhere. The infarct was small compared with the ischemic penumbra on the CT perfusion study obtained prior to treatment. There was no evidence of hemorrhagic transformation. Aspirin 81 mg daily was commenced following the MRI. Echocardiography was performed to rule out a cardioembolic source, given her history of rheumatic heart disease and mitral stenosis. This demonstrated a dilated left atrium, moderate mitral stenosis, and mild to moderate mitral regurgitation. There was no evidence of patent foramen ovale or septal defect, and no thrombus. Given her history, she was started on warfarin prior to discharge. Blood pressure control was optimized. She was discharged home (modified Rankin scale [mRS] of 0), at 4 days following her presentation and intervention.

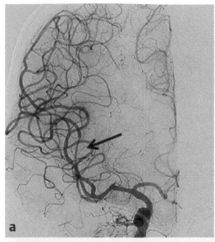
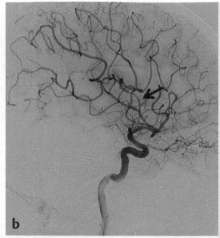
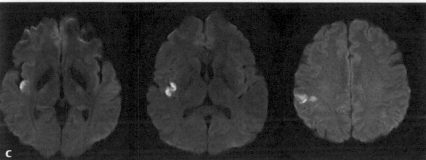

Fig. 15.8 Following single-pass thrombectomy, control angiography in frontal (**a**) and lateral (**b**) projections shows complete recanalization of the occluded branch and reperfusion of the entire distal territory, including the posterior parietal and angular branches. There is mild spasm seen in the M2 branch at the site where stent retriever was deployed (**a**, **b**, *arrows*). MRI and axial diffusion-weighted images obtained 24 hours postprocedure (**c**) show a small region of restricted diffusion involving the posterior third of the right insular cortex, extending to involve right precentral gyrus, with no evidence of diffusion restriction elsewhere.

15.3 Discussion

15.3.1 Background

The MCA is one of the terminal branches of the ICA, together with the ACA. Embryologically, at approximately ninth week of fetal life, the MCA develops from the fusion of several ACA perforators of the lateral striate group in response to the significant growth of the cerebral hemispheres that constitute the telencephalon. The first segment, denominated M1, is usually constituted by a single trunk with a diameter of approximately 3 mm, which courses laterally parallel to the floor of the middle cranial fossa. Distal to the main trunk, the artery typically (78% of cases) divides into two divisions (termed superior and inferior); less commonly there are three (12%) or greater than three divisions (10%). There is some controversy regarding the location of the transition point of the M1 and M2 segments. The traditional transition point described by Fischer (1938) was considered to occur when the artery performs a 90-degree turn to enter the vertical portion of the Sylvian fissure; thus, the M1 segment would include a pre- and post-bifurcation segment. This does not, however, have practical relevance. A more practical concept is to consider that the M1 segment ends when the main trunk bifurcates, a definition which is now also used in the recent consensus statement regarding recommendations on angiographic revascularization grading standards for acute ischemic stroke.

Mechanical thrombectomy is now the standard of care for acute ischemic stroke with occlusion of the M1 segment of MCA. The M1 segment of MCA was the most common location of intracranial arterial occlusion in the recently published randomized controlled trials which showed benefit for endovascular treatment in large artery occlusive stroke. For example, in MR CLEAN, M1 occlusion accounted for 66.1% of cases in the interventional group and 62% of cases in the control group. Similarly in the ESCAPE trial, M1 or effective M1 occlusions accounted for 68.1% of cases in the interventional group and 71.4% of cases in the control group, while in EXTEND-IA M1 occlusions accounted for 57% of cases in the interventional and 51% of cases in the control groups.

There are a number of important anatomical considerations in M1 segment of MCA occlusion, which can have a significant impact on patient outcome, the most important being the lenticulostriate arteries. The lenticulostriate arteries are a group of small caliber perforators arising from the proximal segments of the ACA and MCA. The following groups can be identified: from the ACA the recurrent artery of Heubner and the medial lenticulostriate arteries, and from the MCA the lenticulostriate arteries can be divided into a smaller medial group and a larger lateral group. There is a broad range of variations related to these perforating arteries. Most commonly, the lenticulostriate arteries of the MCA arise from the posterosuperior aspect of the M1 segment, although in approximately 20% of cases they can originate from the superior or inferior divisions of MCA, or less commonly from an early cortical branch of MCA. The medial group of lenticulostriate arteries from MCA are in equilibrium with the medial lenticulostriate arteries from the ACA and the recurrent artery of Heubner. Territory includes the anteroinferior portion of the head of caudate nucleus, the anterior third of the putamen, the anterior limb of internal capsule, the anterolateral edge of the globus pallidus, the medial aspect of the anterior commissure, and the anterior part of the hypothalamus. Territory of the lateral group of lenticulostriate arteries includes the upper portion of the head and body of caudate nucleus, the putamen, the lateral segment of globus pallidus, the lateral half of the anterior commissure, and the superior segments of both limbs of the internal capsule. The blood supply to the structures lateral to the putamen, including the claustrum and external capsule, is derived from perforators arising from the insular branches of the MCA.

As the lenticulostriates are end arteries, thrombus in the M1 segment of MCA can occlude the ostium of these perforating arteries resulting in infarction in their territory of supply. Proximal occlusions of the M1 segment of the MCA incorporating the lenticulostriate perforator origins are associated with a poorer clinical outcome than distal M1 occlusions that spare these perforators.

Another important anatomical consideration is that, similar to carotid terminus occlusion, there is no possibility of antegrade collateral supply to the distal territory in M1 segment of MCA occlusion. Therefore, collateral supply to the distal territory, if it exists, must be retrograde due to filling of leptomeningeal collaterals from the ipsilateral ACA or posterior cerebral artery (PCA) territory. Various grading schemes have been applied to assess collateral supply to the occluded MCA territory in M1 occlusive stroke. Good collateral supply to the occluded territory has been shown to be an independent predictor of good functional outcome following interventional treatment in M1 occlusive stroke.

Finally, in terms of anatomical considerations, while true anomalies of the MCA are rare and less frequent than anomalies of other intracranial arteries given the relatively recent phylogenetic ancestry of this artery, anomalous anatomy and variations in branching patterns can be encountered, and must be recognized. These will be discussed later in more detail, but briefly encompass the duplicated/accessory MCA, fenestration of the M1 segment, early bifurcation of the M1 segment, variation in branching pattern/division of the M1 segment, and variation in dominance of the M2 trunks.

15.3.2 Workup and Diagnosis

Patient History

At the time of admission, a detailed and complete history should be collected by an experienced stroke neurologist, whenever possible with the help of collateral history from family, friends, or witnesses of the event. It is important, however, that this be obtained rapidly and with a view to achieving the following:

- Confirm a sudden neurologic event compatible with an acute stroke and anticipate on the basis of the symptoms/history the vascular territory most probably involved.
- Determine the exact time of symptom onset.
- Identify vascular risk factors.
- Access previous functional status and comorbidities of the patient as well as current medication.
- Evaluate eligibility for intravenous thrombolytic therapy.
- Evaluate eligibility for endovascular therapy.

Examination and Investigation

Findings on physical examination in patients presenting with acute stroke due to M1 occlusion will depend on the hemisphere involved, location of occlusion, and degree of collateral supply. The aim of the examination is to determine severity of stroke symptoms and neurological deficits should be assessed and graded using the NIHSS scale. Examination should also evaluate for any atypical features, which may help exclude a stroke mimic.

Emergency imaging should be obtained as quickly as possible in the setting of suspected acute stroke before any treatment-related decision is made. Following the recent 2015 AHA/ASA Focused Update of the 2013 Guidelines for the Early Management of Patients with Acute Ischemic Stroke Regarding Endovascular Treatment, the following imaging recommendations were made: First, in most instances a nonenhanced CT of the brain will provide the necessary information to make decisions regarding emergency treatment. Second, if endovascular therapy is contemplated, a noninvasive intracranial vascular study is strongly recommended during the initial imaging evaluation but should not delay administration of intravenous tPA if it can be given. Third, the benefits of additional imaging beyond CT and CTA or MR and MRA, such as CT perfusion, or diffusion- and perfusion-weighted imaging for selecting patients for endovascular therapy are as yet unknown.

The objectives of noncontrast CT are to exclude hemorrhage, or other stroke mimics (e.g., tumor or extra-axial hematoma with mass effect), and assess for evidence of early or established ischemic change and extent of same. The ASPECTS score can be applied to determine the extent of change. It may also be possible to identify the location of a proximal thrombus as a linear hyperdensity in the expected region of the M1 segment (hyperdense MCA sign), or focus of hyperdensity within an M2 branch in the sylvian fissure (hyperdense dot sign).

Noninvasive vascular imaging (usually CTA) should ideally be obtained from the aortic arch up to the high cerebral convexity. This allows reliable identification of the exact location of the thrombus, and provides further important information regarding arterial access (such as the presence of bovine arch or vascular tortuosity) as well as identifying any associated extracranial disease, such as ipsilateral ICA stenosis or occlusion.

MRI/MRA studies are a valid option to CT/CTA and some centers have adapted their workflow and logistics to use these techniques as a screening tool in acute stroke. The basic MRI-stroke protocol can be relatively fast and usually includes an axial diffusion-weighted imaging (DWI), axial T2*/susceptibility weight imaging, and axial fluid-attenuated inversion recovery, as well intracranial time of flight (TOF) MRA and avoids radiation. It is imperative, however, that using MRI over CT does not introduce unnecessary delay in time to treatment, and its use in hyperacute stroke requires streamlined processes where patients can be screened for safety issues and imaged without delay. A downfall of obtaining TOF MRA is its limited utility in assessing the extracranial arterial system. Nevertheless, gadolinium-enhanced MRA can be performed additionally instead in cases suspected of an extracranial stenosis/occlusion/dissection, though at the expense of time.

Advanced imaging investigations, such as CT/MR perfusion, dynamic and multiphase CTA, can be used for the determination of penumbra and collateral status, respectively. Although their benefits are not well known and still lack standardization, they have potential to act as more refined selection tools, particularly in cases of unknown time of onset/time of onset more than 6 hours and/or a lower ASPECTS score.

15.3.3 Imaging Findings

In the acute phase of stroke, loss of gray-white matter differentiation and subtle low attenuation change on nonenhanced CT or restricted diffusion on MRI usually corresponds to already established "core" infarction. It is important in M1 occlusion to scrutinize the basal ganglia, and capsular regions for evidence of early ischemic change related to lenticulostriate artery occlusion. The size of core infarct at admission has been shown to be negatively correlated with patient outcome.

It is important to bear in mind that a "normal" nonenhanced CT scan does not rule out an ischemic stroke, particularly in the first hours. DWI presents a higher sensitivity for hyperacute stroke, and is superior than CT in delineating early infarction. Nevertheless, its sensitivity does not reach 100%. Furthermore, it is now known that some diffusion restricting lesions can regress.

CTA depicts thrombus as a filling defect or "cut-off" of contrast at the site of occlusion. When thrombus is present in the M1 segment, location should be further localized as proximal (i.e., involving the proximal half of the M1 and thus frequently occluding the lenticulostriate vessels) or distal (i.e., involving the distal half of the M1 segment and possibly sparing the lenticulostriate vessels). Use of multiplanar reformats and maximum intensity projection (MIP) images can be helpful in determining the site of occlusion, particularly in MCA occlusion beyond the M1 segment, or in situations where there is variant anatomy present. Coronal reconstructions in particular are helpful in identifying location of thrombus and its relationship to and patency of lenticulostriate arteries.

Leptomeningeal collateral supply to the distal MCA territory in M1 occlusion can be assessed on CTA. Collaterals are best demonstrated on axial MIP images, and collateral grade/score is determined by assessing the extent of contrast opacification of MCA branches ipsilateral to the occlusion, typically using the contralateral "normal" hemisphere as a comparison. If collateral supply to the occluded territory is good then contrast on CTA can retrogradely fill MCA branches back to the level of the distal point of the thrombus, allowing an estimation of thrombus length. However, there is not, as yet, a uniform way of scoring leptomeningeal collaterals on CTA across studies, and several different grading systems have been proposed varying from 2-point (good or bad collateral supply) to 6-point grading scales. More recently, collateral assessment on three-phase CTA has been proposed. In this grading system, collaterals are assessed on a 6-point scale based on extent and prominence of branches filling in the territory of the occluded vessel in combination with delay across CTA phases. This is of benefit as fast acquisition of single-phase CTA on modern scanners can underestimate degree of collateral filling.

The noninvasive vascular imaging study obtained, whether CTA or MRA, will act as a roadmap to guide intervention, and should be scrutinized for other vascular abnormalities or anatomical variations that might hinder endovascular treatment (e.g., unfavorable arch anatomy), introduce greater risk to the procedure (e.g., M1 fenestration), or prevent direct access to the occluded segment (e.g., ipsilateral ICA occlusion).

15.3.4 Decision-Making Process

Where thrombus is located either proximally or distally in the M1 segment, current updated AHA/ASA guidelines clearly recommend mechanical thrombectomy in selected patients (age: ≥ 18 years, NIHSS: ≥ 6, and ASPECTS score: ≥ 6), if treatment can be initiated (groin puncture) within 6 hours (*Class 1; level of evidence A*).

Whenever a thrombus is located in a M2 or M3 segment of the MCA, endovascular treatment can still be considered in carefully selected patients if performed within the first 6 hours, although with a lower level of evidence (*Class IIb; level of evidence C*). Nevertheless, this level of evidence is similar to the level of evidence described for acute strokes with causative thrombus on the ACAs, PCAs, vertebral arteries, and basilar artery.

The five recently published randomized clinical trials of endovascular stroke using primarily stent retrievers for thrombectomy have all included patients with M2 occlusions, although the numbers are relatively low (varying from 3.7% of all cases treated endovascularly in the ESCAPE study to 11% in the EXTENDED-IA study). Recent studies have specifically evaluated the risks and outcomes of mechanical thrombectomy in this particular location, and in their series, the procedure was safe and associated with greater chance for a good angiographic and clinical result as compared with M1 occlusions.

Less straightforward cases benefit from multidisciplinary discussion, which must be undertaken as an emergency without introducing significant delay, and may require advanced multimodal imaging for ultimate decision making.

15.3.5 Management

Medication

Currently, in accordance with the aforementioned updated 2019 guidelines from the AHA/ASA, all eligible patients should still receive intravenous tPA even if endovascular treatments are being considered. Further studies will be required to investigate whether tPA infusion can be skipped if a proximal thrombus is depicted and a mechanical thrombectomy anticipated.

Treatment

From the updated 2019 guidelines from the AHA/ASA, current standard of care in eligible cases of M1 segment of MCA occlusion is emergent mechanical thrombectomy (*Class I; level of evidence A*). The current level of evidence is mainly for thrombectomy with stent retriever, as this was the device most commonly used in the recent randomized controlled trials including MR CLEAN, ESCAPE, SWIFT PRIME, and EXTEND-IA. Use of salvage technical adjuncts including intra-arterial fibrinolysis may be reasonable to achieve the angiographic results (TICI 2b/3), if completed within 6 hours of symptom onset (*Class IIb; level of evidence B-R*).

Aspiration thrombectomy, using the penumbra aspiration system, is also an option, particularly if the clot is proximal, as is the case with occlusion of M1 segment of MCA. The two techniques, that is, stent retriever thrombectomy and penumbra system aspiration, can also be combined, for example if one technique alone fails to recanalize the artery, or for more distal MCA occlusions, for example M2 occlusion where flow arrest in the ICA and aspiration from the level of the carotid can potentially be ineffective.

Postprocedure Care

A basic neurologic examination is usually performed at the end of the procedure, often when the patient is still on the angiography table to assess for any immediate changes of neurological status and NIHSS score. Patients should then be cared for in a dedicated stroke unit/high dependency unit/ICU as appropriate to their level of needs.

A CT scan is recommended 24 hours after the procedure (or earlier in case of clinical deterioration) to assess for hemorrhagic transformation or developing malignant infarction with mass effect.

Postprocedure care after mechanical thrombectomy also includes groin inspection and evaluation of temperature and distal pulses of the lower limbs.

Instigation of measures for secondary stroke prevention is critical, with identification and correction of vascular risk factors and determination of stroke etiology. One common classification system used for determining stroke etiology is the TOAST classification system. If no evident etiology for the episode was found on admission, an extensive investigation should be performed in the subacute setting, particularly in young patients, in order to correctly classify the subtype of acute ischemic stroke.

15.3.6 Literature Synopsis

The lenticulostriate arteries arising from the MCA range between 6 and 20 per hemisphere and are usually divided into lateral and medial groups. Nevertheless, in 60% of cases, an exact separation between groups cannot be clearly made.

Although these vessels usually arise from the posterosuperior aspect of the M1 segment, it is important to bear in mind that they may emerge from different MCA segments or even early cortical branches.

Different patterns of origin of the lenticulostriates can also be present, namely, a single stem (candelabra artery), a number of common stems that further divide into many branches or alternatively numerous small branches that arise directly from the parent MCA vessel. After penetrating the anterior perforated substance, the primary vessels give rise to two to four secondary branches, each of which leads to tertiary branches, at the terminals of which are small precapillary arteriole envelopes.

In digital subtraction angiography (DSA), the lenticulostriate arteries are better visualized in anteroposterior projections and typically present a superior direction, being proximally laterally concave and then laterally convex. Although DSA remains superior, CTA and MRA can also be useful in the evaluation of these vessels.

As previously stated, the lenticulostriate arteries of the MCA (particularly the medial group) are in balance with other perforating arteries of the ACA/recurrent artery of Heubner, as well as perforating branches of the anterior communicating artery, the posterior communicating artery, the anterior choroidal artery, and posterior choroidal arteries.

The medial and lateral lenticulostriate arteries together with the recurrent artery of Heubner are responsible for the vascularization of specific territories that are relatively consistent with little left–right asymmetry. In terms of overall supply, the lack of anastomoses between major vessels supplying the striatum implies that hemodynamically, the three corticostriatal zones have independent vascular beds. Therefore, occlusion of a given parental vessel would cause damage largely restricted to a specific corticostriatal zone of the striatum. Large infarcts involving the lateral lenticulostriates, medial lenticulostriates, and recurrent artery of Heubner parental vessels affect primarily sensorimotor, associative, and limbic zones, respectively. Thus, occlusion of the lateral lenticulostriates would produce largely motor (sensorimotor) signs, whereas vascular disease affecting the recurrent artery of Heubner would lead to predominantly emotional and motivational (limbic) symptoms.

In patients with acute stroke secondary to proximal vessel occlusion, the lenticulostriate territory can be involved by different mechanisms, depending on the location of the thrombus: in cases of occlusion of the ICA by distal embolism and/or hemodynamic changes; in cases of proximal M1 segment involvement by occlusion of their ostium (the most frequent occurrence) or an artery-to-artery embolism.

Occlusion in the proximal M1 segment usually results in involvement of first-order perforator branches and thus seems to lead to nucleocapsular infarcts with a larger volume, in contrast to the smaller volume (< 15 mm) lacunar-type infarcts which correspond to occlusion of third-order vessels.

In the diagnosis and treatment of large artery occlusive stroke involving MCA, it is important to be aware of the possible variant anatomy and anomalies of the MCA itself. One of the variants of the M1 segment is the so-called early division or bifurcation, characterized by a division of the main trunk of the MCA within less than 10 mm from the origin (which usually occurs within 12–16 mm). This condition should be distinguished from the "false early bifurcations." Indeed, the fact that early temporal branches increase in size as their origin comes closer to the ICA bifurcation can eventually lead to the misinterpretation of the localization of the main bifurcation. These branches usually arise at right angles to the main trunk of the MCA, different from the post-bifurcation M2 arteries that run initially nearly parallel and diverge after the genu.

True anomalies of the MCA are rare and less frequent than anomalies of other intracranial arteries given the relatively recent phylogenetic ancestry of this artery, and include fenestration and duplicated/accessory MCA. Both are related to a variant persistence of different transient embryological vessels, giving rise to diverse possible patterns of the final arterial tree.

As the MCA develops from the fusion of several ACA perforators of the lateral striate group, a disposition may arise where two perforators remain dominant, thus resulting in the "accessory MCA." There are therefore two distinct arteries that run parallel in the sylvian fissure with separate origins and no distal convergence. The accessory vessel is, in fact, a hypertrophied recurrent artery of Heubner, a medial ACA perforator, or another perforator-like vessel. To qualify as an MCA, the vessel must have cortical territory. Different authors have developed variable classifications in order to summarize this topic. According to Teal's classification, a duplicated MCA is distinguished from an accessory MCA in that the former originates from the ICA bifurcation and the latter from the ACA. Manelfe's classification considers only the term "accessory MCA," dividing this variant into three types according to their origin: type 1, the smaller of the two branches coming from the ICA (thus corresponding to a duplicated MCA according to Teal's classification), type 2 originating from the proximal A1 segment, and type 3 from the distal A1 segment. Lasjaunias et al have simplified this classification, considering only a proximal type (including both types 1 and 2 of Manelfe's classification) and a distal type (corresponding to type 3 of Manelfe's classification) accessory MCA. This classification adds value regarding the prediction of origin of the lenticulostriate arteries (which in the end is the most important consideration), as it considers that in the proximal type of accessory MCA, the more cranial vessel gives rise to all the perforators, while the true MCA is purely cortical. However, in the case of a distal-type accessory MCA (which in fact corresponds to an enlarged recurrent artery of Heubner), the lenticulostriate arteries can arise from both arteries.

Finally, a "triplicated" appearance of the MCA can also be present if a true recurrent artery of Heubner is present in association with an accessory MCA.

Fenestrations, in contrast, are seen as a division of a single-artery lumen into distinctly separate channels, each with its own endothelial and muscular layers, while the adventitia may be shared. The artery will have a single origin. The two limbs of the fenestration converge distally. Most fenestrations of the MCA occur in the M1 segment and are unilateral, although their prevalence remains very low (around 0.2% at angiography and 1% in autopsy series).

It is thus crucial to carefully examine the anatomy of all the segments of the MCA before and during a mechanical thrombectomy in an attempt to identify any of the possible variants/anomalies of the MCA and to methodically plan the procedure. If an accessory MCA is present, it is important to verify in which artery the thrombus is located. It is also essential to assess the specific origin of the lenticulostriates. Another interesting aspect which may influence the outcome of these patients is that the presence of an accessary MCA could provide leptomeningeal collateral blood supply to the occluded portion of the territory.

Galimanis et al published in 2011 their large series of 623 patients with anterior circulation stroke treated with intra-arterial thrombolysis, mechanical revascularization techniques, or both and found that the more distal the MCA occlusion, the more favorable the patient outcome. In their series, a good score of mRS (0–2) at 3 months was obtained in 52.2% of patients with M1 occlusions and this percentage increased to 64.1% for M2 occlusions and to 74.1% for M3/4 occlusions.

More recently, Behme et al evaluated whether the specific localization of an M1 occlusion (distal vs. proximal) might predict an unfavorable outcome after a successful mechanical thrombectomy. In their study, they were able to show a statistically significant difference between successfully recanalized proximal and distal M1 occlusions regarding a disability-free early outcome (mRS score of 0 or 1) at discharge ($p = 0.03$) and at 90 days ($p = 0.04$). Interestingly, these findings did not go along with significant differences in baseline NIHSS, age, or time from symptom onset to revascularization, well-known predictors of outcome. It was the exact anatomical location of the clot in the M1 in relation to the perforators that played a key role for the outcome. There was a statistically significant difference between the two groups ($p < 0.0001$) regarding the presence of an acute basal ganglia infarct involving the internal capsule on the CT scan performed at 24 hours postprocedure. In their series, a proximal M1 occlusion reached a positive predictive value of 83% for the prediction of a persistent disability. The study shows that proximal occlusions of the M1 segment of the MCA incorporating the lenticulostriate perforators are associated with a poorer clinical outcome than distal M1 occlusions that spare these perforators.

Interestingly, MCA curvature may also influence the results of mechanical thrombectomy with stent retrievers. Schwaiger et al published a study evaluating 159 patients with carotid terminus or MCA occlusion and measuring different arterial angles (ICA/M1 angle, M1/M1 angle, and M1/M2 angles) in standard anteroposterior angiograms. Angles in patients with successful versus unsuccessful recanalization were then compared. Patients with unsuccessful recanalization (TICI 0–2a) of an ICA/proximal M1 occlusion had significantly larger ICA/M1 ($p < 0.001$) and M1/M1 ($p = 0.001$) angles than patients with successful recanalization. Larger M1/M2 angles were also associated with unsuccessful recanalization in cases of distal M1 or proximal M2 occlusions ($p = 0.006$).

Finally, while the efficacy of mechanical thrombectomy for M1 occlusion, and effective M1 occlusion, has been clearly demonstrated recently through randomized controlled trials, the efficacy and safety of mechanical thrombectomy for isolated M2 occlusions has also now recently been demonstrated through a post hoc meta-analysis of the STAR, SWIFT, and SWIFT PRIME studies.

15.3.7 Pearls and Pitfalls

- Mechanical thrombectomy is now the standard of care for acute ischemic stroke with occlusion of the M1 segment of MCA.
- A knowledge of MCA normal anatomy and variants is important when considering endovascular treatment of patients with M1 occlusion.
- Effort should be made to identify the origin of the lenticulostriate arteries and their relation to the location of the thrombus.
- As the lenticulostriates are end arteries, thrombus in the M1 segment of MCA can occlude the ostium of these perforating arteries resulting in infarction in their territory of supply.
- Proximal M1 thrombus, contrary to distal thrombus, more commonly involves the lenticulostriate artery origins, and is therefore more commonly associated with accompanying basal ganglia infarction.
- Proximal occlusions of the M1 segment of the MCA incorporating the lenticulostriate perforators are associated with a poorer clinical outcome than distal M1 occlusions that spare these perforators.

Further Readings

Behme D, Kowoll A, Weber W, Mpotsaris A. M1 is not M1 in ischemic stroke: the disability-free survival after mechanical thrombectomy differs significantly between proximal and distal occlusions of the middle cerebral artery M1 segment. J Neurointerv Surg. 2015; 7(8):559–563

Berkhemer OA, Fransen PS, Beumer D, et al. MR CLEAN Investigators. A randomized trial of intraarterial treatment for acute ischemic stroke. N Engl J Med. 2015; 372 (1):11–20

Campbell BC, Mitchell PJ, Kleinig TJ, et al. EXTEND-IA Investigators. Endovascular therapy for ischemic stroke with perfusion-imaging selection. N Engl J Med. 2015; 372(11):1009–1018

Saver JL, Goyal M, Bonafe A, et al. SWIFT PRIME Investigators. Stent-retriever thrombectomy after intravenous t-PA vs. t-PA alone in stroke. N Engl J Med. 2015; 372(24):2285–2295

Goyal M, Demchuk AM, Menon BK, et al. ESCAPE Trial Investigators. Randomized assessment of rapid endovascular treatment of ischemic stroke. N Engl J Med. 2015; 372(11):1019–1030

Coutinho JM, Liebeskind DS, Slater LA, et al. Mechanical thrombectomy for isolated M2 occlusions: a post hoc analysis of the STAR, SWIFT, and SWIFT PRIME studies. AJNR Am J Neuroradiol. 2016; 37(4):667–672

Decavel P, Vuillier F, Moulin T. Lenticulostriate infarction. Front Neurol Neurosci. 2012; 30:115–119

Dorn F, Lockau H, Stetefeld H, et al. Mechanical thrombectomy of M2-occlusion. J Stroke Cerebrovasc Dis. 2015; 24(7):1465–1470

Feekes JA, Cassell MD. The vascular supply of the functional compartments of the human striatum. Brain. 2006; 129(Pt 8):2189–2201

Flores A, Tomasello A, Cardona P, et al. Catalan Stroke Code and Reperfusion Consortium Cat-SCR. Endovascular treatment for M2 occlusions in the era of stentrievers: a descriptive multicenter experience. J Neurointerv Surg. 2015; 7 (4):234–237

Galimanis A, Jung S, Mono ML, et al. Endovascular therapy of 623 patients with anterior circulation stroke. Stroke. 2012; 43(4):1052–1057

Lasjaunias P, Berenstein A, terBrugge KG. Surgical Neuroangiography. Vol. 1, 2nd ed. Berlin: Springer; 2006

Powers WJ, Derdeyn CP, Biller J, et al. American Heart Association Stroke Council. 2015 American Heart Association/American Stroke Association Focused Update of the 2013 Guidelines for the Early Management of Patients With Acute Ischemic Stroke Regarding Endovascular Treatment: A Guideline for Healthcare Professionals From the American Heart Association/American Stroke Association. Stroke. 2015; 46(10):3020–3035

Schwaiger BJ, Gersing AS, Zimmer C, Prothmann S. The curved MCA: influence of vessel anatomy on recanalization results of mechanical thrombectomy after acute ischemic stroke. AJNR Am J Neuroradiol. 2015; 36(5):971–976

Sheth SA, Yoo B, Saver JL, et al. UCLA Comprehensive Stroke Center. M2 occlusions as targets for endovascular therapy: comprehensive analysis of diffusion/perfusion MRI, angiography, and clinical outcomes. J Neurointerv Surg. 2015; 7(7):478–483

Shi ZS, Loh Y, Walker G, Duckwiler GR, MERCI and Multi-MERCI Investigators. Clinical outcomes in middle cerebral artery trunk occlusions versus secondary division occlusions after mechanical thrombectomy: pooled analysis of the Mechanical Embolus Removal in Cerebral Ischemia (MERCI) and Multi MERCI trials. Stroke. 2010; 41(5):953–960

Zaidat OO, Yoo AJ, Khatri P, et al. Cerebral Angiographic Revascularization Grading (CARG) Collaborators, STIR Revascularization working group, STIR Thrombolysis in Cerebral Infarction (TICI) Task Force. Recommendations on angiographic revascularization grading standards for acute ischemic stroke: a consensus statement. Stroke. 2013; 44(9):2650–2663

Fischer E. Die Lageabweichungen der vorderen Hirnarterie im Gefäßbild. Zentralbl Neurochir. 1938(3):300–313

Teal JS, Rumbaugh CL, Bergeron RT, et al. Anomalies of the middle cerebral artery: accessory artery, duplication, and early bifurcation. Am J Roentgenol. 1973; 118 (3):567–575

16 Basilar Artery Occlusion

16.1 Case Description

16.1.1 Clinical Presentation

A 66-year-old male presented to the hospital in the early morning, with fluctuating right-sided weakness, right gaze preference and right facial droop, bilateral legs ataxia, slurred speech, and drowsiness. National Institute of Health Stroke Scale (NIHSS) score was 13. His wife recalled that the patient was talking somewhat slowly the night before. They slept in different rooms and, in the morning, she found him on the ground.

16.1.2 Imaging Workup and Investigations

On noncontrast CT, there was no evidence of established infarctions. A CT angiography (CTA) demonstrated a basilar artery (BA) filling defect extending in bilateral posterior cerebral arteries (PCAs). CT perfusion demonstrated a significant cerebral blood flow (CBF)/time to peak (TTP) mismatch in the territory of the BA and to a lesser extent of the PCAs bilaterally (▶ Fig. 16.1a).

16.1.3 Diagnosis and Treatment

Acute basilar artery occlusion (BAO). Intravenous tissue plasminogen activator (IV-tPA) was not given due to the long time since last known well. The patient was brought to the angiography suite for endovascular treatment (EVT).

16.1.4 Technique

- Right common femoral artery puncture with placement of an 8-Fr short vascular access sheath into the common femoral artery.
- A 6-Fr guide catheter placed in the left vertebral artery, which was of sufficient caliber to allocate a large catheter. A digital subtraction angiography run demonstrated the known distal BAO (▶ Fig. 16.1b).
- A large-bore aspiration catheter was advanced into the right vertebral artery over a 1.8-Fr microcatheter and a 0.014-in microwire.
- The aspiration catheter was parked with the tip adjacent to the proximal end of the thrombus, and the microcatheter was removed.
- The aspiration catheter was connected to the suction device and aspiration was carried out for 5 minutes.

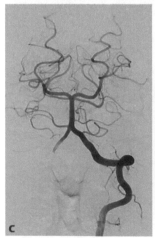
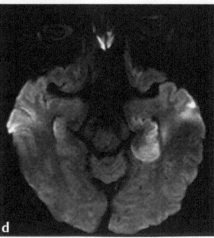
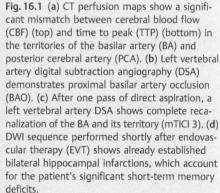
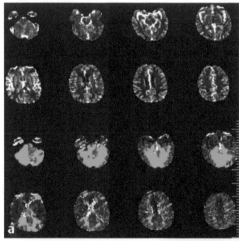
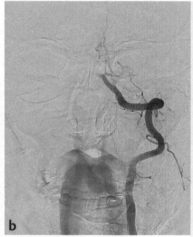

Fig. 16.1 (a) CT perfusion maps show a significant mismatch between cerebral blood flow (CBF) (top) and time to peak (TTP) (bottom) in the territories of the basilar artery (BA) and posterior cerebral artery (PCA). (b) Left vertebral artery digital subtraction angiography (DSA) demonstrates proximal basilar artery occlusion (BAO). (c) After one pass of direct aspiration, a left vertebral artery DSA shows complete recanalization of the BA and its territory (mTICI 3). (d) DWI sequence performed shortly after endovascular therapy (EVT) shows already established bilateral hippocampal infarctions, which account for the patient's significant short-term memory deficits.

- After 5 minutes, the aspiration catheter was pulled under continuous aspiration and manual sucrion from the guiding catheter.
- A postaspiration angiographic run demonstrated complete recanalization with a modified treatment in cerebral ischemia (mTICI) score of 3 (▶ Fig. 16.1c). Time from puncture to recanalization was 23 minutes.

16.1.5 Postprocedural Care and Outcome

The patient was transferred to the stroke unit. Postoperative investigations identified a previously undiagnosed atrial fibrillation, for which treatment was initiated.

The patient had full recovery of his motor, cognitive, and speech function, with a residual deficit in short-term memory, and was discharged after 10 days. An MRI a few days after treatment demonstrated bilateral, left-greater-than-right hippocampal infarctions (▶ Fig. 16.1d). At the 4-month clinic follow-up, the patient still had remarkable short-term memory deficits, which caused him significant anxiety and depression.

16.2 Companion Case

16.2.1 Clinical Presentation

Shortly after midnight, a 57-year-old male was emergently brought by ambulance to the emergency department after suffering a syncopal event while drinking with some friends at a bar. On arrival he was pale and diaphoretic and had multiple episodes of vomiting. His NIHSS score was 13, with right-sided weakness and facial droop, right-sided neglect, and aphasia.

16.2.2 Imaging Workup and Investigations

On noncontrast CT, there was no evidence of established infarctions. A CTA demonstrated a nonocclusive thrombus in the proximal BA (▶ Fig. 16.2a). CT perfusion demonstrated a significant CBF/TTP mismatch in the cerebellum. Neck images demonstrated significant tortuosity of the aortic arch (type 3) and of bilateral vertebral arteries.

16.2.3 Diagnosis and Treatment

Acute basilar artery subocclusion. IV-tPA was given and the patient was referred for EVT.

16.2.4 Technique

- Right common femoral artery puncture with placement of an 8-Fr short vascular access sheath into the common femoral artery.
- A 6-Fr guide catheter placed in the left subclavian artery and the left vertebral artery was catheterized with an aspiration catheter and a microcatheter. A run confirmed subocclusion of the BA. An extremely tight bend in the V2 segment made impossible the navigation of the devices; therefore, this approach was aborted (▶ Fig. 16.2b).

- The extreme tortuosity of the arch made impossible the catheterization of the right vertebral artery, despite multiple attempts with Simmons 2 and 3 catheters and normal and shapeable glidewires.
- A 6-Fr dedicated sheath was inserted in the right radial artery and a 0.071-in catheter was advanced into the right vertebral artery until another sharp turn (▶ Fig. 16.2c).
- The turn was negotiated with a soft-tipped 5-Fr distal access catheter and a 0.18-in microcatheter over a 0.014-in microwire (▶ Fig. 16.1c).
- The distal access catheter was parked at the V2–V3 junction and the microcatheter was navigated through the occlusion and positioned in the right PCA.
- A 4 × 30 mm stent retriever was deployed over the thrombus and left in place for 5 minutes, after which it was removed under aspiration from the distal access catheter.
- A postaspiration angiographic run demonstrated complete recanalization with an mTICI score of 3. There was an underlying stenosis of the proximal BA of 50%, which was not treated given its noncritical features (▶ Fig. 16.2d). Puncture to reperfusion time was 90 minutes.

16.2.5 Postprocedural Care and Outcome

The patient was transferred to the stroke unit. Postoperative echocardiography identified a patent foramen ovale.

The patient had complete recovery of his motor, cognitive, and speech function, with residual homonymous hemianopia and imbalance. An MRI prior to discharge demonstrated bilateral cerebellar and occipital lobe infarctions. At the 4-month clinic follow-up, the patient was completely independent and only endorsed minimal visual symptoms.

16.2.6 Background

Posterior circulation strokes are less frequent than their anterior counterparts, and account for approximately 15 to 20% of the total ischemic strokes. BAO is an even rarer event and represents 1 to 4% of all strokes.[1]

Due to the particular anatomical and physiological characteristics of the BA, its occlusion can be difficult to diagnose clinically. The condition carries an extremely high mortality, with multiple large cohort studies quoting rates between 85 and 95% if left untreated.[2,3,4]

The BA originates at the pontomedullary junction from the union of the vertebral arteries. The vessel measures an average diameter of 3.74 mm,[5] courses along the anterior surface of the brainstem, and eventually divides in the bilateral PCAs at its tip. The vessel gives the anterior inferior cerebellar arteries (AICAs), the superior cerebellar arteries (SCAs), multiple brainstem and thalamic perforators and has been schematically divided in proximal, middle, and distal segments. The proximal segment goes from the vertebrobasilar junction to the origin of the AICAs, the middle from the AICAs to the SCAs, and the distal from the SCAs to the basilar tip. Besides supplying a large portion of the cerebellum, the BA is the main feeder for some of the most critical areas of the brainstem. The proximal and middle segments and their branches supply the pons, while the

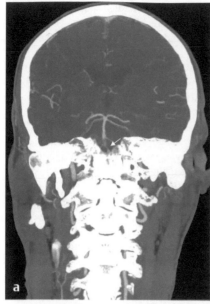

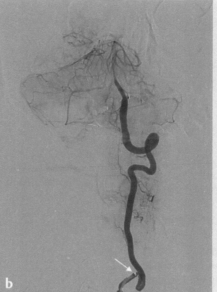

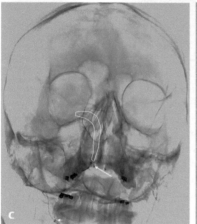

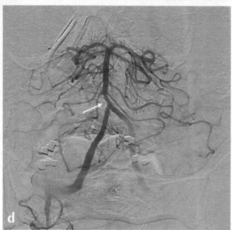

Fig. 16.2 (**a**) CTA coronal MIP showing subtotal occlusion of the proximal basilar artery (*arrow*), with preserved flow in the distal vessel and in the PCAs. (**b**): Left vertebral artery digital subtraction angiography (DSA) run demonstrating the proximal basilar artery (BA) subtotal occlusion. Note the extreme tortuosity of the vessel with a turn that could not be negotiated despite multiple attempts (*arrow*). (**c**) Single-shot DSA with a 5-Fr intermediate catheter at the V2–V3 junction (*short arrow*) and a microcatheter in the distal right V4 segment (*long arrow*). The *white line* shows the deployed 4 × 30 mm stent retriever, with the distal end in the right posterior cerebral artery (PCA). (**d**) Postthrombectomy DSA showing mTICI 3 reperfusion of the basilar artery with a residual stenosis of approximately 50% of the vessel lumen (*arrow*).

distal segment and its branches, including the PCAs, supply the midbrain, thalami, and hippocampi. The basilar tip gives multiple critical perforators to the thalamus and midbrain.[1]

Clinically, the manifestations of BAOs are manifold, depending on multiple factors such as location and extent of the thrombus, collateral circulation (including anastomoses between perforators), and etiology of the occlusion.[6] In general, reduced consciousness is a clinical hallmark of BAO.[7] Symptoms include the following: (1) various degrees of motor deficits, from facial or bland hemiparesis to tetraplegia; (2) dysarthria; (3) headache; (4) visual impairment; (5) vertigo, nausea, and vomiting; and (6) loss of consciousness and coma. Symptom onset is as well variable, going from vague, nonspecific prodromal symptoms like vertigo or nausea to sudden loss of consciousness and coma. Especially if the emergence of symptoms is insidious, the syndrome can mimic a nonstroke condition, thus delaying a referral to neurology and a timely diagnosis and appropriate treatment. This is particularly evident in patients with a preexisting atherosclerotic stenosis of the BA, which, by virtue of having developed rich collateral network, can develop a BAO and show only small ischemic lesions on imaging or very mild clinical manifestations. Once a pontine infarct is established, secondary to a middle segment occlusion, depending on the extent, the patient can present with hemi- or tetraplegia, altered consciousness, and cranial nerve palsies. Extensive pontine infarction is also the most common cause of locked-in syndrome. Distal segment and basilar tip occlusions can result in nuclear and supranuclear symptoms, tetraparesis/plegia, and thalamic syndromes with or without amnesia and behavioral abnormalities. Depending on the conformation of the circle of Willis, symptoms can involve one or both PCAs, with possible visual symptoms and hippocampal infarctions, as shown in the first case.

The most common causes of posterior circulation occlusion are cardiac and large-artery embolism, arterial dissection, and atherosclerotic stenotic disease. In general, patients with atherosclerotic BA occlusions are in the sixth or seventh decade, while those with embolic stroke are younger.[6] Underlying intracranial atherosclerosis with significant stenosis (>70%) has been reported in as high as 24% of patients with BAO.[4]

After having ruled out a hemorrhage with a plain head CT, CTA, or MRI angiography, provide the final diagnosis of BAO. The hyperdense BA sign on noncontrast CT, although relatively specific in cases with high pretest probability of BAO, is seen only in 50 to 70% of patients.[8]

Similar to what has been developed in anterior circulation strokes, a 10-point posterior circulation Acute Stroke Prognosis

Early CT (pc-ASPECTS) score was developed and validated to quantify early ischemia. This score is reportedly most effective if calculated on source images of a CTA.[9]

While, in general, DWI sequences are the gold standard for the detection of acute infarction, it has been shown that 6 to 10% of all strokes are initially DWI negative—this rate being higher in the posterior circulation, particularly in the early period after occlusion.[10]

EVT in BAO can be carried out by stent retrieval, aspiration, or by a combination thereof. Given the relatively small caliber of the vertebral arteries, a large bore guiding catheter cannot be placed in this vessel most of the times and needs to be left in the subclavian artery. An intermediate, aspiration-capable distal access catheter can be then navigated in the vertebral artery over a microcatheter and J-tipped microwire. Depending on the technique of choice, the aspiration catheter can be positioned at the proximal end of the thrombus/embolus or the microcatheter can be used to gently pass the occlusion and advanced until the tip is in one of the PCAs prior to deployment of a stent retriever. The technique for EVT of BAO does not differ from that used in anterior circulation occlusions. As shown in the second case described earlier, particularly tortuous anatomies can require a radial access. In this instance, given the maximum radial sheath diameter of 6 Fr, smaller guide and aspiration catheters need to be used. In cases with an underlying atherosclerotic stenosis, angioplasty with or without stenting might be necessary to consolidate the results of the procedure. The technical aspects of these procedures are described in other sections of the book. Deployment of a stent in the acute setting will require emergent institution of dual-antiplatelet therapy to avoid acute thrombosis. At our institution, we use a loading dose of 325 mg of aspirin associated with 300 mg of clopidogrel or 180 mg of ticagrelor. We also routinely use a weight-based continuous IV drip of eptifibatide as a bridging therapy, to be stopped 6 hours after administration of the oral dual-antiplatelet agents.

16.2.7 Discussion

Spontaneous recanalization rates after BAO are not known but are thought to be low and not higher than 20% at most. Due to the varied and often waxing and waning nature of the symptoms, most patients seek medical attention many hours after the embolic event and out of the traditional time window for IV-tPA. Given the exceptionally high morbidity and mortality of this condition, patients are often treated, both medically and endovascularly, regardless of when last known well, with reported treatment delays up to 48 hours after symptom onset.[11,12] In most case series, IV-tPA has been given up to 6 hours and mechanical thrombectomy has been performed well beyond 8 hours. Similarly to what led to the modern approach to anterior circulation stroke, the most consistent predictor of a bad clinical outcome appears to be the extent of infarction at the time of treatment, with higher pc-ASPECTS scores associated with better outcomes. In general, it appears that the good outcome of recanalization is less time dependent in BAO than in anterior circulation strokes.[3,9] This is potentially secondary to the particular vascular supply to the BA and its territory: depending on the site of the occlusion and on the patient's anatomy, blood flow can still reach patent portions of

the vessel either through the vertebral arteries or the posterior communicating arteries. Moreover, there are strong collateral connections between the three paired cerebellar arteries and between brainstem perforators. These collaterals can give at least partial supply the brainstem and keep tissue viable, thus extending the therapeutic window. This rich anastomotic network could also account for the somewhat erratic nature of the symptoms, which could depend in variable measures by the patient's pressure, collateral circulation, thrombus buildup, and potential migration of the clot. As shown in the second case, it is also possible to have a subocclusive clot, hence with persistence of minimal antegrade and perforator flow in the BA.[3]

While the safety and efficacy of EVT in anterior circulation occlusions have been widely studied and analyzed through multiple randomized trials, the role for endovascular therapy in BAO has been investigated less systematically. The first multicentric randomized trial designed to compare EVT and IV-tPA in BAO was the "Acute Basilar Artery Occlusion: Endovascular Interventions vs Standard Medical Treatment (BEST)" study. It showed that thrombectomy was superior to best medical therapy in the treatment of BAO in terms of achievement of a good clinical outcome, considered as a modified Rankin scale (mRS) of 0 to 3, at 90 days and was stopped, as it had happened to similar studies on anterior circulation large-vessel occlusions, due to loss of equipoise between the two treatment arms.[13]

A recent large multicentric retrospective study demonstrated how EVT for BAO leads to reperfusion in 90% of cases and to an mRS of 0 to 2 at 90 days in 45% of cases. This study showed a 13% mortality rate and a rate of procedural complications of 4.2%. Hemorrhagic infarction and parenchymal hematomas were associated with worse clinical outcomes. Younger age, absence of diabetes mellitus, and lower NIHSS at admission were all predictors of better outcomes.[2] The results of this study were overall more positive, perhaps due to different patient selection criteria, than that of two recent meta-analyses that showed overall recanalization rates around 80%, and a mortality of 30%.[14,15]

In terms of technique, a recent meta-analysis of five studies that compared operative times, reperfusion rates, and clinical outcomes between first-line aspiration and stent retrieval demonstrated that aspiration is more likely to achieve an mTICI 2b–3 recanalization with shorter procedural times and a smaller risk of new territory embolizations. Clinical outcomes, hemorrhagic complications, and mortality, however, do not significantly differ between the two techniques.[16]

The location of the BAO could be a predictor of the presence of an underlying atherosclerotic stenosis. In these instances, revascularization can be more technically challenging and there might be the need for a rescue angioplasty with or without stenting. Multiple studies have demonstrated how the majority (73%) of BAO superimposed on a preexistent stenosis happen in the proximal and middle segments of the BA, while the vast majority (92%) of purely embolic ones are in its distal segment. These works have demonstrated a safe and effective profile of acute angioplasty with or without stenting in BAO with an underlying atherosclerotic stenosis, recanalization rates between 90 and 100%, and favorable clinical outcomes as high as 65%.[4]

16.2.8 Pearls and Pitfalls

- A randomized multicentric study confirms prior data that show superiority of EVT on medical therapy alone for BAO.
- Particularly tortuous subclavian anatomies might require radial access.
- Aspiration first appears to lead to recanalization faster and with less unwanted embolization than stent retrieval, without a significant difference in clinical outcomes.
- Rescue angioplasty with and without stenting is safe and effective in those patients with underlying intracranial atherosclerotic stenosis of the BA.

References

[1] Mattle HP, Arnold M, Lindsberg PJ, Schonewille WJ, Schroth G. Basilar artery occlusion. Lancet Neurol. 2011; 10(11):1002–1014

[2] Kang DH, Jung C, Yoon W, et al. Endovascular thrombectomy for acute basilar artery occlusion: a multicenter retrospective observational study. J Am Heart Assoc. 2018; 7(14):1–9

[3] Lindsberg PJ, Pekkola J, Strbian D, Sairanen T, Mattle HP, Schroth G. Time window for recanalization in basilar artery occlusion: speculative synthesis. Neurology. 2015; 85(20):1806–1815

[4] Lee YY, Yoon W, Kim SK, et al. Acute basilar artery occlusion: differences in characteristics and outcomes after endovascular therapy between patients with and without underlying severe atherosclerotic stenosis. AJNR Am J Neuroradiol. 2017; 38(8):1600–1604

[5] Smoker WR, Price MJ, Keyes WD, Corbett JJ, Gentry LR. High-resolution computed tomography of the basilar artery: 1. Normal size and position. AJNR Am J Neuroradiol. 1986; 7(1):55–60

[6] Demel SL, Broderick JP. Basilar occlusion syndromes: an update. Neurohospitalist. 2015; 5(3):142–150

[7] Laureys S, Owen AM, Schiff ND. Brain function in coma, vegetative state, and related disorders. Lancet Neurol. 2004; 3(9):537–546

[8] Mortimer AM, Saunders T, Cook JL. Cross-sectional imaging for diagnosis and clinical outcome prediction of acute basilar artery thrombosis. Clin Radiol. 2011; 66(6):551–558

[9] Puetz V, Khomenko A, Hill MD, et al. Basilar Artery International Cooperation Study (BASICS) Group. Extent of hypoattenuation on CT angiography source images in basilar artery occlusion: prognostic value in the Basilar Artery International Cooperation Study. Stroke. 2011; 42(12):3454–3459

[10] Nagel S, Herweh C, Köhrmann M, et al. MRI in patients with acute basilar artery occlusion - DWI lesion scoring is an independent predictor of outcome. Int J Stroke. 2012; 7(4):282–288

[11] Smith WS. Intra-arterial thrombolytic therapy for acute basilar occlusion: pro. Stroke. 2007; 38(2) Suppl:701–703

[12] Lindsberg PJ, Mattle HP. Therapy of basilar artery occlusion: a systematic analysis comparing intra-arterial and intravenous thrombolysis. Stroke. 2006; 37(3):922–928

[13] World Stroke Congress Abstracts. Late breaking submissions. Int J Stroke. 2018; 13:225–244

[14] Phan K, Phan S, Huo YR, Jia F, Mortimer A. Outcomes of endovascular treatment of basilar artery occlusion in the stent retriever era: a systematic review and meta-analysis. J Neurointerv Surg. 2016; 8(11):1107–1115

[15] Gory B, Eldesouky I, Sivan-Hoffmann R, et al. Outcomes of stent retriever thrombectomy in basilar artery occlusion: an observational study and systematic review. J Neurol Neurosurg Psychiatry. 2016; 87(5):520–525

[16] Ye G, Lu J, Qi P, Yin X, Wang L, Wang D. Firstline a direct aspiration first pass technique versus firstline stent retriever for acute basilar artery occlusion: a systematic review and meta-analysis. J Neurointerv Surg. 2019; 11(8):740–746

17 ADAPT Technique for Acute Ischemic Stroke Thrombectomy

17.1 Case Description

17.1.1 Clinical Presentation

An 86-year-old man presented to the emergency department (ED) at 6 a.m. after being found by his wife at approximately 5:30 a.m. His was last seen normal at 10 p.m. the night before. He presented with dysarthria, left hemiplegia, right gaze preference, left lower quadrant cut, and a mild left-sided neglect. Examination in the ED was consistent with a right middle cerebral artery (MCA) syndrome, and his National Institutes of Health Stroke Scale (NIHSS) score was 12. He has a past medical history of coronary artery disease, hypertension, hyperlipidemia (HLD), gastroesophageal reflux disease, benign prostatic hyperplasia, chronic kidney disease, sick sinus syndrome, and idiopathic pulmonary fibrosis.

17.1.2 Imaging Workup and Investigations

- Noncontrast CT of the head performed at 6:15 a.m. demonstrated loss of the differentiation in the right basal ganglia; ASPECTS score was 9 (▶ Fig. 17.1).
- CTA demonstrated a complete occlusion of the right internal carotid artery (ICA) at the bifurcation and isolated right hemispheric circulation with no opacification of the intracranial ICA or MCA (▶ Fig. 17.2). Subsequent imaging demonstrated opacification of the ICA ophthalmic segment via sphenopalatine artery collaterals with tandem occlusion of the carotid terminus.
- CT perfusion demonstrated a small core infarct in the right basal ganglia but a large area of prolonged mean transit time (MTT) and preserved cerebral blood volume (CBV)

throughout the right MCA distribution consistent with a large area of ischemic penumbra.

17.1.3 Diagnosis

- Acute ischemic stroke secondary to right ICA and MCA occlusion with large area of ischemic penumbra.

17.1.4 Treatment

- The patient was outside the time window for intravenous tissue plasminogen activator (IV-tPA; 4.5 hours), given his last known normal was 8 hours prior to presentation.
- Endovascular therapy was considered to be the best available therapy for the extensive clot burden of the MCA and carotid occlusion.
- The patient was quickly transferred to the angiography suite and groin puncture was performed at 7:15 a.m. and complete recanalization was achieved in 39 minutes.

17.1.5 Materials and Endovascular Treatment

- Anesthesia:
  - Local, lidocaine 2%.
  - No sedation, conscious or otherwise, was utilized.
- Groin access:
  - 18 g Cook needle, 9 Fr pinnacle sheath.
- Right common carotid artery access:
  - 6-Fr 088 Neuron Max sheath (Penumbra Inc., Alameda, CA) over a 5-Fr Berenstein insert (Penumbra Inc.) and 0.038 Terumo (Terumo, Tokyo, Japan) Glidewire. Angiography

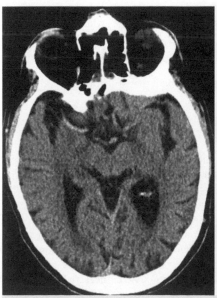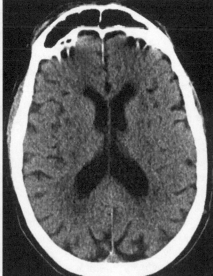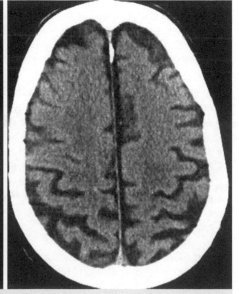

Fig. 17.1 Noncontrast CT demonstrates right MCA hyperdense sign and a small core infarct of the right putamen.

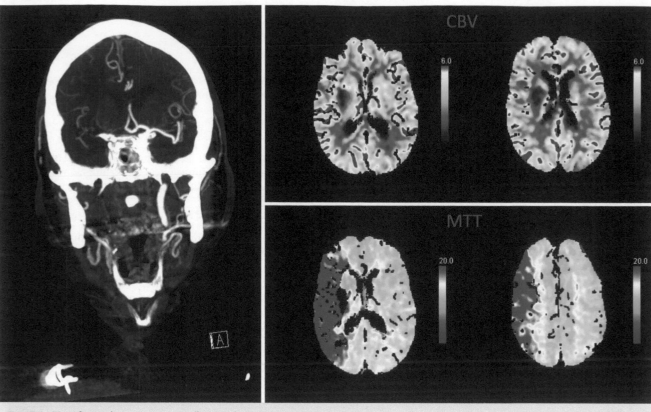

Fig. 17.2 CT perfusion demonstrates a small core infarct in the right putamen (CBV) with a large area of penumbra in the region of the right MCA distribution (MTT) secondary to a right ICA and MCA occlusion (CTA MIP).

demonstrated complete occlusion of the internal carotid origin with partial reconstitution of the ICA ophthalmic segment via sphenopalatine artery collaterals. There was a tandem occlusion of the carotid terminus.

- Right common carotid artery angioplasty and stenting:
  - The carotid occlusion was crossed with a velocity microcatheter (Penumbra Inc.) and a 0.016 Fathom guidewire. This was exchanged for a 4 mm × 20 mm Apex balloon (Boston Scientific, Nantucket, MA) over a 0.014 Transend (Boston Scientific) exchange microwire for Percutaneous transluminal angioplasty (PTA) of the bifurcation. Subsequently, a 10 mm × 40 mm Cordis Precise ProRx stent (Cordis, Miami Lakes, FL) was deployed to maintain vessel patency (▶ Fig. 17.3, ▶ Fig. 17.4, ▶ Fig. 17.5). At the time of stent deployment, 20 mg of ReoPro was administered intravenously and 600 mg of Plavix and 650 of ASA were given orally at the conclusion of the procedure.
- Right ICA and MCA thrombectomy:
  - The Neuron Max sheath was advanced across the carotid bifurcation into the distal cervical ICA. Repeat angiography demonstrates occlusion of the ICA at the level of the posterior communicating artery. A 5 MAX ACE reperfusion catheter (Penumbra Inc.) was advanced over a Velocity microcatheter and a 0.016 Fathom guidewire into the carotid terminus. The velocity microcatheter was removed and the 5 MAX ACE reperfusion catheter was slowly advanced across the carotid terminus and proximal right MCA M1 segment under direct aspiration (▶ Fig. 17.5, ▶ Fig. 17.6, ▶ Fig. 17.7, ▶ Fig. 17.8). When flow (in tubing)

was noted to be stagnant, the catheter was removed. A clot of 5 cm was present in the catheter tip (▶ Fig. 17.9). Final control angiography demonstrated complete recanalization of the right ICA and right MCA (▶ Fig. 17.10).

17.1.6 Outcome

- The patient returned to baseline on the table (NIHSS 1).
- CT of the head performed on postoperative day1 demonstrated a small core infarct in the right posterior basal ganglia (▶ Fig. 17.11).
- Patient was discharged on postoperative day 4 at a mRS score of 1 and a NIHSS of 1.
- At 90-day follow-up, the patient was still at mRS 1 and NIHSS 1 (for mild dysarthria).

17.1.7 Discussion

Direct aspiration thrombectomy or ADAPT (A Direct Aspiration first Pass Technique for acute stroke thrombectomy) is a standardized approach to stroke thrombectomy made possible by the development of large bore (054–064) catheters, such as the Penumbra 072 JET7, ACE 068, 5 MAX, 4 MAX, and 3 MAX reperfusion catheters that retain high trackability and are easily navigated into the intracranial circulation. It has been demonstrated by some groups that the direct aspiration technique can be fast, efficacious, safe, and cost-effective. Two clinical trials have compared contact aspiration to stent retriever as first line approach for mechanical thrombectomy. Both trials showed similar

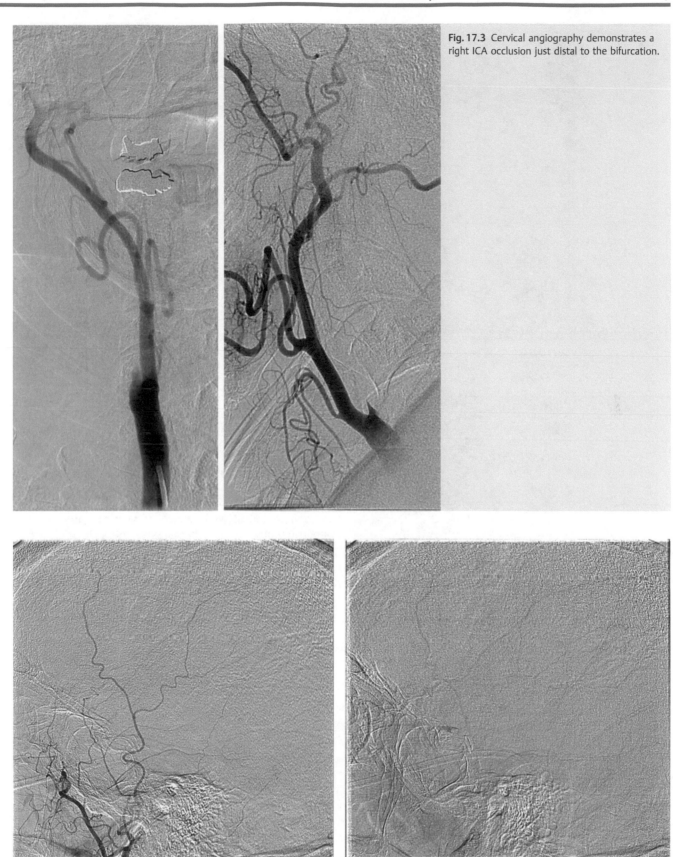

Fig. 17.3 Cervical angiography demonstrates a right ICA occlusion just distal to the bifurcation.

Fig. 17.4 Delayed image from right CCA angiography centered over the head demonstrates a tandem occlusion of the ICA terminus/MCA.

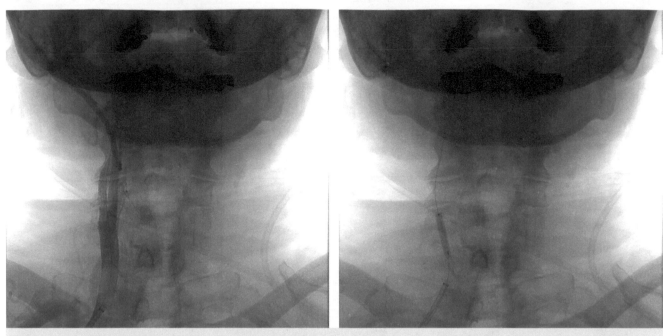

Fig. 17.5 Angioplasty and stenting of ICA origin to preserve patency of the vessel.

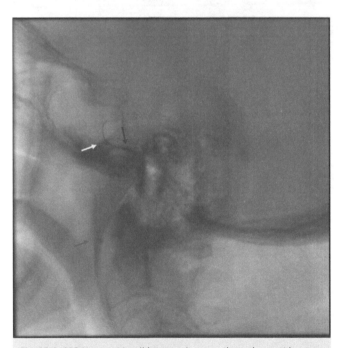

Fig. 17.6 088 Neuron Max (*blue arrow*) access through carotid stent over 3 Max (*red arrow*) and 5 MAX ACE (*yellow arrow*).

efficacy and safety profile of direct aspiration when compared to stent retriever. Importantly, the COMPAS trial, showed significant cost reduction when direct aspiration was used as first line compared to first line stent retriever.

This standardized approach uses a uniform setup for every case. An example of a standardized setup for stroke utilizes a 9-Fr short Pinnacle sheath for femoral access which allows anesthesia to "slave" an arterial line and an 088 Neuron Max with a 5.6-Fr Berenstein insert to navigate into either the ICA or the dominant vertebral artery. The goal is to place the 088

Neuron Max into the petrous ICA or around the C2 vertebral artery turn. This provides a stable platform from which the largest bore aspiration catheter is advanced into the target vessel. For the ICA and MCA M1 segment, a large bore aspiration catheter such as 072 JET7, ACE 068, or 5 MAX ACE catheter over either a 3 MAX or a Velocity microcatheter and a 0.016 Fathom guidewire is utilized. The coaxial system reduces the "ledge effect" of a large bore catheter catching on the ophthalmic artery origin and allows for easier and safer navigation into the carotid terminus or MCA. In many instances, the 5 MAX ACE will advance into the MCA M2 segment. A 4 MAX or a 3 MAX can also be utilized for the MCA M2 segment and distally. The goal is to advance the largest aspiration catheter possible proximal to the clot face and under aspiration slowly advance the catheter distally over the clot 5 to 7 mm. At the distal aspect of the clot, the catheter remains in place for approximately 30 seconds while watching the aspiration tubing. In some instances, the clot will be "ingested" and flow will be seen in the aspiration tubing. If flow is not demonstrated in the aspiration tubing after 90 seconds, the catheter is slowly withdrawn. While removing the catheter, if flow is not seen it is likely that the clot is engaged in the catheter tip and the catheter should be removed while under continuous aspiration. While removing the catheter if the catheter is withdrawn proximal to the clot face and flow is seen in the aspiration tubing, it is possible that either the clot was ingested or the clot was not removed and a follow-up control angiography may be performed at this time to demonstrate vessel patency. When this technique is successful, it eliminates the need to introduce a stent retriever or penumbra separator leading to an overall lower procedure device cost. Direct aspiration thrombectomy utilizing this process can be performed three to five times before utilizing adjunct devices at the operator's discretion.

We found this technique can provide efficient and efficacious revascularization. In a multicenter experience, Turk et al

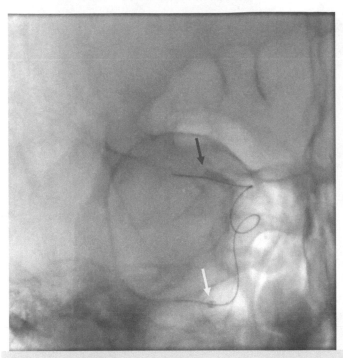

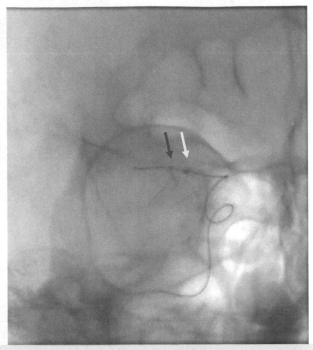

Fig. 17.7 Triaxial support for intracranial access: 088 Neuron max (not visualized) in the distal cervical segment. The 5 MAX ACE (*yellow arrow*) is advanced over the 3 MAX (*red arrow*) and a 0.016-in Fathom wire.

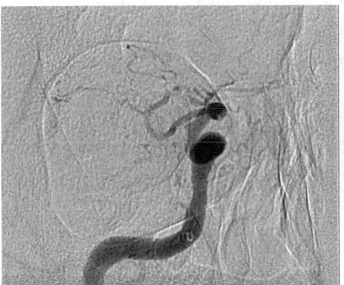

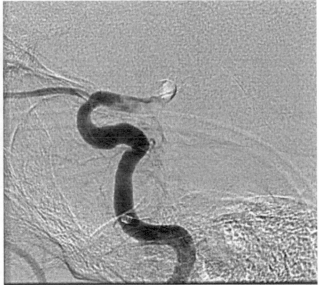

Fig. 17.8 Postangioplasty/stenting of the right ICA demonstrates persistent occlusion of the right ICA communicating segment extending to the MCA.

demonstrated an overall successful revascularization rate (TICI 2b–3) of 95% utilizing direct aspiration and other adjunctive devices when aspiration alone failed; the aspiration component of the ADAPT technique alone was successful in achieving revascularization of the occluded vessel 78% of the time. These rates of revascularization are comparable to those demonstrated in many of the stent retriever studies—STAR (85%), NASA (76%), MR CLEAN, and ESCAPE. Direct aspiration also yielded recanalization in an expedient manner. In a retrospective review of all stroke cases performed at the Medical University of South Carolina, Turk et al demonstrated that with the original penumbra-separator aspiration system the average time to successful recanalization was 87.7 minutes, while utilizing a "Solumbra" technique it was 46.8 minutes ($p < 0.0001$) and with direct aspiration the average time to recanalization was 37.1 minutes ($p < 0.001$); in addition, there were higher rates of final TICI 2b–3 recanalization in the direct aspiration group, 79, 83, and 95%, respectively. The significance of this improved procedure time should not be downplayed, as it is improvement in catheter technology that allows these current generation aspiration catheters to be navigated easily to the intracranial circulation with minimal discomfort to the patient.

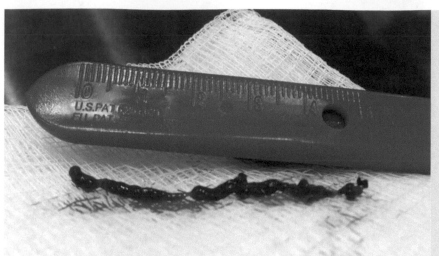

Fig. 17.9 Postaspiration thrombectomy demonstrates removal of 5 cm of thrombus.

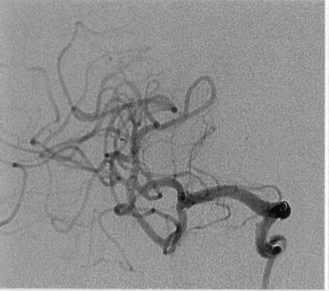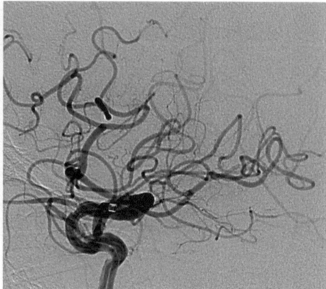

Fig. 17.10 TICI 3 recanalization 30 minutes from groin puncture.

Turk et al demonstrated that the average total cost for patients treated with the ADAPT technique was significantly lower than those patients treated with the penumbra separator system ($p < 0.0001$) and those treated with Solumbra ($p = 0.0008$). The average total cost for these patients when the primary device was successful at achieving TICI 2b or 3 revascularization was $47,673 for the penumbra separator system, $46, 735 for Solumbra, and $31, 716 for direct aspiration ($p = 0.007$). While these approaches overall had similar final TICI 2b or 3 recanalization rate, the direct aspiration group had relatively high rate of primary recanalization with aspiration alone and low need for the use of adjunctive devices which increase the overall cost of the procedure.

Direct aspiration has been shown in multiple single-center experiences to be a cost-effective first-line approach to stroke thrombectomy.

17.1.8 Pearls and Pitfalls

- Use large stable guide sheath: Neuron Max 088.
- Use the largest aspiration catheter possible for target vessel to maximize aspiration forces.
- Use of a coaxial system reduces the "ledge effect" which aids in navigation of the catheters around the ophthalmic turn.
- Slowly advance catheter over clot under aspiration to help ingest or cork clot.

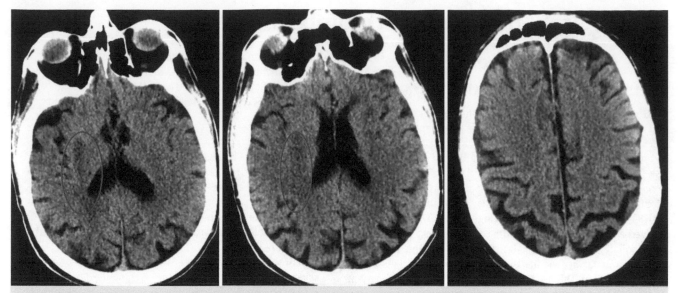

Fig. 17.11 Postoperative day 4 follow-up CT of the head demonstrates small core infarct of putamen, unchanged from initial CT of the head. Patient was discharged at an NIHSS score of 1.

- Procedure maybe repeated three to five times before use of adjunctive devices to help lower overall cost of the procedure.

Further Reading

Turk AS, Turner R, Spiotta A, et al. Comparison of endovascular treatment approaches for acute ischemic stroke: cost effectiveness, technical success, and clinical outcomes. J Neurointerv Surg. 2015; 7(9):666–670

Turk AS, Frei D, Fiorella D, et al. ADAPT FAST study: a direct aspiration first pass technique for acute stroke thrombectomy. J Neurointerv Surg. 2014; 6(4):260–264

Zaidat O, Castonguay A, Gupta R, et al. Post-marketing revascularisation and clinical outcome results as compared to the SWIFT and TREVO-2 clinical trials. Neuro Intervent Surg. 2013; 5:A51

Pereira VM, Gralla J, Davalos A, et al. Prospective, multicenter, single-arm study of mechanical thrombectomy using Solitaire Flow Restoration in acute ischemic stroke. Stroke. 2013; 44(10):2802–2807

Alawieh A, Chatterjee AR, Vargas J, et al. Lessons learned over more than 500 stroke thrombectomies using ADAPT with increasing aspiration catheter size. Neurosurgery. 2018; doi: 10.1093/neuros/nyy444. [Epub ahead of print]

Turk AS, Siddiqui A, Fifi JT, et al. Aspiration thrombectomy versus stent retriever thrombectomy as first-line approach for large vessel occlusion (COMPASS): a multicentre, randomised, open label, blinded outcome, non-inferiority trial. Lancet. 2019; 393(10175):998–1008

Laperge B, Blanc R, Gory B, et al. Effect of Endovascular Contact Aspiration vs Stent Retriever on Revascularization in Patients With Acute Ischemic Stroke and Large Vessel Occlusion: The ASTER Randomized Clinical Trial. JAMA. 2017; 318(5):443–452

18 General Anesthesia in Thrombectomy

18.1 Case Description

18.1.1 Clinical Presentation

A 76-year-old female developed right hemiparesis and aphasia and was last known well at 9:30 p.m. Emergent medical services arrived at her home at 10:30 p.m. and she was transferred to an outside hospital. She had no significant ischemic stroke risk factors and was on a daily dose of 81 mg of aspirin. Intravenous tissue plasminogen activator (IV-tPA) was administered at 11:58 p.m. Her National Institutes of Health Stroke Scale (NIHSS) score was 15. A CT angiography (CTA) of the head showed a left M1 segment middle cerebral artery (MCA) occlusion (collateral score 3, clot burden score 6). She was transferred to our facility via life flight, arriving at the angiography suite at 1:54 a.m. Due to aphasia, agitation, anticipated patient discomfort, and increased procedural complexity from motion artefact, she was rapidly intubated and groin puncture was performed at 2:05a.m. At 2:23 a.m., she was completely revascularized consistent with thrombolysis in cerebral infarction (TICI) 3.

18.1.2 Imaging Workup and Investigations

A noncontrast computed tomography (NCCT) of the brain demonstrated early changes concerning for acute ischemia in the caudate nucleus and putamen. There was no evidence of hemorrhage. CTA demonstrated an occlusion of the mid M1 segment of the left MCA (▶ Fig. 18.1a, b). There was excellent collateralization to the MCA territory (collateral score: 3, clot burden score: 6).

18.1.3 Diagnosis

Left M1 segment MCA occlusion.

18.1.4 Treatment

Due to persistent neurological deficit despite IV-tPA, presentation within a favorable time window (4 hours and 24 minutes from last known well), presence of large vessel occlusion on CTA, and excellent collateral supply to the occluded territory, the patient was deemed an excellent candidate for mechanical thrombectomy.

Initial Management

Full dose IV-tPA was administered at the outside hospital.

Mechanical Thrombectomy

Devices

- 8-Fr short vascular femoral sheath.
- NeuronMax guide catheter (Penumbra).
- Berenstein select catheter (Penumbra).
- 0.035 Glidewire (Terumo).
- Sofia intermediate catheter (MicroVention).
- 0.027 Marksman microcatheter (Medtronic).
- 0.014 Synchro-2 Standard microwire (Stryker).
- 6 × 40 mm Solitaire stent retriever (Medtronic).
- 8-Fr Angio-Seal closure device (St. Jude Medical).

Technique

- The patient was brought into the angiography suite and placed on the table. Her identity was confirmed using two identifiers and a time-out was performed. The patient was intubated simultaneously to prepping and draping of both femoral regions in usual sterile fashion, and an 8-Fr short vascular sheath was placed in the right common femoral artery (CFA).
- A NeuronMax guide catheter was navigated over a Berenstein select catheter and a 0.035 Glidewire and used to selectively catheterize the left internal carotid artery (ICA). In triaxial fashion, a Sofia aspiration catheter was navigated over a 0.027 Marksman microcatheter and a 0.014 Synchro-2 Standard, and used to selectively catheterize the superior division of the left M2 MCA segment (▶ Fig. 18.1c, d).
- Placement was confirmed with a microcatheter run in the left M2. A 6 × 40 mm Solitaire device was introduced and deployed from the M2 to the supraclinoid ICA. After waiting for 5 minutes, the mechanical thrombectomy device was retrieved with aspiration on the Sofia. The device was inspected and an organized thrombus was seen.
- The postthrombectomy run showed complete revascularization (TICI 3). The diagnostic catheter was brought back up and a three-vessel diagnostic angiogram was completed. At the end of the procedure, the diagnostic catheter and NeuronMax were removed and the arteriotomy site was closed with Angio-Seal.

18.1.5 Postprocedure Care/Outcome

The patient was extubated at the end of the procedure. At the time, her right hemiparesis had partially resolved. Her subsequent course in hospital was uneventful. A brain MRI the next day showed infarction in the left basal ganglia without hemorrhagic transformation (▶ Fig. 18.1e, f). She was diagnosed with atrial fibrillation and discharged to rehabilitation on Apixaban. At 90 days she had returned to her baseline functional status and scored 0 on the modified Rankin Scale (mRS) without objective neurological deficit.

18.2 Discussion

Mechanical thrombectomy using modern stroke devices such as stent retrievers and large bore aspiration catheters has proven to be a safe and effective form of treatment for large vessel acute ischemic strokes of the anterior circulation in several recent randomized controlled clinical trials and meta-analyses up to 24 hours from stroke onset.[1,2,3,4,5,6,7,8,9] Mechanical thrombectomy may be performed in an intubated patient under general anesthesia or under conscious sedation without intubation. While general consensus exists about the benefits of

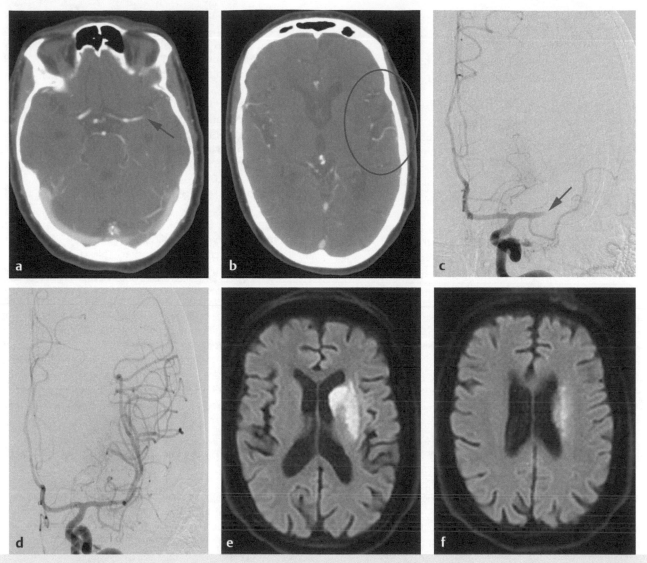

Fig. 18.1 (a,b) CT angiography of the head showing occlusion of the mid M1 segment of the left middle cerebral artery (MCA) (*red arrow*: occlusion; *red cycle*: collaterals distal to the occlusion); (c,d) Digital subtraction angiogram pre- and postthrombectomy with complete recanalization of the left M1 MCA segment (*red arrow*: occlusion); (e,f) Diffusion-weighted MRI of the brain the day after thrombectomy showing infarction of the left basal ganglia.

mechanical thrombectomy, the choice of sedation and airway management remains controversial. The literature reports a significant discrepancy between prospective and retrospective data. While several retrospective studies and meta-analyses of observational studies indicate that conscious sedation may lead to superior functional outcomes,[10,11,12,13] prospective trials failed to show an advantage for conscious sedation over general anesthesia in terms of outcome.[5,14,15,16,17]

18.2.1 Early Retrospective Studies

In 2006, Abou-Chebl et al published a case series reporting on the application of coronary interventional techniques, including stenting and angioplasty, for cerebral large vessel occlusion strokes. Most cases (37/40) were performed under conscious sedation. The remaining three patients received general anesthesia due to deafness, severe agitation, and patient

movement in acute stroke. The authors advocated for conscious sedation, as it may allow for earlier detection of intraprocedural complications.[18] Van den Berg et al performed a retrospective analysis of 348 patients undergoing intra-arterial treatment including mechanical thrombectomy and intra-arterial thrombolysis for large vessel occlusion stroke of the anterior circulation. A total of 278 patients received conscious sedation, while only 70 underwent the procedure under general anesthesia. The authors concluded that patients undergoing conscious sedation were significantly more likely to have good outcomes than patients receiving general anesthesia.[19] However, after adjusting for prespecified prognostic factors, statistical significance was no longer present.

At this point, it has to be considered that retrospective studies are always at risk for selection bias, as severely ill patients with poor prognosis in the first place may be more likely to receive general anesthesia instead of conscious sedation.

18.2.2 Prospective Studies and Randomized Controlled Trials

The Sedation versus Intubation for Endovascular Stroke Treatment (SIESTA) trial, a recent single-center randomized controlled trial conducted in Germany, investigated the improvement of NIHSS 24 hours after intervention as primary outcome parameter. A total of 73 patients were randomized into the general anesthesia group, while a total of 77 were randomized into the conscious sedation group. Eleven (14.3%) patients randomized into the conscious sedation group required conversion to general anesthesia due to severe agitation (7 patients), apnea from sedation bolus,[2] respiratory insufficiency,[1] and direct puncture of ICA.[1]

The study did not find a statistically significant difference in NIHSS improvement between general anesthesia (−3.2 points) and conscious sedation (−3.6 points). Postthrombectomy complications were more frequent in the general anesthesia group for postoperative hypothermia (32.9 vs. 9.1%, $p < 0.01$), delayed extubation (49.3 vs. 6.5%, $p < 0.01$), and pneumonia (13.7 vs. 3.9%, $p < 0.05$). The unadjusted 3-month results showed a higher functional independence among the patients treated with mechanical thrombectomy under general anesthesia versus conscious sedation (37 vs. 18.2%, $p < 0.01$). However, it warrants mention that the SIESTA trial was primarily designed to evaluate short-term outcomes.[15]

Comparable results were reported by Loewhagen et al in a randomized controlled trial named the AnStroke trial,[16] as well as in a non-randomized prospective study by Slezak et al[17] The primary outcome measure of both studies was the mRS 90 days after mechanical thrombectomy. While Slezak at al found that patients receiving general anesthesia had higher NIHSS scores at 24 hours postprocedure (14 vs. 9, $p < 0.01$), and were more prone to develop pneumonia (25.3 vs. 16.5%, $p < 0.05$), the functional outcomes at three months were equivalent. The AnStroke trial described no statistical difference in any of the measured outcome parameters but reported a higher incidence of pneumonia in the general anesthesia group.[16] A recently published post hoc analysis of the Solitaire with the Intention for Thrombectomy as Primary Endovascular Treatment (SWIFT-PRIME) trial focused on the outcomes of different anesthesia techniques used in mechanical thrombectomy. Primary outcomes included 90 days mRS, time to treatment initiation, and rates of successful recanalization. The study reported lower rates of functional independence after 90 days and higher incidence of pneumonia in the general anesthesia group ($p = 0.05$), while successful revascularization rates and the time to treatment initiation were comparable.[3,20] The recent General or Local Anesthesia in Intra-arterial Therapy (GOLIATH) trial investigated the infarct growth on serial MRI 48 to 72 hours after mechanical thrombectomy as primary endpoint. Prior to data collection, authors hypothesized that patients under conscious sedation would have less infarct growth compared to patients undergoing general anesthesia before mechanical thrombectomy. After 72 hours, no statistically significant difference was found ($p = 0.10$). The general anesthesia group had a volume growth of 8.2 mL (2.2–38.6), while the conscious sedation group had a growth rate of 19.4 mL (2.4–79.0). The successful reperfusion rate, on the other hand, was significantly higher in the general anesthesia group (76.9 vs. 60.3%; $p = 0.04$).

Currently, there are several ongoing randomized controlled studies with the aim to compare the outcomes of conscious sedation and general anesthesia. The Sedation versus General Anesthesia for Endovascular Therapy in Acute Ischemic Stroke (SEGA) trial has a planned enrollment of 260 patients. The primary outcome parameter of this study is 90-day mRS. This study is expected to be completed by the end of 2020.[21] Another ongoing randomized controlled trial primarily investigating the 90-day mRS is the General Anesthesia versus Sedation during intra-arterial treatment for Stroke (GASS) trial. This study is enrolling 350 patients with an estimated completion date of December 2019.[22]

The Anesthesia Management in Endovascular Therapy for Ischemic Stroke (AMETIS) trial is primarily assessing neurological outcome at day 90 post–mechanical thrombectomy or serious complication within 7 days postprocedure after general anesthesia versus conscious sedation. This study is enrolling 270 participants and is planned to be completed in January 2020.

The majority of recently published prospective and randomized controlled trials showed comparable outcomes for both anesthesia techniques in terms of 24-hour NIHSS improvement and 90-day functional independence. However, a consistent complication of general anesthesia was the development of pneumonia. While this complication did not appear to affect the overall functional outcomes or mortality of patients, it should be considered when making a decision for a sedation technique.

18.2.3 Meta-analyses

The outcomes of these prospective studies strongly contradict the findings of previous retrospective studies and meta-analyses. Brinjikji et al performed two meta-analyses to evaluate the impact of anesthesia techniques on the outcomes of patients undergoing mechanical thrombectomy for large vessel occlusion strokes. One meta-analysis published in 2015 included nine retrospective studies released between 2010 and 2014 with a total of 1,956 patients, of which 814 received general anesthesia and 1,142 received conscious sedation for mechanical thrombectomy for large vessel occlusion stroke. The results of this meta-analysis indicated that general anesthesia may lead to worse outcomes after mechanical thrombectomy in terms of mortality, respiratory complications, and functional outcomes compared to conscious sedation, while no difference in procedural time was observed.[19] Similar findings were reported by McDonald et al in a meta-analysis showing that in-hospital mortality, pneumonia, hospital costs, and length of stay were also reduced in conscious sedation compared to general anesthesia.[13]

In 2017, Brinjikji et al performed another meta-analysis including 22 articles with 3 randomized controlled trials and 19 observational studies published between 2010 and 2017 including 4,716 patients (1,819 underwent general anesthesia and 2,897 non-general anesthesia). After adjusting for the baseline NIHSS scores, the general anesthesia group was associated with lower odds of good clinical outcome (odds ratio [OR], 0.59; 95% confidence interval [CI], 0.29–0.94). Interestingly, when looking at studies that solely used stent retriever or aspiration techniques instead of stenting and balloon dilation techniques, there was no significant difference in good clinical outcome (OR, 0.84; 95% CI, 0.67–1.06).[23]

18.2.4 Decision Making

Since there are currently no distinct guidelines recommending a specific anesthetic type available, a variety of individual factors should be considered before deciding whether mechanical thrombectomy for acute ischemic stroke of the anterior circulation should be performed under conscious sedation or general anesthesia. Both techniques have their advantages and limitations.

18.2.5 Airway Protection

Major indications for general anesthesia include vomiting, decreased consciousness, agitation, or bulbar dysfunction, such as impaired gag reflex, compromising the airway.[15,24] Although a frequently mentioned concern about general anesthesia is the increased risk of pneumonia,[25] which was apparent in several studies, it did not affect the functional outcome or the overall mortality of patients receiving general anesthesia for mechanical thrombectomy.[15,16,17] In some cases, a conversion from conscious sedation to general anesthesia may be necessary due to increased agitation or intraprocedural complications.[16,17] Aside from delays of procedural time, these conversions always involve the known risks associated with emergent intubation such as airway injury or aspiration.[26,27]

18.2.6 Compliance and Patient Movement

The presence of sensory or global aphasia also warrants special precaution, as compliance of these patients will be compromised due to their impaired ability to understand and follow instructions provided to them during the procedure by the interventionalist.[11] Another argument in favor of general anesthesia is substantial reduction of movement in agitated or noncompliant patients. This can potentially lead to motion artifacts[28] and subsequently to compromised safety, and prolonged interventional procedures. It is hypothesized that head motion during the interventional procedure may increase the risk of vascular injury by vessel perforation, leading to intracranial hemorrhages or dissections.[29,30] To overcome these limitations, Janssen et al advocated for head immobilization using a standard cervical collar during mechanical thrombectomy under conscious sedation.[11]

18.2.7 Time from Symptom Onset to Effective Treatment

Another aspect to consider is the timing from stroke onset until recanalization. It is known that timing is crucial in acute ischemic stroke, as ischemic time is proportional to the loss of functional brain tissue.[31] While this appears to vary among different institutions, some authors report a significant delay if general anesthesia is used.[11,32] On the contrary, several large prospective randomized controlled trials did not show a difference in timing between general anesthesia and conscious sedation.[15,16] In a post hoc analysis of the SIESTA trial, it was found that the time from groin puncture to final angiographic result

was reduced in patients under general anesthesia compared to conscious sedation,[14] possibly due to reduced motion artifact. However, these times may be dependent on the primarily used method at the individual institution. If the anesthesia team and the interventionalists are more experienced in performing endovascular interventions under general anesthesia than under conscious sedation or vice versa, this may influence the time required for these procedures.

18.2.8 Hemodynamic Complications under General Anesthesia

One of the main concerns of general anesthesia during endovascular treatment is the risk of intraprocedural hypotension. Loewhagen et al previously showed that a fall in mean arterial pressure (MAP) of more than 40% is associated to poor neurological outcome.[33] Stead et al described that wide fluctuation of blood pressures within the first hours of a large vessel occlusion stroke are associated with increased 90-day mortality. Furthermore, certain anesthetic gases cause cerebral vasodilation which leads to shunting of blood flow from ischemic areas to unaffected areas of the brain, thus worsening the ischemic damage. This phenomenon has been described as the "reverse Robin Hood syndrome."[34] On the other hand, there are several studies suggesting potential neuroprotective effects of inhaled anesthetics due increased brain tissue pO_2.[35,36] This controversial data on the choice of the right anesthetic agent may be a possible explanation for the heterogeneity among recent randomized controlled trials. The AnStroke trial reported the use of a combination of volatile inhaled and intravenous anesthetic agents,[16] while only intravenous anesthesia was used in the GOLIATH trial.[37] In the study protocol of the SIESTA trial, it was stated that the choice of the anesthetic agent was made individually based on the judgment of the anesthesiologist.[15]

Hypocapnia from hyperventilation during anesthesia leads to cerebral vasoconstriction, compromises the cerebral perfusion, and can facilitate the development of vasospasm in the setting of impaired autoregulation due to large vessel occlusions.[33,38,39] These risks can be overcome by the right choice of anesthetic agents as well as more aggressive management and close monitoring of mean arterial pressure and arterial CO_2. Due to these risk factors, the authors of the AnStroke trial changed their institutional guidelines for hemodynamic management and anesthesia in large vessel occlusion stroke patients. The protocol included close monitoring of blood pressure and CO_2 as well as aggressive management of hypotension and hypocapnia. As a result, a mean arterial pressure of 91 ± 8 mm Hg and normocapnia was achieved in all patients. These changes were reflected by successfully minimized complications in general anesthesia and comparable outcomes to conscious sedation.[16]

18.2.9 Monitoring of Complications

Intraprocedural monitoring of neurological deficits is hypothesized to be another potential benefit of conscious sedation. In an awake patient, a possible embolization may be detected early due to apparent neurological deficits, which could not be observed immediately in an intubated patient under general anesthesia. Early postinterventional complications such as acute vessel occlusion may also be detected earlier in a patient in an alert state after conscious sedation.[38] Therefore, it is recommended to extubate the patient as early as possible, which is also known to reduce the risk of pneumonia.[40]

18.3 Conclusion

Most recent data show equivalent clinical results for both anesthesia techniques, leading to the conclusion that both conscious sedation and general anesthesia are justifiable in patients undergoing mechanical thrombectomy for large vessel occlusion of the anterior circulation. The most recent American Heart Association/American Stroke Association guidelines for the early stroke management recommend that the decision for the right anesthetic technique during mechanical thrombectomy should be made individually, based on patient risk factors, technical feasibility, and clinical characteristics. However, this recommendation is based on moderate evidence, indicating that more randomized controlled trial data are required.[24]

However, since a variety of independent factors are to be considered, the decision for the right sedation method should always be made on an individual basis. While there are certain criteria making general anesthesia necessary, special attention should be paid to the abovementioned caveats in terms of hypocapnia and drops of fluctuations in mean arterial pressure in order to minimize complications and optimize outcomes. When performing a mechanical thrombectomy under conscious sedation, it should also be considered that the procedure exposes the patient to considerable discomfort at the groin puncture site as well as during retraction of the stent retriever. This may not be tolerated by every patient and can lead to increased intraprocedural movement and decreased compliance. Furthermore, the decision for the safest method depends on the priorities and the experience of the interventionalist and the anesthesiologist. The choice for the right sedation method should always be based on individual patient factors such as neurological and mental status, agitation, ability to cooperate, and the need for airway protection. Ultimately, the decision depends on the judgement of the interventionalist and the anesthesiologist to choose the right sedation technique, providing the most comfort and safety for each individual patient.

18.4 Pearls and Pitfalls

- General anesthesia may be considered in patients with severe agitation, complete aphasia, or impaired gag reflex.
- During general anesthesia, special attention should be paid to avoid hypocapnia and hypotension.
- Conscious sedation is helpful for intraprocedural monitoring of complications.
- Substantial patient movement during conscious sedation can be overcome by head immobilization with a standard cervical collar.
- Time from symptom onset to effective treatment is not significantly different in any anesthetic technique and mostly based on physician and institutional experience.
- The ultimate decision for an anesthetic technique should be based on individual patient factors as well as on the confidence of interventionalist and anesthesiologist.

References

[1] Goyal M, Menon BK, van Zwam WH, et al. HERMES Collaborators. Endovascular thrombectomy after large-vessel ischaemic stroke: a meta-analysis of individual patient data from five randomised trials. Lancet. 2016; 387(10029):1723–1731

[2] Jovin TG, Chamorro A, Cobo E, et al. REVASCAT Trial Investigators. Thrombectomy within 8 hours after symptom onset in ischemic stroke. N Engl J Med. 2015; 372(24):2296–2306

[3] Saver JL, Goyal M, Bonafe A, et al. SWIFT PRIME Investigators. Stent-retriever thrombectomy after intravenous t-PA vs. t-PA alone in stroke. N Engl J Med. 2015; 372(24):2285–2295

[4] Campbell BCV, Mitchell PJ, Kleinig TJ, et al. EXTEND-IA Investigators. Endovascular therapy for ischemic stroke with perfusion-imaging selection. N Engl J Med. 2015; 372(11):1009–1018

[5] Ilyas A, Chen C-J, Ding D, et al. Endovascular mechanical thrombectomy for acute ischemic stroke under general anesthesia versus conscious sedation: a systematic review and meta-analysis. World Neurosurg. 2018; 112:e355–e367

[6] Goyal M, Demchuk AM, Menon BK, et al. ESCAPE Trial Investigators. Randomized assessment of rapid endovascular treatment of ischemic stroke. N Engl J Med. 2015; 372(11):1019–1030

[7] Berkhemer OA, Fransen PSS, Beumer D, et al. MR CLEAN Investigators. A randomized trial of intraarterial treatment for acute ischemic stroke. N Engl J Med. 2015; 372(1):11–20

[8] Nogueira RG, Jadhav AP, Haussen DC, et al. DAWN Trial Investigators. Thrombectomy 6 to 24 hours after stroke with a mismatch between deficit and infarct. N Engl J Med. 2018; 378(1):11–21

[9] Albers GW, Marks MP, Kemp S, et al. DEFUSE 3 Investigators. Thrombectomy for stroke at 6 to 16 hours with selection by perfusion imaging. N Engl J Med. 2018; 378(8):708–718

[10] Brinjikji W, Murad MH, Rabinstein AA, Cloft HJ, Lanzino G, Kallmes DF. Conscious sedation versus general anesthesia during endovascular acute ischemic stroke treatment: a systematic review and meta-analysis. AJNR Am J Neuroradiol. 2015; 36(3):525–529

[11] Janssen H, Buchholz G, Killer M, Ertl L, Brückmann H, Lutz J. General anesthesia versus conscious sedation in acute stroke treatment: the importance of head immobilization. Cardiovasc Intervent Radiol. 2016; 39 (9):1239–1244

[12] Abou-Chebl A, Zaidat OO, Castonguay AC, et al. North American SOLITAIRE stent-retriever acute stroke registry: choice of anesthesia and outcomes. Stroke. 2014; 45(5):1396–1401

[13] McDonald JS, Brinjikji W, Rabinstein AA, Cloft HJ, Lanzino G, Kallmes DF. Conscious sedation versus general anaesthesia during mechanical thrombectomy for stroke: a propensity score analysis. J Neurointerv Surg. 2015; 7(11):789–794

[14] Pfaff JAR, Schönenberger S, Nagel S, et al. Effect of general anesthesia versus conscious sedation for stroke thrombectomy on angiographic workflow in a randomized trial: a post hoc analysis of the SIESTA trial. Radiology. 2018; 286 (3):1016–1021

[15] Schönenberger S, Uhlmann L, Hacke W, et al. Effect of conscious sedation vs general anesthesia on early neurological improvement among patients with ischemic stroke undergoing endovascular thrombectomy: a randomized clinical trial. JAMA. 2016; 316(19):1986–1996

[16] Löwhagen Hendén P, Rentzos A, Karlsson J-E, et al. General anesthesia versus conscious sedation for endovascular treatment of acute ischemic stroke: the AnStroke trial (Anesthesia During Stroke). Stroke. 2017; 48(6):1601–1607

[17] Slezak A, Kurmann R, Oppliger L, et al. Impact of anesthesia on the outcome of acute ischemic stroke after endovascular treatment with the solitaire stent retriever. AJNR Am J Neuroradiol. 2017; 38(7):1362–1367

[18] Abou-Chebl A, Krieger DW, Bajzer CT, Yadav JS. Intracranial angioplasty and stenting in the awake patient. J Neuroimaging. 2006; 16(3):216–223

[19] van den Berg LA, Koelman DLH, Berkhemer OA, et al. MR CLEAN Pretrial Study Group, Participating Centers. Type of anesthesia and differences in clinical outcome after intra-arterial treatment for ischemic stroke. Stroke. 2015; 46(5):1257–1262

[20] Eker OF, Saver JL, Goyal M, et al. SWIFT PRIME Investigators. Impact of anesthetic management on safety and outcomes following mechanical thrombectomy for ischemic stroke in SWIFT PRIME cohort. Front Neurol. 2018; 9:702

[21] SEdation Versus General Anesthesia for endovascular therapy in acute ischemic stroke - full text view - ClinicalTrials.gov [Internet]. [cited 2018

Nov 18]. Available at: https://clinicaltrials.gov/ct2/show/NCT03263117. Accessed September 20, 2019

[22] General Anesthesia versus Sedation During Intra-arterial Treatment for Stroke - full text view - ClinicalTrials.gov [Internet]. [cited 2018 Nov 18]. Available at: https://clinicaltrials.gov/ct2/show/NCT02822144. Accessed September 20, 2019

[23] Brinjikji W, Pasternak J, Murad MH, et al. Anesthesia-related outcomes for endovascular stroke revascularization: a systematic review and meta-analysis. Stroke. 2017; 48(10):2784–2791

[24] Powers WJ, Rabinstein AA, Ackerson T, et al. American Heart Association Stroke Council. 2018 guidelines for the early management of patients with acute ischemic stroke: a guideline for healthcare professionals from the American heart association/American stroke association. Stroke. 2018; 49(3): e46–e110

[25] Hassan AE, Chaudhry SA, Zacharatos H, et al. Increased rate of aspiration pneumonia and poor discharge outcome among acute ischemic stroke patients following intubation for endovascular treatment. Neurocrit Care. 2012; 16(2):246–250

[26] Li J, Murphy-Lavoie H, Bugas C, Martinez J, Preston C. Complications of emergency intubation with and without paralysis. Am J Emerg Med. 1999; 17 (2):141–143

[27] Jabre P, Avenel A, Combes X, et al. Morbidity related to emergency endotracheal intubation–a substudy of the KETAmine SEDation trial. Resuscitation. 2011; 82(5):517–522

[28] Rossitti S, Pfister M. 3D Road-mapping in the endovascular treatment of cerebral aneurysms and arteriovenous malformations. Interv Neuroradiol. 2009; 15(3):283–290

[29] Brekenfeld C, Mattle HP, Schroth G. General is better than local anesthesia during endovascular procedures. Stroke. 2010; 41(11):2716–2717

[30] Soize S, Kadziolka K, Estrade L, Serre I, Bakchine S, Pierot L. Mechanical thrombectomy in acute stroke: prospective pilot trial of the solitaire FR

device while under conscious sedation. AJNR Am J Neuroradiol. 2013; 34 (2):360–365

[31] Saver JL. Time is brain–quantified. Stroke. 2006; 37(1):263–266

[32] Li F, Deshaies EM, Singla A, et al. Impact of anesthesia on mortality during endovascular clot removal for acute ischemic stroke. J Neurosurg Anesthesiol. 2014; 26(4):286–290

[33] Löwhagen Hendén P, Rentzos A, Karlsson J-E, et al. Hypotension during endovascular treatment of ischemic stroke is a risk factor for poor neurological outcome. Stroke. 2015; 46(9):2678–2680

[34] Alexandrov AV, Sharma VK, Lao AY, Tsivgoulis G, Malkoff MD, Alexandrov AW. Reversed Robin Hood syndrome in acute ischemic stroke patients. Stroke. 2007; 38(11):3045–3048

[35] Sivasankar C, Stiefel M, Miano TA, et al. Anesthetic variation and potential impact of anesthetics used during endovascular management of acute ischemic stroke. J Neurointerv Surg. 2016; 8(11):1101–1106

[36] Hoffman WE, Charbel FT, Edelman G, Ausman JI. Thiopental and desflurane treatment for brain protection. Neurosurgery. 1998; 43(5):1050–1053

[37] Simonsen CZ, Yoo AJ, Sørensen LH, et al. Effect of general anesthesia and conscious sedation during endovascular therapy on infarct growth and clinical outcomes in acute ischemic stroke: a randomized clinical trial. JAMA Neurol. 2018; 75(4):470–477

[38] Wang A, Abramowicz AE. Role of anesthesia in endovascular stroke therapy. Curr Opin Anaesthesiol. 2017; 30(5):563–569

[39] Takahashi CE, Brambrink AM, Aziz MF, et al. Association of intraprocedural blood pressure and end tidal carbon dioxide with outcome after acute stroke intervention. Neurocrit Care. 2014; 20(2):202–208

[40] Nikoubashman O, Schürmann K, Probst T, et al. clinical impact of ventilation duration in patients with stroke undergoing interventional treatment under general anesthesia: the shorter the better? AJNR Am J Neuroradiol. 2016; 37 (6):1074–1079

19 Conscious Sedation in Thrombectomy

19.1 Case Description

19.1.1 Clinical Presentation

An 80-year-old male presents to the emergency department (ED) at 8 a.m. after waking up with a dense left hemiparesis, left-sided facial droop, and a left hemisensory loss. Although moderately drowsy, he is awake and able to follow basic commands. He was last seen normal at 3 a.m. The patient's National Institutes of Health Stroke Scale (NIHSS) score was 17.

Two days prior to admission, he presented to the ED with left-sided amaurosis fugax. Computed tomography angiography (CTA) at that time demonstrated a new occlusion of the right internal carotid artery (ICA; ▶ Fig. 19.1). He was discharged after a 24-hour observation period with a new prescription for Lovenox.

Past medical history is significant for coronary artery disease, congestive heart failure, atrial fibrillation, hypertension, hyperlipidemia, sleep apnea, and a remote history of nonaneurysmal subarachnoid hemorrhage (SAH).

19.1.2 Imaging Workup and Investigations

- Noncontrast computed tomography (NCCT) of the head demonstrates a hyperdense clot in the right middle cerebral artery (MCA; ▶ Fig. 19.2a).
- CTA demonstrates an occlusive clot in the right M1 (▶ Fig. 19.2b) as well as recanalization of the right ICA consistent with an artery-to-artery embolus (▶ Fig. 19.2c).
- CT perfusion (CTP) demonstrates decreased cerebral blood volume (CBV) isolated to the basal ganglia (▶ Fig. 19.2d) and markedly diminished cerebral blood flow (CBF) in the

entirety of the right MCA territory consistent with a small core and large ischemic penumbra (▶ Fig. 19.2e, f).

19.1.3 Diagnosis

Acute ischemic stroke secondary to right MCA M1 occlusion.

19.1.4 Treatment

Initial Management

- Patient is not a tissue plasminogen activator (tPA) candidate due to time of onset, recent use of anticoagulation, and prior history of SAH.
- Due to the large ischemic penumbra and small infarct core, he was considered a candidate for endovascular recanalization.
- The patient was immediately transferred to the angio suite. Conscious sedation was given in the form of 25 µg of fentanyl and 5 mg of midazolam. No airway support was necessary and the patient was kept on his nasal cannula.

Endovascular Treatment

Material

- Micropuncture set.
- 5-Fr sheath.
- 5-Fr Simmons 2 glide catheter.
- 6-Fr Shuttle.
- Transcend guidewire (0.014 in).
- 5 Max Catheter (5 Fr).
- Rebar 18 (0.021 microcatheter).
- Solitaire 4 × 20 device.
- Penumbra aspiration device.

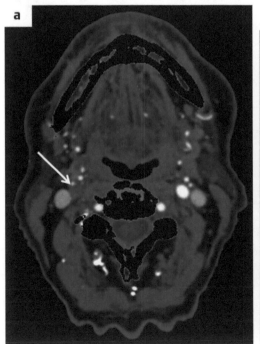

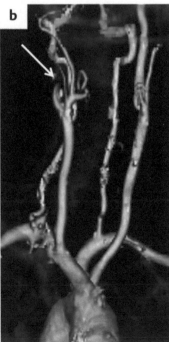

Fig. 19.1 (a) Axial CTA image demonstrates occlusion of the right internal carotid artery (ICA) (*arrow*). (b) 3D reconstructed image demonstrates the occlusion of the right ICA (*arrow*).

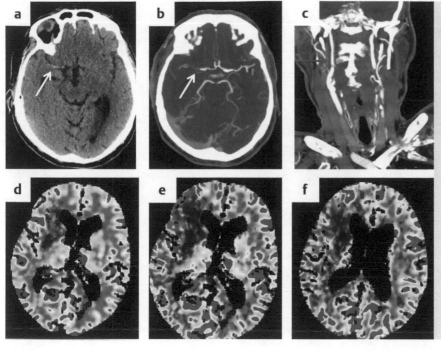

Fig. 19.2 a Noncontrast CT of the head demonstrates a hyperdense MCA (*arrow*). (**b**) CTA demonstrates a thrombus in the right MCA. (**b**) Coronal-reformatted CTA image demonstrates a patent right ICA. Two days prior the right ICA was occluded (▶ Fig. 19.1); thus, this is consistent with an artery-to-artery embolus. (**d**) CT perfusion image CBV map demonstrates decreased CBV in the right basal ganglia. (**e,f**) CBF maps demonstrate decreased CBF in the entirety of the right MCA territory.

Technique

- Micropuncture set was used to access the right common femoral artery (CFA) and a 5-Fr sheath was placed in the right CFA.
- 5-Fr Simmons 2 glide catheter was then placed in the right common carotid artery where digital subtraction angiography was performed. The Simmons catheter was used due to the patient's tortuous aortic arch.
- Angiography demonstrated a patent right ICA and occlusion of the proximal right M1 (▶ Fig. 19.3a, b).
- Using exchange technique, the system was upsized to a 6-Fr Shuttle which was placed in the right ICA. An attempt was made to aspirate the clot with a 5-Max Catheter; however, the catheter could not be advanced.
- The microcatheter tip was advanced to an M2 branch of the right MCA. A 4 × 20 Solitaire device was deployed in the M1 segment. The microcatheter and Solitaire were removed but there was some persistent clot in the M1 segment (▶ Fig. 19.3c).
- As the patient was under conscious sedation, we were able to examine him during the procedure. He was able to move his left arm. However, he suddenly re-lost function in his left upper extremity.
- A second run demonstrated reocclusion of the right MCA (▶ Fig. 19.3d).
- Using coaxial technique, a 5-Max catheter was advanced to the site of the residual thrombus. Aspiration thrombectomy was then performed using the 5-Max catheter to aspirate the remainder of the clot. Final control angiogram demonstrated near-total restoration of flow with thrombolysis in cerebral infarction (TICI) 2b flow (▶ Fig. 19.3e, f).

Outcomes

- At 24 hours, the patient's NIHSS score was 8.
- The patient had some mental status changes 3 days postrecanalization. NCCT of the head demonstrated some increased mass effect and a small punctate hemorrhage in the right basal ganglia.
- Patient was discharged to a rehabilitation unit, and was able to ambulate with a cane and had only trace weakness in his left upper and lower extremities1 month following treatment.

19.2 Companion Case

19.2.1 Clinical Presentation

An 84-year-old man presented to the ED 1 hour after developing a left MCA syndrome. His initial NIHSS score was 25.

19.2.2 Imaging Workup and Investigations

Initial advanced stroke imaging demonstrated no evidence of early ischemic change and a left M1 thrombus. The patient was given intravenous (IV) tPA and brought to the angiography lab for mechanical thrombectomy. The procedure was performed with conscious sedation. Initial angiography confirmed the M1 occlusion, but the image was severely motion degraded (▶ Fig. 19.4) due to agitation and inability to follow commands on account of global aphasia. The patient was given more sedation and was held still, while a 5-Max Ace was used to aspirate the clot with TICI 3 reperfusion achieved in 14 minutes. As seen by the completion angiography (▶ Fig. 19.4), with increased sedation it was possible to keep the patient still; however, he was now too drowsy for reassessment during and straight after the procedure.

19.2.3 Outcome

Patient had a NIHSS score of 0 at 24 hours and only a tiny infarct in the left insula.

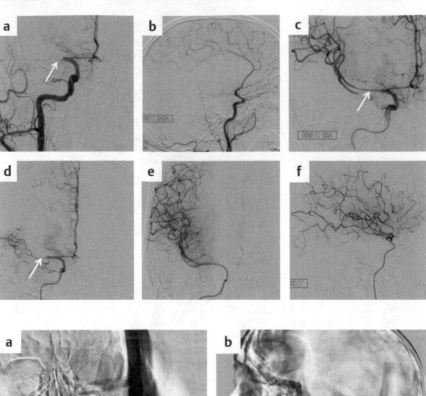

Fig. 19.3 (**a,b**) Right CCA injection demonstrates an occlusion of the right M1 branch (*arrow*). (**c**) Post–stent-retriever deployment image demonstrates partial recanalization of the right M1 occlusion (*arrow*) with filling of MCA branch vessels. (**d**) Second run post–stent-retriever deployment demonstrates persistent thrombus in the right MCA (*arrow*). A 5-Max catheter was then advanced to the site of the thrombus and the clot was aspirated. (**e,f**) Post–suction thrombectomy run demonstrates recanalization of the right MCA with TICI 2B flow.

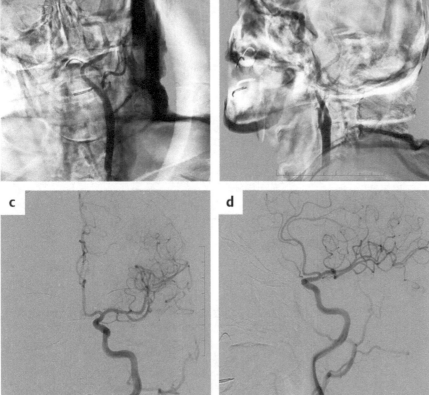

Fig. 19.4 (**a**) AP and (**b**) lateral CCA injections performed once the Neuron Max was navigated into the left CCA. As evidenced by the motion artefact, the patient was moving significantly at the time making the smart mask unusable for navigation. The patient was more heavily sedated while the 5-Max Ace was navigated to the clot face and thromboaspiration was performed. This resulted in good-quality images obtained post attainment of TICI 3 reperfusion (**c,d**).

19.2.4 Case Discussion: Anesthesia Choices in Stroke Intervention

There are a number of challenges in the anesthetic management of patients receiving intra-arterial therapy for acute ischemic stroke. Similar to the patient in the first vignette, stroke patients are generally elderly and suffer from multiple medical comorbidities such as hypertension, coronary artery disease, cardiac arrhythmias, and congestive heart failure. Both the anesthesiologist and neurointerventionalist must consider a number of important factors in deciding how to manage these patients, including choice of anesthetic method (general endotracheal anesthesia versus conscious sedation), ability of the patient to protect his or her airway, ability of the patient to follow commands and stay still, patient volume status and blood pressure management, and intraoperative management of any medical comorbidities such as hyperglycemia or dysrhythmias. Ultimately, decisions regarding the choice of anesthetic agents in patients receiving intra-arterial therapy for acute ischemic stroke should not be taken lightly.[1]

Anesthetic choice for patients receiving endovascular recanalization procedures for treatment of acute ischemic stroke has historically been a topic of great controversy.[2,3,4] Many practitioners view general endotracheal anesthesia as advantageous when compared to conscious sedation due to perceptions that general endotracheal anesthesia eliminates intraoperative movement (seen in the supplementary case performed with conscious sedation), thereby improving procedural safety, intraoperative time, and efficacy.[2]

As stroke intervention requires navigation of microcatheters and microguidewires in the cerebrovasculature, using road map images, accurate superimposition of the live fluoroscopic images on the road map image is essential in ensuring that devices are placed in the correct location. Any degree of patient movement following creation of the road map can negatively affect the ability of the neurointerventionalist to properly navigate the microcatheter and microguidewire. In addition, patient movement could limit the ability of the neurointerventionalist to identify X-ray markers of catheters, mechanical devices, and wires.[2] In the worst case scenario, this could lead to vessel perforation or dissection (see Chapter 36). It is because of perceptions of increased procedural efficiency, efficacy, and safety that general endotracheal anesthesia remains widely used in the intra-arterial treatment of acute ischemic stroke.[5,6]

However, recent evidence has emerged to suggest that, in many cases, the use of general endotracheal anesthesia may be associated with poorer clinical outcomes and lower recanalization rates when compared to conscious sedation or local anesthesia. One meta-analysis of nearly 2,000 patients demonstrated that patients receiving general endotracheal anesthesia encountered higher rates of death, respiratory complications, good neurological outcomes, and recanalization.[7] Many of the major concerns regarding the risks of conscious sedation (i.e., higher risk of wire perforation or vascular injury, risks of intraprocedural intubation, and decreased procedural efficiency) have not been borne out. To date, there is no conclusive evidence demonstrating higher rates of dissection or wire perforation among patients receiving conscious sedation or local anesthesia.[7] Furthermore, there is no conclusive evidence to suggest that there is any difference in procedure length or time to reperfusion among patients receiving general anesthesia or conscious sedation. Finally, while emergent intubation is associated with higher rates of airway trauma, aspiration, and death, the use of this technique among patients receiving conscious sedation for neurointerventional procedures is low.[8]

Conscious sedation has a number of physiologic advantages when compared to general endotracheal anesthesia. First, dynamic cerebral autoregulation is generally preserved with midazolam which results in decreased volatility in intraprocedural cerebral perfusion.[9] Meanwhile, inhaled anesthetic agents, including N_2O and the fluorinated ethers, are associated with a higher risk of cerebral hypoperfusion and are even thought to be neurotoxic. There is evidence to suggest that such general anesthetic agents cause vasodilatation of the nonischemic territories, thus resulting in a steal phenomenon.[9,10] In addition, significant hemodynamic changes are known to occur during the induction and recovery phases of general anesthesia which can compromise cerebral perfusion pressures.[11] General anesthesia is also associated with higher rates of intraprocedural hypotension which can compromise cerebral perfusion pressures.[12] Conscious sedation also allows the team to evaluate the patient while awake in order to monitor for any improvement or worsening of the patient's clinical deficit. In this case, for example, the patient recovered some function when partial recanalization was achieved with the stent retriever, but shortly lost function secondary to reocclusion of the MCA. Finally, general endotracheal anesthesia has been shown to be associated with higher rates of respiratory complications secondary to aspiration and airway trauma.[13]

There are still a number of unanswered questions regarding anesthesia management in patients receiving endovascular treatment for acute ischemic stroke. First, the exact reasons behind the improved outcomes associated with conscious sedation are unknown. As mentioned above, intraprocedural hypotension (defined by some as SBP < 140 mm Hg) is more likely to occur with general anesthesia than conscious sedation.[12] Typically, the target blood pressure range for patients with acute ischemic stroke is 20 to 30% above the patient's baseline pressure.[9] However, there is no evidence to date to suggest that there is any benefit in pharmacologically increasing blood pressure in patients who are hemodynamically stable.[1,9] Managing intraprocedural hypertension is also difficult and typically requires the use of short acting antihypertensives such as sodium nitroprusside or esmolol. Immediate postrecanalization hypertension could result in a higher risk of postprocedure hemorrhage; so, it is important to monitor and manage this in order to avoid this complication. Ideal protocols for fluid management have also yet to be established. In general, patients presenting with acute ischemic stroke are elderly with decreased cardiac reserves, anemic, and often hypovolemic. While hypovolemia is typically thought to be associated with poorer outcomes, aggressive intravenous hydration could result in dramatic lowering of the patient's hematocrit, thus decreasing cerebral oxygen delivery.[1,9]

Ultimately, there is a growing consensus based on a growing body of evidence that conscious sedation is the anesthetic method of choice during endovascular management of acute ischemic stroke patients. However, before each procedure, communication between the neurointerventionalist and anesthesia team is essential in order to determine the ideal management strategy for each patient. There are certainly cases where general anesthesia should be considered, especially in cases where there is a high likelihood that the patient will be agitated and unable to keep still, and in cases where the patient will be unable to maintain his or her airway.

19.2.5 Pearls and Pitfalls

- Conscious sedation is the anesthesia method of choice in managing patients receiving endovascular therapy for acute ischemic stroke, based on evidence suggesting higher rates of recanalization and long-term good neurological outcome.
- General anesthesia is associated with greater fluctuations of hemodynamic parameters, cerebral steal phenomenon from

the ischemic vascular territory, and higher rates of respiratory complications.

- Contraindications to conscious sedation include inability of the patient to maintain his or her airway, and agitation limiting the ability of the patient to hold still during the procedure.

- It is important to keep in mind that patients may not be able to follow commands due to inability to comprehend, which may be the result of receptive or global aphasia from stroke or language barriers.

- Restraints such as straps around the torso, arms and legs, and taping the head can assist in keep a patient still during the procedure.

- Standard projections and knowledge of normal anatomy in these projections allows the operator to navigate through occluded vessels even when the road map is degraded by motion or not available.

References

[1] Lee CZ, Litt L, Hashimoto T, Young WL. Physiologic monitoring and anesthesia considerations in acute ischemic stroke. J Vasc Interv Radiol. 2004; 15(1, Pt 2):S13–S19

[2] Brekenfeld C, Mattle HP, Schroth G. General is better than local anesthesia during endovascular procedures. Stroke. 2010; 41(11):2716–2717

[3] Gupta R. Local is better than general anesthesia during endovascular acute stroke interventions. Stroke. 2010; 41(11):2718–2719

[4] Molina CA, Selim MH. General or local anesthesia during endovascular procedures: sailing quiet in the darkness or fast under a daylight storm. Stroke. 2010; 41(11):2720–2721

[5] McDonagh DL, Olson DM, Kalia JS, Gupta R, Abou-Chebl A, Zaidat OO. Anesthesia and sedation practices among neurointerventionalists during acute ischemic stroke endovascular therapy. Front Neurol. 2010; 1:118

[6] McDonald JS, Brinjikji W, Rabinstein AA, et al. Conscious sedation versus general anesthesia during mechanical thrombectomy for stroke: a propensity score analysis. J Neurointerv Surg. 2014; 7(11):789–794

[7] Brinjikji W, Murad MH, Rabinstein AA, et al. Conscious sedation versus general anesthesia during endovascular acute ischemic stroke treatment: a systematic review and meta-analysis. AJNR Am J Neuroradiol. 2014; 36 (3):525–529

[8] Hassan AE, Akbar U, Chaudhry SA, et al. Rate and prognosis of patients under conscious sedation requiring emergent intubation during neuroendovascular procedures. AJNR Am J Neuroradiol. 2013; 34(7):1375–1379

[9] Lee CZ, Young WL. Anesthesia for endovascular neurosurgery and interventional neuroradiology. Anesthesiol Clin. 2012; 30(2):127–147

[10] Petersen KD, Landsfeldt U, Cold GE, et al. Intracranial pressure and cerebral hemodynamic in patients with cerebral tumors: a randomized prospective study of patients subjected to craniotomy in propofol-fentanyl, isoflurane-fentanyl, or sevoflurane-fentanyl anesthesia. Anesthesiology. 2003; 98 (2):329–336

[11] Rosenberg M, Weaver J. General anesthesia. Anesth Prog. 1991; 38(4–5):172–186

[12] Davis MJ, Menon BK, Baghirzada LB, et al. Calgary Stroke Program. Anesthetic management and outcome in patients during endovascular therapy for acute stroke. Anesthesiology. 2012; 116(2):396–405

[13] Hassan AE, Chaudhry SA, Zacharatos H, et al. Increased rate of aspiration pneumonia and poor discharge outcome among acute ischemic stroke patients following intubation for endovascular treatment. Neurocrit Care. 2012; 16(2):246–250

20 Endovascular Therapy for Patients with an Isolated M2 Occlusion

20.1 Case Description

20.1.1 Clinical Presentation

A 64-year-old female with a past medical history significant for hypertension and idiopathic thrombocytopenic purpura presented to the emergency department (ED) of a thrombectomy capable hospital with global aphasia. National Institutes Health Stroke Scale (NIHSS) score was 4. The patient did not have a definitive last time known well and as such was not eligible for intravenous (IV) thrombolysis.

20.1.2 Imaging Workup and Investigations

- Noncontrast computed tomography (NCCT) performed in the ED demonstrated early left insular changes; her ASPECTS score was 9 (▶ Fig. 20.1).
- CT angiogram (CTA) demonstrated an occlusion of the left middle cerebral artery (MCA)'s proximal inferior division (M2; ▶ Fig. 20.2).

20.1.3 Diagnosis

Left M2 inferior division occlusion with minimal changes on NCCT.

20.1.4 Management

- The patient had no definitive last time known well. As such, the patient was not eligible for IV thrombolysis.
- The patient was taken to the catheterization laboratory for urgent neurointervention.

20.1.5 Endovascular Treatment

Materials

- 6-Fr short vascular access sheath.
- Davis 5 Fr diagnostic catheter.
- 90-cm Neuron Max 88 guide catheter.
- Terumo guidewire.
- Rosen exchange length wire.
- Penumbra ACE 60 reperfusion catheter.
- 3 Max reperfusion catheter.
- Velocity microcatheter.
- Sychro-2 soft microwire.
- Solitaire 4 mm × 40 mm stent retriever.

20.1.6 Technique

- The procedure was performed awake, with minimal conscious sedation. A 6-Fr short sheath was placed in the right groin.
- A 5-Fr Davis diagnostic catheter was used to obtain rapid access to the left common carotid artery. An exchange maneuver was performed over an exchange length Rosen wire, and a 90-cm Neuron Max 88 guide catheter was placed in the proximal left internal carotid artery (ICA).
- The procedure was performed on a monoplane machine. When working with monoplane angiography for acute stroke of the anterior circulation, we found that oblique angiograms allow for optimal navigation of the intracranial vasculature. Furthermore, the oblique view should ideally show the guide catheter in order to detect early guide prolapse.
- Initial oblique angiograms showed a proximal cutoff of the inferior division of the left MCA. Also, there was some non–flow-limiting, catheter-induced spasm. This spasm has in our local experience replicated a mild flow arrest without the use of a balloon guide (▶ Fig. 20.3).
- A velocity microcatheter over a Synchro-2 microwire within an ACE 60 catheter was advanced under fluoroscopic

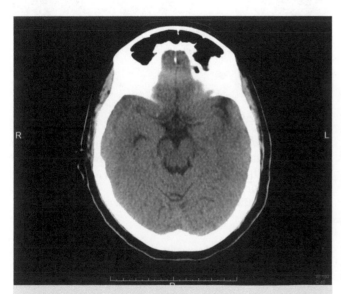

Fig. 20.1 NCCT demonstrating early changes in the left insular cortex.

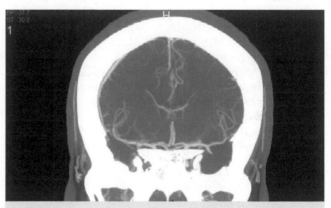

Fig. 20.2 Coronal CTA MIPS showing a left inferior division M2 occlusion.

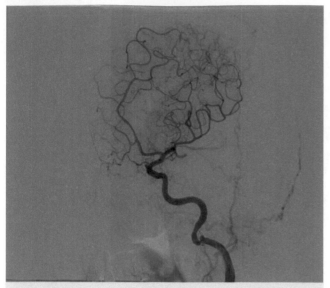

Fig. 20.3 Oblique projection neurointervention on a monoplane machine for ease of navigation in the anterior circulation (and concomitant visualization of the guide catheter). Note the acute left M2 inferior division occlusion, and the catheter-induced spasm in the proximal left ICA.

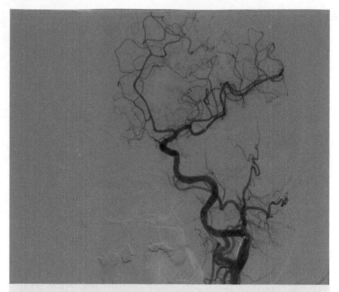

Fig. 20.4 First pass showing reperfusion of the target vessel with persistence of non–flow-limiting thrombus.

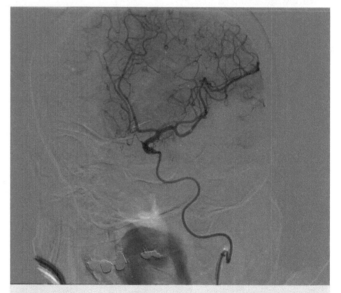

Fig. 20.5 Microcatheter injection via the 3 MAX reperfusion catheter demonstrating persistence of the non–flow-limiting thrombus despite treatment with IV Integrilin.

guidance. The lesion was crossed with the microwire and the velocity placed distal to the lesion.

- The microwire was removed and subtle back bleeding was observed through the microcatheter, indicating a position likely distal to the clot. A Solitaire 4 × 40 stent retriever was deployed and allowed to integrate into the clot for several minutes.
- In order to avoid embolization to new territory, suction was used and the clot was "sandwiched" via the ACE 60 suction catheter to the stent retriever. With suction applied to the Neuron Max 88 via a 60-mL syringe, the construct was removed.
- Repeat angiography in the same oblique plane was performed. This demonstrated reperfusion of the target vessel with a non–flow-limiting amount of thrombus still in the left inferior division M2 (▶ Fig. 20.4).
- At this juncture, we initiated an Integrilin drip of 25% of the cardiac dosage for both bolus and infusion (NYU-BK NIR Integrilin protocol). While the bolus was being administered, a 3 Max suction catheter was prepared and navigated over the Synchro-2 soft microwire.
- Repeat angiography through the 3 Max showed persistence of the nonocclusive thrombus in the target vessel (▶ Fig. 20.5).
- The microwire was reintroduced and a suction thrombectomy was performed in the inferior M2 branch. Repeat angiography showed complete thrombolysis in cerebral infarction (TICI) 3 reperfusion (▶ Fig. 20.6).
- On the table, the patient began to follow commands consistently, while still having an expressive aphasia.

20.1.7 Postprocedural Care

- The patient was transferred to the medical intensive care unit (ICU) for monitoring with every 1-hour neurochecks.
- 12 hours postprocedure, the patient had an NIHSS score of 0, with resolution of her aphasia.
- MRI obtained the next day demonstrated an infarct of the left insular region (▶ Fig. 20.7).

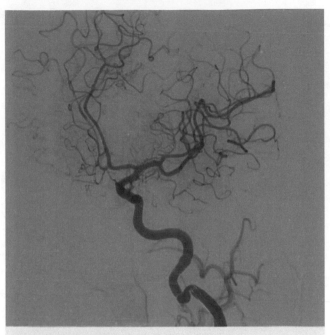

Fig. 20.6 TICI 3 reperfusion of the target vessel.

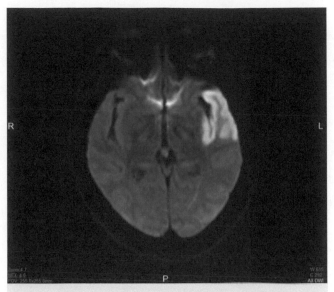

Fig. 20.7 MRI demonstrating left insular diffusion restriction.

20.1.8 Outcome

- Resolution of symptoms with successful thrombectomy.
- Discharged to home with a modified Rankin scale (mRS) score of 0.

20.1.9 Tips and Tricks

- Use of monoplane angiography in thrombectomy capable centers can greatly reduce time to reperfusion, since no time is wasted in transfer.

- On monoplane machines oblique, demagnified views can allow for one plane navigation of the anterior circulation with the ability to monitor the guide catheter for prolapse.
- Local spasm in the proximal ICA can be possibly helpful when not using a balloon guide catheter (in favor of a more navigable device) to create decreased flow during thrombectomy.
- After removal of the microwire, gentle back bleeding in the microcatheter can be highly suggestive in our experience of a location distal to the clot.

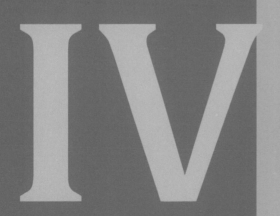

Part IV

Advanced Techniques

IV

21 Percutaneous Radial Arterial Access for Thrombectomy

21.1 Case Description

21.1.1 Clinical Presentation

A 77-year-old male patient presented to the emergency department 45 minutes after sudden onset of vertigo and nausea followed by progressive decreased level of consciousness and coma. At the moment of the clinical examination, the patient was already intubated.

21.1.2 Imaging Workup and Investigations

- Computed tomography angiography (CTA) of arch to vertex and noncontrast computed tomography (NCCT) of brain was immediately performed. CTA of the circle of Willis demonstrated occlusive thrombus in the proximal to midsegment basilar artery (▶ Fig. 21.1). NCCT of the brain showed no signs of hemorrhage (▶ Fig. 21.2).
- CTA at the level of the aortic arch demonstrated a type III aortic arch (▶ Fig. 21.3), as well as moderate tortuosity of the right vertebral artery origin (not demonstrated).

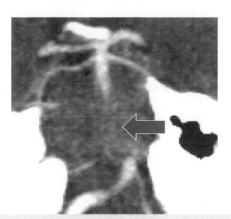

Fig. 21.1 CTA demonstrating complete midbasilar occlusion.

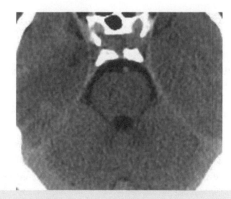

Fig. 21.2 Noncontrast CT confirming absence of intracranial hemorrhage.

21.1.3 Diagnosis

Acute basilar artery thrombosis.

21.1.4 Treatment

The patient was transferred immediately to the neuroangiography suite for an emergency mechanical thrombectomy. Given the difficult arch anatomy and vertebral tortuosity, a right radial access was used.

Materials

- Radial access kit (Terumo Medical, Somerset, NJ).
- Hydrophilic 10-cm 6-Fr vascular sheath (Glidesheath Slender Terumo Medical, Somerset, NJ).
- 5-Fr Berenstein catheter (Performa, Merit Medical, South Jordan, UT).
- Soft-tipped Bentson guidewire (Cook Medical, Bloomington, IN).
- 0.035 Terumo guidewire (Terumo Medical, Somerset, NJ).
- ACE 60 aspiration catheter (Penumbra, Alameda, CA).
- Velocity microcatheter (Penumbra, Alameda, CA).
- Transend microwire (Stryker Neurovascular, Fremont, CA).
- Statseal, Biolife (Sarasota, Florida).
- Safeguard Radial compression device (Merit Medical, South Jordan, UT).

Technique

- Patency of the ulnopalmar arterial arcade was assessed using the modified, bedside Barbeau test.[1] Anesthesia was

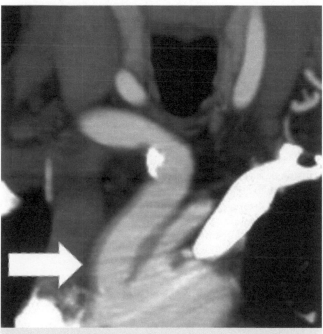

Fig. 21.3 Arch CT angiography demonstrating a type III, which often heralds difficult femoral access.

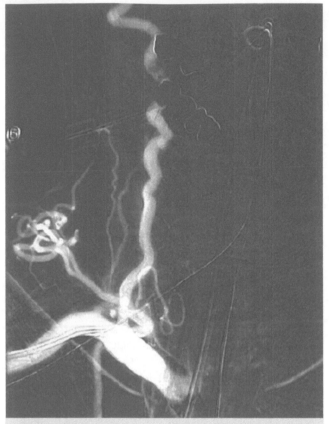

Fig. 21.4 Digital subtraction angiography demonstrating right vertebral artery tortuosity.

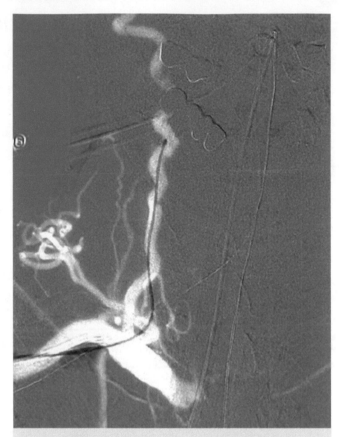

Fig. 21.5 Right vertebral access with a Terumo guidewire and diagnostic catheter.

performed by administering a mixture of lidocaine 1% and 100 µg nitroglycerin into the subcutaneous tissues surrounding the radial artery under ultrasound guidance.

- The radial artery was punctured at 45 degrees, approximately 1 to 2 cm proximal to the wrist crease, with a 22G short bevel micropuncture needle from a radial access kit.
- A guidewire was advanced through the needle, with the wire position confirmed using ultrasound. A hydrophilic 10-cm 6-Fr vascular sheath was then advanced over the wire, without making a skin nick, by removing the guidewire and dilator.
- A 20-mL syringe containing 2.5-mg verapamil, 2,000 international units unfractionated heparin, and 200 µg nitroglycerin was attached to the sheath sidearm with blood aspirated back into the syringe. This admixture of blood and fluid containing the three medications was then slowly instilled back through the sheath intra-arterially over 1 minute to augment local arterial vasodilation and minimize potential arterial spasm and/or thrombosis.
- A 5-Fr Berenstein catheter was advanced through the radial sheath over a soft-tipped Bentson guidewire (Cook Medical, Bloomington, IN). The roadmap confirmed the moderate right vertebral artery tortuosity (▸ Fig. 21.4).
- The right vertebral artery origin was easily passed with a Terumo guidewire and the diagnostic catheter was placed in the distal V2 segment (▸ Fig. 21.5).
- Control angiography confirms the proximal basilar artery occlusion (▸ Fig. 21.6). After an exchange maneuver, a coaxial system of an ACE 60 aspiration catheter and Velocity

microcatheter was advanced over a Transend microwire up to the level of the basilar artery occlusion (▸ Fig. 21.6).
- After one pass of aspiration, there was complete recanalization of the basilar artery with no distal emboli (▸ Fig. 21.7).

21.1.5 Postprocedural Care

- Statseal and Safeguard Radial Compression Device were applied after which the arterial sheath was removed.
- Patent hemostasis was confirmed by compressing the ulnar artery and assessing for radial artery patency using a pulse oximeter, followed by removal of the band after gradual deflation of the balloon tamponade.

21.1.6 Outcome

- After extubation, the patient made a complete recovery (modified Rankin Scale: 0).

21.1.7 Background

Radial artery access has become an established approach for many cardiac interventionalists due to the significant decrease in access site complications and decreased mortality.[2] Since it was first introduced in 1989,[3] the improved time to patient mobilization postprocedure and low incidence of access site complications has made it particularly appealing, especially in

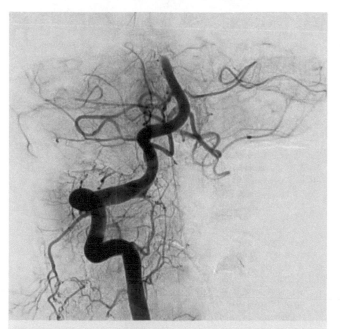

Fig. 21.6 Digital subtraction angiography confirmation of unchanged basilar occlusion.

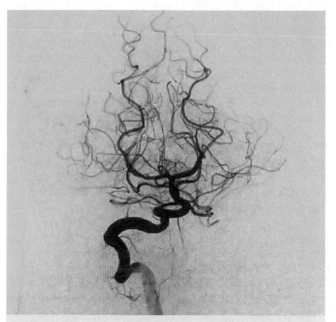

Fig. 21.7 Complete basilar recanalization on digital subtraction angiography.

situations where same-day discharge is preferable.[4] More recently, it has been adopted by many interventional radiology practices.[5] Where posterior fossa intervention is planned, access to the posterior circulation may be facilitated by this technique in the setting of challenging access from a traditional transfemoral arterial route, marked tortuosity of the vertebral arteries (including hostile origin access), or even considered an alternative to "routine" transfemoral route, either due to patient or operator preference.[6] Aortic arch anatomy may be challenging or unfamiliar to navigate from an upper extremity approach, particularly for left vertebral and left common carotid cannulation from right-sided access. This has delayed the adoption of radial artery access for standard diagnostic cerebral catheter angiography. However, difficult arch anatomy and severe abdominal aortic disease may represent a situation where upper extremity access is preferable over a conventional femoral approach.

21.1.8 Discussion

While radial access has been utilized by peripheral interventional radiologists and cardiologists for many years, this practice has not been routinely used or described by many neurointerventionalists. When considering upper extremity access, radial artery access is significantly less challenging and has a lower associated risk than brachial artery access. Madden et al found in their series a 10% complication rate of percutaneous brachial artery access.[7]

Accessing the brachial artery above its bifurcation has a significantly higher complication rate than accessing the radial artery at the wrist.[7] In addition, the radial artery is superficial and never requires surgical cut down or closure. Snelling et al were recently one of the first to describe, in a series of 148 cerebral angiograms, how safety and efficacy can be preserved while transitioning from femoral to transradial approach.[8]

With a less than 1% risk of access site hematoma, radial artery access has a significantly lower risk of access site complications compared to lower extremity (femoral) artery access.[9] This may be especially important in the setting of anticoagulation or in vasculopathic patients in whom thrombolytic medications have been administered.[10] Jolly et al reported a reduction of 73% in major bleeding when radial access was compared to femoral access in a systemic review and meta-analysis of randomized controlled trials.[11] Another advantage of the radial access technique it the optimization of patient positioning postintervention, as patients are not required to stay in a supine position for several hours which is the case in femoral artery access.

Ultrasound of the radial artery is critical to procedure planning. A radial artery diameter of less than 2 mm (measured at the site of proposed puncture after application of topical nitroglycerin) can be accessed provided they are not overstretched by the sheath or catheter. However, we recommend not accessing vessels less than 2 mm during the learning curve, so as to avoid spasm and potential occlusion. Smaller diameter vessels may tolerate smaller sheaths but this may limit the ability to perform certain procedures due to restriction in size of guiding catheters.

Radial artery anatomic variants are extensively described in the cardiology literature. Early and distal divisions of the radial artery are not uncommon. Even with the use of preprocedural ultrasound, small muscular/cutaneous branches will occasionally be encountered when advancing a guidewire without image guidance. This may be particularly problematic if an angled hydrophilic guidewire is utilized in the forearm without fluoroscopy, as these wires tend to be overselective in the forearm. Our practice is to stop advancing the guidewire when resistance is encountered. At our institution, we increase the heparin dose to 5,000 IU in cases where aberrant radial artery bifurcation anatomy is encountered, as these patients have a higher incidence of radial artery thrombosis. However, depending on the clinical indication for the interventional neuroradiologic procedure being performed, this may not be appropriate (i.e., mechanical stroke thrombectomy with/without administration of systemic thrombolytic medication). A radial artery loop is an important variant to be aware of and should be assessed when performing the initial planning ultrasound.[12] In these cases, care must be taken to advance slowly through the loop under fluoroscopic guidance and not advance if resistance is encountered.

The most likely cause of resistance in the radial artery will be arterial spasm, with forceful advancement of the catheter, in this context, risking avulsion of the radial artery.[13] Multiple catheter exchanges will also increase the likelihood of arterial spasm and the interventionalist should remain cognizant of this risk whenever a new catheter is advanced.

Radial artery thrombosis is described as occurring in between 1 and 10% of cases, but in the majority of patients, the intact palmar arch renders this complication of no clinical significance.[11] The implications for future radial catheterization attempts are perhaps more significant, given the frequent lack of clinical symptoms and improved outcomes associated with radial approach.[14],[15] As discussed, this complication can be secondary to aberrant anatomy and may be avoided by administration of a higher heparin dose as well as optimization of local vasodilation. Hemostatic technique is also critical to avoiding thrombosis, and patent hemostasis should be ensured as much as possible during use of the compression band.

21.1.9 Pearls and Pitfalls

- Radial artery access is an alternative to femoral access in case of difficult arch anatomy and/or vessel tortuosity.
- Established technique within the cardiology community, gaining in popularity with body interventionalists.
- No skin nick needed.
- Administration of "cocktail" of 2.5 mg verapamil, 2,000 IU unfractionated heparin, and 200 μg nitroglycerin mixed with autologous blood through the vascular sheath to reduce the risk of vasospasm.
- Being aware of the anatomic variants of the vessels in the forearm.
- Radial access can be used for a variety of interventional neuroradiology procedures.

References

[1] Barbeau GR, Arsenault F, Dugas L, Simard S, Larivière MM. Evaluation of the ulnopalmar arterial arches with pulse oximetry and plethysmography: comparison with the Allen's test in 1010 patients. Am Heart J. 2004; 147 (3):489–493

[2] Valgimigli M, Frigoli E, Leonardi S, et al. MATRIX Investigators. Radial versus femoral access and bivalirudin versus unfractionated heparin in invasively managed patients with acute coronary syndrome (MATRIX): final 1-year results of a multicentre, randomised controlled trial. Lancet. 2018; 392 (10150):835–848

[3] Campeau L. Percutaneous radial artery approach for coronary angiography. Cathet Cardiovasc Diagn. 1989; 16(1):3–7

[4] Jolly SS, Yusuf S, Cairns J, et al. RIVAL Trial Group. Radial versus femoral access for coronary angiography and intervention in patients with acute coronary syndromes (RIVAL): a randomised, parallel group, multicentre trial. Lancet. 2011; 377(9775):1409–1420

[5] Posham R, Biederman DM, Patel RS, et al. Transradial approach for noncoronary interventions: a single-center review of safety and feasibility in the first 1,500 cases. J Vasc Interv Radiol. 2016; 27(2):159–166

[6] Oselkin M, Satti SR, Sundararajan SH, Kung D, Hurst RW, Pukenas BA. Endovascular treatment for acute basilar thrombosis via a transradial approach: initial experience and future considerations. Interv Neuroradiol. 2018; 24(1):64–69

[7] Madden NJ, Calligaro KD, Zheng H, Troutman DA, Dougherty MJ. Outcomes of brachial artery access for endovascular interventions. Ann Vasc Surg. 2019; 56:81–86

[8] Snelling BM, Sur S, Shah SS, Marlow MM, Cohen MG, Peterson EC. Transradial access: lessons learned from cardiology. J Neurointerv Surg. 2018; 10 (5):487–492

[9] Valgimigli M, Gagnor A, Calabró P, et al. MATRIX Investigators. Radial versus femoral access in patients with acute coronary syndromes undergoing invasive management: a randomised multicentre trial. Lancet. 2015; 385 (9986):2465–2476

[10] Kolkailah AA, Alreshq RS, Muhammed AM, Zahran ME, Anas El-Wegoud M, Nabhan AF. Transradial versus transfemoral approach for diagnostic coronary angiography and percutaneous coronary intervention in people with coronary artery disease. Cochrane Database Syst Rev. 2018; 4(4):CD012318

[11] Jolly SS, Amlani S, Hamon M, Yusuf S, Mehta SR. Radial versus femoral access for coronary angiography or intervention and the impact on major bleeding and ischemic events: a systematic review and meta-analysis of randomized trials. Am Heart J. 2009; 157(1):132–140

[12] Charalambous MA, Constantinides SS, Talias MA, Soteriades ES, Christou CP. Repeated transradial catheterization: feasibility, efficacy, and safety. Tex Heart Inst J. 2014; 41(6):575–578

[13] Kristić I, Lukenda J. Radial artery spasm during transradial coronary procedures. J Invasive Cardiol. 2011; 23(12):527–531

[14] Kotowycz MA, Dzavík V. Radial artery patency after transradial catheterization. Circ Cardiovasc Interv. 2012; 5(1):127–133

[15] Gupta S, Nathan S. Radial artery use and reuse. Cardiac Interv Today. 2015 (9):49:56

22 Percutaneous Transcarotid Endovascular Thrombectomy for Acute Ischemic Stroke

22.1 Case Description

22.1.1 Clinical Presentation

An 87-year-old male patient presented to the emergency department with a right hemispheric syndrome consisting of left-sided hemiplegia, left hemineglect, and a forced gaze deviation to the right.

22.1.2 Imaging Workup and Investigations

- Noncontrast computed tomography (NCCT) of the head (► Fig. 22.1) demonstrated a "hyperdense" right middle cerebral artery (MCA) sign, representing a thromboembolic occlusion. Low-attenuation changes, representing evolving perforator infarcts, were seen in the posterior aspect of the right lentiform nucleus as well as the right caudate body. No abnormalities in the right insula, or the remaining right cerebral cortex, were seen (ASPECTS score of 8).
- Computed tomography angiography (CTA) of the arch to vertex confirmed an occlusive thrombus in the right M1 segment, as well as considerable tortuosity of the proximal right common carotid artery (CCA; ► Fig. 22.2).

22.1.3 Diagnosis

Acute right MCA ischemic stroke due to right M1 thromboembolic occlusion.

22.1.4 Treatment

The patient was transferred immediately to the neuroangiography suite for angiography and emergency mechanical thrombectomy. An initial attempt at mechanical thrombectomy was conducted via a conventional right transfemoral arterial approach. Given the marked right common carotid arterial tortuosity, stable deployment of a stent retriever, or positioning of an aspiration catheter, at the level of the thromboembolic occlusion could not be carried out. A percutaneous right common carotid arterial puncture was then performed (► Fig. 22.3).

Materials

- 5-Fr micropuncture kit.
- 6-Fr 45-cm straight Destination sheath (Terumo Medical, Somerset, NJ).
- Rotating Tuohy Borst hemostatic valve (Merit Medical, South Jordan, UT) ACE 68 aspiration catheter (Penumbra, Alameda, CA).
- 3 Max aspiration catheter (Penumbra, Alameda, CA).
- Fathom 16 microwire (Boston Scientific, Fremont, CA).
- Vascular closure device (Angio-Seal, Terumo Medical, Somerset, NJ).

Technique

- Sedation support for the patient was provided on an emergent basis by the anesthesia department.
- Ultrasound of the neck was performed using a high-resolution linear probe (preferably a vascular access "hockey stick" type).
- Percutaneous access to the right CCA was achieved using a 5-Fr micropuncture kit, with puncture done using an approach that avoids passing through the sternocleidomastoid muscle as well as the right internal jugular vein.
- A guidewire was advanced through the needle, and wire position was confirmed by using ultrasound and fluoroscopy. The 2-Fr inner cannula from the micropuncture set was then advanced over the guidewire, and angiography was performed.
- Wire access was directed into the right internal carotid artery (ICA), using the roadmapping technique, with subsequent readvancement of the 5-Fr micropuncture cannula into the right ICA.
- An Amplatz extra stiff guidewire was placed in the right ICA, with removal of the 5-Fr micropuncture cannula, and placement of a 6-Fr 45-cm straight Destination sheath.
- The detachable sheath valve was replaced by a rotating hemostatic valve, with the sheath placed on continuous flush, and sidearm access provided for performing angiography.
- Control angiography confirmed the proximal right MCA occlusion (► Fig. 22.4a). A coaxial system of an ACE 68 aspiration catheter and 3 Max aspiration catheter was advanced over a Fathom 16 microwire to the level of the right M1 occlusion.
- After one pass of aspiration with the ACE 68 aspiration catheter in combination with aspiration on the Destination sheath sidearm, there was complete recanalization of the right MCA (thrombolysis in cerebral infarction [TICI] 3) with no distal emboli (► Fig. 22.4b).

22.1.5 Postprocedure Care

- A 6-Fr vascular closure device was deployed for hemostasis.
- CT of the head was performed immediately following the intervention as well as 24 hours later, showing no procedure-related complications or hemorrhagic transformation of the infarcts.

22.1.6 Outcome

- The patient was significantly better 24 hours postprocedure, with resolution of her fixed gaze deviation, and partial recovery of her left arm and leg strength. At 3 months, she made an excellent recovery with no residual deficits (modified Rankin scale [mRS]: 0).

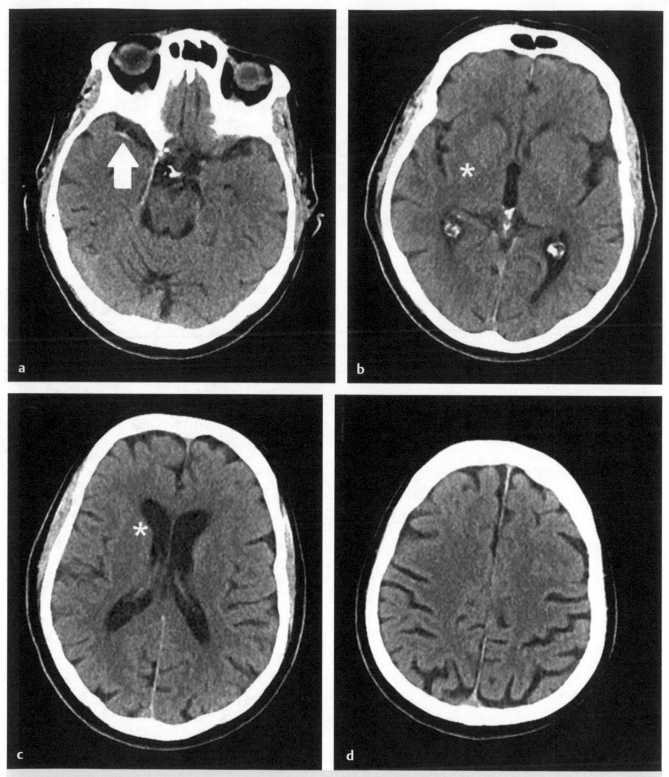

Fig. 22.1 Noncontrast CT of the head in an 87-year-old patient with a right hemispheric syndrome showing (**a**) hyperdense right MCA sign (*white arrow*), (**b**) evolving perforator infarcts in the posterior right lentiform nucleus (*), (**c**) evolving perforator infarcts in the right caudate body (*), and (**d**) no abnormalities in the remaining right cerebral cortex (ASPECTS score of 8).

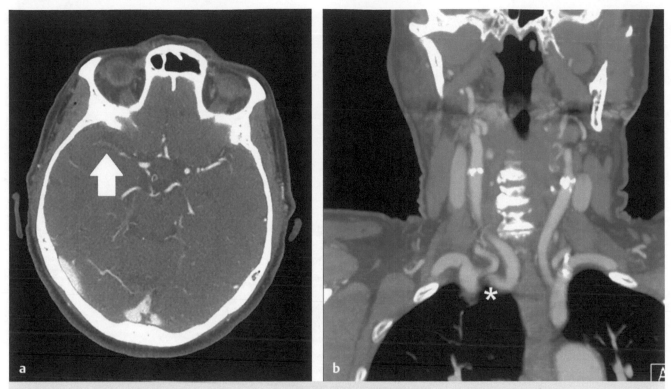

Fig. 22.2 CT angiography arch to vertex in an 87-year-old patient with a right hemispheric syndrome showing (a) occlusive thrombus in the right M1 segment (*white arrow*). (b) Considerable tortuosity of the proximal right common carotid artery (*).

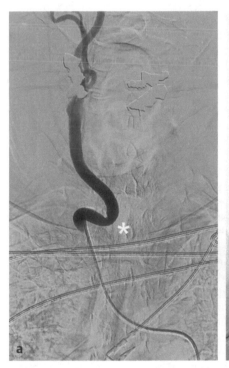
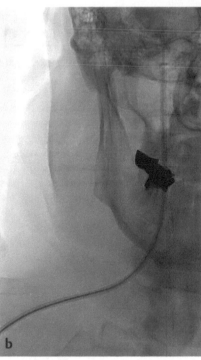

Fig. 22.3 Anteroposterior right common carotid origin angiogram in an 87-year-old patient with a right hemispheric syndrome. (a) Considerable tortuosity of the proximal right common carotid artery (*). (b) Fluoro image of the coaxial ACE 68 aspiration catheter and 3 MAX microcatheter in the internal carotid artery after direct right common carotid artery puncture.

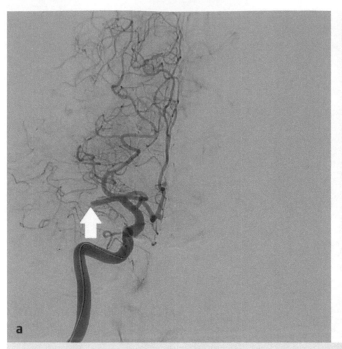 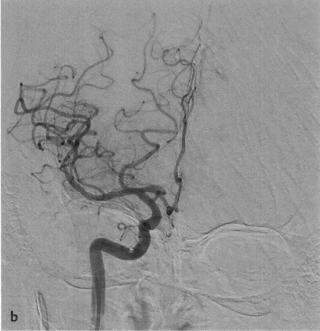

Fig. 22.4 Anteroposterior right internal carotid artery angiography in an 87-year-old patient with a right hemispheric syndrome. **(a)** Occlusive thrombus in the right M1 segment (*white arrow*). **(b)** Complete right MCA recanalization (TICI 3) with no distal emboli.

22.2 Background

Although transfemoral arterial access is almost always the first-line approach for performing mechanical thrombectomy in acute ischemic stroke, situations may arise where this may not be possible or appropriate. Difficult aortic arch anatomy (e.g., type 3), marked tortuosity of the common carotid arteries, severe thoraco-abdominal aortic disease, or aorto-iliac/femoral steno-occlusive disease may represent situations where percutaneous carotid arterial access may be considered over a conventional femoral approach.

22.3 Discussion

The concept of accessing the carotid arterial circulation directly by performing cerebral angiography was first introduced in 1927 by Egas Moniz. However, this approach was eventually replaced by the currently used transfemoral arterial route. For procedures being performed in the cerebral circulation supplied by the carotid arteries, the transfemoral arterial approach offers distinct advantages of very low access site-related complications, ability to catheterize the right or left carotid arterial circulation, and possession of virtually all of the current interventional neuroradiology equipment designed with this access in mind. However, situations may arise where difficult aortic arch anatomy (ex: Type 3), marked tortuosity of the common carotid arteries, severe thoracoabdominal aortic disease, or aortoiliac/femoral steno-occlusive disease is encountered. Percutaneous carotid arterial access may be considered to ensure successful performance of the procedure in question. Blanc et al first published direct cervical arterial access for performing intracranial endovascular treatment in 2006, with Sfyroeras et al publishing their large series of open surgical arteriotomy for transcarotid

stent placement in 2013. Since then, several case reports and case series have been published on percutaneous transcarotid endovascular thrombectomy for acute ischemic stroke. Fjetland and Roy most recently described their experience with seven transcarotid thrombectomy procedures. Reperfusion grading 2b or 3 on the TICI scale was achieved. One patient developed a neck hematoma in need of treatment and two patients died. In the remaining patients, clinical outcome was graded as a mRS score of 3 or less. Despite the relative ease of obtaining access to the carotid arterial circulation using ultrasound guidance, there remain several areas of concern. Patients may be experiencing stroke syndromes which do not permit them to cooperate through their procedure, especially with interventions being considered around the neck region. Although some may be able to undergo the transcarotid procedure without sedation, early consideration to escalated patient support, through monitored anesthesia care, or even endotracheal intubation and general anesthesia, should be given. The choice of sheath placed in the carotid artery is also not standard. Ideally, shorter length sheaths with lumens supporting the use of modern-day aspiration catheters, having hemostatic rotating valves, would be available. Current radial arterial access sheaths, although allowing for larger lumen-to-sheath rations, may kink at their entry point into the carotid circulation due to their thin wall structure. Sheaths with dilators tapering to 0.018 in would allow for smooth transitioning from the initial micropuncture access. A key area of concern is hemostasis following completion of the procedure. Although some authors have advocated for manual compression following removal of the vascular sheath, there remains a risk of sustained hemostasis, especially in the setting of uncooperative patients turning or lifting their heads, or when thrombolytic medications have been administered. Currently, there are no vascular closure devices licensed for use in the carotid region, and all have their shortcomings. Strong consideration should be given to surgical closure of the arteriotomy site, especially during the early days of operators performing this access, or when there is concern that other methods may fail.

22.3.1 Pearls and Pitfalls

- Common carotid artery access is an alternative to femoral access in case of difficult arch anatomy and/or vessel tortuosity, as well as in severe steno-occlusive disease involving the aortoiliac/femoral circulation
- High degree of comfort with ultrasound-guided vascular access is required
- Carotid arterial puncture can be performed using micropuncture technique, taking care to avoid passing through the sternocleidomastoid muscle, with cranial angulation of the puncture to optimize vascular sheath trajectory
- The procedure may require sedation or general anesthetic with endotracheal intubation in order to insure patient cooperation
- Achieving successful hemostasis following vascular sheath removal remains the biggest issue, with a range of techniques used (manual compression, deployment of vascular closure devices not currently indicated for carotid arterial closure, or open surgical closure).

23 Distal Access Catheter Technique without Balloon Assistance

23.1 Case Description

23.1.1 Clinical Presentation

An 80-year-old female with a past medical history of hypertension, diabetes mellitus type II, kidney tumor, atrial fibrillation, and peripheral arterial disease was transferred to the hospital after she became suddenly unresponsive, was unable to speak, and experienced a right-sided weakness. She received tissue plasminogen activator 3 hours following symptom onset.

At presentation, the patient's Glasgow Coma Scale was 6, withdrawing bilaterally to pain, less on the right side, and was not opening her eyes to verbal stimulus. The National Institutes of Health Stroke Scale (NIHSS) score was 19. She was intubated in the emergency department.

23.1.2 Imaging Workup and Investigations

- Noncontrast computed tomography (NCCT), performed at 4 hours 50 minutes, demonstrated no signs of stroke (▶ Fig. 23.1a).
- CT angiography showed suspected left M2 occlusion (▶ Fig. 23.1b).
- Perfusion imaging was not conducted as patient was taken for mechanical thrombectomy.

23.1.3 Diagnosis

Left M2 occlusion in the setting of atrial fibrillation.

23.1.4 Treatment

Initial Management

- Alteplase was administered 3 hours following symptom onset.

Endovascular Management

- The right groin was prepped and draped in the usual sterile manner. Eight-French sheath was placed in the right femoral artery.
- A NeuronMax catheter was placed in the left internal carotid artery (ICA), and target vessel occlusion in the left M2 was confirmed (▶ Fig. 23.2). Sofia plus catheter was placed over the microwire into the proximal left middle cerebral artery.
- A 3-mm Trevo microcatheter was advanced over a 0.014-in microwire and placed past the M2 occlusion.
- The clot was removed in the first pass under aspiration through the Sofia catheter.
- Left ICA digital subtraction angiography demonstrated recanalization of the target M2 occlusion, with complete reperfusion (▶ Fig. 23.3)
- Overall, TICI 3 reperfusion was demonstrated.

23.1.5 Progress

- Postprocedure, the patient was moving all four extremities with mild weakness on the right side. She was extubated on the following day. Aphasia gradually improved and the patient was oriented to herself and to place.
- NCCT at 24 hours showed no signs of acute infraction.

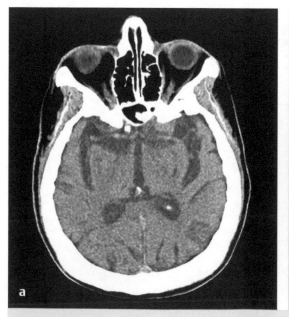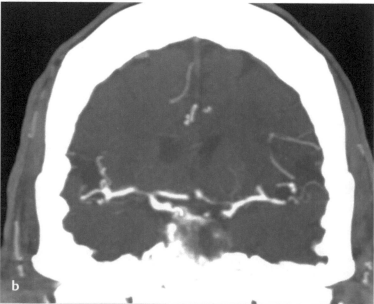

Fig. 23.1 (a) Noncontrast CT showed no ischemic stroke (b), while CT angiography showed signs of left M2 occlusion.

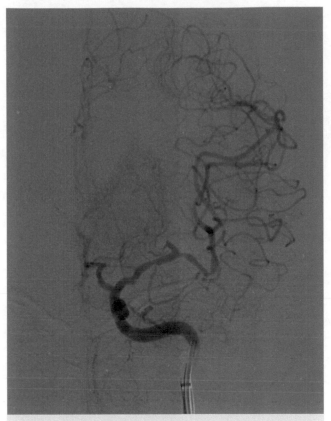

Fig. 23.2 Preprocedure digital subtracted angiography confirmed the presence of complete left M2 occlusion.

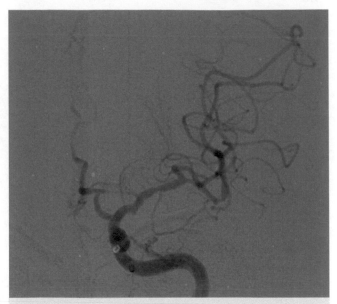

Fig. 23.3 Postprocedure digital subtracted angiography showed complete reperfusion of the previously occluded left M2.

- The patient was started on aspirin 81 mg.
- The patient was discharged to a skilled nursing facility.

23.1.6 Discussion

Mechanical thrombectomy underwent rapid development in the past few years after being proven superior to medical treatment for the management of ischemic stroke. MERCI retriever was one of the first devices to be used for that purpose.[1,2] The distal access catheter (DAC) is the largest catheter that can be easily tracked into an anterior intracranial vessel, such as the M1 or A1 segments. Multiple studies evaluated the utility of DAC in different endovascular procedures, including embolization of cerebral aneurysms, arteriovenous malformation, and mechanical thrombectomy.[1,3,4,5,6,7,8,9,10,11,12,13] The use of DAC during mechanical thrombectomy was originally developed to compliment the MERCI retriever and facilitate faster and safer deployment, distal support, trackability and accessibility to cerebral arterial clots at the time of thrombectomy, with the goal of achieving a higher clot retrieval rate.[3] The principle is to provide distal support to the microcatheter and align the pulling force on the clot in line with the vessel toward the DAC, thereby achieving safer and more effective clot retrieval.

The same concept of distal access with a large-bore catheter was originally provided by aspiration catheters, like the Penumbra, until DACs facilitated the application of a very similar principle to stent retrievers.[14] In our case, a Sofia catheter was used as DAC to facilitate Trevo access for clot retrieval. The advantage of having a large inner lumen and shorter length is to increase the effective flow rate out of the catheter according to the Hagen Poiseuille equation.[3] Kalia et al compared the use of DAC with the largest Penumbra reperfusion catheter. They found that DAC had 1.5 times greater flow when compared to Penumbra, which may be related to the lumen diameter and shorter length of the DAC.[3] Currently, DAC catheters are used alone as aspiration catheters or in conjunction with stent retrievers to improve access to tortuous anatomy or aid retrieval with joint aspiration.

References

[1] Spiotta AM, Chaudry MI, Hui FK, Turner RD, Kellogg RT, Turk AS. Evolution of thrombectomy approaches and devices for acute stroke: a technical review. J Neurointerv Surg. 2015; 7(1):2–7

[2] Smith WS, Sung G, Saver J. Mechanical thrombectomy for acute ischemic stroke: final results of the Multi MERCI trial. Stroke. 2008; 39(4) 1205–1212

[3] Kalia JS, Zaidat OO. Using a distal access catheter in acute stroke intervention with penumbra, merci and gateway. A technical case report. Interv Neuroradiol. 2009; 15(4):421–424

[4] Colby GP, Lin L-M, Huang J, Tamargo RJ, Coon AL. Utilization of the Navien distal intracranial catheter in 78 cases of anterior circulation aneurysm treatment with the Pipeline embolization device. J Neurointerv Surg. 2013; 5 Suppl 3:iii16–iii21

[5] Colby GP, Lin L-M, Xu R, et al. Utilization of a novel, multi-durometer intracranial distal access catheter: nuances and experience in 110 consecutive cases of aneurysm flow diversion. Intervent Neurol. 2017; 6(1–2):90–104

[6] Binning MJ, Yashar P, Orion D, et al. Use of the outreach distal access catheter for microcatheter stabilization during intracranial arteriovenous malformation embolization. AJNR Am J Neuroradiol. 2012; 33(9):E117–E119

[7] Hauck EF, Tawk RG, Karter NS, et al. Use of the outreach distal access catheter as an intracranial platform facilitates coil embolization of select intracranial aneurysms: technical note. J Neurointerv Surg. 2011; 3(2):172–176

[8] Lin L-M, Colby GP, Huang J, Tamargo RJ, Coon AL. Ultra-distal large-bore intracranial access using the hyperflexible Navien distal intracranial catheter for the treatment of cerebrovascular pathologies: a technical note. J Neurointerv Surg. 2014; 6(4):301–307

[9] Janssen H, Killer-Oberpfalzer M, Patzig M, Buchholz G, Lutz J. Ultra-distal access of the M1 segment with the 5 Fr Navien distal access catheter in acute (anterior circulation) stroke: is it safe and efficient? J Neurointerv Surg. 2017; 9(7):650–653

[10] Spiotta AM, Hussain MS, Sivapatham T, et al. The versatile distal access catheter: the Cleveland Clinic experience. Neurosurgery. 2011; 68(6):1677–1686, discussion 1686

[11] Shallwani H, Shakir HJ, Rangel-Castilla L, et al. Safety and efficacy of the Sofia (6f) plus distal access reperfusion catheter in the endovascular treatment of acute ischemic stroke. Neurosurgery. 2018; 82(3):312–321

[12] Mokin M, Waqas M, Nagesh SVS, et al. Assessment of distal access catheter performance during neuroendovascular procedures: measuring force in three-dimensional patient specific phantoms. J Neuro Interventional Surg.. 2018; 11(6):2018–014468

[13] Chartrain AG, Kellner CP, Morey JR, et al. Aspiration thrombectomy with off-label distal access catheters in the distal intracranial vasculature. J Clin Neurosci. 2017; 45:140–145

[14] Lee H-C, Kang D-H, Hwang Y-H, Kim Y-S, Kim Y-W. Forced arterial suction thrombectomy using distal access catheter in acute ischemic stroke. Neurointervention. 2017; 12(1):45–49

Part V

Complex Cases

V

24 Tandem Lesions

24.1 Case Description

24.1.1 Clinical Presentation

A 60-year-old male patient presented to an outside center with severe right hemiparesis, neglect, and speech disturbance. Initial National Institutes of Health Stroke Scale (NIHSS) score was 17. He was transferred as a code stroke to a regional stroke center for further evaluation and treatment. At the time of assessment, he was three hours from symptom onset, with resolution of some symptoms. The NIHSS score improved to 2 and then 0. Past medical history was significant for prior ischemic heart disease with coronary artery bypass graft, hypertension, and dyslipidemia. Medications included aspirin 81 mg daily.

24.1.2 Imaging Workup and Investigations

Noncontrast computed tomography (NCCT) of the brain (▶ Fig. 24.1a, b) demonstrated subtle loss of gray-white matter differentiation in the region of the insular ribbon on left (ASPECTS score of 9). No other early or established ischemic change was seen. There was no evidence of hemorrhage. CT angiography (CTA) performed from the level of the aortic arch demonstrated occlusion of the M1 segment of left middle cerebral artery (MCA) immediately beyond the anterior temporal branch origin with excellent collateralization to the distal MCA territory (▶ Fig. 24.1c, d). There was evidence of atherosclerotic disease in the region of the left carotid bulb, with mixed calcific

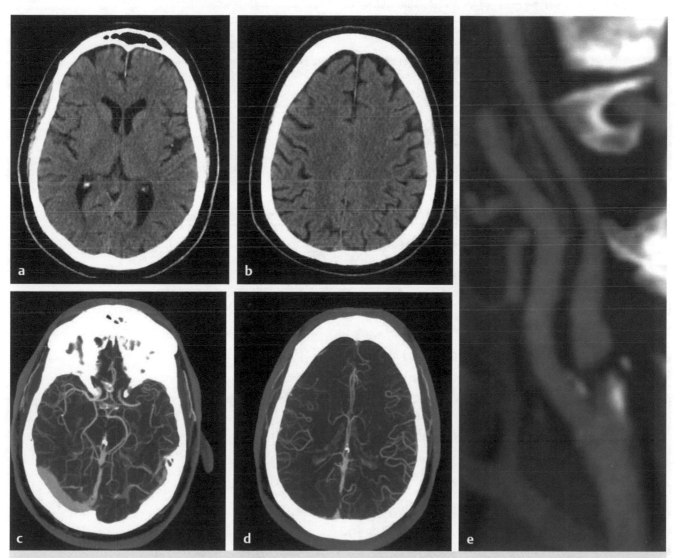

Fig. 24.1 NCCT brain demonstrating subtle loss of gray white matter differentiation in the region of the insular ribbon on left (ASPECTS score 9; a,b). CTA occlusion of the M1 segment of left MCA immediately beyond the anterior temporal branch origin with excellent collateralization to the distal MCA territory (c,d) is depicted. There was evidence of atherosclerotic disease in the region of the left carotid bulb with mixed calcific and soft plaque present and resultant severe, greater than 90%, luminal stenosis (e).

and soft plaque present, and resultant severe, greater than 90%, luminal stenosis (▶ Fig. 24.1e).

CT perfusion demonstrated significant mismatch with prolonged time to peak (TTP) within the left MCA territory (▶ Fig. 24.2a), and preservation of relative cerebral blood volume (rCBV; ▶ Fig. 24.2b).

In light of the presence of tandem disease and the possibility that carotid stenting and antiplatelet medication might be required, an urgent MRI was performed to assess established infarction, as this would help with assessing hemorrhagic risk. Diffusion weighted imaging showed a small area of diffusion restriction involving the left insular ribbon, and in the left frontal deep white matter (▶ Fig. 24.3a, b). T2 gradient echo imaging showed relatively long length of thrombus in the M1 to M2 segment of left MCA (▶ Fig. 24.3c, d).

24.1.3 Diagnosis

Tandem disease: left M1 segment of MCA occlusion, and tandem left internal carotid artery (ICA) severe stenosis.

24.1.4 Treatment

Although the patient had demonstrated significant clinical improvement, there was a concern that, given the CTA findings, he would later deteriorate, and limited available literature for this group of patients suggests they perform poorly in the long-term without treatment. Following discussion with the stroke physician, patient decision was made to proceed with treatment and intervention.

Initial Management

Full-dose intravenous tissue plasminogen activator (IV-tPA) was administered.

Endovascular Treatment

Materials

- 8-Fr short angiographic sheath.
- 8-Fr balloon guide catheter.

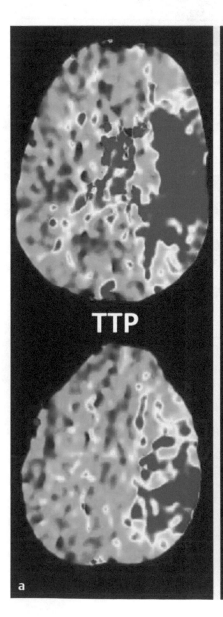
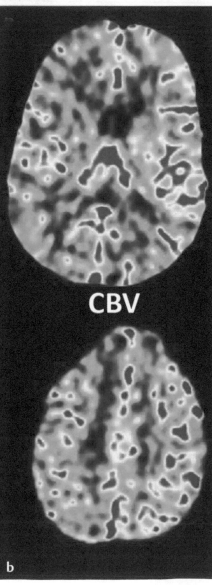

Fig. 24.2 CT perfusion demonstrated significant mismatch with prolonged TTP within the left MCA territory (**a**), and preservation of rCBV (**b**).

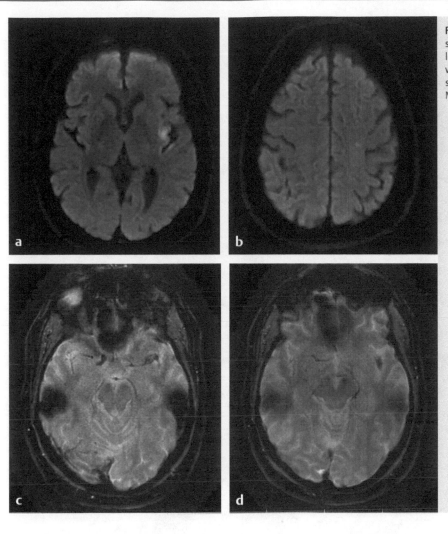

Fig. 24.3 Diffusion weighted imaging showed a small area of diffusion restriction involving the left insular ribbon, and in the left frontal deep white matter (**a,b**). T2 gradient echo imaging showed relatively long length of thrombus in the M1 to M2 segment of left MCA (**c,d**).

- 5-Fr VTK slip catheter.
- 0.035-angled hydrophilic wire.
- Aviator Plus PTA balloon catheter 4 mm × 20 mm.
- Synchro 14 microguidewire.
- 5-Fr H1 slip catheter.
- Trevo 18 microcatheter.
- Trevo XP Provue 4 × 20 mm stent retriever.
- 8-Fr Angioseal closure device

Technique

Intervention was performed with conscious sedation and local anesthetic. A single-wall right common femoral artery (CFA) puncture was performed, and the 8-Fr short vascular access sheath inserted. 2,500 IU heparin was administered intravenously following puncture. The 8-Fr balloon guide catheter was advanced to the left common carotid artery (CCA) over a 5-Fr VTK slip catheter, with the aid of an angled Terumo guidewire using roadmap guidance. Left common carotid angiography confirmed the presence of severe, more than 90% stenosis of the left ICA in the region of the carotid bulb (▶ Fig. 24.4a, b). The caliber of the ICA beyond the occlusion was reduced, suggesting near occlusion. Angiography also confirmed persistent left M1 occlusion (▶ Fig. 24.4c), which was distal to the origin of lenticulostriate perforators and the anterior temporal branch origin. The left anterior cerebral artery (ACA) territory filled normally, and collateralization to the left MCA territory from ACA was seen in the later phases of angiography.

Left CCA angioplasty was performed with the intention of dilating the stenosis to a degree which would allow the guide catheter to pass and mechanical thrombectomy to be performed. A Synchro 14 guidewire was used to cross the left ICA stenosis, and navigated into the ICA beyond the narrowing. Over this, using a rapid exchange maneuver, a 4 mm × 20 mm Aviator Plus PTA balloon catheter was advanced and placed across the stenosis. Gentle balloon angioplasty was performed; the stenosis was purposefully underdilated, and the balloon was underinflated to less than 4 mm diameter. Initial waisting of the balloon, observed at the start of inflation, was no longer evident by the end of the inflation, and control angiogram showed improved caliber at the level of the stenosis to approximately 50% luminal narrowing (▶ Fig. 24.4d, e). This appeared sufficient to allow passage of the guide catheter. An angled 0.038 Terumo guidewire was used to cross the residual stenosis, a 5-Fr H1 slip catheter was advanced over the Terumo, and the 8-Fr balloon guide catheter was then advanced to the level of midcervical ICA over the slip-cath/wire combination. Control angiography showed good antegrade flow in the ICA, with some contrast stasis below the distal end of the guide, presumably as the guide was partially occlusive at the level of the stenosis.

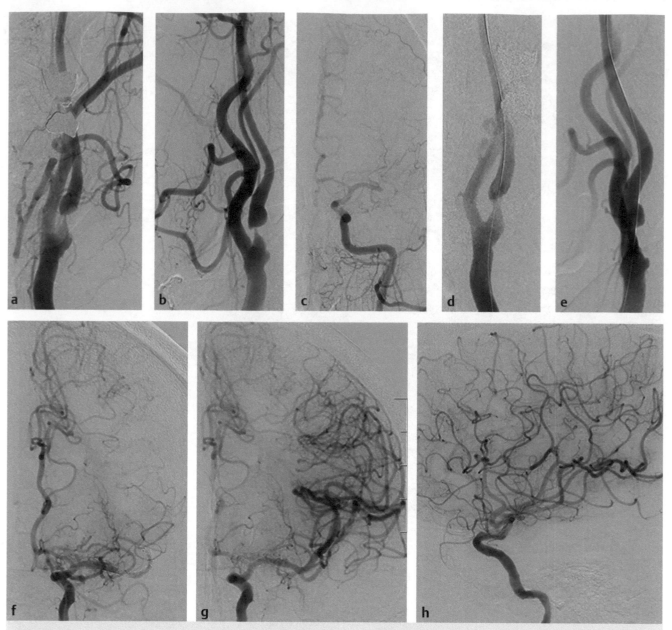

Fig. 24.4 Left common carotid angiography confirmed the presence of severe, > 90% stenosis of the left ICA in the region of the carotid bulb (a,b). Angiography confirmed persistent left M1 occlusion (c), which was distal to the origin of lenticulostriate perforators and the anterior temporal branch origin. DSA control angiogram showed improved caliber at the level of the stenosis to approximately 50% luminal narrowing after angioplasty(d,e). Angiogram with the stent retriever in situ showed some filling of the occluded vessel with filling defects consistent with the thrombus in the stent (f). Following a single pass, the control angiogram showed complete recanalization of the M1 segment and M2 branches and complete reperfusion of the distal MCA territory (g,h).

A Trevo microcatheter was rapidly navigated into the left M1 segment of MCA with the aid of a Synchro 14 guidewire. The wire was advanced through the left M1 thrombus and placed distally in the inferior division M2 branch. A 4 mm × 20 mm Trevo XP Provue stent retriever was then deployed from the inferior division back into the distal M1 segment across the thrombus. Control angiography with the stent retriever in situ showed some filling of the occluded vessel, with filling defects consistent with the thrombus in the stent (► Fig. 24.4f). The stent retriever was left in position for 5 minutes to allow interaction with thrombus before retrieval. Retrieval was performed with flow arrest and continuous manual aspiration through the

8-Fr balloon guide catheter. A long length of clot was retrieved in the Trevo stent. Following this single pass, the control angiogram showed complete recanalization of the M1 segment and M2 branches, and complete reperfusion of the distal MCA territory (► Fig. 24.4g, h).

The synchro wire was advanced through the 8-Fr guide catheter into the left ICA to maintain access across the ICA stenosis and the guide catheter was pulled back into the distal CCA. Control angiography showed that the left ICA remained patent, with approximately 50% residual narrowing at the level of the previously severe stenosis (► Fig. 24.5a, b). As the patient had received full-dose IV-tPA and was on aspirin, a decision

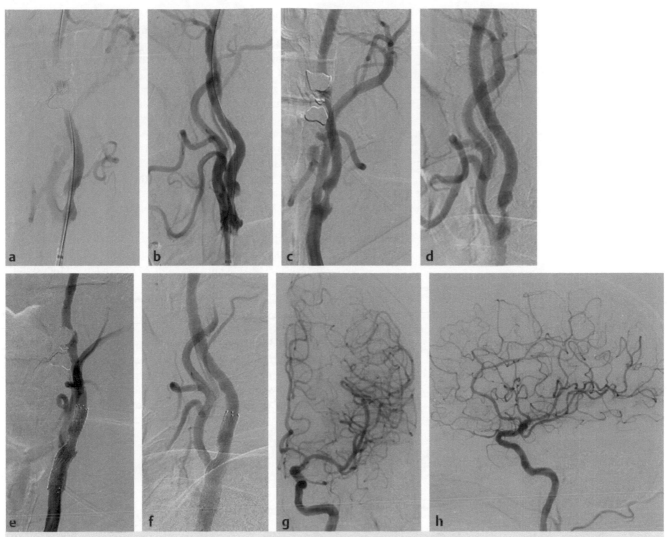

Fig. 24.5 Control angiography showed that the left ICA remained patent, with approximately 50% residual narrowing at the level of the previously severe stenosis (a,b). Angiography confirmed persistent left ICA stenosis involving the carotid bulb, and corresponding to approximately 50% luminal narrowing (c,d). A single balloon inflation was performed with good opening of the stent. Control angiography showed very mild residual narrowing/waisting of the stent at the level of the previous stenosis (e,f). Final control intracranial run demonstrated no evidence of thromboembolic complication (g,h).

was made not to place a stent, as this would require additional antiplatelet therapy in the form of either a Reopro bolus or a loading dose of 300 mg po clopidogrel. Definitive treatment of the ICA (presumably unstable) plaque and residual stenosis was therefore deferred to the non-hyperacute setting. All devices were retrieved. An 8-Fr Angioseal closure device was placed in the right CFA.

Postprocedure Care/Outcome

The patient's clinical condition remained unchanged throughout the procedure, with no change in neurological status pre and postprocedure. In view of the tandem disease and ICA angioplasty, strict blood pressure control was maintained postprocedure for 24 hours, with systolic blood pressure maintained below 140 mm Hg in order to avoid hyperperfusion injury.

The patient remained well. He was loaded with 300 mg clopidogrel on the day following thrombectomy once NCCT

demonstrated no hemorrhage, and was maintained on 75 mg clopidogrel daily thereafter. Aspirin 81 mg daily was continued as well.

On day 3 postthrombectomy, elective stenting of the left ICA was performed. This was performed with conscious sedation and full-systemic heparinization. A 6-Fr 80-cm-long shuttle sheath was advanced to the left CCA. Angiography confirmed persistent left ICA stenosis involving the carotid bulb, corresponding to approximately 50% luminal narrowing (▶ Fig. 24.5c, d), and which appeared similar to the degree of stenosis following M1 thrombectomy and ICA angioplasty 3 days previously. Using roadmap guidance, the ICA stenosis was crossed with an Angioguard RX distal embolic protection device with 6 mm basket. This was deployed in a straight portion of the distal cervical ICA. Using a rapid exchange maneuver, an 8 to 6 mm × 40 mm PROTEGE RX tapered stent was deployed across the stenosis from the level of the distal carotid bulb to CCA. Fluoroscopy showed mild narrowing of the stent at the level of the stenosis. Using a rapid exchange maneuver, poststenting dilatation was performed with a 4 mm × 15 mm Aviator Plus PTA balloon catheter. Prior to performing angioplasty, a bolus of 0.2 mg glycopyrrolate was given intravenously, as prophylaxis against bradycardia/asystole. A single balloon inflation was performed with good opening of the stent. Control angiography showed very mild residual narrowing/waisting of stent at the level of the previous stenosis (▶ Fig. 24.5e, f). The Angioguard distal embolic protection device was retrieved. Final control intracranial run demonstrated no evidence of thromboembolic complication (▶ Fig. 24.5g, h). There were no angiographic features to suggest hyperperfusion of the distal territory. The patient was well postprocedure, with no new neurological deficit, and was discharged home the following day on dual antiplatelet medication.

24.2 Companion Case

24.2.1 Clinical Presentation

A 66-year-old male presented with a 6-hour history of right hemispheric stroke symptoms; his NIHSS score was 9. NCCT of the brain showed hyperdensity of the M1 segment of right MCA (▶ Fig. 24.6a), with occlusion of the right M1 segment on CTA (▶ Fig. 24.6b). The cervical right ICA appeared occluded. There existed evidence of developing ischemic change in the right parietooccipital watershed territory (▶ Fig. 24.7), without early change elsewhere in the right MCA territory. The patient was

outside the time window for intravenous thrombolysis and was brought for endovascular treatment (▶ Fig. 24.6c) Left carotid angiography showed filling of the right ACA across the A Comm, with filling of the right carotid termination, and cut off in the proximal right M1 segment. The right A1 segment was hypoplastic. Late arterial phase of angiography showed leptomeningeal collateralization to the right MCA territory. Right common carotid injection at the level of the carotid bifurcation showed near occlusion of the right ICA. An 8-Fr guide catheter was placed in the right CCA. The stenosis was crossed and a PRECISE stent was deployed in the right carotid. A Rebar 18 microcatheter was then navigated through the ICA and across the right M1 occlusion, and a Solitaire 4 × 20 mm stent was deployed from the right M1 segment of MCA to the supraclinoid ICA. The stent was left in situ for 5 minutes and then retrieved. The guide catheter remained in the right CCA. During retrieval, the Solitaire became entangled in the carotid stent and spontaneously detached. A second PRECISE stent was placed to jail the Solitaire against the carotid wall. Control angiography showed antegrade flow through the right ICA, and demonstrated successful recanalization of the right MCA. There was, however, reduced flow through the stents, with filling defects within the stents suggestive of developing thrombus. Intravenous aspirin had been administered during the procedure, and the patient was loaded with 300 mg Plavix via nasogastric tube. Follow-up CTA 5 days later showed the right CCA was occluded with no contrast opacification of the lumen within the stent. MRI of the brain

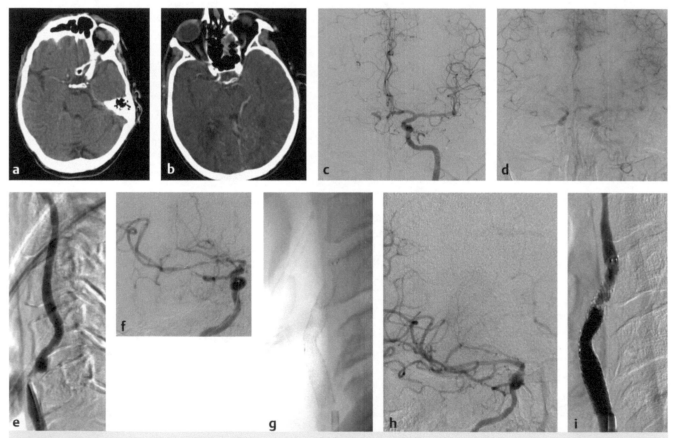

Fig. 24.6 NCCT brain showed hyperdensity of the M1 segment of right MCA (**a**), with occlusion of the right M1 segment on CT angiography (**b**). Narrative DSA images illustrate thrombectomy (▶ Fig. 24.6 [c–i]).

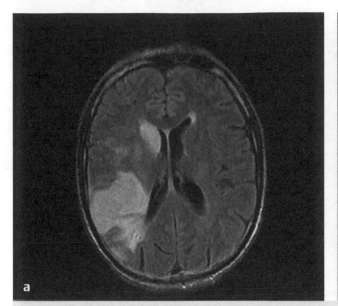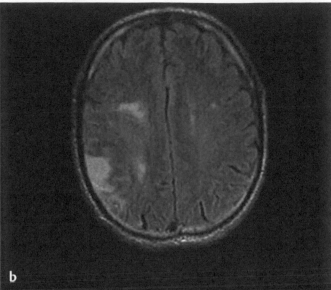

Fig. 24.7 MRI brain showed completion of infarction in the right posterior parietal and temporal region, in the right head of caudate nucleus, and small volume infarcts in the centrum semiovale with preservation otherwise of right MCA territory.

showed completion of infarction in the right posterior parietal and temporal region, right head of caudate nucleus, and small volume infarcts in the centrum semiovale with preservation otherwise of right MCA territory (▶ Fig. 24.7). The patient had demonstrated some on-table improvement at the end of the procedure with improved power in the left upper and lower limb; on day 7, modified Rankin scale (mRS) score was 1, and it was 0 on the 30-day clinical follow-up.

24.2.2 Discussion

Background

ICA stenoses are most commonly atherosclerotic in etiology. Extracranial ICA stenosis accounts for 15 to 25% of ischemic stroke, with an incidence that may be as high as 10% in patients older than 80 years. Ipsilateral high-grade ICA stenosis or occlusion is present in approximately 10 to 20% of patients presenting with acute large vessel occlusion stroke, which further complicates endovascular access and may lead to a delay in recanalization of the target vessel occlusion.

In patients with occlusion of the extracranial carotid artery and intracranial large arteries (tandem occlusions), a favorable outcome largely depends on timely restoration of flow in the occluded ICA, especially in patients with poor collaterals. The presence of an extracranial carotid stenosis or occlusion is a risk factor for poor outcome after interventional stroke treatment. It has been shown in the literature that, if untreated, acutely symptomatic carotid artery occlusion leads to severe neurological morbidity and death in up to 70 and 55% of patients, respectively. Due to high-clot burden and slow-distal flow, occlusion of the ICA combined with distal intracranial occlusion is a predictor of poor response to IV thrombolysis alone, with low rates of recanalization and high rates of unfavorable outcomes.

24.2.3 Workup and Diagnosis

Patient History

In an acute setting, it may be difficult for the neurointerventionalist to gather information regarding relevant medical history expeditiously. This information may already have been obtained by the emergency or neurology department staff. Patients with carotid disease (or their family members) may report a history of prior stroke or transient ischemic attacks, either from thromboemboli or related hypoperfusion of watershed regions. Since atherosclerosis is a systemic disease, a history of coronary artery disease or peripheral vascular disease may also be elicited.

Risk factors contributing to atherosclerotic disease may be present, including smoking, diabetes, hypertension, and hyperlipidemia.

Examination and Investigation

Findings on physical examination in patients presenting with acute stroke will manifest in relation to the ischemic or hypoperfused territory and/or neurologic deficits from previously infarcted territory. A bruit may be heard on auscultation over the cervical ICA.

CTA in the workup of the acute stroke patient should be performed from the level of the aortic arch, allowing assessment of both the extracranial as well as intracranial arterial system. In this way, ICA stenosis will be identified as well as any intracranial arterial occlusion, i.e., it allows identification of "tandem disease." Accurate estimation of the degree of luminal narrowing and characterization of the plaque may be performed with CTA or magnetic resonance angiography (MRA); however, CTA has a higher spatial resolution than MRA and will more reliably depict calcifications. As a modality, CT is usually more accessible than MRI in the acute setting, is quicker to perform, and does not require the extensive patient safety screening of MRI. In addition, MRA occasionally suffers from inability to reliably differentiate slow flow or critical stenosis from a complete occlusion. It should be noted that flow related artifacts are less common with contrast-enhanced than time-of-flight MRA.

In a nonemergency setting, the use of precontrast T1 carotid wall imaging can identify intraplaque hemorrhage which may be helpful in risk stratification of patients regardless of percentage ICA stenosis.

Although advances in noninvasive CTA and MRA imaging have eliminated routine use of digital subtraction angiography (DSA) for carotid stenosis quantification in the nonemergent setting, when endovascular therapy is being considered in the acute setting (e.g., mechanical thrombectomy or carotid angioplasty or stenting), DSA remains the gold standard for measurement of percentage stenosis.

Carotid Doppler ultrasonography is of limited utility in the acute setting. It should be reserved as a screening tool for carotid disease in the nonemergent setting, as it suffers from interoperator variability, artifacts due to calcified atherosclerotic plaques, and difficulties distinguishing pseudo-occlusion from complete occlusion.

24.2.4 Imaging Findings

Noncontrast CT or MRI of the head may demonstrate old or recent embolic infarcts in the territory of the ipsilateral anterior circulation or in the MCA–posterior cerebral artery (PCA) and/or MCA–ACA watershed regions.

CTA from the aortic arch to the vertex of the skull performed as part of the hyperacute stroke workup will demonstrate ICA stenosis as an area of caliber narrowing in the artery. It can also give additional information regarding plaque characteristics, such as allowing differentiation between calcified and non-calcified plaque, and identification of low/"fatty" attenuation within plaque suggestive for lipid rich content. A potential downfall can, however, occur with CTA if the ICA stenosis is adequately severe to limit flow, causing a slow-flow situation. In this setting, contrast passage is delayed, and may give the false impression that the artery is occluded (pseudo-occlusion/false occlusion sign). The potential for "false occlusion" on CTA is an important consideration, as occlusion length has been shown to be an important determinant of the efficacy and complication rates of mechanical thrombectomy. This can be overcome by performing either multiphase CTA or by acquiring a delayed CT following the initial CTA, thereby definitively distinguishing a true ICA occlusion from a severe ICA stenosis.

MRA will also show an area of luminal narrowing; however, MRA can overestimate the degree of stenosis, and will also be affected by delayed passage of contrast through a severely stenosed artery, misleading the reader into thinking the ICA is occluded just beyond the stenosis (i.e., pseudo-occlusion). Performing contrast-enhanced MRA as an arterial followed by delayed phase can overcome this issue.

Patients presenting with acute stroke, and intracranial large artery occlusion with significant ICA stenosis, will demonstrate CT perfusion asymmetry (with elevated time to peak [TTP]/mean transit time [MTT], decreased regional cerebral blood flow [rCBF], and preserved or reduced rCBV) or MR perfusion map asymmetry in the arterial territory distal to the intracranial arterial occlusion, and can also have additional generalized perfusion abnormality in the entire hemisphere. In the absence of an intracranial arterial occlusion, CT perfusion imaging in ICA stenosis can show wedge-shaped areas of perfusion abnormality in the MCA–PCA and/or MCA–ACA watershed territories, with preservation of rCBV if the territory is ischemic, or reduced rCBV if the territory is already infarcted. If there is poor collateralization to the carotid territory, for example, if there is an incomplete circle of Willis, then the perfusion abnormality seen may affect the whole hemisphere in a similar manner.

If an extracranial carotid occlusion is present, no contrast will be seen distal to the occlusion on CTA. The proximal extent of the intracranial and/or extracranial occlusion may be then difficult to determine on CTA, as the slow or stagnant contrast column within the ipsilateral ICA will not opacify the face of the clot.

DSA remains the gold standard in the diagnosis of ICA stenosis or occlusion, and differentiation from pseudo-occlusion. Percentage stenosis should be calculated according to the formula set forth in the North American Symptomatic Carotid Endarterectomy Trial (NASCET): % ICA stenosis = (1 – [narrowest ICA diameter/diameter normal distal cervical ICA]) × 100.

A critical stenosis may be identified by as "string sign" or a small thread of contrast visible within a stenosis, in association with a diffusely and smoothly narrowed caliber of the remainder of the extracranial ICA, due to downregulation. In the setting of a critical stenosis, percentage stenosis calculated using NASCET criteria will be "falsely" lowered due to the smaller caliber of the distal ICA, resulting in a smaller denominator. It is helpful to look at the contralateral extracranial ICA for more accurate estimation of the true ICA diameter.

On DSA, patients with long-standing severe or critical ICA stenosis may demonstrate well-developed pial-pial collaterals in the ACA–MCA and/or MCA–PCA watershed regions of the brain.

24.2.5 Decision-Making Process

The presence of a high-grade stenosis or occlusion of the ICA or vertebral artery (VA) poses a unique challenge in the setting of large vessel occlusion acute ischemic stroke. In these situations, quick and direct access to the intracranial thrombus may not be possible without first addressing the extracranial stenosis/occlusion. Several approaches to this situation may be considered and the appropriate course of action should be determined by the characteristics of the upstream lesion.

High-Grade Stenosis Due to Atherosclerotic Plaque

The diameter inside a high-grade stenosis is usually smaller than the 3 or 4 mm diameter of a stent retriever. In addition, positioning a balloon guide catheter in the ICA for proximal flow arrest and aspiration, or passing a distal access catheter intracranially to allow effective aspiration during clot removal, is very important when using stent retrievers. Therefore, the proximal lesion must be dilated in order to safely and effectively perform a mechanical thrombectomy.

Dilation of the extracranial stenosis can be performed with angioplasty alone, or with carotid stenting with or without angioplasty, or by using the Dotter technique (crossing the stenosis over a wire using an inner dilator placed inside the guide catheter). No strict guidelines or consensus exists with regard to which of these treatment options is superior. Angioplasty alone or angioplasty with stenting should result in an increase in vessel diameter, although stenting will likely to be more efficacious and more durable than angioplasty alone. Use of angioplasty without stenting allows for more rapid access to the intracranial thrombus, and also allows for both carotid endarterectomy and stenting as potential revascularization options after thrombectomy. In addition, placement of a stent requires loading and maintenance doses of antiplatelet agents, which increase the risk of hemorrhagic conversion. At our institution, we prefer, if possible, performing angioplasty alone for tandem disease, and perform either carotid endarterectomy (CEA) or stenting within the next 2 weeks, depending on the indication, patient, and lesion characteristics.

If carotid stenting is performed, a distal embolic protection device should be used if possible. After carotid stenting, the balloon occlusion guide catheter or distal access catheter must be placed beyond the stent for two reasons: inflating a balloon guide catheter in the ICA with flow arrest or performing effective aspiration through an intracranially placed distal access catheter (DAC) increases the chance of successful mechanical thrombectomy when using stent retrievers. In addition, the operator should avoid contact with the carotid stent struts during withdrawal of a deployed stent retriever, as the stent retriever may become entangled in the carotid stent (as shown in the companion case presented here).

High-Grade Stenosis Due to Dissection

Angioplasty of a dissected vessel may worsen or extend the dissection. There is also risk of worsening a dissection injury by crossing a dissection with a microcatheter or guide catheter. It is reasonable in these cases to perform carotid stenting of the dissection first, with or without the placement of a distal embolic protection device. After successful stenting, gentle angioplasty may be necessary to reduce a residual high-grade narrowing and allow an appropriately sized guide catheter to pass beyond the stent.

Tandem Occlusion

No clear consensus exists on the sequence of proximal versus distal revascularization. The advantages of proximal recanalization followed by distal revascularization are improved blood flow to the entire territory and improved collateralization to the territory of the intracranial occlusion. Proximal revascularization also prevents a recurrent occlusion of the intracranial vessels from slow or stagnant flow. It also allows access to the intracranial lesion with larger guide catheters.

A possible advantage of revascularizing the intracranial occlusion, first, would be quicker restoration of cerebral blood flow to the intracranial area by prioritizing treatment of the distal lesion and possibly reducing cerebral ischemia. There should, however, be a route pertaining to collateralization for intracranial filling, for example, through the circle of Willis.

There are case reports which concern the attempts to recanalize the intracranial occlusion across the anterior communicating artery; however, this puts the contralateral hemisphere at risk. In addition, luminal compromise of the anterior communicating artery can further decrease the collateral supply to the occluded vascular territory.

24.2.6 Management

Medication

Medical management of tandem disease in acute ischemic stroke includes blood pressure management to a goal that maintains cerebral perfusion, and volume repletion with IV fluids.

tPA may be given, if the patient presents within 4.5 hours of last seen normal and no contraindications are present.

After groin access and sheath insertion, the patient should be heparinized to a target activated clotting time (ACT) of 250 to 300 seconds or 2 to 2.5 × higher than the baseline ACT. If the patient has recently received IV-tPA, or tPA is still infusing, then either a lower dose (e.g., 2,000–3,000 units) of heparin can be given, or procedure can be performed without heparin, particularly if there is a perceived high risk of hemorrhagic conversion.

For patients in whom carotid stenting is performed, if one is not already on dual-antiplatelet regimen, then he or she should be loaded with aspirin and clopidogrel orally or via an emergently placed nasogastric tube. There are other routes available for aspirin administration which may be preferable in the acute situation, either PR or IV, although intravenous aspirin is not available in some countries. Minimum loading doses should be 300 mg of each.

If balloon angioplasty of the carotid bulb is performed, the patient may be given glycopyrrolate to prevent bradycardia or asystole.

Angioplasty

In most cases, a 0.014-in microwire can be passed beyond the ICA or VA stenosis or occlusion. Gentle angioplasty is performed to, at least, a diameter and that allows safe passage of guide catheter or DAC beyond the stenosis. In the case of an occlusion, the microcatheter is then placed distal to the upstream lesion, and contrast is injected to confirm location and differentiate between a dissection and an atherosclerotic lesion. The microcatheter injection is also helpful in delineating the extent of the lesion, and confirming location within a true lumen prior to mechanical thrombectomy.

Stenting with or without Angioplasty

Rapid stenting of the extracranial stenosis may be performed. The use of distal embolic protection device is left to operator preference but should be used whenever possible. Pre- and/or poststenting balloon angioplasty may be necessary to allow the catheter to cross the stenosis.

As outlined already, if carotid stenting is performed first, then the guide catheter or DAC must be advanced through and beyond the deployed stent to prevent entanglement of the stent retriever during retrieval.

If intracranial thrombectomy is performed first, then the guide or DAC should be advanced beyond the stenosis. This may require angioplasty. Another option may be passage of catheters in a telescoping fashion over a microwire/microcatheter/DAC in order to obtain access beyond the stenosis. Access beyond the stenosis is essential to avoid pulling the open stent retriever through the stenosis, which might result in dissection or loss of thrombus distally. The disadvantage is that, when passed, the distal access or guide catheter may be occlusive in the narrowed lumen.

24.2.7 Postprocedure Care

Groin access site bleeding risk is greater in patients in whom a stent is placed because of several factors such as larger sheath placement, heparinization is not reversed at end of procedure, and dual antiplatelets. If possible, a closure device should be used to achieve hemostasis at the puncture site. 1% Lidocaine with epinephrine may be injected after groin closure if there is bleeding from soft tissues. An external compression device, such as a Femostop device, may be helpful in maintaining hemostasis if closure device fails or cannot be inserted. If a closure device is not used, then consideration can be given to leaving the sheath in situ until tPA/heparin is no longer in the system and then obtaining hemostasis with manual pressure.

Blood pressure management postcarotid stenting and/or angioplasty is critical to preventing hyperperfusion injury and hemorrhagic conversion of infarcted brain tissue. Patients should be managed in a dedicated stroke unit, high-dependency unit (HDU), or intensive care unit (ICU).

24.2.8 Literature Synopsis

Ipsilateral high-grade ICA stenosis is present in approximately 10 to 20% of patients presenting with acute large vessel occlusion stroke. Due to high-clot burden, slow flow, and poor collaterals, patients with tandem disease do not respond well to IV thrombolysis alone, with rates of recanalization as low as 23% and unfavorable outcomes seen in 82 to 100% of patients in the literature.

There are several case reports and series on the use of acute endovascular intervention in tandem occlusion. Recently published cohort studies in the stent-retriever era indicate that tandem occlusions of the ICA and MCA can be treated with acute stenting of the extracranial ICA and stent-retriever mechanical thrombectomy in the MCA or basilar artery with a reasonable risk profile. The recanalization rates in these studies reported [3] TICI 2B distal reperfusion in 61 to 100% of patients. Hemorrhagic conversion of infarcts was seen in 13 to 36% of patients. At 90-day follow-up, 41 to 72% of patients had an mRS score less than 2 and 14% of patients died.

Some of the randomized controlled clinical trials published in 2015 (MR CLEAN, ESCAPE, REVASCAT), showing benefit for mechanical thrombectomy in large artery occlusive stroke, allowed inclusion of patients with proximal cervical carotid stenosis. In addition, all but one trial allowed inclusion of patients with complete atherosclerotic cervical ICA occlusion (SWIFT PRIME). The number of patients with cervical ICA occlusion or stenosis and specifics of management were not consistently reported across all the trials. In the REVASCAT trial, 18.6% of patients had tandem disease, and 9/19 patients with ICA occlusion were stented. In the MR CLEAN trial, 146 (29%) patients with intracranial large artery occlusion also had an additional extracranial ICA stenosis or occlusion. The treatment effect in this subgroup was in favor of thrombectomy (OR: 1.43, 95% CI:

0.78–2.64). In the interventional arm, 30 of 75 patients with carotid stenosis or occlusion underwent carotid artery stenting.

Regarding the use of distal protection devices in the acute situation, Puri et al utilized a distal embolic protection device in 21.4% of large artery occlusive stroke patients with extracranial occlusions. No distal emboli occurred in cases when using a distal protection device (6 patients), whereas distal emboli were seen in 3 of 22 patients (13.7%) treated without a distal protection device.

Although thrombectomy for patients with intracranial large artery occlusion and tandem carotid occlusion/stenosis is indicated by the available data, the optimal management of the underlying carotid disease is not clear. There are several potential advantages and disadvantages for angioplasty and stenting at the time of thrombectomy. Although immediate revascularization may reduce the risk of recurrent stroke, urgent stenting generally requires dual antiplatelet therapy, which is associated with an increased incidence of intracranial hemorrhage. In addition, there is some risk for thromboembolic stroke at the time of stenting. Further studies on the definitive management of symptomatic extracranial carotid stenosis in patients undergoing emergent mechanical thrombectomy are required.

24.2.9 Pearls and Pitfalls

- Tandem pathology is present in approximately 10 to 20% of patients presenting with acute large vessel occlusion stroke, which further complicates endovascular access and may lead to a delay in recanalization of the target vessel occlusion.
- The presence of an extracranial carotid stenosis or occlusion is a risk factor contributing to poor outcome, even when IV thrombolysis is administered.
- Several approaches to the situation may be considered and the appropriate course of action should be determined by the characteristics of the upstream lesion (stenosis, occlusion, presence of a dissection). No clear consensus exists on the sequence of proximal extracranial versus distal intracranial revascularization.
- Recently published cohort studies in the stent-retriever era indicate that tandem occlusions of the ICA and MCA can be treated with acute stenting of the extracranial ICA and stent-retriever mechanical thrombectomy in the MCA with a reasonable risk profile. Further evaluation of these treatment strategies is warranted.

Further Readings

[1] Grau AJ, Weimar C, Buggle F, et al. Risk factors, outcome, and treatment in subtypes of ischemic stroke: the German stroke data bank. Stroke. 2001; 32 (11):2559–2566
[2] Rubiera M, Ribo M, Delgado-Mederos R, et al. Tandem internal carotid artery/middle cerebral artery occlusion: an independent predictor of poor outcome after systemic thrombolysis. Stroke. 2006; 37(9):2301–2305
[3] Endo S, Kuwayama N, Hirashima Y, Akai T, Nishijima M, Takaku A. Results of urgent thrombolysis in patients with major stroke and atherothrombotic occlusion of the cervical internal carotid artery. AJNR Am J Neuroradiol. 1998; 19(6):1169–1175
[4] Berkhemer OA, Fransen PS, Beumer D, et al. MR CLEAN Investigators. A randomized trial of intraarterial treatment for acute ischemic stroke. N Engl J Med. 2015; 372(1):11–20
[5] Vagal AS, Khatri P, Broderick JP, Tomsick TA, Yeatts SD, Eckman MH. Time to angiographic reperfusion in acute ischemic stroke: decision analysis. Stroke. 2014; 45(12):3625–3630

[6] Cohen JE, Gomori JM, Rajz G, Itshayek E, Eichel R, Leker RR. Extracranial carotid artery stenting followed by intracranial stent-based thrombectomy for acute tandem occlusive disease. J Neurointerv Surg. 2015; 7(6):412–417

[7] Maurer CJ, Joachimski F, Berlis A. Two in one: endovascular treatment of acute tandem occlusions in the anterior circulation. Clin Neuroradiol. 2014; 25(4)–397–402

[8] Lescher S, Czeppan K, Porto L, Singer OC, Berkefeld J. Acute stroke and obstruction of the extracranial carotid artery combined with intracranial tandem occlusion: results of interventional revascularization. Cardiovasc Intervent Radiol. 2015; 38(2):304–313

[9] Dababneh H, Bashir A, Hussain M, et al. Endovascular treatment of tandem internal carotid and middle cerebral artery occlusions. J Vasc Interv Neurol. 2014; 7(4):26–31

[10] Stampfl S, Ringleb PA, Möhlenbruch M, et al. Emergency cervical internal carotid artery stenting in combination with intracranial thrombectomy in acute stroke. AJNR Am J Neuroradiol. 2014; 35(4):741–746

[11] Puri AS, Kühn AL, Kwon HJ, et al. Endovascular treatment of tandem vascular occlusions in acute ischemic stroke. J Neurointerv Surg. 2015; 7(3):158–163

[12] Papanagiotou P, Roth C, Walter S, et al. Carotid artery stenting in acute stroke. J Am Coll Cardiol. 2011; 58(23):2363–2369

[13] Spiotta AM, Lena J, Vargas J, et al. Proximal to distal approach in the treatment of tandem occlusions causing an acute stroke. J Neurointerv Surg. 2015; 7(3):164–169

[14] Khatri P, Yeatts SD, Mazighi M, et al. IMS III Trialists. Time to angiographic reperfusion and clinical outcome after acute ischaemic stroke: an analysis of data from the Interventional Management of Stroke (IMS III) phase 3 trial. Lancet Neurol. 2014; 13(6):567–574

[15] Jovin TG, Chamorro A, Cobo E, et al. REVASCAT Trial Investigators. Thrombectomy within 8 hours after symptom onset in ischemic stroke. N Engl J Med. 2015; 372(24):2296–2306

25 Pseudo-occlusion

25.1 Case Description

25.1.1 Clinical Presentation

A 59-year-old female was transferred to our regional stroke center with a 90-minute history of sudden onset aphasia, right hemiplegia, and neglect. National Institutes of Health Stroke Scale (NIHSS) score was 28. She had known atrial fibrillation, and anticoagulation was on hold in view of a recent surgical procedure. In addition to the history of atrial fibrillation comorbidities included hypertension, which was controlled on medication. There were no other cardiovascular risk factors.

25.1.2 Imaging Workup and Investigations

Noncontrast enhanced computed tomography (NCCT) of the brain (▶ Fig. 25.1a) demonstrated some loss of gray-white matter differentiation in the left lentiform nucleus and insular region. Elsewhere, the gray-white matter differentiation was preserved. There was hyperdensity which was consistent with thrombus in the left carotid termination and proximal middle cerebral artery (MCA; ▶ Fig. 25.1b).

Computed tomography angiography (CTA), single-phase study performed from the level of the aortic arch, showed filling of the left common carotid artery (CCA), and very proximal left internal carotid artery (ICA; ▶ Fig. 25.1c, d). There was, however, no contrast opacification of the left ICA beyond the level of the carotid bulb (▶ Fig. 25.1e). The same applied to the left intracranial ICA, ICA termination, and M1 segment of MCA (▶ Fig. 25.1f–h). The left A1 segment and more distal left anterior cerebral artery (ACA) appeared patent on CTA. Left MCA branches in the sylvian fissure filled through leptomeningeal collaterals (not shown). Subsequent catheter angiogram performed for purposes of endovascular stroke treatment showed that the left cervical and proximal intracranial ICA was, in fact, patent; injection of the left cervical ICA demonstrated slow filling of the ICA to the level of the supraclinoid segment where there was abrupt "cut-off" of contrast filling in keeping with left carotid terminus occlusion (▶ Fig. 25.2a–d).

25.1.3 Diagnosis

Left cervical and proximal intracranial ICA "pseudo-occlusion" in the setting of left carotid terminus occlusion.

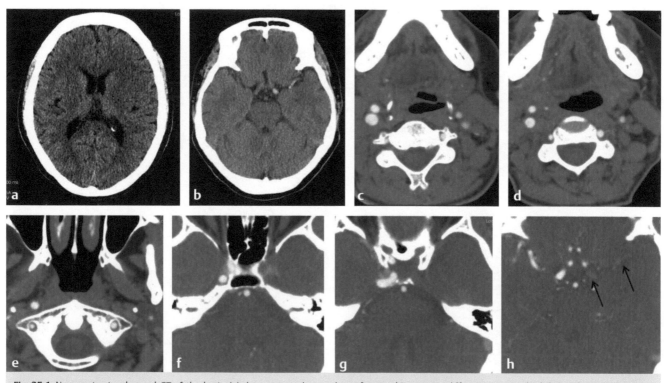

Fig. 25.1 Non-contrast enhanced CT of the brain (a) demonstrated some loss of gray-white matter differentiation in the left lentiform nucleus and insular region. Elsewhere, gray-white matter differentiation was preserved. There was hyperdensity consistent with thrombus in the left carotid termination and proximal MCA (b). CTA, single-phase study performed from the level of the aortic arch, showed filling of the left CCA and very proximal left ICA (c,d). There was, however, no contrast opacification of the left ICA beyond the level of the carotid bulb (e), and no contrast opacification of the left intracranial ICA, ICA termination, or M1 segment of MCA (f–h). The left A1 segment and more distal left ACA appeared patent on CTA.

25.1.4 Treatment

Initial Management

Intravenous thrombolysis was contraindicated in view of the recent surgery and therefore not administered. The patient was transferred directly to the neurointerventional suite.

Endovascular Treatment

Materials

- 8-Fr short angiographic sheath.
- 8-Fr MERCI balloon guide catheter.
- 5-Fr VTK slip catheter.
- 0.035 Terumo angled guidewire.
- Trevo 18 microcatheter.
- Synchro 14 microguidewire.
- Trevo ProVue 4 × 20 mm stent retriever.
- 8-Fr Angio-Seal closure device.

Technique

Endovascular treatment was performed with conscious sedation and local anesthetic. Heparin was not administered. A single-wall common femoral artery (CFA) puncture was performed, and an 8-Fr short vascular access sheath inserted. An 8-Fr balloon guide catheter was advanced to the cervical portion of the left ICA over a 5-Fr VTK slip catheter with the aid of an angled Terumo guidewire using roadmap guidance. Left ICA angiography showed slow filling of the left carotid artery to the level of the supraclinoid segment, where there was a sharp cut-off with meniscus sign at the proximal clot face (▶ Fig. 25.2a–d). There was no anterograde flow and no opacification of the MCA or ACA. Contrast stagnation and layering was noted in the cervical and supraclinoid ICA. A Trevo 18 microcatheter was navigated across the occluded carotid terminus and left M1 segment of MCA and into the superior division of MCA. Microcatheter injection confirmed position distal to thrombus in a good caliber M2 branch. A Trevo ProVue 4 × 20 mm stent retriever device was then deployed from the proximal M2 segment back to the supraclinoid segment of the ICA (▶ Fig. 25.2e).

Control angiography with the stent in situ showed some anterograde flow through the deployed stent with filling defect consistent with thrombus in the supraclinoid ICA and carotid terminus region (▶ Fig. 25.2e). The stent was left in situ for 5 minutes to allow incorporation of thrombus and then retrieved using flow arrest and continuous aspiration. Clot fragments were retrieved in the stent, and on aspiration of the guide

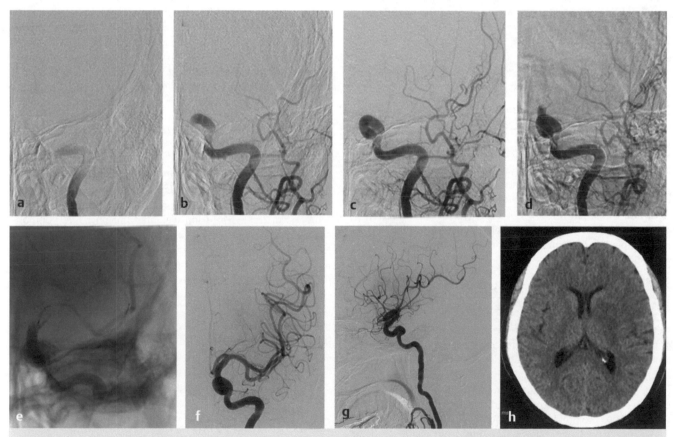

Fig. 25.2 DSA showed that the left cervical and proximal intracranial ICA was, in fact, patent; injection of the left cervical ICA demonstrated slow filling of the ICA to the level of the supraclinoid segment, where there was abrupt "cut-off" of contrast filling in keeping with left carotid terminus occlusion (a–d). Control angiography with the stent in situ showed some antegrade flow through the deployed stent with filling defect consistent with thrombus in the supraclinoid ICA and carotid terminus region (e). Clot fragments were retrieved in the stent, and on aspiration of the guide catheter. Control angiography showed complete recanalization of the left ICA, MCA, and now filling of left ACA from the carotid injection (f, g). Noncontrast CT of the head performed 24 hours postprocedure (h) demonstrated infarction in the left lentiform nucleus, caudate, insula and small volume patchy left frontal lobe infarction, with no evidence of hemorrhage.

catheter. Control angiography showed complete recanalization of the left ICA, MCA, and the filling of the left ACA from the carotid injection (▶ Fig. 25.2f, g). There was complete reperfusion of the distal territory (TICI 3), with no evidence of thromboembolic complication. Some mild vasospasm of the left cervical ICA was seen postretrieval which did not require treatment.

All devices were removed. An 8-Fr Angio-Seal was inserted for hemostasis at the femoral artery puncture site.

Postprocedure Care/Outcome

The patient demonstrated on-table improvement following clot retrieval with improved power in the right arm and leg, along with some improvement of aphasia and neglect. She was transferred to the neuro high-dependency unit (HDU) for further monitoring and care.

NCCT of the head performed 24 hours postprocedure (▶ Fig. 25.2h) demonstrated infarction in the left lentiform nucleus, caudate, insula, and small volume patchy left frontal lobe infarction, with no evidence of hemorrhage.

Following CT, the patient was commenced on intravenous heparin infusion for anticoagulation. Anticoagulation with apixaban was later commenced.

On 3-month follow-up in clinic, the patient was well, with no residual significant symptoms or deficit (modified Rankin scale [mRS] of 0).

25.2 Companion Case

25.2.1 Clinical Presentation

A 58-year-old man was admitted through the emergency department with right-sided hemiparesis and expressive dysphasia. He was last seen well 4 hours previously. The NIHSS score was 23. Cardiovascular risk factors included a long history of cigarette smoking (0.5 pack/day for 38 years). There was also a positive family history of stroke, with his brother having experienced a stroke at the age of 60 years. In addition, the patient had a 10-month history of T4M1 goblet cell carcinoma of appendix, which was being treated with surgery and chemotherapy. The prestroke mRS score was 0.

25.2.2 Imaging Workup and Investigations

NCCT demonstrated subtle early ischemic changes with loss of gray–white matter differentiation in the region of the left caudate nucleus, insula, and left superior frontoparietal region with an Alberta Stroke Program Early CT (ASPECTS) score of 6 (▶ Fig. 25.3a–c). No evidence of hemorrhage was seen. Hyperdense vessel sign was seen extending from the midportion of the left M1 to the proximal M2 (not shown).

CTA performed as single-phase study from the level of the aortic arch showed filling defects consistent with partially occlusive thrombus in the left distal M1 segment of MCA and proximal M2 branches (▶ Fig. 25.3d). In the neck, there was filling of the left CCA and left external carotid artery (ECA); however, the left ICA appeared occluded (▶ Fig. 25.3e). On correlation with axial source images, soft plaque/thrombus was

noted at the origin of the left ICA, with only a small focus of contrast opacification of the left ICA in the region of the carotid bulb (▶ Fig. 25.3f). More distally in the neck, there was no contrast opacification of the ICA (▶ Fig. 25.3g, h). Distally, there was reconstitution of the distal ICA via the left posterior communicating artery (not shown).

Subsequent MRI and gadolinium-enhanced MRA on the day following presentation demonstrated that the left ICA was patent; however, there was severe, more than 90%, stenosis of the left ICA origin (▶ Fig. 25.4a).

25.2.3 Diagnosis

Partially occlusive left M1–M2 thrombus, with left cervical ICA "pseudo-occlusion" in the setting of severe left ICA origin stenosis.

25.2.4 Treatment

As the patient was within the 4.5 hour window from onset of symptoms, intravenous tissue plasminogen activator (tPA) was administered. The NIHSS score decreased to 14 within 30 minutes of initiation of the tPA infusion.

Endovascular therapy was discussed; however, the decision was taken to not proceed in view of a combination of the following factors: already established early infarction with ASPECTS score of 6, the presence of partially occlusive thrombus with some contrast opacification around the thrombus, improvement with tPA to an NIHSS score that probably reflected the already established infarction, and the presence of an ICA pseudo-occlusion which would likely require acute intervention with angioplasty with or without stenting and acute initiation of antiplatelet therapy.

Further Care/Outcome

Follow-up imaging with MRI and gadolinium-enhanced MRA demonstrated patency of the left ICA with severe, more than 90%, stenosis of the left ICA origin and recanalization of the left MCA (▶ Fig. 25.4a). Diffusion-weighted imaging (DWI) demonstrated diffusion restriction in keeping with infarction in the left caudate nucleus, insula, anterior temporal lobe, frontal and parietal lobes, as well as left posterior watershed territory (▶ Fig. 25.4b–d). There was no evidence of hemorrhagic transformation.

Lipid lowering medication and antiplatelet therapy was commenced. The patient demonstrated further interval improvement to NIHSS score of 6 during his hospital stay. He was discharged to stroke rehabilitation center 5 days following admission. He subsequently underwent left carotid endarterectomy for the management of the left ICA stenosis.

25.3 Discussion

25.3.1 Background

The phenomenon of "pseudo-occlusion" had been described on CTA as early as 2001. Since then, radiologists and interventionalists have gained progressive awareness of this potential imaging pitfall. Pseudo-occlusion is an imaging phenomenon that

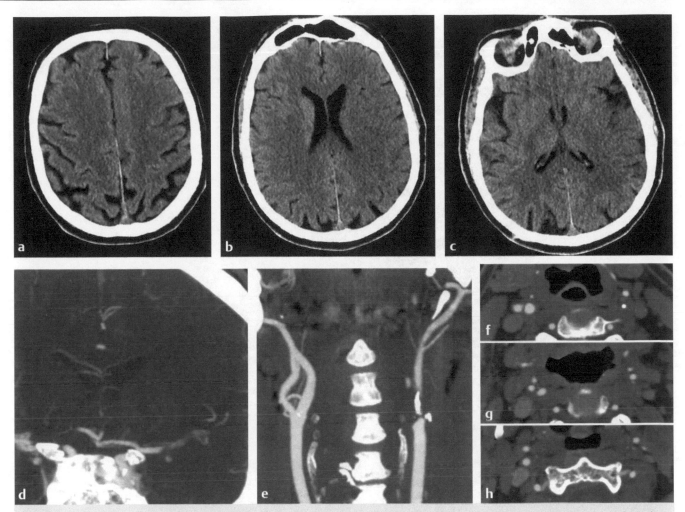

Fig. 25.3 Noncontrast CT demonstrated subtle early ischemic changes with loss of gray–white matter differentiation in the region of the left caudate nucleus, insula, and left superior frontoparietal region with ASPECTS score of 6 (**a–c**). CTA performed as single-phase study from the level of the aortic arch showed filling defects consistent with partially occlusive thrombus in the left distal M1 segment of MCA and proximal M2 branches (**d**). In the neck, there was filling of the left CCA and left ECA; however, the left ICA appeared occluded (**e**). On correlation with axial source images, soft plaque/thrombus was noted at the origin of the left ICA, with only a small focus of contrast opacification of the left ICA in the region of the carotid bulb (**f**). More distally in the neck, there was no contrast opacification of the ICA (**g,h**).

can be encountered on single-phase CTA or MRA whenever an artery appears "falsely" occluded, and which occurs in two main situations: first, in the setting of an intracranial occlusion with associated slow flow or stasis in the proximal vessel (as demonstrated by the first case presented here);second, when there is a significant flow-limiting proximal stenosis and simulating a total arterial occlusion (as depicted in the presented companion case). The entity is most commonly recognized in the setting of carotid terminus (carotid T) occlusion and/or proximal cervical ICA stenosis, both of which can lead to a false occlusion sign of the cervical and intracranial ICA. However, pseudo-occlusions are not limited to the anterior circulation, and can also occur in cases of vertebral artery proximal stenosis and/or distal occlusion. Furthermore, a thrombus in any other proximal intracranial vessel, such as the M1 segment, might also appear totally occlusive based on a CTA/MRA evaluation but seen to be only partially occlusive on catheter angiography.

The most common cause of severe proximal carotid stenosis leading to a possible pseudo-occlusion phenomenon is atherosclerotic disease. Indeed, approximately 10 to 25% of all ischemic strokes are thought to be related to carotid atherosclerosis. Luminal narrowing remains the standard parameter used to report the severity of carotid atherosclerotic disease. The risk of stroke increases with the degree of stenosis, and the international guidelines tend to focus on this aspect when recommending cutoffs for surgical or endovascular treatment of carotid disease. Acute stroke may occur secondary to plaque rupture and subsequent luminal thrombus formation with local sudden occlusion and/or embolic events. The other possible mechanism is hemodynamic compromise which is typically associated with watershed infarcts. Three of the recent positive randomized controlled trials that showed benefit for mechanical thrombectomy in acute large artery occlusive stroke provide specific information regarding the percentage of patients with ipsilateral extracranial carotid occlusion, which varied between 12.7% in ESCAPE, 18.6% in REVASCAT, and 32.2% in MR CLEAN.

Regarding the specific occurrence of a carotid terminus ("T") occlusion, it varied between 16% in the SWIFT-PRIME and 27.6% in ESCAPE. Among patients with occlusions of the intracranial ICA or the first segment of the MCA (or both),

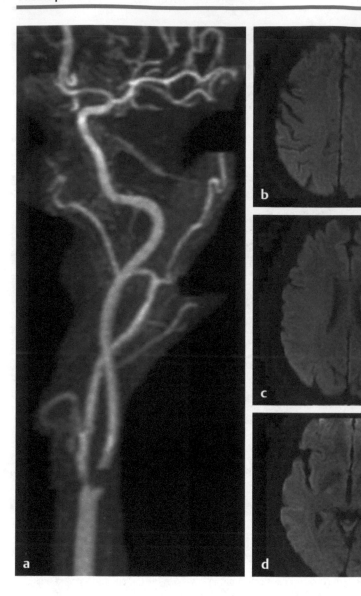

Fig. 25.4 Subsequent MRI and gadolinium-enhanced MRA on the day following presentation demonstrated that the left ICA was patent; however, there was severe, >90%, stenosis of the left ICA origin (a). DWI demonstrated diffusion restriction in keeping with infarction in the left caudate nucleus, insula, anterior temporal lobe, frontal and parietal lobes, as well as left posterior watershed territory (b–d). There was no evidence of hemorrhagic transformation.

intravenous tPA results in early reperfusion in 13 to 50%, depending on additional factors such as constitution and length of thrombus. Accordingly, these are the ideal candidates for mechanical thrombectomy, according to current guidelines of American Heart Association (AHA)/American Stroke Association (ASA).

Regardless of the location of thrombus or stenosis, pseudo-occlusion is an important entity to recognize, as misinterpretation can impact on decision making and treatment approach in the setting of acute stroke.

25.3.2 Workup and Diagnosis

Patient History

Patients with carotid stenosis may have a history of prior episodes of transient ischemic attack (TIA). While a TIA leaves no immediate impairment, the distinction between TIA and ischemic stroke has become less important in recent years, as affected individuals have a high risk for future ischemic events, particularly in the days and weeks immediately after symptom resolution. Correspondingly, the most recent AHA/ASA guidelines for examination/investigation and preventive approaches are similar for both conditions.

In cases of severe proximal stenosis due to large artery atherosclerosis, TIA/stroke events are most frequently embolic from unstable plaque. Less commonly, TIA/stroke etiology may be secondary to hemodynamic compromise, which will typically affect watershed territories.

As previously noted, atherosclerosis is the most common etiology of severe proximal carotid stenosis, and as it is usually part of a more diffuse process, signs and symptoms of associated peripheral artery disease and/or coronary heart disease are frequently observed in these patients.

Workup and Investigations

Fast and oriented clinical evaluation at admission includes confirmation of a neurologic event compatible with a stroke, identification of the time of onset of symptoms, evaluation of the severity of the neurological deficits (NIHSS score), and collection of a past medical and surgical history (including medications) in order to assess eligibility of the patient for acute treatment (including recombinant tPA infusion or mechanical thrombectomy).

Initial medical and neurological assessment should then be promptly followed by a diagnostic imaging protocol.

25.3.3 Imaging Findings

In the setting of acute stroke, plain CT scan and/or conventional MRI with DWI are required in order to assess the brain parenchyma for evidence of evolving infarction and exclusion of hemorrhagic stroke. Regardless of the chosen imaging modality, the most important message is to obtain satisfactory imaging without delaying the most appropriate treatment.

The pattern and distribution of acute lesions can help in identifying the most probable mechanism of stroke: watershed-distribution infarcts suggest hemodynamic compromise secondary to a severe proximal stenosis; cortical–subcortical and deep nuclei infarcts in the territory of one or more branches of a single large artery (such as the ICA) are more consistent with artery to artery embolism; and the presence of infarcts in multiple vascular territories suggests cardioembolic source.

Noninvasive vascular imaging, with either CTA or MRA, should be obtained as quickly as possible in order to identify any intracranial arterial occlusion and, if appropriate, plan for emergency mechanical thrombectomy. This should not delay the administration of intravenous rtPA if indicated. Imaging should be performed from the level of the aortic arch to include the intracranial circulation, as this will not only identify site of occlusion but also assess the degree of collateralization, suggest etiology of the occlusion, and evaluate the route of access if endovascular revascularization is required. For this purpose, CTA is a convenient, fast, widely available, usually easily accessible and nonoperator dependent technique for the evaluation of the supra-aortic and intracranial vessels. CTA also allows superior assessment of collateral supply over MRA, particularly in the setting of carotid T and MCA occlusions where collateralization is retrograde through leptomeningeal collaterals. One of the main pitfalls of CTA when performed as a single-phase study is the possible phenomenon of "pseudo-occlusion" as illustrated by the representative cases in this chapter. Pseudo-occlusion is a consequence of the static nature of CTA, which gives a snapshot in time and does not allow for evaluation of the arterial flow itself. As new multidetector CT scanners provide very fast imaging times, when images are acquired it may be too early to see contrast passage through a tight proximal stenosis or if a distal thrombus is present. The absence of contrast material in an artery will then simulate a true arterial occlusion. Contrast-enhanced MRA also suffers from similar pitfalls, while time-of-flight MRA is of inferior quality to contrast-enhanced MRA when assessing the extracranial supra-aortic circulation.

True proximal occlusions cannot therefore be confidently separated from a significant proximal stenosis on a single-phase CTA protocol, and delayed images are required to evaluate for slow filling of the distal artery. Similarly, delayed imaging is required to avoid the pitfall of misinterpreting a focal intracranial arterial occlusion as an occlusion of the whole proximal artery, as can be seen with carotid terminus occlusion where the entire ICA can be devoid of contrast material on single-phase CTA as a consequence of slow flow or stasis. To overcome these limitations, different options are available. The most common approach is to perform multiphase CTA as standard of care in the assessment of the acute stroke patients.

Although multiphase CTA increases radiation dose, it simultaneously allows a better assessment of intracranial collaterals (which are often underestimated in single-phase CTA) and can also be used as an estimate of core infarct. Multiphase CTA thus represents more than a snapshot evaluation of flow, adding a dynamic component to the study. Other options include close monitoring of all CTA studies, and immediately repeating the scan from the level of the skull base without additional contrast in selective cases, whenever the four supra-aortic vessels are not seen filling in the neck. While this might protect patients from unnecessary radiation, it is time consuming and not practical in high-volume centers. Alternatively, differentiation between a complete and a partial occlusion can be made with a time-resolved CTA derived from CT perfusion data sets, which is often obtained as part of a multimodel CT protocol in the setting of an acute stroke. This 4D CT technique provides time-resolved images of the arterial, parenchymal, and venous phases and can also be used for both thrombus and collateral status assessment. In fact, the presence of antegrade contrast opacification across a partially occlusive thrombus (angiographically termed the "clot outline sign") can be depicted with this technique and separated from collateral flow with excellent sensitivity and specificity. The main drawbacks of time-resolved CTA are related to postprocessing, which is both time consuming and nonstandardized.

Correlation of noninvasive angiographic imaging findings with the diagnostic angiograms obtained at time of stroke intervention usually provides the final diagnosis. Nevertheless, even on digital subtraction angiography (DSA), acquisition of delayed images is often necessary to differentiate between true occlusions and "pseudo-occlusions."

25.3.4 Decision-Making Process

If facing the dilemma of distinguishing a pseudo-occlusion from a true occlusion, one has to consider the angiographic imaging technique used. For example, if a multiphase CTA has been obtained, then the initial and delayed images should be scrutinized in an effort to establish the correct diagnosis before intervention is considered. If only a single-phase CTA is obtained, then additional clues such as hyperdensity of the carotid terminus on NCCT of the head showing a carotid terminus occlusion, calcification of the common carotid bifurcation/carotid bulb indicating atherosclerosis, and a gradual fade out of contrast in the cervical ICA on CTA are all valuable indicators to raise suspicion for a possible pseudo-occlusion. If single-phase CTA studies are monitored, either by the radiologist or technologist conducting the study, and four arteries (i.e., two ICAs and two vertebral arteries) are not seen filling in the neck, then immediately rescanning the patient without administration of additional contrast can help distinguish a true from a false occlusion.

Correct identification of the phenomenon of "pseudo-occlusion" through noninvasive angiographic techniques allows better delineation of occlusive clot burden. This is important, as clot burden and thrombus length are not only known determinants of the efficacy and complication rates of mechanical thrombectomy but also predictors of final clinical outcome.

Accurate information on extent of thrombus is also important for treatment planning, as precise definition of the target lesion, that is, the occluding thrombus, is desirable when performing an endovascular procedure. It also allows the neurointerventionalist to anticipate any potential issues regarding gaining access to the occluded arteries; for example, in the case of significant flow limiting carotid stenosis, where prethrombectomy angioplasty with or without stenting may be required in order to access the ICA and allow for thrombectomy. Advanced knowledge of such issues will ultimately save valuable time and increase the likelihood of success of the procedure.

In cases of intracranial pseudo-occlusion (e.g., where a thrombus in a proximal intracranial artery, such as the M1 segment, appears totally occlusive, based on a CTA/MRA evaluation, but is seen to be only partially occlusive on DSA), the depiction of antegrade contrast opacification theoretically represents a lesser degree of ischemia to the distal vascular territory, potentially increasing the time window to allow revascularization procedures to be performed. Evidence in this area is, however, lacking.

Overall, it is important that one possesses the awareness of the potential phenomenon of pseudo-occlusion. The appearance of an apparently occluded ICA or vertebral artery on single-phase CTA or MRA should not be allowed to weigh too heavily into decision making in the acute stroke patient with an intracranial arterial occlusion, high NIHSS score, and lack of early changes on initial NCCT of the head. In cases where there is doubt, the initial DSA performed prethrombectomy will confirm/exclude the diagnosis. It is, however, important to consider that early angiographic runs from a proximal position may suffer from the same pitfall as CTA/MRA, due to the presence of a column of nonopacified blood within the distal artery. In the setting of a distal vertebral/basilar occlusion, the proximal vertebral may fill poorly on subclavian injection, and in the setting of carotid terminus occlusion, the proximal ICA may fill poorly on a common carotid injection. In such cases, the exact extent of clot can only be determined after selective cannulation and injection of either the vertebral artery or ICA, respectively.

25.3.5 Management

In the setting of an acute stroke due to a carotid terminus thrombus or other proximal intracranial occlusion, mechanical thrombectomy is now the standard of care. This is independent of an associated "pseudo-occlusion" phenomenon/severe stenosis/true occlusion in the proximal ICA, as long as the remaining inclusion and exclusion criteria required for these procedures are fulfilled. Standard of care includes administration of intravenous thrombolysis within 4.5 hours of symptom onset unless contraindicated.

In cases of symptomatic severe carotid stenosis, a revascularization procedure (either carotid angioplasty and stenting [CAS] or carotid endarterectomy) is recommended within the first 2 weeks. The particular acute management of tandem lesions is addressed in a separate chapter of the book.

Revascularization is not recommended in patients with chronic proximal carotid occlusions.

Secondary prevention measures must be undertaken, such as commencement of antiplatelet therapy or anticoagulation as necessary, and also identification of modifiable risk factors such as hypertension, dyslipidemia, diabetes, and smoking, among others.

25.3.6 Postprocedure Care

Postprocedure care involves early identification of possible complications associated with stroke treatment such as hemorrhagic transformation of the ischemic infarct or development of new areas of infarction due to distal embolic events/fragmentation of thrombus, or complications specific to mechanical thrombectomy such as development of groin hematoma. Patient's neurological condition should be closely monitored using scales such as the Glasgow Coma Scale (GCS) and the NIHSS score. NCCT of the head should be obtained at 24 hours poststroke treatment (including intravenous thrombolysis alone, or mechanical thrombectomy) or earlier if neurological deterioration occurs.

In cases where carotid stenting is performed either during the thrombectomy procedure, or in subsequent days, additional subacute complications may occur such as hyperperfusion/reperfusion syndrome or in-stent thrombosis. Therefore, additional close monitoring over a longer time frame is required in such patients.

25.3.7 Literature Synopsis

Although single-phase CTA provides excellent anatomic detail of the supra-aortic and intracranial vessels, it is limited to providing information from a single time point during the passage of a contrast bolus. This limitation can result in the phenomenon of "pseudo-occlusion," as presented here in the provided cases, where slow flow due to a severe proximal stenosis or a distal occlusion leads to absence of contrast opacification of an artery, which may be erroneously interpreted as a complete occlusion.

On noninvasive angiographic imaging, diagnosis of a true carotid occlusion requires a multiphase or time-resolved study. The NCCT scan as well as source images and maximal intensity projections of both initial and delayed CTA acquisitions should all be reviewed carefully, paying particular attention to the extracranial as well as intracranial circulation.

In addition to differentiating pseudo-occlusions from true occlusions, it is also important to identify other conditions that may present a similar appearance on CTA, such as arterial hypoplasia or agenesis, dissection, and near occlusion where an artery is of significantly reduced caliber distal to a severe chronic stenosis. In cases of true occlusion of the cervical ICA, the ascending pharyngeal artery can be mistaken for a "string sign"/carotid near occlusion. Awareness of the course of the ascending pharyngeal and identification of this artery as a small ascending vessel, which is adjacent but separate to the expected course of the collapsed/occluded ICA, is important.

Attention to the collaterals is also important; in the case of carotid pseudo-occlusions due to significant proximal carotid stenosis, there is often a significant and well-developed network of collaterals, either through the leptomeningeal route intracranially or the ECA–ICA anastomoses with associated reconstitution of the ICA from the cavernous/supraclinoid segments. This is usually not the scenario in case of a pseudo-occlusion due to a carotid terminus thrombus or a sudden occlusion. In vertebral disease, collaterals from ascending and deep cervical arteries, or through the ECA, can be seen in cases of significant vertebral stenosis/chronic occlusion.

25.3.8 Pearls and Pitfalls

- In all cases of presumed carotid occlusion, delayed angiographic images are required to seek a late, slow flow in the distal ICA and thus to exclude a phenomenon of pseudo-occlusion. This can be achieved with multiphase CTA.
- The most common causes of pseudo-occlusion are carotid terminus occlusion and/or proximal severe cervical ICA stenosis.
- Pseudo-occlusion is not limited to the carotid, and can also be seen in cases of vertebral artery proximal stenosis and/or distal occlusion.
- A correct diagnosis of pseudo-occlusion is necessary for correct delineation of the occlusive clot burden, which is an imaging predictor for size of infarct core, NIHSS at baseline, efficacy of reperfusion therapies, and final outcome.
- Awareness of the potential phenomenon of pseudo-occlusion is important. The appearance of an apparently occluded ICA or vertebral artery on single-phase CTA or MRA should not be allowed to weigh too heavily into decision making in the acute stroke patient with an intracranial arterial occlusion, high NIHSS score, and lack of early changes on initial NCCT of the head. In cases where there is doubt, the initial DSA performed prethrombectomy will allow differentiation of a true from a false occlusion.

Further Readings

Lev MH, Farkas J, Rodriguez VR, et al. CT angiography in the rapid triage of patients with hyperacute stroke to intraarterial thrombolysis: accuracy in the detection of large vessel thrombus. J Comput Assist Tomogr. 2001; 25(4):520–528

Power S, McEvoy SH, Cunningham J, et al. Value of CT angiography in anterior circulation large vessel occlusive stroke: imaging findings, pearls, and pitfalls. Eur J Radiol. 2015; 84(7):1333–1344

Frölich AM, Psychogios MN, Klotz E, Schramm R, Knauth M, Schramm P. Antegrade flow across incomplete vessel occlusions can be distinguished from retrograde collateral flow using 4-dimensional computed tomographic angiography. Stroke. 2012; 43(11):2974–2979

van den Wijngaard IR, Boiten J, Holswilder G, et al. Impact of collateral status evaluated by dynamic computed tomographic angiography on clinical outcome in patients with ischemic stroke. Stroke. 2015; 46(12):3398–3404

Goyal M, Menon BK, Hill MD, Demchuk A. Consistently achieving computed tomography to endovascular recanalization < 90 minutes: solutions and innovations. Stroke. 2014; 45(12):e252–e256

Goyal M, Demchuk AM, Menon BK, et al. ESCAPE Trial Investigators. Randomized assessment of rapid endovascular treatment of ischemic stroke. N Engl J Med. 2015; 372(11):1019–1030

Saver JL, Goyal M, Bonafe A, et al. SWIFT PRIME Investigators. Stent-retriever thrombectomy after intravenous t-PA vs. t-PA alone in stroke. N Engl J Med. 2015; 372(24):2285–2295

Campbell BCV, Mitchell PJ, Kleinig TJ, et al. EXTEND-IA Investigators. Endovascular therapy for ischemic stroke with perfusion-imaging selection. N Engl J Med. 2015; 372(11):1009–1018

Jovin TG, Chamorro A, Cobo E, et al. REVASCAT Trial Investigators. Thrombectomy within 8 hours after symptom onset in ischemic stroke. N Engl J Med. 2015; 372 (24):2296–2306

Berkhemer OA, Fransen PSS, Beumer D, et al. MR CLEAN Investigators.. A randomized trial of intraarterial treatment for acute ischemic stroke. N Engl J Med. 2015; 372:11–20

Powers WJ, Derdeyn CP, Biller J, et al. on behalf of the, American Heart Association Stroke Council. 2015 AHA/ASA focused update of the 2013 guidelines for the early management of patients with acute ischemic stroke regarding endovascular treatment. A guideline for professionals from the American Heart Association/ American Stroke Association. Stroke. 2015; 46(10):3020–3035

26 Underlying Intracranial Stenosis

26.1 Case Description

26.1.1 Clinical Presentation

A 59-year-old male with hypertension and smoking history presented with severe dysarthria, right-sided weakness, and altered level of consciousness (LOC). He was last known well at 16:00 hours. He called his partner at 03:40 hours, but only breathing noises were audible and the patient was not able to talk. His family rushed to his home and found him on the couch, unable to speak, and unable to move his right arm. He was moving his lower limbs, left more so than right. Emergency medical service (EMS) was called and he was brought to the stroke center as a code stroke at 04:38 hours.

National Institutes of Health Stroke Scale (NIHSS) score was 14 for severe dysarthria, right-arm weakness, bilateral lower limb weakness, and ataxia. He was also found to have altered LOC.

26.1.2 Imaging Workup and Investigations

- Noncontrast computed tomography (NCCT) done shortly after presentation to the emergency department (about 80 minutes after discovery of symptom onset) revealed hyperdense basilar artery (▶ Fig. 26.1a).
- CT angiography (CTA) revealed long-segment occlusion of the basilar artery (▶ Fig. 26.1b).
- CT perfusion (CTP) showed increased mean transit time (MTT) of the pons and the cerebellum with reduced cerebral blood volume (CBV) and cerebral blood flow (CBF). It was uncertain if it was truly infarcted tissue or an artifact due to photon starvation and streak artifact (▶ Fig. 26.1c).

26.1.3 Diagnosis

Basilar artery long-segment occlusion with significant streak artifact over the pons, limiting the assessment of early infarction. Corresponding abnormal tissue perfusion tissue of the posterior fossa.

26.1.4 Management

- Due to uncertainty of time of onset, tissue plasminogen activator (tPA) was not given.
- Patient was intubated in the emergency department prior to transfer to the angiography suite.

26.1.5 Endovascular Treatment

Materials

- 8-Fr short vascular access sheath.
- 6-Fr Neuron MAX 088 access catheter (Penumbra, Inc.).
- HH1 Impress hydrophilic catheter (Merit, Inc.).
- Terumo guidewire
- 5 MAX ACE 68 aspiration catheter (Penumbra, Inc.).
- 3 MAX aspiration catheter (Penumbra, Inc.).
- Transend EX soft tip microguidewire.
- Trevo XP ProVue microcatheter.
- Synchro 14 microwire.
- Trevo XP ProVue 4 × 20 mm stent retriever.

Technique

- Procedure performed under general anesthesia.
- As tPA was not provided, heparin was given to keep the activated clotting time (ACT) between 250 and 300 throughout the course of the procedure.
- Right common femoral artery (CFA) puncture with placement of an 8-Fr short vascular access sheath into the CFA.
- The 6-Fr Neuron MAX 088 access catheter (Penumbra, Inc.) and the HH1 Impress hydrophilic catheter were prepared and connected to a continuous flush. The system was then used to catheterize the left vertebral artery using roadmap technique with the aid of the Terumo guidewire. The Neuron MAX was advanced to the C2 level, and the HH1 and guidewire were removed.
- Diagnostic hand injections in both anteroposterior (AP) and lateral showed long segment occlusion of the basilar artery trunk (▶ Fig. 26.2a).

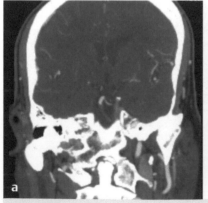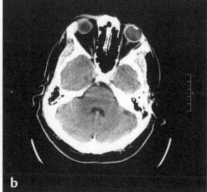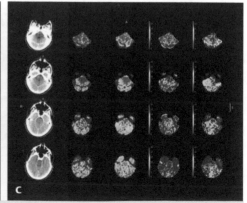

Fig. 26.1 CT/CTA/CTP. (a) NCCT showing hyperdense basil artery. (b) Long-segment basilar occlusion. (c) Decreased CBF and CBV of the pons.

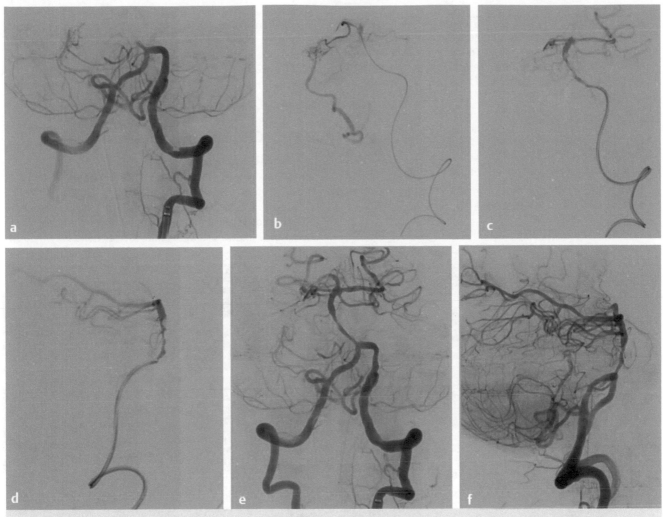

Fig. 26.2 CT/CTA/CTP. (a) NCCT showing hyperdense basil artery. (b) Long-segment basilar occlusion. (c) Decreased CBF and CBV of the pons.

- The 5 MAX ACE 68 aspiration catheter and the 3 MAX aspiration catheter were prepared and connected to continuous flush. Under fluoroscopic guidance with roadmaps, both catheters were navigated coaxially through the Neuron MAX, with the aid of a Transend EX soft tip microguidewire, until the proximal clot margin.
- The 3 MAX and the Transend wire were removed.
- The 5 MAX ACE 68 aspiration catheter was connected to the penumbra aspiration pump with the connecting tubing, and the pump was primed. When optimal negative pressure was achieved, the connecting tubing valve was opened.
- Some blood was seen sucked back into the catheter followed by almost immediate flow arrest. After 90 seconds the 5 MAX was pulled gradually; however, due to the acute angle of the V4 it was difficult to keep the clot engaged.
- Hand injection after the 5 MAX removal showed minimal recanalization.
- The Trevo XP ProVue microcatheter was prepped and connected to a continuous flush and was then navigated with the aid of a Synchro microwire through the 5 MAX distal to the clot.

- Hand injection revealed a micro arteriovenous malformation (AVM) and the intravascular location of the catheter (▶ Fig. 26.2b).
- A 4 × 20 mm Trevo stent retriever was deployed along the length of the basilar trunk and first flow was achieved (▶ Fig. 26.2c, d).
- Microinjection confirmed the location of the Trevo micro catheter with no perforation.
- The 5 MAX was advanced to the proximal aspect of the clot to wedge it and connect it to the Penumbra aspiration pump.
- Both the Trevo stent retriever and the 5 MAX were pulled as a unit under aspiration. Clot fragments were retrieved.
- Hand injections through the Neuron Max showed the basilar almost completely recanalized with focal midbasilar narrowing. There was less opacification of the right posterior cerebral artery (PCA) with poor visualization of the distal branches (TICI 2b; ▶ Fig. 26.2e, f).
- 2 mg of intra-arterial (IA) tPA was given through the Neuron Max.
- After confirmation of proper puncture site, the sheath was removed and an 8-Fr Angio-seal device used for hemostasis.

26.1.6 Postprocedure Care

The patient was transferred to the intensive care unit (ICU). The systolic blood pressure was kept < 180 mm Hg. Dual antiplatelets were started the day after thrombectomy. Atorvastatin 80 mg PO/NG was started daily.

26.1.7 Outcome

- The patient remained intubated and did not improve clinically. He was comatose with ocular bobbing and absence of horizontal gaze movements. There were minimal corneal reflexes, with pupils 2 mm and sluggishly reactive. Decerebrating posturing was observed after tactile stimuli.
- Repeat CTA showed reocclusion of the basilar artery (▶ Fig. 26.3), and magnetic resonance imaging (MRI) showed

massive posterior circulation infarctions involving the pons, cerebellum and the left occipital lobe (▶ Fig. 26.4). The patient developed "locked in" syndrome. He was kept on mechanical ventilation in the cardiac care unit (CCU), and ultimately the family asked to withdraw life support. He died peacefully.

26.2 Companion Case

26.2.1 Clinical Presentation

- A 40-year-old woman was transferred as a code stroke, presenting with right hemiparesis inability to speak, and a NIHSS score of 16. Computed tomography (CT)/CTA/CTP of head demonstrated a mid to distal basilar artery occlusion. She was not a tPA candidate, given the uncertain onset of symptoms, and was sent for endovascular therapy.

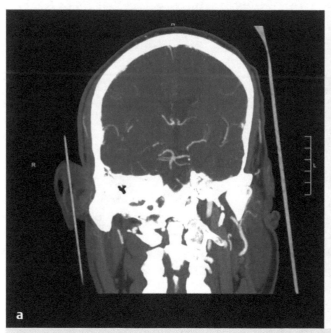
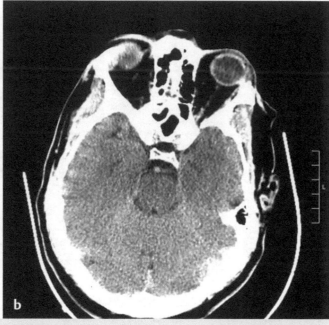

Fig. 26.3 Postthrombectomy day 1. (a) NCCT showing hyperdense basilar artery and hypodense pons. (b) CTA showing reoccluded basilar artery.

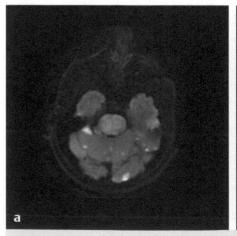
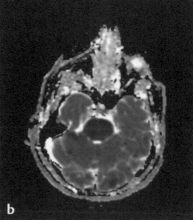
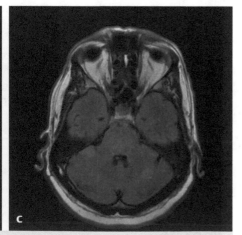

Fig. 26.4 MRI day 1 postthrombectomy. (a) DWI demonstrates multiple foci of diffusion restriction in the cerebellum as well as diffuse pontine diffusion restriction. (b) ADC map shows corresponding low ADC. (c) FLAIR shows corresponding hyperintensities.

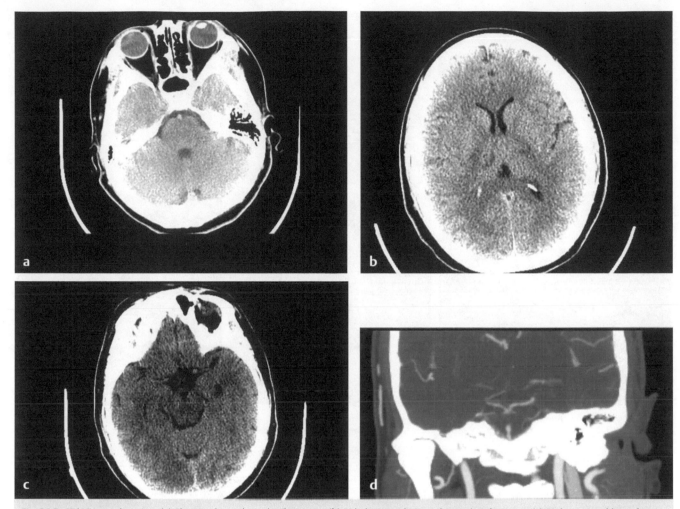

Fig. 26.5 CT/CTA at admission. (**a**) Showing hyperdense basilar artery. (**b**) Bithalamic and internal capsule infarctions. (**c**) Right occipital loss of gray–white differentiation. (**d**) Basilar occlusion.

26.2.2 Imaging Workup and Investigations

- NCCT performed shortly after presentation to the emergency department revealed hyper dense basilar artery and hypodensities of the bilateral thalami and the right occipital lobe. (▶ Fig. 26.5)
- CTA revealed mid to distal basilar artery occlusion (▶ Fig. 26.5).

MRI

- Scattered foci of diffusion restriction in the posterior circulation, involving both thalami, midbrain, pons, and right occipital lobe (▶ Fig. 26.6)

26.2.3 Management

- Given the patient's young age, the stroke team agreed to take the patient to the angiography suite for mechanical thrombectomy, and informed consent was obtained from the family.

26.2.4 Endovascular Treatment

Materials

- 5-Fr and 6-Fr short vascular access sheaths.
- 5-Fr Bernstein diagnostic catheter.
- 6-Fr Envoy DA catheter.
- Trevo 18 microcatheter.
- TrevoXP ProVue 4 × 20 mm stent retriever.
- Terumo guidewire.
- Transend EX soft tip microguidewire.
- Solitaire 4 mm × 30 mm stent retriever.
- 6-Fr Angio-seal.

Technique

- The procedure was performed under general anesthesia with the patient intubated.
- Bilateral CFA punctures were performed with placement of 6-Fr short vascular access sheath into the right CFA and 5-Fr sheath in the left.
- The 5-Fr Bernstein diagnostic catheter was navigated into the right common carotid artery (CCA) and internal carotid artery

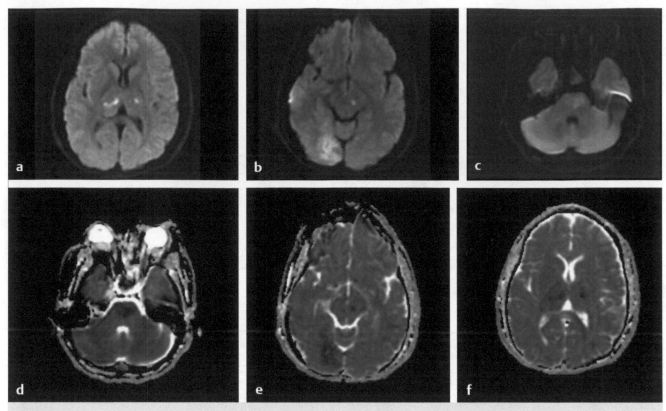

Fig. 26.6 MRI prior to thrombectomy confirming the presence of multiple posterior circulations infarcts.

(ICA) to assess the posterior communicating artery and the PCA.

- The 6-Fr Envoy DA catheter was navigated into the left vertebral artery. AP and lateral runs showed distal basilar occlusion with midbasilar artery diameter change, large left extracranial origin of posterior inferior cerebellar artery (PICA), duplicated left anterior inferior cerebellar artery (AICA), right AICA/PICA, and a small accessory right AICA.
- Double-catheter simultaneous runs showed good roadmap for mechanical thrombectomy (▶ Fig. 26.7).
- Trevo 18 microcatheter was navigated into the left P1 with the aid of a Transend EX soft tip microguidewire. Superselective run confirmed intravascular positioning.
- TrevoXP ProVue 4 × 20 mm stent retriever was deployed and incubated for 5 minutes before retrieval. Repeat left vertebral artery run showed partial recanalization to left P1.
- Similar steps were performed for the right P1.
- Repeat left vertebral artery run showed partial recanalization of bilateral P1 s and superior cerebellar arteries (SCAs). The flow was not robust, with severe stenosis at distal basilar trunk, so a decision was taken to deploy Solitaire stent across the severe stenosis.
- Microcatheter was advanced to the left distal PCA.
- Solitaire 4 × 30 mm stent was deployed across basilar stenosis and detached.
- Working projection runs showed improved flow from distal basilar trunk to PCAs and SCAs. A small filling defect just proximal to right SCA origin was visualized.
- ReoPro loading dose was given and infusion continued while in ICU.

- Final AP, lateral runs from left vertebral and right internal carotid showed no other complications.
- Catheters were removed, and a 6-Fr Angio-Seal was used for hemostasis.

26.2.5 Postprocedure Care

- She was admitted to the ICU, under stroke team for ongoing management.
- She was eventually transferred to the ward in stable condition and had an uncomplicated stay in the stroke unit.
- The cause of her stroke was not established even after an extensive workup.
- Follow up CT/CTA showed no new infarction. The stent was patent as well as the posterior circulation vasculature (▶ Fig. 26.8).

26.2.6 Outcome

- She was discharged to rehabilitation center.
- Atorvastatin 40 mg PO daily, ASA 81 mg PO daily, and Plavix 75 mg PO daily were started during admission and continued after discharge.
- When visiting the clinic for 90-day follow-up, she was cognitively intact and feeling well. Her functional status was improved, although she continued to walk with a cane due to right-sided leg weakness. She also experienced a numbness on the left side of her face, arm, and leg, but no change in temperature sensation. On examination, she felt decreased sensation to light touch in the left cranial nerve (CN) V2/V3

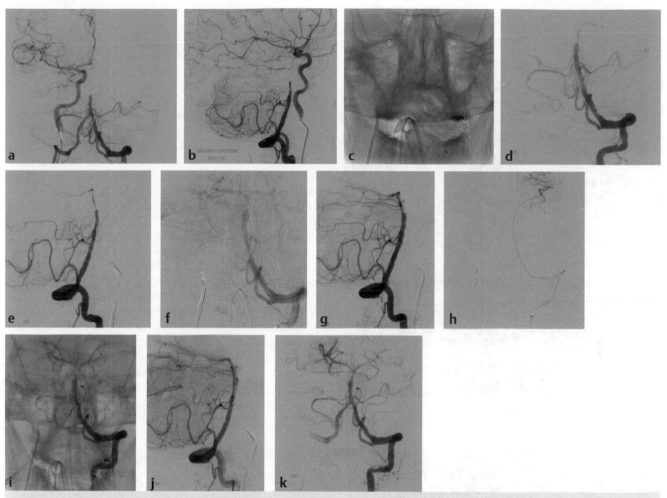

Fig. 26.7 Thrombectomy angiography. **(a,b)** AP and lateral dual catheter angiography showing the basilar occlusion in addition to both PCA and SCA **(c)** Trevo stent deployed in the left PCA **(d,e)** AP and lateral left vertebral artery injection shown partial recanalization of the left PCA and the basilar tip. **(f)** right PCA thrombectomy. **(g)** Better opacification of the basilar artery and its branches postthrombectomy **(h)** Microinjection into the left PCA in preparation for Solitaire stent placement. **(i–k)** Post–Solitaire stent deployment and detachment.

regions of her face; V1 was intact. The left upper visual field appeared to be restricted. There was a subtle spastic catch in her left arm. Strength was 5/5 in all four limbs. Proprioception was intact.

- Follow-up MRI/MRA in 6 months showed evolution of the known infarcts with patency of the stent (▶ Fig. 26.9).

26.3 Discussion

26.3.1 Background

There exist limited data on the prevalence of asymptomatic intracranial atherosclerotic stenosis (ICAS).[1] ICAS is one of the leading causes of stroke and accounts for 5 to 10, 15 to 29, and 30 to 50% of all acute ischemic strokes among white, black, and Asian populations, respectively.[2,3] The landmark WASID trial in 2005 studied medical management for patients with symptomatic large vessel ICAS of 50 to 99% within the preceding 90 days before randomization.[4] The clinical significance of underlying ICAS in acute ischemic stroke is not well understood, and therefore the optimal treatment strategy is not known.

The definition of ICAS in the setting of acute ischemic stroke is inconsistent. Many authors have used the technique described in the WASID trial to calculate the degree of stenosis.[4] Several studies calculate the degree of stenosis on the first angiographic run after endovascular thrombectomy (EVT) and confirm ICAS again 3 to 5 minutes after IA vasodilator injection.[5,6] Other authors report the same stenosis calculation without the administration of IA vasodilators.[7]

The success of EVT depends on the underlying etiology of the stroke, with atherothrombosis presenting the greatest challenge for reperfusion.[8] Recent studies have presented evidence that angioplasty with or without stenting is a safe and feasible treatment option for refractory occlusion/stenosis after EVT in the setting of ICAS.[5,6,7,9,10,11]

26.3.2 Discussion

We first present a case of acute basilar thrombosis with clear evidence of residual stenosis after EVT. The patient unfortunately developed reocclusion of the basilar artery hours after the procedure. Hwang et al showed that instant or delayed

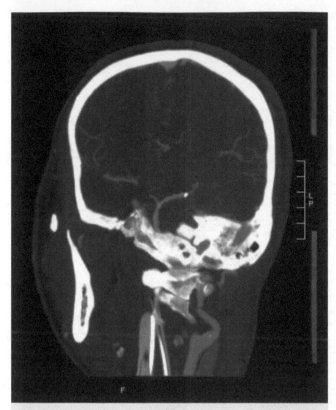

Fig. 26.8 Follow-up CTA showing patent stent.

reocclusion in the setting of ICAS is common and was associated with a low probability of favorable 3-month outcome.[7] Mosimann et al also showed that early reocclusion (within 48 hours) was common for patients with residual stenosis at the EVT site.[12] This evidence has prompted several investigators to consider angioplasty with/without stenting and IA infusion of blood thinners when residual stenosis is present at the thrombectomy site. Yoon et al showed that angioplasty and stenting, when possible, was safe, effective, and associated with high-rate of good outcome.[6] Kang et al demonstrated safety and efficacy of angioplasty with/without stenting, and IA infusion of antiplatelet medication, in 140 patients with acute large vessel occlusion due to underlying ICAS.[13] They found no difference in outcome between the two treatment groups and concluded that both were effective and safe.

Our second case is an example of basilar artery stenting for severe residual stenosis following EVT. Once the decision was made to stent the residual basilar artery stenosis, a ReoPro loading dose was given followed by infusion. Some groups use a dual antiplatelet loading dose (325 mg ASA and 600 mg Plavix) via NG during the procedure. Other authors report not giving any antiplatelets until a postoperative CT scan is done to ensure no intracranial hemorrhage, and starting the patient on antiplatelet medication at that point. Gao et al examined 30 patients with acute basilar artery stroke undergoing EVT. Of the 30 patients, 13 received combined EVT, angioplasty, and stent placement. They loaded patients with 300 mg ASA and 300 mg Plavix via NG intraoperatively. They reported efficacy and safety of

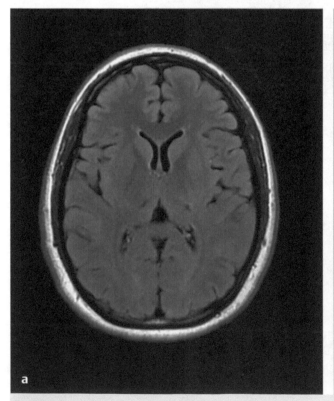

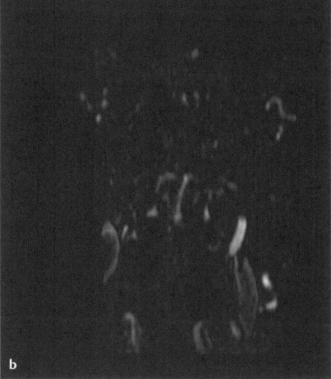

Fig. 26.9 Six-month follow-up MRI/MRA showing evolution of the known infarctions and patency of the basilar stent with optimal vascular opacification

EVT combined with angioplasty and stenting for basilar occlusions with underlying severe ICAS.[9] IA antiplatelet drug delivery is another option for patients with underlying ICAS and severe residual stenosis after EVT. Kang et al[14] used the following strategy to manage cases with in situ thrombo-occlusion: if following successful recanalization there was residual stenosis at the occlusion site, additional angiographic runs every 10 minutes for 30 minutes were acquired. If any of those runs showed reocclusion, a repeat recanalization was performed using mechanical thrombectomy. Head CT was then performed in the angiography suite to rule out hemorrhage. Once bleeding was excluded, a low-dose IA tirofiban infusion was given (0.5 mg of tirofiban diluted with 8 mL of normal saline, at a rate of 1 mL/min; the dose ranged from 0.5 to 1.0 mg). Refractory cases were treated by rescue stenting with angioplasty. With the low dose of tirofiban, the rate of symptomatic ICH was not significantly elevated in this study. In comparison, Kellert et al[15] reported that when tirofiban was initially infused at 0.4 µg/kg/min over 30 minutes, followed by a continuous infusion of 0.1 µg/kg/min for 48 hours (e.g., 18 mg for a 60-kg adult), it resulted in higher rates of fatal ICH with no improvement in the recanalization rate.

26.3.3 Pearls and Pitfalls

- Compared to those with embolic occlusion, ICAS-related occlusion has relatively poor functional outcomes post-EVT.[16]
- Different strategies have been described for managing such lessons such as angioplasty, stenting, dual-antiplatelet therapy, heparin infusion, warfarin or glycoprotein-IIb/IIIa inhibitor, or combination of these.
- One should have a low threshold to reimage early post-EVT to detect and manage worsening stenosis or reocclusion with ICAS.
- The balance between the risks of reocclusion versus ICH should always be kept in mind.

References

[1] Bang OY. Intracranial atherosclerosis: current understanding and perspectives. J Stroke. 2014; 16(1):27–35

[2] Holmstedt CA, Turan TN, Chimowitz MI. Atherosclerotic intracranial arterial stenosis: risk factors, diagnosis, and treatment. Lancet Neurol. 2013; 12 (11):1106–1114

[3] Qureshi AI, Feldmann E, Gomez CR, et al. Intracranial atherosclerotic disease: an update. Ann Neurol. 2009; 66(6):730–738

[4] Chimowitz MI, Lynn MJ, Howlett-Smith H, et al. Warfarin-Aspirin Symptomatic Intracranial Disease Trial Investigators. Comparison of warfarin and aspirin for symptomatic intracranial arterial stenosis. N Engl J Med. 2005; 352(13):1305–1316

[5] Kim GE, Yoon W, Kim SK, et al. Incidence and clinical significance of acute reocclusion after emergent angioplasty or stenting for underlying intracranial stenosis in patients with acute stroke. AJNR Am J Neuroradiol. 2016; 37 (9):1690–1695

[6] Yoon W, Kim SK, Park MS, Kim BC, Kang HK. Endovascular treatment and the outcomes of atherosclerotic intracranial stenosis in patients with hyperacute stroke. Neurosurgery. 2015; 76(6):680–686, discussion 686

[7] Hwang YH, Kim YW, Kang DH, Kim YS, Liebeskind DS. Impact of target arterial residual stenosis on outcome after endovascular revascularization. Stroke. 2016; 47(7):1850–1857

[8] Matias-Guiu JA, Serna-Candel C, Matias-Guiu J. Stroke etiology determines effectiveness of retrievable stents. J Neurointerv Surg. 2014; 6(2):e11

[9] Gao F, Lo WT, Sun X, Mo DP, Ma N, Miao ZR. Combined use of mechanical thrombectomy with angioplasty and stenting for acute basilar occlusions with underlying severe intracranial vertebrobasilar stenosis: preliminary experience from a single Chinese center. AJNR Am J Neuroradiol. 2015; 36 (10):1947–1952

[10] Jia B, Feng L, Liebeskind DS, et al. EAST Study Group. Mechanical thrombectomy and rescue therapy for intracranial large artery occlusion with underlying atherosclerosis. J Neurointerv Surg. 2018; 10(8):746–750

[11] Lee YY, Yoon W, Kim SK, et al. Acute basilar artery occlusion: differences in characteristics and outcomes after endovascular therapy between patients with and without underlying severe atherosclerotic stenosis. AJNR Am J Neuroradiol. 2017; 38(8):1600–1604

[12] Mosimann PJ, Kaesmacher J, Gautschi D, et al. Predictors of unexpected early reocclusion after successful mechanical thrombectomy in acute ischemic stroke patients. Stroke. 2018; 49(11):2643–2651

[13] Kang DH, Yoon W, Kim SK, et al. Endovascular treatment for emergent large vessel occlusion due to severe intracranial atherosclerotic stenosis. J Neurosurg.:(e-pub ahead of print 2008)

[14] Kang DH, Kim YW, Hwang YH, Park SP, Kim YS, Baik SK. Instant reocclusion following mechanical thrombectomy of in situ thromboocclusion and the role of low-dose intra-arterial tirofiban. Cerebrovasc Dis. 2014; 37(5):350–355

[15] Kellert L, Hametner C, Rohde S, et al. Endovascular stroke therapy: tirofiban is associated with risk of fatal intracerebral hemorrhage and poor outcome. Stroke. 2013; 44(5):1453–1455

[16] Lee JS, Lee SJ, Yoo JS, et al. Prognosis of acute intracranial atherosclerosis-related occlusion after endovascular treatment. J Stroke. 2018; 20(3):394–403

27 Intracranial Dissection

27.1 Case Description

27.1.1 Clinical Presentation

A 26-year-old woman with no significant medical history developed right-side weakness in association with headache and deviation of the eyes to the left. She arrived at a peripheral hospital 105 minutes after the onset of the symptoms, with National Institutes of Health Stroke Scale (NIHSS) and Glasgow Coma Scale (GCS) scores of 9 and 10, respectively. She immediately underwent plain CT that demonstrated diffuse subarachnoid hemorrhage (SAH) and left frontal intraparenchymal hematoma (▶ Fig. 27.1). CT angiography (CTA) showed complete occlusion of the left internal carotid artery (ICA) at the level of the supraclinoid segment. The patient was promptly transferred to the main hospital; during the transportation, one episode of generalized seizure occurred. On arrival, her neurological status worsened (GCS 8) and she was intubated.

27.1.2 Imaging Workup and Investigations

- Noncontrast CT was performed at 120 minutes. This did not demonstrate hypodensity, but diffuse SAH and left frontal hematoma (▶ Fig. 27.1).
- CTA revealed a left ICA occlusion at the ophthalmic segment.

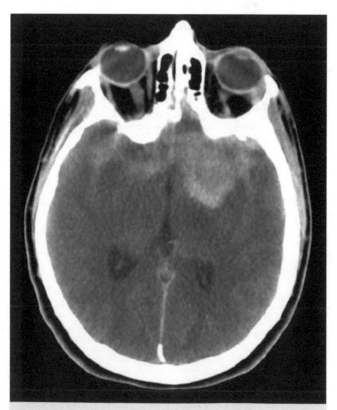
Fig. 27.1 Diffuse SAH and left frontal hematoma.

- Digital subtraction angiography (DSA; performed at 170 minutes from the onset) confirmed the complete occlusion of the left ICA and excellent collaterals via anterior communicating artery with no significant venous delay (< 2 seconds; ▶ Fig. 27.2).

27.1.3 Diagnosis

Intracranial dissection of the left ICA (ophthalmic segment).

27.1.4 Treatment

Given the chance of spontaneous recanalization of the dissected segment and consequent second bleeding, considering the excellent collaterals via anterior communicating artery, we decided to coil the ICA proximal to the dissection. An Envoy 6 Fr was parked in the cervical segment of the left ICA, and we catheterized the ICA with an Echelon 10 microcatheter in conjunction with a Traxcess .014 microwire. Ten coils were detached and the complete occlusion of the artery was ensured.

27.1.5 Posttreatment Management

After treatment, the patient was transferred to the neurological intensive care unit (ICU) to maintain the stability of the vital parameters. A plain CT performed at 24 hours did not show evidence of rebleeding or ischemic signs; also, paroxysmal eye movement (PEM) and electroencephalography (EEG) had no abnormalities. When sedation was reduced for a neurological evaluation, the patient's GCS score was 7.

The patient remained stable for the following 4 days, then the transcranial Doppler (TCD) was suspicious for vasospasm, and CT/CTA/CT perfusion (CTP) were performed (▶ Fig. 27.3). No evidence of ischemic signs or vasospasm was found, but there was a diffuse increase of mean transit time (MTT) on CTP with no ischemic core.

On day 6, a significant increase of IP was noted along with abnormal TCD findings; the decision to skip CT and go directly to the angiography suite was taken the same day. The images showed severe vasospasm of the left anterior cerebral artery (ACA) and middle cerebral artery (MCA), and selective injection of nimodipine was carried out through the anterior communicating artery (▶ Fig. 27.4). Despite this treatment, the patient developed a large ischemic stroke due to vasospasm and died on day 12 after a decompressive craniotomy was performed (▶ Fig. 27.5).

27.1.6 Comments

A surgical superficial temporary artery–MCA bypass should have probably been considered when patient was still asymptomatic for vasospasm. There is no doubt that an attempt of recanalization of the ICA would have led to massive bleeding, and coiling the ICA to ensure the arterial occlusion was the right therapeutic option.

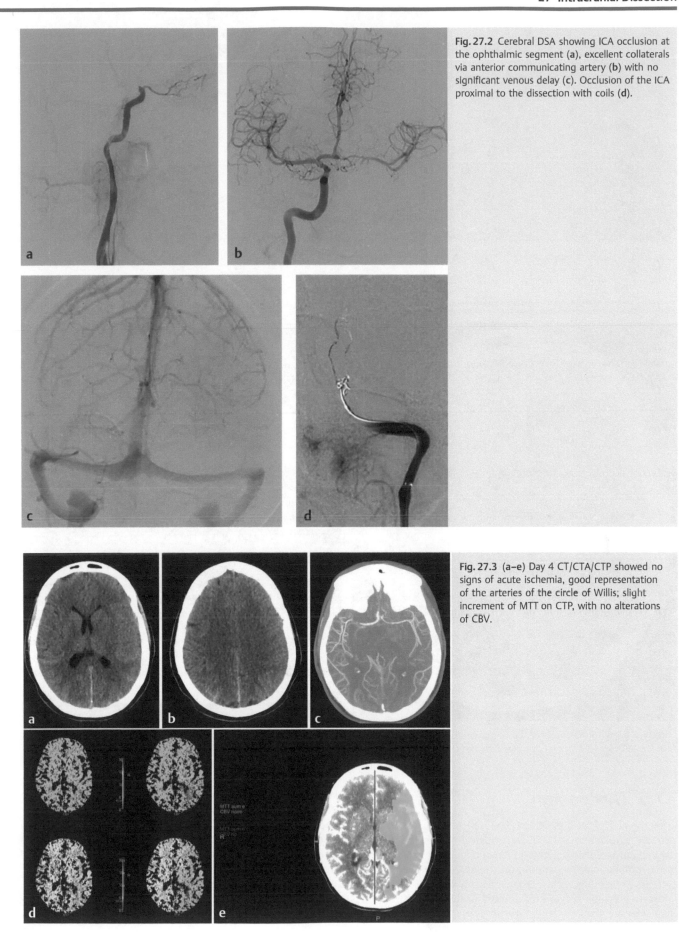

Fig. 27.2 Cerebral DSA showing ICA occlusion at the ophthalmic segment (**a**), excellent collaterals via anterior communicating artery (**b**) with no significant venous delay (**c**). Occlusion of the ICA proximal to the dissection with coils (**d**).

Fig. 27.3 (**a–e**) Day 4 CT/CTA/CTP showed no signs of acute ischemia, good representation of the arteries of the circle of Willis; slight increment of MTT on CTP, with no alterations of CBV.

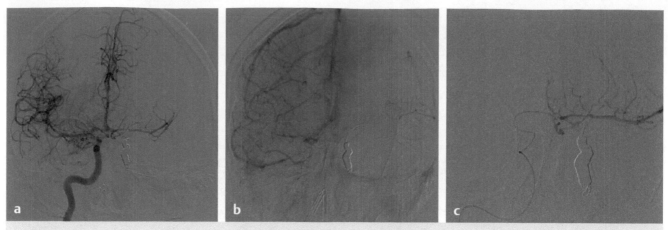

Fig. 27.4 Evidence of severe vasospasm on day 6 (**a,b**) and selective injection of nimodipine into the left hemisphere via anterior communicating artery (**c**).

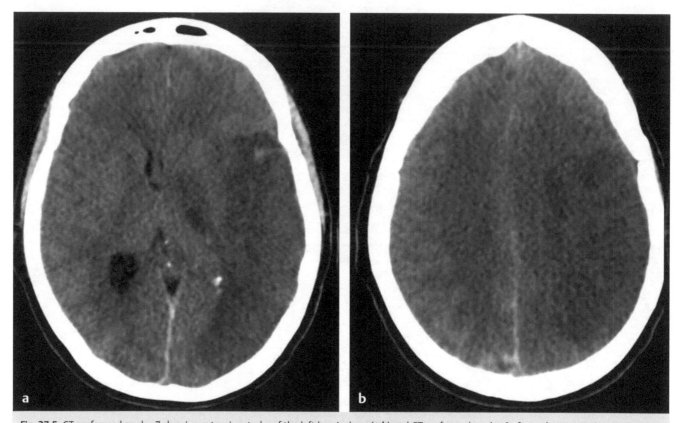

Fig. 27.5 CT performed on day 7 showing extensive stroke of the left hemisphere (**a,b**) and CT performed on day 8 after a decompressive craniectomy was carried out (**c**).

27.2 Discussion

Intracranial arterial dissections (IAD) are a rare cause of acute ischemic stroke and SAH. Epidemiological studies suggest that the incidence of IAD is higher in Asian populations than in European populations. Depending on the study, the mean age of patients presenting with IAD ranges from 45 to 60 years old.[1] Interestingly, men are two times more likely to suffer from IAD than women. To date, there are no systematic epidemiologic studies examining the risk factors contributing to IAD. Trauma has anecdotally been associated with this disease as have connective tissue diseases such as Loeys-Dietz, polycystic kidney disease, and segmental arterial mediolysis. The role of hypertension in IAD is still unclear.[1] Overall, it is generally assumed that there is a genetic component involved due to the ethnic differences in disease prevalence.

IADs differ substantially from cervical arterial dissections (CADs) in a number of ways. The presentation of CAD is typically neck pain, headache and acute ischemic stroke, while IAD typically presents with SAH or acute ischemic stroke. In addition, IAD is much more likely to occur in the posterior circulation, while cervical artery dissection is more likely to occur in the anterior circulation.[2] The higher rates of bleeding associated with IAD can be explained by the structural differences in the cervical versus intradural arteries. Intradural arteries have a robust internal elastic lamina; when compared to the cervical arteries, they are lacking in elastic fibers in the tunica media and external elastic lamina and have little adventitial tissue. Thus, the intradural arteries are more prone to subadventitial dissection and SAH.[1] Two mechanisms have been proposed for IADs. IADs presenting with ischemia are thought to result from dissection between the internal elastic lamina and the media, with pushing of the internal elastic lamina toward the vessel lumen resulting in vessel occlusion or narrowing. Meanwhile, dissection, resulting in SAH, is believed to occur due to dissection within the tunica media or adventitia with disruption of the vessel wall.[3,4]

The natural history and outcomes of IAD depend heavily on the presentation. Patients who present with SAH have high mortality rates when left untreated (20–50%),[5] while those who present with stroke or headache have early mortality rates (0–5%).[5] Patients who present with SAH have rebleeding rates of up to 50%, generally within the first week of the initial event. At the same time, patients who present with acute ischemic stroke experience recurrent stroke rates of about 10%, generally within the first 2 to 3 years following the initial event.[5] In general, patients with posterior circulation dissections show a poorer prognosis compared to those with anterior circulation dissections.[6] Among patients who present without stroke or SAH (i.e., asymptomatic or headache), clinical deterioration rates are exceedingly low ranging from 2 to 3%.[7]

On imaging, IAD has a wide range of manifestations including aneurysmal dilatation, focal stenosis, and occlusion.[8] In general, it is thought that fusiform aneurysmal dilatations and pearl-and-string lesions are associated with SAH, while a focal narrowing or occlusion is associated with stroke. A focal stenosis or occlusion in the setting of SAH can be suggestive of an IAD,[8,9] like in the case presented. Studies on the serial imaging of untreated IADs have shown that these lesions heal in multiple ways, including focal aneurysmal dilatation, persistent stenosis or occlusion, or recanalization and normalization of vessel caliber.[10] The exact time course for these structural changes is unknown.

Treatment of IADs depends on the clinical presentation of the lesion. IADs which present without SAH are treated medically unless they are associated with mass effect.[11] There are a few case reports on the use of intra-arterial and intravenous thrombolysis in patients with IAD-related stroke; however, the safety and efficacy of these treatments in this setting have yet to be systematically studied.[12,13] Patients with cerebral ischemia are typically treated with anticoagulation or antiplatelet therapy, but this has yet to be studied in a clinical trial.[11] Studies on treatment of CAD have demonstrated no difference in anticoagulation and antiplatelet therapy.[11,14] Some caution against the use of anticoagulation in IAD is because of the potential risk for SAH.[15] As IAD without stroke or SAH is known to have a benign course, conservative management without antiplatelet or antithrombotic therapy has been advocated.[7]

Currently, the most favored method of treatment of ruptured dissecting aneurysms is endovascular therapy. Endovascular techniques for treating ruptured dissecting aneurysms can be divided into deconstructive and reconstructive techniques. Deconstructive techniques involve sacrifice of the parent vessel through occlusion and trapping of the aneurysm. With the advent of stents and flow diverters, reconstructive techniques, allowing for parent artery preservation, have been increasingly used. To date, there are no randomized clinical trials studying the efficacy and safety of deconstructive and reconstructive techniques. However, one recently published meta-analysis on the topic found that deconstructive techniques were associated with higher rates of long-term complete occlusion (88 vs. 81%).[16] While this meta-analysis found that deconstructive techniques were associated with higher rates of perioperative morbidity, long-term good neurological outcome rates were similar, about 90% for both groups.[16] One of the major limitations of endovascular techniques is in the treatment of posterior inferior cerebellar artery (PICA)-involving lesions. Deconstructive techniques are associated with high rates of stroke and subsequent mass effect in the treatment of PICA lesions. In a series of 72 patients treated with deconstructive techniques, Kashiwazaki et al found two cases of spinal cord infarction and seven cases of Wallenberg syndrome, secondary to occlusion of PICA dissecting aneurysms.[17] However, reconstruction of PICA-involving lesions requires the aneurysm sac to be left partially open to ensure adequate PICA flow, thus placing the patient at a higher risk of recanalization and hemorrhage. Thus, for these types of lesions, bypass surgery has traditionally been advocated.[18]

References

[1] Debette S, Compter A, Labeyrie MA, et al. Epidemiology, pathophysiology, diagnosis, and management of intracranial artery dissection. Lancet Neurol. 2015; 14(6):640–654

[2] Medel R, Starke RM, Valle-Giler EP, Martin-Schild S, El Khoury R, Dumont AS. Diagnosis and treatment of arterial dissections. Curr Neurol Neurosci Rep. 2014; 14(1):419

[3] Yonas H, Agamanolis D, Takaoka Y, White RJ. Dissecting intracranial aneurysms. Surg Neurol. 1977; 8(6):407–415

[4] Kocaeli H, Chaalala C, Andaluz N, Zuccarello M. Spontaneous intradural vertebral artery dissection: a single-center experience and review of the literature. Skull Base. 2009; 19(3):209–218

[5] Santos-Franco JA, Zenteno M, Lee A. Dissecting aneurysms of the vertebrobasilar system. A comprehensive review on natural history and treatment options. Neurosurg Rev. 2008; 31(2):131–140, discussion 140

[6] Yoshimoto Y, Wakai S. Unruptured intracranial vertebral artery dissection. Clinical course and serial radiographic imagings. Stroke. 1997; 28(2):370–374

[7] Kobayashi N, Murayama Y, Yuki I, et al. Natural course of dissecting vertebrobasilar artery aneurysms without stroke. AJNR Am J Neuroradiol. 2014; 35(7):1371–1375

[8] Rahme RJ, Aoun SG, McClendon J, Jr, El Ahmadieh TY, Bendok BR. Spontaneous cervical and cerebral arterial dissections: diagnosis and management. Neuroimaging Clin N Am. 2013; 23(4):661–671

[9] Pfefferkorn T, Linn J, Habs M, et al. Black blood MRI in suspected large artery primary angiitis of the central nervous system. J Neuroimaging. 2013; 23(3):379–383

[10] Mizutani T. Natural course of intracranial arterial dissections. J Neurosurg. 2011; 114(4):1037–1044

[11] Arauz A, Ruiz A, Pacheco G, et al. Aspirin versus anticoagulation in intra- and extracranial vertebral artery dissection. Eur J Neurol. 2013; 20(1):167–172

[12] Moon Y, Lee JH, Cho HJ, et al. Intravenous thrombolysis in a patient with acute ischemic stroke attributable to intracranial dissection. Neurologist. 2012; 18(3):136–138

[13] Huded V, Kamath V, Chauhan B, et al. Mechanical thrombectomy using solitaire in a 6-year-old child. J Vasc Interv Neurol. 2015; 8(2):13–16

[14] Markus HS, Hayter E, Levi C, Feldman A, Venables G, Norris J, CADISS Trial Investigators. Antiplatelet treatment compared with anticoagulation treatment for cervical artery dissection (CADISS): a randomised trial. Lancet Neurol. 2015; 14(4):361–367

[15] Metso TM, Metso AJ, Helenius J, et al. Prognosis and safety of anticoagulation in intracranial artery dissections in adults. Stroke. 2007; 38(6):1837–1842

[16] Sönmez Ö, Brinjikji W, Murad MH, Lanzino G. Deconstructive and reconstructive techniques in treatment of vertebrobasilar dissecting aneurysms: a systematic review and meta-analysis. AJNR Am J Neuroradiol. 2015; 36(7):1293–1298

[17] Kashiwazaki D, Ushikoshi S, Asano T, Kuroda S, Houkin K. Long-term clinical and radiological results of endovascular internal trapping in vertebral artery dissection. Neuroradiology. 2013; 55(2):201–206

[18] Park W, Ahn JS, Park JC, Kwun BD, Kim CJ. Occipital artery-posterior inferior cerebellar artery bypass for the treatment of aneurysms arising from the vertebral artery and its branches. World Neurosurg. 2014; 82(5):714–721

28 Hyperacute Extracranial Angioplasty and Stenting: When and How

28.1 Case Description

28.1.1 Clinical Presentation

A 69-year-old male presented initially to the emergency department of an outside center with chest pain, dyspnea, and right arm pain. He was diagnosed with bilateral pulmonary emboli on computed tomography pulmonary angiography (CTPA), and was also noted to be in atrial fibrillation. Oral aspirin had already been administered in view of presentation with chest pain. Anticoagulation with low molecular weight heparin was commenced. Later in the same day, there was a sudden onset of left hemiparesis including left facial weakness and dysarthria. Noncontrast computed tomography (NCCT) of brain was performed, but no evidence of hemorrhage was found.

The patient was transferred as a code stroke to our regional stroke center for further evaluation and treatment. At the time of assessment, he was 2 hours from symptom onset. The left hemiparesis had improved significantly during transfer, with residual mild left upper limb drift, mild left facial weakness, and mild dysarthria remaining (National Institutes of Health Stroke Scale [NIHSS] score of 3).

Past medical history was significant for cigarette smoking, and dyslipidemia treated with lipid-lowering medication. There were no other known cardiovascular risk factors at the preadmission stage, and the only regularly administered preadmission medication was rosuvastatin 5 mg once daily.

28.1.2 Imaging Workup and Investigations

NCCT of brain (► Fig. 28.1a–c) demonstrated subtle loss of gray-white matter differentiation in the right basal ganglia. No other early or established ischemic change was observed. There was no evidence of hemorrhage. Computed tomography angiography (CTA) performed from the level of the aortic arch demonstrated right carotid artery (RCA) stenosis with soft ulcerated plaque (► Fig. 28.1d). The caliber of the right internal carotid artery (ICA) distal to the stenosis was reduced compared to the contralateral side, indicating critical stenosis. A small nonocclusive thrombus was visualized in the midportion of the right M1 segment, along the superior wall of the vessel (► Fig. 28.1e, f). No other intracranial thrombus or intracranial arterial occlusion was observed on CTA. A patent anterior communicating artery

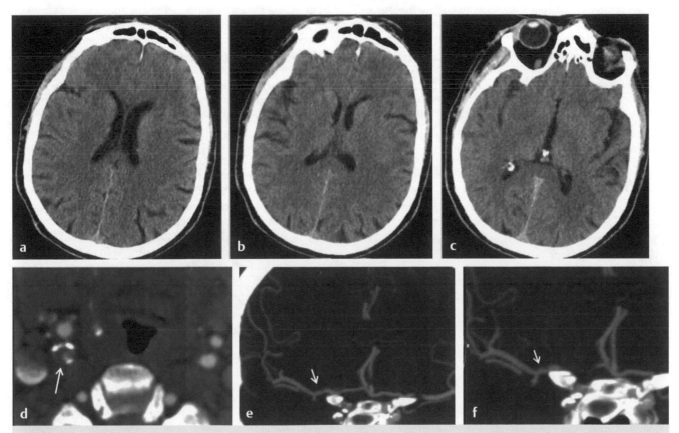

Fig. 28.1 Noncontrast enhanced CT of the brain (a–c) demonstrated subtle loss of gray-white matter differentiation in the right basal ganglia. CT angiography performed from the level of the aortic arch demonstrated RCA stenosis, with soft ulcerated plaque (d). A small nonocclusive thrombus was visualized in the midportion of the right M1 segment, along the superior wall of the vessel (e,f).

(AComm) was identified on the CTA (▶ Fig. 28.1e, f), while a right-sided posterior communicating artery (PComm) could not be appreciated.

28.1.3 Diagnosis

Right ICA critical stenosis.

28.1.4 Treatment

Intravenous (IV) tissue plasminogen activator was contraindicated, as therapeutic dose of low molecular weight heparin had been recently administered. The patient had demonstrated significant clinical improvement (NIHSS score of 3). An emergency multidisciplinary discussion took place regarding the best approach to management. As the right M1 thrombus was very small and nonocclusive, it was felt that immediate endovascular intervention and mechanical thrombectomy was not required. Supporting this, there was already loss of gray-white matter differentiation in the basal ganglia, suggesting early infarction. It was considered very likely, given the configuration of the carotid plaque and the degree of stenosis, that the intracranial thrombus was embolic from the ICA rather than cardioembolic related to the atrial fibrillation. There was consensus that the RCA should be urgently revascularized. Risks and benefits of carotid stenting versus urgent endarterectomy were discussed, in particular taking into consideration the already administered antiplatelet agent, low molecular weight heparin, and the diagnosis of bilateral pulmonary emboli which would require continuation of anticoagulation treatment. Following discussions, a decision was taken to proceed with urgent carotid stenting.

Initial Treatment

Once decision was made to proceed with stenting, a loading dose of 300 mg Plavix was administered, as well as 162 mg aspirin, and the patient was transferred to the neurointerventional suite.

Endovascular Treatment

Materials

- 8-Fr short angiographic sheath.
- 6-Fr 80-cm Shuttle sheath.
- 5-Fr Berenstein catheter.
- 0.035 angled hydrophilic wire.
- Angioguard RX Emboli Capture Guidewire System.
- Synchro 14 microguidewire.
- Mini Trek RX PTA balloon catheter 2 mm × 15 mm.
- Mini Trek RX PTA balloon catheter 3 mm × 15 mm.
- Aviator Plus PTA balloon catheter 5 mm × 20 mm.
- Carotid WALLSTENT 9 mm × 40 mm.
- 8-Fr Angio-Seal closure device.

Technique

Intervention was performed with conscious sedation and systemic heparinization. Local anesthetic was administered at the puncture site. A single-wall, right common femoral artery (CFA) puncture was performed. An 8-Fr short angiographic sheath was placed for vascular access. A 6-Fr 80-cm Shuttle was advanced to the right common carotid artery (CCA) over a 5-Fr Berenstein catheter. Right common carotid angiography confirmed the presence of irregular ulcerated plaque involving the ICA bulb, with stenosis of the right ICA just beyond its origin. The external carotid artery (ECA) led over the ICA. Distally, the cervical portion of the ICA was patent, but of reduced caliber, in keeping with a critical stenosis (▶ Fig. 28.2a).

Based on the caliber of the distal vessel, a 5-mm Angioguard distal protection device was chosen. Predilation of the stenosis was necessary to allow passage of the Angioguard. The stenosis was crossed with a Synchro-14 microguidewire using roadmap guidance (▶ Fig. 28.2b). Over this, a 2 mm × 15 mm Mini Trek balloon dilatation catheter was advanced and placed across the stenosis. Angioplasty with the 2-mm balloon was not sufficient to allow passage of the Angioguard across the stenosis, therefore a second single inflation angioplasty was performed with a 3 mm × 15 mm Mini Trek balloon dilatation catheter. Following this, the Angioguard device was successfully advanced across the stenosis, and deployed in a straight segment of distal cervical ICA (▶ Fig. 28.2c, *arrow*). Angioguard deployment resulted in further reduction of flow in the ICA, and the following steps were rapidly undertaken: A 9 × 40 mm carotid Wallstent was chosen. Further presenting angioplasty was required to allow passage of the stent, and this was performed using a 5 mm × 20 mm Aviator Plus balloon, utilizing rapid exchange maneuver. The Wallstent was then optimally positioned and deployed across the stenosis (▶ Fig. 28.2d, e). A weight-calculated bolus of ReoPro (0.25 mg/kg) was administered immediately once the stent was deployed to bridge, while the administered antiplatelet agents achieved full effect. The Angioguard distal protection device was then recaptured uneventfully and removed.

Poststenting angiography (▶ Fig. 28.2f, g) showed improved caliber of the ICA, with mild residual waisting at the level of the stenosis, improved distal flow in the ICA, and improved perfusion of the right hemisphere, with ICA now leading over ECA. The previously noted filling defect in the M1 segment of middle cerebral artery (MCA) was no longer evident (▶ Fig. 28.3a). A right MCA distal branch occlusion with slow flow, and distal cutoff observed in an inferior parietal M3 branch was noted, possibly representing distal passage of the small right M1 segment thrombus (▶ Fig. 28.3b). This was too distal for stent-retriever thrombectomy, and in the late arterial to parenchymal phase, leptomeningeal collaterals could be seen filling the territory of the occluded branch. The patient was examined, and since the clinical condition was unchanged from the start of the procedure, no further intervention was performed. All devices were retrieved, and an 8-Fr Angio-Seal closure device placed in the right CFA for hemostasis.

Postprocedure Care/Outcome

The patient's clinical condition remained unchanged throughout the procedure, with no change in neurological status pre- and postprocedure. Strict blood pressure control was maintained postprocedure for 24 hours, with systolic blood pressure (SBP) maintained below 140 mm Hg in order to avoid hyperperfusion injury.

The patient remained well and continued with an oral dose of 75 mg clopidogrel and 81 mg aspirin daily. In view of the

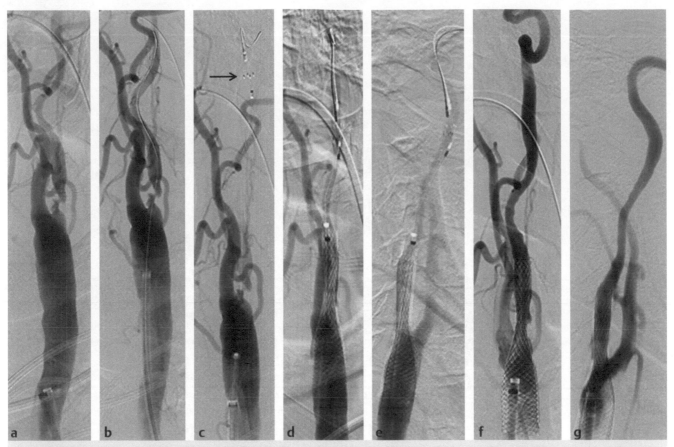

Fig. 28.2 Distally, the cervical portion of the ICA was patent, but of reduced caliber, in keeping with a critical stenosis (**a**). The stenosis was crossed with a Synchro-14 microguidewire using roadmap guidance (**b**). The Angioguard device was successfully advanced across the stenosis, and deployed in a straight segment of distal cervical ICA (**c**). The Wallstent was then optimally positioned and deployed across the stenosis (**d,e**). Poststenting angiography (**f,g**) showed improved caliber of the ICA, with mild residual waisting at the level of the stenosis, improved distal flow in the ICA, and improved perfusion of the right hemisphere with ICA now leading over ECA.

diagnosis of bilateral pulmonary emboli and atrial fibrillation, anticoagulation was continued, initially with low-molecular-weight heparin, with subsequent transition to apixaban 2.5 mg orally twice daily on discharge.

NCCT of the brain was performed 24 hours postprocedure (▶ Fig. 28.4a, b). This demonstrated evolving infarct in the right basal ganglia, with a small region of central petechial hemorrhagic change and without significant mass effect, and also no evidence of infarction elsewhere. The patient showed further neurological improvement, with left upper limb returning to normal power. He was discharged home 6 days postprocedure with mild residual left facial weakness and mild dysarthria remaining.

28.2 Discussion

28.2.1 Background

ICA stenoses are most commonly atherosclerotic in etiology. Extracranial ICA stenosis accounts for 15 to 25% of ischemic stroke, with an incidence that may be as high as 10% in patients older than 80 years. Ipsilateral high-grade ICA stenosis or occlusion is present in approximately 10 to 20% of patients presenting with acute large vessel occlusion stroke which further complicates endovascular access and may lead to a delay in

recanalization of the target vessel occlusion. The risk of stroke in patients with extracranial ICA stenosis is associated with the degree of narrowing; for asymptomatic patients with less than 75% stenosis, the risk of stroke is less than 1%/year, but the risk increases to 2 to 5%/year for patients with greater than 75% stenosis. In symptomatic patients (previous transient ischemic attack [TIA] or stroke), the risk is considerably higher; nearly 10% in the first year and 30 to 35% over the next 5 years for patients with stenoses larger than 70%. Currently, the three major treatments for extracranial ICA stenosis are medical management, carotid endarterectomy (CEA), and carotid angioplasty with stenting.

28.2.2 Workup and Diagnosis

Patient History

In an acute setting, it may be difficult for the neurointerventionalist to gather information regarding relevant medical history expeditiously. This information may already have been obtained by emergency department staff or the stroke physician/neurologist. Patients with carotid disease (or their family members) may report a history of prior stroke or TIAs either as a result of thromboemboli or related hypoperfusion of watershed regions. Since atherosclerosis is a systemic disease, a

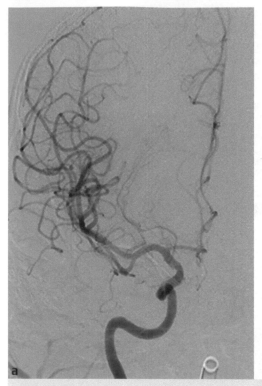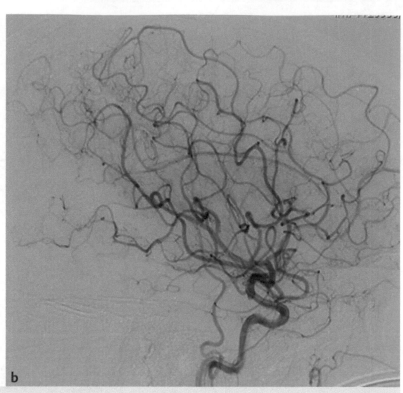

Fig. 28.3 The previously noted filling defect in the M1 segment of MCA was no longer evident (**a**). A right MCA distal branch occlusion with slow flow and distal cut off seen in an inferior parietal M3 branch was noted, possibly representing distal passage of the small right M1 segment thrombus (**b**).

history of coronary artery disease or peripheral vascular disease may also be elicited.

Risk factors for atherosclerotic disease may be present, including smoking, diabetes, hypertension, and hyperlipidemia.

Examination and Investigations

Findings on physical examination will depend on the ischemic or hypoperfused territory. Neurologic deficits may also be present from previously infarcted territories. A bruit may be heard on auscultation over the cervical ICA.

ICA stenosis will be apparent on CTA performed in the hyperacute or acute stroke workup; therefore, it should be performed from the level of the aortic arch. Accurate estimation of the degree of stenosis and characterization of the plaque may be performed with CTA and/or MRA. CTA has the benefit of higher spatial resolution than MRA and will more reliably depict calcifications. In addition, MRA occasionally also suffers from inability to reliably differentiate slow flow or critical stenosis from a complete occlusion. Flow-related artifacts are less common with contrast-enhanced MRA compared to time-of-flight (TOF) MRA. In the nonacute setting, the use of precontrast, T1-weighted, high-resolution MRI of the carotid wall at 3 Tesla may also identify intraplaque hemorrhage, which can be helpful in risk stratification of patients regardless of percentage of stenosis.

Although advances in noninvasive CTA and MRA imaging have eliminated routine use of digital subtraction angiography (DSA) for carotid stenosis quantification in the nonemergent setting, when endovascular therapy is being considered in the acute setting (e.g., mechanical thrombectomy, carotid angioplasty, or stenting), DSA remains the gold standard for measurement of percentage stenosis.

Carotid Doppler ultrasongraphy is of limited utility in the acute setting. It should be reserved as a screening tool in the nonemergent setting, as it suffers from interoperator variability, artifacts due to calcified atherosclerotic plaques, and difficulties distinguishing pseudo-occlusion from complete occlusion.

28.2.3 Imaging Findings

NCCT or MRI of the head may demonstrate old or recent embolic infarcts in the territory of the ipsilateral anterior circulation or infarcts in the MCA–posterior cerebral artery (PCA) and/or anterior cerebral artery (ACA)–MCA watershed regions. CTA from the aortic arch to the vertex of the skull, which is performed as part of hyperacute stroke workup, will demonstrate ICA stenosis as an area of caliber narrowing in the artery. MRA will also show an area of narrowing; however, MRA suffers from lower spatial resolution and may overestimate the degree of stenosis. Furthermore, in the setting of critical ICA stenosis, the slow flow of contrast beyond the stenosis may result in absence of signal distal to the stenosis, and mislead the reader into thinking the ICA is occluded just beyond the stenosis (pseudo-occlusion). Maximum-intensity projections and multiplanar reconstructions are helpful in evaluating the morphology and extent of stenosis. The presence and size of the AComm and PComm arteries should be noted. MRI of carotid plaques may also demonstrate high-risk features such as the presence of intraplaque hemorrhage, inflammation, large lipid core, and/or ulcerations.

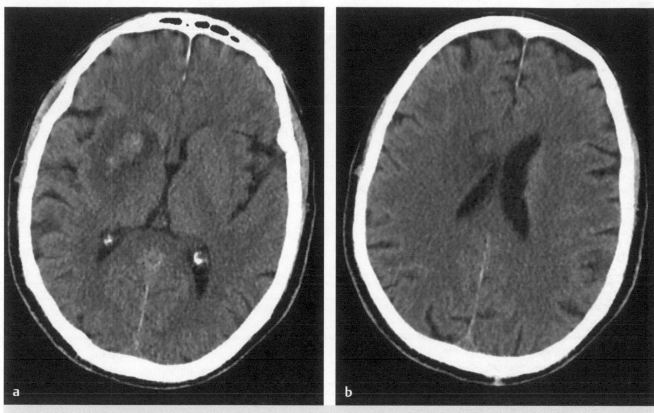

Fig. 28.4 Noncontrast CT of the brain performed 24 hours postprocedure (**a, b**) demonstrated evolving infarct in the right basal ganglia, petechial hemorrhagic change without significant mass effect.

Patients presenting with significant ICA stenosis may demonstrate CT perfusion asymmetry (with elevated time to peak/ mean transit time, decreased relative cerebral blood flow, and preserved or reduced relative cerebral blood volume) in the arterial territory distal to the stenosis, or confined to the ACA–MCA and/or MCA–PCA watershed regions. If an extracranial carotid occlusion is present, no contrast will be seen distal to the occlusion on CTA. The proximal extent of the intracranial and/or extracranial occlusion may be difficult determine on CTA, as the slow or stagnant contrast column within the ipsilateral ICA may not opacify the face of the clot.

DSA remains the gold standard in the diagnosis of ICA stenosis or occlusion, differentiation from pseudo-occlusion, and characterization of extent and morphology of the stenosis. Percentage stenosis should be calculated according to the formula set forth in the North American Symptomatic Carotid Endarterectomy Trial (NASCET): % ICA stenosis = (1– [narrowest ICA diameter/diameter normal distal cervical ICA]) × 100. A critical stenosis may be identified as "string sign," or a small thread of contrast, visible within a stenosis in association with a diffusely and smoothly narrowed caliber of the remainder of the extracranial ICA due to downregulation. In the setting of a critical stenosis, percentage stenosis calculated using NASCET criteria will be "falsely" lowered due to the smaller caliber of the distal ICA, resulting in a smaller denominator. It is helpful to look at the contralateral extracranial ICA for more accurate estimation of the true ICA diameter. Normally, the ICA should fill before the ECA territories when CCA injections are performed. On DSA, patients with long-standing severe or critical ICA stenosis may demonstrate well-developed, pial-pial collaterals in the ACA–MCA and/or MCA–PCA watershed regions of the brain on angiography.

28.2.4 Decision-Making Process

A number of randomized controlled trials published in 2015 have proven to be beneficial for endovascular intervention over medical treatment alone in large artery occlusive stroke. The clinical presentation and imaging findings in this case would not fit the inclusion criteria for these trials. The patient's presenting symptoms had improved to a NIHSS score of 3 and there was no large vessel occlusion on the CTA. Immediate mechanical thrombectomy was thus not indicated.

Urgent revascularization is, however, indicated, given the presence of a significant stenosis of the extracranial carotid artery and the presenting stroke. In general, patients with pre-occlusive carotid stenosis, as in this case, are considered for emergency intervention, whereas those with lesser degrees of stenosis could initially be managed medically with urgent, but not emergency intervention. A number of randomized clinical trials have demonstrated the benefit of carotid revascularization within the first 2 weeks after stroke or TIA. Numerous clinical trials have compared CEA versus carotid artery stenting (CAS). Based on the results of these trials, as discussed further in later sections, current combined consensus statements from neurosurgical, neurology, interventional neuroradiology, cardiology, and vascular surgery societies state that in a majority of cases where there is a need for revascularization of symptomatic extracranial carotid stenosis, CEA is recommended over CAS unless contraindications to surgery are present, or in other specific situations as outlined later in the discussion section.

In the present case, the patient had been anticoagulated with low-molecular-weight heparin for the treatment of acute pulmonary emboli. Furthermore, anticoagulation would also be needed after revascularization for the medical management of atrial fibrillation. The need for anticoagulation places the patient at higher surgical risk for neck hematoma from CEA. In addition, data from a pooled analysis of the three major CEA trials demonstrated no significant benefit of CEA with near occlusion of the ICA, as with this patient, where the absolute risk reduction was negative. Proceeding with CAS is justified on the basis of these considerations.

28.2.5 Management

Conservative

Medical management of extracranial carotid atherosclerotic disease is by far the most commonly used treatment and includes aspirin 81 to 325 mg PO daily. It is the only modality that is considered an essential aspect of management for any patient with a noncardioembolic acute infarct, and is used either alone or in conjunction with more invasive treatments. However, aspirin generally should not be given for the first 24 hours following treatment with IV or IA thrombolytic therapy. Alternatives to aspirin for patients with aspirin intolerance include clopidogrel or ticlopidine, although the effectiveness of these antiplatelets in acute stroke setting is not established. The use of dual-antiplatelet therapy remains largely unproven, with the exception that short-term treatment with clopidogrel plus aspirin appears to be beneficial for high-risk TIA and minor stroke in Asian populations.

Beyond the acute phase of an acute ischemic stroke or TIA, long-term antiplatelet therapy for secondary stroke prevention should be continued.

Major treatable atherosclerotic stroke risk factors including hypertension, diabetes, smoking, and dyslipidemia should also be addressed.

Surgical Treatment

CEA is performed by surgical exploration of the carotid bifurcation, temporary occlusion of flow with or without bypass, arteriotomy, and dissection of plaque. Patching of the ICA may reduce the perioperative risk of stroke. Eversion technique does not alter incidence of stroke but lowers risk of restenosis or occlusion.

Carotid Angioplasty and Stenting

In the nonemergent setting, the patient should be preloaded with dual-antiplatelet therapy, usually aspirin and clopidogrel, for at least 3 days prior to the procedure.

In the acute setting, a decision must be made whether to perform angioplasty of the stenosis without stenting, or stenting with or without angioplasty. The placement of a stent requires administration of antiplatelet agents. In the acute setting, aspirin can be administered intravenously (if available) or via

perrectal or oral routes. The only route of administration for clopidogrel is oral. Typical loading dose would be 300 to 650 mg of aspirin and 300 mg of clopidogrel. If there is concern regarding dysphagia in the acute setting, or the patient is sedated or obtunded, then a nasogastric tube can be placed and antiplatelet agents administered via this. A loading bolus of Abciximab 0.25 mg/kg IV may be administered after stent deployment, as a bridge while antiplatelet agents achieve full effect. Stenting is usually performed with full systemic heparinization (after groin access, target activated clotting time 2–2.5 × baseline or greater than 250 seconds), unless contraindicated.

Compared with carotid angioplasty without stenting, insertion of a stent reduces the risk of embolization, thrombosis, carotid artery recoil, and long-term restenosis.

A self-expanding stent should be used. Percutaneous transluminal angioplasty (PTA) by itself and balloon-mounted stents no longer play a role in extracranial carotid artery disease. Tapered stents are considered more suitable if the proximal and distal diameters of the vessel differ significantly because they reduce the radial outward force distally, while still maintaining sufficient wall apposition proximally. Untapered stents, on the other hand, are more suitable for stenoses in which the proximal and distal diameters of the vessel are similar.

Stenting of the carotid artery stenosis may be performed with or without a distal embolic protection device. Proximal protection with balloon occlusion is also an option. Prestenting balloon angioplasty may be necessary to allow a distal protection device and/or stent to cross the stenosis. If balloon angioplasty of carotid bulb is being performed, the patient can be given prophylactic glycopyrrolate to prevent bradycardia or asystole. Intravenous atropine can be administered for induced bradycardia or reflex asystole if needed. Following stent insertion, post–stenting balloon angioplasty may be necessary to achieve adequate reduction in the degree of stenosis, and improve wall apposition of the stent.

28.2.6 Postprocedure Care

Groin access site bleeding risk is greater in patients in whom a stent is placed because of several factors: larger sheath placement, heparinization is not reversed following the procedure, and the patient is usually on dual antiplatelets. For this reason, unless contraindicated, a femoral artery closure device will be placed at the end of the procedure for hemostasis. If a closure device is contraindicated, then the sheath can be left in situ until heparin has left the system, following which the sheath can be removed and hemostasis achieved with manual pressure. Mixture of 1% lidocaine and epinephrine can be administered subcutaneously after groin closure if there is continued oozing from the soft tissues. An external femoral artery compression device, such as a femostop device, can be considered to maintain hemostasis if a closure device cannot be placed, or the closure device fails.

Blood pressure management post–carotid stenting and/or angioplasty is critical to prevent hyperperfusion injury and intracranial hemorrhage. Patients require close monitoring and should be admitted to appropriate level of postprocedure care, such as a stroke unit, high-dependency unit (HDU), or intensive care unit (ICU).

There is some variation in the literature and between centers regarding the management of antiplatelet medication following carotid stenting. Dual-antiplatelet therapy should, however, be continued for at least 1 month postprocedure, and preferably up to 6 months, after which aspirin alone should continue, often indefinitely.

Delayed restenosis may occur in up to 6% of patients after CAS. Follow-up ultrasonography to evaluate stent patency is recommended at 1 month, 6 months, 12 months, and yearly thereafter. Once patency has been established over an extended period of time, longer follow-up intervals may be appropriate.

28.2.7 Literature Synopsis

The following randomized controlled trials have addressed the treatment of patients with symptomatic extracranial ICA stenosis: the NASCET, the European Carotid Surgery Trial (ECST), and the Veterans Affairs Cooperative Studies Program Trial. A pooled analysis of these three trials clearly demonstrated the benefits of surgery versus medical treatment in the group with stenosis greater than 70%; an absolute risk reduction of 16% was noted after 5 years of follow-up. Patients with moderate stenosis (50–69%) still benefitted from surgery, although the overall gains were more modest, with an absolute risk reduction of 4.6% after 5 years. In patients with mild stenosis (≤50%), the risks incurred during CEA outweighed the benefits of surgery.

The benefit of CEA versus best medical treatment in asymptomatic patients with stenosis was also evaluated in three major trials: the Veterans Affairs Cooperative Studies Program Trial, the Asymptomatic Carotid Atherosclerosis Study (ACAS), and the Asymptomatic Carotid Surgery Trial (ACST). These studies demonstrated that CEA is beneficial for patients younger than 75 years with asymptomatic stenosis greater than 70% because it approximately halves the net 5-year stroke risk from 12% down to 6%.

The timing of treatment for a symptomatic patient has also been evaluated. Increasing evidence from observational and epidemiologic studies shows that the risk for subsequent stroke in patients with carotid stenosis is highest in the first few weeks after the qualifying event, and this risk declines rapidly thereafter. A post hoc analysis of the NASCET and ECST data revealed that the 30-day perioperative risk for stroke and death was unrelated to time since the last symptomatic event and was not increased in patients operated on 2 weeks after nondisabling stroke. In contrast, the risk for ipsilateral ischemic stroke in the medical group fell rapidly with time since the event, as did the absolute benefit of surgery. This decline in benefit is more pronounced in women than in men. It is therefore suggested that the revascularization should occur within 2 weeks following a qualifying event. Observational evidence suggests that CEA in the first 48 hours after symptom onset is associated with increased risk compared with CEA performed 3 to 14 days after symptom onset.

The previous studies have established the role of CEA in the invasive management of symptomatic carotid stenosis and have also established its role in asymptomatic patients. Several prospective randomized controlled trials have compared CEA to CAS with mixed results. The Carotid Artery Vertebral Artery Trial of Angioplasty and Stenting (CAVATAS) randomized 504 patients and found no difference in stroke or death at 30 days (10.3 vs. 10.4%) and no significant difference in outcomes at 3 years between CEA and CAS. The Stenting and Angioplasty with

Protection in Patients with High Risk for Endarterectomy (SAPPHIRE) trial randomized 310 high-risk surgical patients with more than 50% symptomatic stenosis or more than 80% asymptomatic stenosis at 29 centers to CEA and CAS. At 30 days and 1 year, the CAS group had a lower rate of stroke, death, myocardial infarction (MI), and cranial nerve injury. A subgroup analysis of this trial also revealed significant benefit of CAS over CEA in diabetic patients (major adverse event rate of 4.8 vs. 25%). The results of the SAPPHIRE trial established the role of CAS in high surgical risk patients.

Several trials have compared CAS with CEA in patients with standard surgical risk, leading to conflicting results. The Endarterectomy Versus Angioplasty in Patients with Symptomatic Severe Stenosis (EVA-3S) trial randomized 527 asymptomatic patients in France with more than 60% stenosis. This trial was stopped early due to safety and futility concerns, with ipsilateral stroke or death occurring in 6.1% of CEA patients versus 11.7% of CAS patients. Major criticisms of this study, however, were that distal embolic protection devices were not used in the majority of cases, and there may have been inadequate training of interventionalists. The Stent-supported Percutaneous Angioplasty of the Carotid artery versus Endarterectomy (SPACE) trial randomized 1,200 patients in Germany and Austria and found no difference between CEA and CAS at 30 days and 2 years in ipsilateral stroke or death. Both EVA-3S and SPACE trial results were interpreted as failing to demonstrate noninferiority of CAS versus CEA, even though the SPACE trial was stopped early because of lack of funding and did not have enough statistical power to assess noninferiority. The interventionalist qualifications were more stringent in the SPACE trial than in EVA-3S; however, only 27% of the CAS patients in the SPACE trial were treated with distal embolic protection devices.

The UK-based International Carotid Stenting Study (ICSS) demonstrated a rather striking advantage of CEA versus CAS in 1,713 patients, with a risk of stroke or death following CAS of 8.5 versus 5.1% after CEA. Once again, the use of an embolic protection device was not mandated in this study. Other criticisms included the lack of blinding in follow-up assessments, the qualifications of stent operators were less rigorous than for surgeons (only 10 stents required, whereas surgeons had at least 50 cases), and two inexperienced stent operators had 5 major strokes in 11 patients. There is, therefore, valid concern that the experience of the interventionalists may have affected the results of trials, with significant differences between rates of stroke or death following CAS in different studies: 4.4% for Carotid Revascularization Endarterectomy versus Stenting Trial (CREST), 6.9% for SPACE, 8.5% for ICSS, and 9.6% for Endarterectomy Versus Angioplasty in Patients with Severe Symptomatic Carotid Stenosis (EVA3S), compared with the rather constant rates of stroke or death for CEA between 4 and 6%. In fact, a subgroup analysis of SPACE demonstrated that centers with low recruitment rates have profoundly (and negatively) affected the results of CAS.

The largest trial, to date, is CREST, which compared CEA and CAS in 2,502 low or standard surgical risk patients with symptomatic (53% of enrolled patients) and asymptomatic stenosis (47%) at 117 sites. Distal embolic protection devices were required in all patients in the CAS arm. In addition, a rigorous credentialing process for interventionalists was required. There was no difference between the two cohorts in the 4-year rates of primary endpoint (stroke, death, or MI). The clinical durability (rate of ipsilateral stroke) was also similar in both groups (2.4% in the CEA group, and 2.0% in the CAS group). CAS tended to show greater efficacy in patients younger than 70 years, while CEA tended to show greater efficacy in those older than 70 years. There was a statistically significant difference in any stroke within 30 days in the stenting group (4.1%) versus the CEA group (1.9%, $p = 0.0019$); however, most of these were minor strokes. There was also a lower rate of MI (2.0 vs. 3.4%, $p = 0.0387$) and cranial nerve injury (0.3 vs. 4.7%) in the CAS group. In addition, the impact of MI, either clinical or by biomarkers alone, was found to be more significant than stroke on increasing risk of subsequent mortality.

Beyond 30 days, the efficacy of CEA versus CAS for stroke prevention, restenosis rates, and need for repeat revascularization was comparable across all trials. Overall, patients younger than 70 years had better outcomes with CAS. CAS is associated with a better quality of life at 2 weeks and 1 month; although at 1 year, there was no difference in quality of life outcomes.

A 2012 Cochrane database meta-analysis of 11 trials pooled patients randomized to CEA versus CAS. In patients with symptomatic carotid stenosis at standard surgical risk, CAS was associated with a higher risk of any stroke or death at 30 days after treatment (primary safety outcome) than CEA. In patients younger than 70 years, however, there was no significant difference in the primary safety outcome. The rate of death or major or disabling stroke did not differ significantly between treatments. Endovascular treatment was associated with lower risks of MI, cranial nerve palsy, and access site hematomas. The combination of death or any stroke up to 30 days after treatment or ipsilateral stroke during follow-up (the primary combined safety and efficacy outcome) also favored CEA, but the rate of ipsilateral stroke after the periprocedural period did not differ between treatments. Restenosis during follow-up was more common in patients receiving CAS than in patients assigned CEA. Among patients not suitable for surgery, the rate of death or any stroke between randomization and end of follow-up did not differ significantly between endovascular treatment and medical care.

Despite the controversy, there are well-accepted indications currently for carotid artery stenting in situations where CEA is contraindicated: previous anterior neck surgery (previous CEA or other neck dissection); previous neck irradiation; clinically significant cardiac, pulmonary, or other disease that would greatly increase the risk of anesthesia and surgery; carotid artery stenosis in hyperacute stroke; a high bifurcation; a long segment of stenosis; or a tandem stenosis. Based on available data, patients with symptomatic carotid stenosis who do not have any of these conditions may be better served by treatment with CEA. In addition, the periprocedural risk of stroke and death with CAS for the operator or center should be less than 6%.

Results of the CREST trial suggest that technical aspects should be taken into account when considering CAS. Vessel tortuosity in the neck, atherosclerotic disease in the aortic arch or proximal great vessels, or even arch elongation (type III aortic arch) significantly increases the risk of the procedure, possibly preventing safe deployment of protection devices or leading to cerebral embolization, while navigating protection devices before their deployment. In these scenarios, CEA or best medical management may be the safest alternative for the patient.

Compared to balloon-expandable stents, self-expanding stents offer several advantages. Self-expanding stents conform better to tortuous carotid anatomy, provide improved lesion scaffolding and coverage given their availability in different sizes and lengths, and are easier to deploy by using the vertebral bodies as landmarks. As a result, self-expandable stents are the stents of choice for CAS. There are two main types of carotid stent constructs: open-cell stents (e.g., Precise [Cordis] and Acculink [Abbott Vascular]), and closed-cell stents (e.g., Wallstent [Boston Scientific], Xact [Abbott Vascular], and NexStent [Boston Scientific]). Open-cell stents have more flexibility and conformability to tortuous anatomy; however, they offer less vessel wall support (scaffolding) and are therefore less protective against plaque debris protruding through the stent tines and migrating distally. In a retrospective analysis of more than 3,000 patients, Bosiers et al found more adverse events associated with open-cell devices and with stents that had a larger open-cell area in symptomatic patients. Their rationale behind the findings was a higher rate of embolic events due to decreased "scaffolding" of the ruptured embologenic plaque by open-cell stent struts. On the other hand, other groups have failed to identify any differences between outcomes with the different types of stents. This controversy highlights the fact that each stent design has specific advantages, and choosing the right stent is an art, similar to choosing the right coil for aneurysm embolization. The desired features of a carotid artery stent include scaffolding strength adequate to control prolapsed plaque, but with acceptable flexibility, conformability, and radial strength to track the lesion, appose the vessel wall, and control recoil. The design of the stent edges must also be carefully considered because the ends tend to induce elevated mechanical stresses and may damage the arterial wall after expansion.

Controversy also exists with regard to the use of a distal embolic protection device. In a secondary analysis of the SPACE trial, Jansen et al found that protection devices did not lead to a significant reduction of ipsilateral strokes. On the other hand, a recent meta-analysis by Garg et al (including more than 10,000 patients undergoing CAS with or without protection) demonstrated a relative risk of 0.59 (95% confidence interval [CI]: 0.47–0.73) for stroke, favoring protected over unprotected CAS ($p < 0.001$). This analysis concluded that the use of protection devices appears to reduce the risk for stroke during CAS by 38% for both symptomatic and asymptomatic patients. In specific subsets of patients, protection devices may not be necessary, for example, in the absence of intraluminal atherosclerotic plaque (extraluminal narrowing due to previous surgery, radiation, or tumor).

Finally, some other questions concerning the technique of CAS may arise. Angioplasty before stenting should, in our opinion, be avoided if possible. If angioplasty is necessary, a protection device should be used. Post–stent placement angioplasty may not always be necessary, depending on the type of stenosis, and angiographic runs should be performed after stenting to decide whether additional angioplasty is necessary. If balloon angioplasty is performed, we recommend an angioplasty technique similar to that used for intracranial stenosis: gentle and slow inflation over a prolonged period rather than rapid or vigorous inflation.

28.2.8 Pearls and Pitfalls

- Extracranial ICA stenosis accounts for 15 to 25% of ischemic strokes and has a high incidence, especially in the elderly population. Patients with symptomatic stenoses and high-grade asymptomatic stenoses benefit from revascularization.
- In general, patients with acute stroke symptoms and preocclusive carotid stenosis are considered for emergency intervention, whereas those with lesser degrees of stenosis could initially be managed medically with urgent, but not emergency intervention. A number of randomized clinical trials have demonstrated the benefit of revascularization within the first 2 weeks after stroke or TIA.
- Meta-analysis of data from several randomized control trials of CAS versus CEA found that CAS was associated with a higher risk of any stroke or death at 30 days after treatment than CEA. In patients younger than 70 years, however, there was no significant difference. Overall, patients younger than 70 years had better outcomes with CAS, and patients older than 70 years had better outcomes with CEA. CEA is associated with higher rates of MI, cranial nerve palsy, and access site hematoma compared to CEA.
- Current well-accepted indications for carotid artery stenting are situations in which CEA is contraindicated:
  ○ Previous anterior neck surgery.
  ○ Previous CEA or other neck dissection.
  ○ Previous neck irradiation.
  ○ Clinically significant cardiac, pulmonary, or other disease that would greatly increase the risk of anesthesia and surgery.
  ○ Carotid artery stenosis in hyperacute stroke.
  ○ A high carotid bifurcation.
  ○ A long segment of stenosis.
  ○ A tandem stenosis.
  The respective experiences of the local treating team of neurointerventionalists and surgeons, as well as the anatomy and pathology of the individual patient, will likely influence what kind of treatment is being offered.
- Periprocedural risk of stroke and death with CAS for the operator or center should be less than 6%; otherwise, the patient will be better served by CEA.
- Use of distal embolic protection devices appears to reduce the risk contributing to stroke during CAS by 38% for both symptomatic and asymptomatic patients.

Further Readings

Attigah N, Külkens S, Deyle C, et al. Redo surgery or carotid stenting for restenosis after carotid endarterectomy: results of two different treatment strategies. Ann Vasc Surg. 2010; 24(2):190–195

Blackshear JL, Cutlip DE, Roubin GS, et al. CREST Investigators. Myocardial infarction after carotid stenting and endarterectomy: results from the carotid revascularization endarterectomy versus stenting trial. Circulation. 2011; 123 (22):2571–2578

Bonati LH, Lyrer P, Ederle J, Featherstone R, Brown MM. Percutaneous transluminal balloon angioplasty and stenting for carotid artery stenosis. Cochrane Database Syst Rev. 2012; 9(9):CD000515

Bosiers M, de Donato G, Deloose K, et al. Does free cell area influence the outcome in carotid artery stenting? Eur J Vasc Endovasc Surg. 2007; 33(2):135–141, discussion 142–143

Brott TG, Hobson RW, II, Howard G, et al. CREST Investigators. Stenting versus endarterectomy for treatment of carotid-artery stenosis. N Engl J Med. 2010; 363 (1):11–23

Cutlip DE, Pinto DS. Extracranial carotid disease revascularization. Circulation. 2012; 126(22):2636–2644

Eckstein HH, Ringleb P, Allenberg JR, et al. Results of the stent-protected angioplasty versus carotid endarterectomy (SPACE) study to treat symptomatic stenoses at 2 years: a multinational, prospective, randomised trial. Lancet Neurol. 2008; 7 (10):893–902

Eller JL, Dumont TM, Sorkin GC, et al. Endovascular advances for extracranial carotid stenosis. Neurosurgery. 2014; 74 Suppl 1:S92–S101

Garg N, Karagiorgos N, Pisimisis GT, et al. Cerebral protection devices reduce periprocedural strokes during carotid angioplasty and stenting: a systematic review of the current literature. J Endovasc Ther. 2009; 16(4):412–427

Jansen O, Fiehler J, Hartmann M, Brückmann H. Protection or nonprotection in carotid stent angioplasty: the influence of interventional techniques on outcome data from the SPACE Trial. Stroke. 2009; 40(3):841–846

Lal BK, Brott TG. The carotid revascularization endarterectomy vs. stenting trial completes randomization: lessons learned and anticipated results. J Vasc Surg. 2009; 50(5):1224–1231

Lanzino G, Rabinstein AA, Brown RD, Jr. Treatment of carotid artery stenosis: medical therapy, surgery, or stenting? Mayo Clin Proc. 2009; 84(4):362–387, quiz 367–368

McClelland S, III. Multimodality management of carotid artery stenosis: reviewing the class-I evidence. J Natl Med Assoc. 2007; 99(11):1235–1242

Millon A, Mathevet JL, Boussel L, et al. High-resolution magnetic resonance imaging of carotid atherosclerosis identifies vulnerable carotid plaques. J Vasc Surg. 2013; 57(4):1046–1051.e2

Rothwell PM, Eliasziw M, Gutnikov SA, et al. Carotid Endarterectomy Trialists' Collaboration. Analysis of pooled data from the randomised controlled trials of endarterectomy for symptomatic carotid stenosis. Lancet. 2003; 361 (9352):107–116

Rothwell PM, Eliasziw M, Gutnikov SA, Warlow CP, Barnett HJ. Sex difference in the effect of time from symptoms to surgery on benefit from carotid endarterectomy for transient ischemic attack and nondisabling stroke. Stroke. 2004; 35 (12):2855–2861

Touzé E, Calvet D, Chatellier G, Mas JL. Carotid stenting. Curr Opin Neurol. 2008; 21 (1):56–63

Sadek M, Cayne NS, Shin HJ, Turnbull IC, Marin ML, Faries PL. Safety and efficacy of carotid angioplasty and stenting for radiation-associated carotid artery stenosis. J Vasc Surg. 2009; 50(6):1308–1313

Schillinger M, Gschwendtner M, Reimers B, et al. Does carotid stent cell design matter? Stroke. 2008; 39(3):905–909

Shin SH, Stout CL, Richardson AI, DeMasi RJ, Shah RM, Panneton JM. Carotid angioplasty and stenting in anatomically high-risk patients: Safe and durable except for radiation-induced stenosis. J Vasc Surg. 2009; 50(4):762–767, discussion 767–768

Siewiorek GM, Finol EA, Wholey MH. Clinical significance and technical assessment of stent cell geometry in carotid artery stenting. J Endovasc Ther. 2009; 16 (2):178–188

Brott TG, Halperin JL, Abbara S, et al. American College of Cardiology Foundation/ American Heart Association Task Force on Practice Guidelines, American Stroke Association, American Association of Neuroscience Nurses, American Association of Neurological Surgeons, American College of Radiology, American Society of Neuroradiology, Congress of Neurological Surgeons, Society of Atherosclerosis Imaging and Prevention, Society for Cardiovascular Angiography and Interventions, Society of Interventional Radiology, Society of NeuroInterventional Surgery, Society for Vascular Medicine, Society for Vascular Surgery. 2011 ASA/ ACCF/AHA/AANN/AANS/ACR/ASNR/CNS/SAIP/ SCAI/SIR/SNIS/SVM/SVS guideline on the management of patients with extracranial carotid and vertebral artery disease: executive summary: a report of the American College of Cardiology Foundation/American Heart Association Task Force on Practice Guidelines, and the American Stroke Association, American Association of Neuroscience Nurses, American. Vasc Med. 2011; 16(1):35–77

U-King-Im JM, Young V, Gillard JH. Carotid-artery imaging in the diagnosis and management of patients at risk of stroke. Lancet Neurol. 2009; 8(6):569–580 van der Vaart MG, Meerwaldt R, Reijnen MM, Tio RA, Zeebregts CJ. Endarterectomy or carotid artery stenting: the quest continues. Am J Surg. 2008; 195(2):259–269

Wardlaw JM, Chappell FM, Best JJ, Wartolowska K, Berry E, Research NHS, NHS Research and Development Health Technology Assessment Carotid Stenosis Imaging Group. Non-invasive imaging compared with intra-arterial angiography in the diagnosis of symptomatic carotid stenosis: a meta-analysis. Lancet. 2006; 367(9521):1503–1512

Wholey MH, Wu WC. Current status in cervical carotid artery stent placement. J Cardiovasc Surg (Torino). 2009; 50(1):29–37

29 Failed Mechanical Thrombectomy: What to Do Next

29.1 Case Description

29.1.1 Clinical Presentation

A 73-year-old male with history of atrial fibrillation presented initially to the emergency department (ED) in an outside hospital following acute kidney injury and urinary retention. He was off his dabigatran for 2 to 3 weeks and was scheduled for transurethral resection of the prostate. While in hospital, the patient subsequently developed global aphasia and right-sided weakness. He was last seen normal at 7:10 p.m.

Noncontrast computed tomography (NCCT) of the brain was performed, with no evidence of acute large vascular territory infarct, acute intracranial hemorrhage, mass, or mass effect. Initial NCCT of the head recorded an ASPECTS score of 10. CT angiography was also performed at the outside hospital, which revealed a left supraclinoid ICA occlusion.

A telestroke consult was requested. The patient was transferred to our stroke center for further evaluation and treatment.

At time of arrival and assessment at our hospital, he was 4 hours from symptom onset. His National Institutes of Health Stroke Scale (NIHSS) score was 26.

29.1.2 Imaging Workup and Investigations

A repeat NCCT of the brain demonstrated no early or established ischemic changes and an ASPECTS score of 10 (▶ Fig. 29.1a). There was no evidence of intracranial hemorrhage. CT angiography performed from the level of the aortic arch to the vertex confirmed occlusion of the left supraclinoid internal carotid artery (ICA) and left posterior cerebral artery (PCA) origin (▶ Fig. 29.1b) with filling of the left middle cerebral artery (MCA) via patent anterior communicating artery (AComm). CT perfusion (CTP) scan was also performed, which revealed no core infarct and a very large area at risk (penumbra) involving the entire left anterior cerebral artery (ACA), MCA, and PCA territories (▶ Fig. 29.1c–e).

29.1.3 Diagnosis

Intracranial left ICA occlusion.

29.1.4 Treatment

As he was within 4.5 hours of symptom onset, the patient received intravenous tissue plasminogen activator (IV-tPA) in the ED. Emergency multidisciplinary discussion took place with clear indications for emergent mechanical thrombectomy due to high NIHSS, the presence of a large vessel occlusion (LVO), and the absence of acute infarct of NCCT. The details of the procedure, risks, and benefits were discussed with the patient's next of kin and written informed consent was obtained.

Endovascular Treatment

Materials

- 8-Fr short angiographic sheath.
- 5-Fr vert catheter 125 cm.
- 0.035 angled Terumo hydrophilic wire.
- Velocity microcatheter.
- Fathom 16 microguidewire.
- ACE 068 aspiration catheter.
- Solitaire Platinum 6 × 40 mm stent retriever.
- Trevo XP 4 × 40 mm stent retriever.
- ACE 060 aspiration catheter.
- 8-Fr FlowGate balloon guide catheter (BGC).
- 8-Fr Angio-Seal closure device.
- 6-Fr Neuron Max 088.

Technique

The procedure was performed with conscious sedation. Local anesthetic (1% lidocaine) was administered at the left groin puncture site. A 19-gauge, single-wall, left common femoral arterial puncture was performed by palpation. An 8-Fr short angiographic sheath was placed for vascular access. A 6-Fr Neuron Max 088 was advanced to the left ICA over a 125-cm 5-Fr Vert catheter over an angled Terumo guidewire. Angiography confirmed the presence of a left ICA terminus thromboocclusion (▶ Fig. 29.2a).

A Penumbra ACE068 aspiration catheter was then prepared with Velocity microcatheter and Fathom 016 microwire.

Under fluoroscopic and roadmap mask guidance, a Penumbra ACE068 aspiration catheter was advanced to the face of the clot in the supraclinoid ICA over a Velocity microcatheter and a Fathom 016 microwire. Aspiration was applied using the Penumbra pump for 4 minutes. During aspiration, no blood flow was seen in the catheter. Aspiration thrombectomy catheter was unsuccessful. Control angiography showed persisting occlusion at the supraclinoid ICA. Aspiration thrombectomy with the ACE068 catheter was repeated a second time, again unsuccessfully. Control angiography showed persisting occlusion at the supraclinoid ICA.

In a third attempt at thrombectomy the left M1 segment MCA was selectively catheterized by the Velocity microcatheter over the Fathom microwire. The Penumbra ACE068 aspiration catheter was brought to the face of the clot over the Fathom microwire and Velocity microcatheter. The wire was removed and a Solitaire Platinum 6 × 40 mm stent was unsheathed into the left M1 MCA and supraclinoid ICA. After 5 minutes had elapsed for clot integration into the stent retriever, aspiration pump suction was applied to the aspiration catheter, and the stent retriever and aspiration catheter were withdrawn as a unit from the patient, while applying suction using a 60-mL syringe to the guide catheter in the ICA. No clot was noted outside the patient. Control angiography showed persisting occlusion at the supraclinoid ICA.

A fourth attempt at thrombectomy was performed, this time using a Trevo stent retriever. The left M1 segment MCA was selectively catheterized by the Velocity microcatheter over the

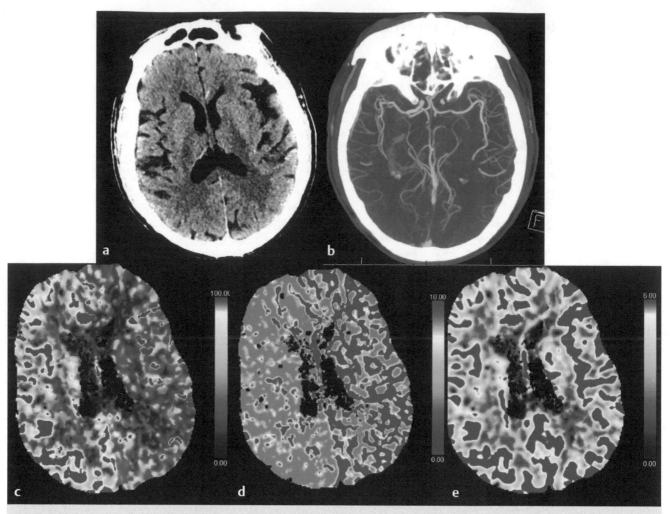

Fig. 29.1 (**a**) Noncontrast CT of the head showing no areas of gray-white dedifferentiation and no acute intracranial hemorrhage. ASPECTS score is 10. (**b**) Maximal intensity projection CT angiography showing occlusion of the left supraclinoid segment ICA, with filling of the left MCA territory via patent anterior communicating artery. CT perfusion mean transit time (MTT) map (**c**) and cerebral blood flow map (**d**) showing a large area of increased MTT and reduced cerebral blood flow, compatible with a large area of ischemia. (**e**) Cerebral blood volume map symmetric indicating no completed infarction at the time of the study, and confirming a large area at risk of infarction.

Fathom microwire. The Penumbra ACE068 aspiration catheter was brought to the face of the clot over the Fathom microwire and Velocity microcatheter. The wire was removed and a Trevo XP 4 × 40 stent retriever was unsheathed into the left M1 MCA and supraclinoid ICA using the "push and fluff" technique. After 5 minutes had elapsed for clot integration into the stent retriever, aspiration pump suction was applied to the aspiration catheter, and the stent retriever and aspiration catheter were withdrawn as a unit from the patient, while applying suction using a 60-mL syringe to the guide catheter in ICA. No clot was noted outside the patient. Control angiography showed persisting occlusion at the supraclinoid ICA.

The Neuron Max 088 guide catheter was then removed.

An 8-Fr Flow Gate was advanced to the left ICA over a 125-cm 5-Fr Vert catheter over an angled Terumo guidewire.

A fifth attempt at thrombectomy was performed using a stent retriever and BGC. Under roadmap mask guidance, the left M1 segment MCA was selectively catheterized with a Velocity microcatheter over a Fathom 016 wire. The wire was removed. A Solitaire Platinum 6 × 40 stent retriever was then unsheathed

into the left M1 MCA and supraclinoid ICA. After 5 minutes, the balloon on the below the guide catheter was inflated and the stent retriever was withdrawn into the guide catheter, while applying suction using a 60-mL syringe to the guide catheter in the ICA. No clot was noted outside the patient. The balloon catheter was deflated. No clot was noted outside the patient. Control angiography showed persisting occlusion at the supraclinoid ICA.

A sixth attempt at thrombectomy was performed using an aspiration catheter and BGC. Under roadmap mask guidance, an ACE060 aspiration catheter was brought to the face of the clot in the supraclinoid ICA over a Terumo guidewire. The wire was removed. With the aspiration catheter remaining in this position, aspiration was applied using the penumbra pump for 5 minutes. Aspiration thrombectomy was then attempted during inflation of the BGC in the cervical ICA, and a 60-mL syringe suction applied to the BGC during aspiration catheter withdrawal into the guide catheter. No clot was noted outside the patient. The balloon catheter was deflated. Control angiography showed persisting occlusion at the supraclinoid ICA.

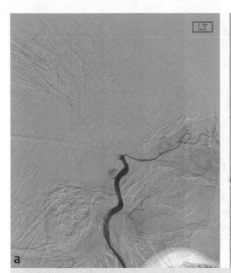 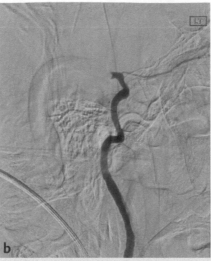 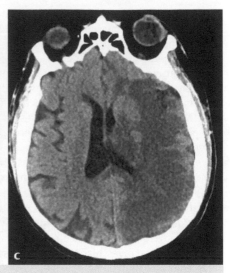

Fig. 29.2 (a) Initial lateral view cerebral angiogram demonstrating occlusion of the left ICA terminus. (b) After seven unsuccessful attempts at mechanical thrombectomy, final lateral view angiogram showing persisting occlusion of the left ICA terminus (mTICI 0). (c) Noncontrast CT of the head 24 hours after the procedure now showing a large acute infarct involving much of the left MCA territory and also portions of the left ACA and PCA territories.

Finally, a seventh attempt at mechanical thrombectomy was made. The left M1 segment MCA was selectively catheterized by the Velocity microcatheter over the Fathom microwire. The Penumbra ACE060 aspiration catheter was brought to the face of the clot over the Fathom microwire and Velocity microcatheter. The wire was removed and a Solitaire Platinum 6 × 40 mm stent was unsheathed into the left M1 MCA and supraclinoid ICA. After 5 minutes had elapsed for clot integration into the stent retriever, aspiration pump suction was applied to the aspiration catheter. The balloon catheter was inflated, and the stent retriever and aspiration catheter were withdrawn as a unit from the patient, while applying suction using a 60-mL syringe to the guide catheter in the ICA. No clot was noted outside the patient. The balloon-guided catheter was deflated. Control angiography showed persisting occlusion at the supraclinoid ICA and modified treatment in cerebral infarction (mTICI) score of 0 (▶ Fig. 29.2b).

At this point, after seven failed attempts at mechanical thrombectomy 3.5 hours into the procedure and approximately 8 hours after symptom onset, further attempts at mechanical thrombectomy were considered to be approaching futility and increased risk. Placement of a detachable stent retriever was considered; however, there was a concern regarding the risk of dual antiplatelet therapy in the setting of potential for hemorrhagic infarct, given the large penumbra on the CTP scan. After discussion with the patient's family, the procedure was aborted.

After an angiographic run of the left common femoral artery (CFA), hemostasis of the left groin was achieved with 8-Fr Angio-Seal closure device.

Postprocedure Care/Outcome

The patient's clinical condition remained unchanged throughout the procedure, with no change in neurological status pre and immediately postprocedure.

During his hospital stay, the patients physical examination revealed gaze preference, global aphasia, homonymous hemianopia, and facial and upper as well as lower extremity right-sided weakness.

NCCT of the brain was performed 24 hours postprocedure (▶ Fig. 29.2c). This demonstrated a large MCA territory infarct involving most of the MCA territory as well as partial ACA infarcts of the paramedian frontal lobe, and partial PCA territory infarction of the occipital lobe and left cerebral peduncle. No hemorrhagic conversion was noted. The patient showed further neurological deterioration in the next 1 to 2 days with development of sluggish left pupil, without new intracranial hemorrhage or significant midline shift. Supportive care was provided to the patient, with the family electing to pursue palliative care shortly afterward.

29.2 Discussion

Much of the clinical benefit of mechanical thrombectomy is accounted for by the effectiveness of the latest generation of stent retrievers and aspiration catheters. Successful reperfusion (defined as mTICI 2b or greater) can routinely be achieved up to 85% of the time with these devices. In recent randomized controlled trials of mechanical thrombectomy, however, 15 to 40% of stent-retriever mechanical thrombectomies failed to achieve substantial reperfusion (mTICI 2b or 3), and 8 to 18% had minimal or no reperfusion (mTICI 0–1).[1,2,3,4,5] Moreover, poor outcomes were still seen in some patients with substantial reperfusion due to delays and/or difficulties encountered during endovascular treatment. These issues highlight the need for further improvements in devices, techniques, and workflows.

From a technical standpoint, mechanical thrombectomy may fail for a variety of reasons: difficult vascular access, thrombus composition, device–thrombus interactions, or the formation of distal emboli.

Anatomical challenges may be encountered anywhere along the course of a catheter in accessing the intracranial clot. Femoral artery access is the traditional method of approach for mechanical thrombectomy procedures. The presence of peripheral artery disease may render femoral artery access more difficult or impossible (aortoiliac occlusive disease). The angle of the origin of the great vessels and the aortic arch often becomes more acute with age. In addition, substantial cervical arterial tortuosity may develop with age, especially in the setting of chronic hypertension.[6] Such anatomical difficulties may render selective catheterization of the great vessels and/or make catheter placement more difficult, requiring different catheter shapes, wires, and exchange techniques, or impossible. Furthermore, in such anatomical configurations, the forces required to navigate intermediate catheters and microcatheters intracranially may cause guide catheter herniation and loss of access.[6] In a study by Ribo et al,[6] predictors of difficult carotid access were older than 75 years, hypertension, dyslipidemia, and left carotid catheterization. Difficult access can cause significant delays in time to revascularization, decreased revascularization rates, and worse outcomes.

Various approaches have been promoted to bypass such scenarios, including direct carotid puncture and radial artery access. Direct carotid access can be safely achieved using ultrasound guidance. In a series of seven patients undergoing direct carotid puncture after multiple unsuccessful femoral attempts lasting from 20 to 90 minutes, carotid access was achieved in 15 minutes or less, and mTICI 2b–3 reperfusion was achieved in 6 (86%) patients within 7 to 49 minutes of access.[7] Achieving hemostasis after thrombectomy, however, is the major drawback, as a closure device for carotid puncture does not exist. Manual compression of a carotid puncture can cause a new thromboembolus to form, and the formation of a large neck hematoma may result in respiratory compromise or cranial nerve injury. Another drawback is the absence of devices with shorter lengths.[8]

Radial artery puncture has been used with increasing frequency; however, this approach may not always allow improved access to aortic arch vessels and does not permit use of larger guide catheters.

Another anatomical obstacle to thrombectomy not infrequently encountered is the presence of a tandem steno-occlusive lesion in the carotid artery. This situation is covered in depth in another chapter of this book. In a retrospective single-center study by Kaesmacher et al, M2 MCA occlusions were at higher risk of reperfusion failure than other clot locations (adjusted OR = 3.36; 95% CI, 1.82–6.21).[9]

Mechanical thrombectomy procedures can also fail due to device–thrombus interactions. Up to 20 to 30% of thrombi may be resistant to removal using current generation retrieval devices. There are a number of forces interacting during mechanical thrombectomy between the device, the thrombus, and the vessel wall, as well as procedural techniques that can influence these forces.

The pressure differential between blood flow at the face of the clot and retrograde blood flow on the distal end of the clot is one such interaction, which may explain the decreased recanalization rates seen in patients with poor collaterals.[10] Another is the combined force of friction and adhesion between the thrombus and the vessel wall. Recent studies have demonstrated decreased revascularization rates of hypodense, fibrin-rich thrombi.[11] In vitro experiments using thrombi of varying fibrin and red blood cell (RBC) proportions have shown that fibrin-rich thrombi (< 20% RBC content) have a significantly higher coefficient of static friction.[12] Furthermore, longer thrombi would be expected to have increased friction and adhesion, given their larger surface area for thrombus–vessel interaction. Some thrombi can be quite hard, making passage of a microwire and/or microcatheter beyond the clot difficult or impossible. In one retrospective series of 72 consecutive patients with failed mechanical thrombectomy, this was seen in 15 of 72 (21%).[13]

Techniques to overcome clot inertia (combined friction/adhesion and impaction forces) include maximizing clot integration by the stent retriever or aspiration catheter. For stent retrievers, device–thrombus interaction is maximized by positioning the device, so that the active element is deployed across the entire length of the thrombus (the proximal marker of a stent retriever should be positioned proximal to the clot). Clot–device interaction can be increased with closed-cell design stent retrievers (Trevo, Stryker) by using the "push and fluff" technique. This involves pushing the wire to deploy the device, rather than unsheathing it, as well as pushing forward on the catheter during deployment to cause the device to expand into the clot[14]. A higher rate of first-pass reperfusion and of complete reperfusion (mTICI 3) was seen using this technique compared to unsheathing of the Trevo.[15]

The ASTER and COMPASS trials have shown that, as a first-line therapy, both ADAPT technique using aspiration catheters and stent retrievers achieve similar rates of successful reperfusion. In the ASTER study, there was a higher rate of conversion to another device or technique with the first-line ADAPT compared to stent retriever (32.8 vs. 23.8%, respectively, p = 0.053).[16]

Use of a cervical BGC, which markedly reduces the pressure head on the face of a thrombus, not only allows for more effective retrieval but also decreases thrombus fragmentation and distal embolization compared to a traditional cervical guide catheter.[17,18] A recent meta-analysis of five nonrandomized studies of 2,022 patients (1,083 BGC group and 939 non-BGC group) was reported by Brinjijki et al.[19] Patients treated with BGCs had higher odds of first-pass recanalization, mTICI 3, mTICI 2b/3, modified Rankin scale (mRS) score of 0 to 2, lower odds of mortality, lower mean number of passes, and shorter procedure times.[19] In ASTER, 92% of the stent-retriever cases utilized a BGC versus none of the ADAPT cases.[20] The ASTER trial results showed no difference in revascularization rates between primary ADAPT approach, primary stent retriever, and BGC; however, the better clinical outcomes for stent retrievers, although not statistically significant, may be related to the decreased frequency of distal emboli with BGC use.[16]

Stent retrievers may also be used in combination with aspiration catheters to maximize clot retrieval forces at both the face of the clot and along the length of the clot. This technique is also advantageous in tortuous intracranial anatomy by optimizing the angle at which the stent retriever is withdrawn ("line of force") and avoiding undesirable traction on the artery itself.[21] Recent studies have emerged combining stent-retriever thrombectomy, local aspiration, and BGC, with promising early results.[22]

Thrombus–device interactions also occur during and after multiple attempts. Static friction is greater than kinetic friction; therefore, once the retrieval is begun, device withdrawal should be steady until the thrombus is removed from the body. Also, each thrombectomy attempt has the potential for causing compression of the thrombus, which also increases the friction between the thrombus and vessel wall, making subsequent retrieval more difficult.[20] In addition, with each subsequent pass, the cumulative risks of the procedure increase, with potential for endothelial damage and vessel perforation.

Intra-arterial thrombolysis was one of the first strategies employed in stroke treatment. Currently, recombinant tPA is sometimes used in combination with mechanical thrombectomy, either initially to "soften" the thrombus or, more commonly, to recanalize distal fragments which were originally present or dislodged during mechanical thrombectomy. There is a theoretical increased risk of postprocedure hemorrhage after intra-arterial tPA (IA-tPA), especially if the patient has been treated with IV thrombolysis or if injecting into an already infarcted territory; however, at low dosages (< 10 mg), there have not been reports of significant increases in hemorrhage rates. Intracranial arterial administration of a GPIIb/IIIa inhibitor is most commonly used in the setting of thromboembolic complications of aneurysm coiling or intracranial stenting.[23] The efficacy, safety, timing, route of administration, and dosage in the setting of stroke thrombectomy needs to be evaluated in larger studies.[24]

Currently, there is no clear data or consensus on which device should be used if the first one or more passes is unsuccessful during mechanical thrombectomy. More complicated techniques may take longer and may be problematic, especially for novice operators. There is no absolute cut-off for the number of passes during mechanical thrombectomy that should be performed prior to aborting the procedure. With each thrombectomy pass, however, there is potential for thrombus compression and increasing difficulty of subsequent retrieval, as well as increased risk of vessel dissection and perforation. Moreover, as the length of the procedure and number of thrombectomy attempts increases, the probability of a good outcome decreases.[25] This can be due to increased clot friction, collateral failure and infarct growth, or increased rate of complications.

Various rescue techniques have been described for refractory cases. Crossing Y-Solitaire thrombectomy technique is one rescue strategy described by Aydin et al in ten cases after three to five unsuccessful attempts.[26] Deployment of two crossing Solitaires into the limb of each M2 branch led to complete recanalization in 80% (after one pass) or 100% of cases (after two passes). Minor-moderate reversible spasm was noted in 50% of cases and minor hemorrhage was noted in 20%. At 90 days, the mRS score was 0 to 3 in all cases. The authors speculate that increased strut surface contact, improved thrombus integration, and engagement of thrombus may contribute to the success of this strategy. Permanent implantation of intracranial stents after multiple failed attempts has also been described in several reports.[27,28,29] This approach is discussed in further detail in a separate chapter in this book.

In some patients, a delay in successful reperfusion can have the same result as a technical failure of clot removal. Delays can be preprocedural or intraprocedural. Preprocedural delays can be caused by patient transfer (initial presentation to a center without thrombectomy capabilities), delayed stroke team activation, placement of a Foley catheter, and unnecessarily waiting for laboratories or next of kin for consent.

Intraprocedural delays may relate to use of general anesthesia, lack of standardized protocols and defined staff roles during mechanical thrombectomy procedures, poor coordination between technologist, nursing, anesthesiologist, neurologist, and/or neurointerventional team members, use of general anesthesia, poor device selection, and catheter incompatibility (see Chapter 6).

Patient outcomes after failed mechanical thrombectomy are poor. Supportive medical therapy should be administered to minimize infarct growth, and recognize and prevent hemorrhagic transformation and malignant edema. Younger patients pose a particular challenge after failed LVO mechanical thrombectomy due to the limited space for cerebral edema. It is also important to discuss the procedural outcome and prognosis with the patient's family after a failed mechanical thrombectomy procedure.

29.2.1 Postprocedure Care

Blood pressure management after failed mechanical thrombectomy is critical to minimize infarct growth, while avoiding hemorrhagic conversion of infarcted brain. Generally, a systolic blood pressure (SBP) below 180 mm Hg is targeted. Patients require close monitoring, and should be admitted to an appropriate level of postprocedural care, such as a stroke unit, high-dependency unit or intensive care unit. After failed mechanical thrombectomy, patients may develop large vascular territory infarcts. In younger patients, a high level of vigilance is required for the possible development of malignant cytotoxic edema within 2 to 3 days, since this can result in life-threatening herniation syndromes. Depending on patient factors and preferences, consideration may be given to decompressive craniectomy in a subset of these patients. In older patients, the combination of more advanced cerebral volume loss and large MCA territory infarcts may not result in significant mass effect. Discussion with family regarding prognosis and resultant significant disability are important. Mortality rates following large vascular territory ischemic stroke are higher, due to increased frequency of complications related to poor airway protection, dysphagia, limited mobility, and institutionalization. The goals of care should be established with next of kin keeping in mind patient's advanced directive or previously expressed wishes.

29.2.2 Pearls and Pitfalls

- In recent randomized controlled trials involving mechanical thrombectomy, however, 15 to 40% of stent-retriever mechanical thrombectomies failed to achieve substantial reperfusion (mTICI 2b or 3), and 8 to 18% had minimal or no reperfusion (mTICI 0–1).
- Mechanical thrombectomy may fail for a variety of reasons: difficult vascular access, thrombus composition, device–thrombus interactions, or the formation of distal emboli.
- Likelihood of successful reperfusion after mechanical thrombectomy may decrease with every pass. Each unsuccessful thrombectomy attempt has the potential for causing compression of the thrombus, which also increases the friction between the thrombus and vessel wall.
- Further improvements in thrombectomy devices, techniques, and workflows are necessary.

References

[1] Berkhemer OA, Fransen PS, Beumer D, et al. MR CLEAN Investigators. A randomized trial of intraarterial treatment for acute ischemic stroke. N Engl J Med. 2015; 372(1):11–20

[2] Campbell BC, Mitchell PJ, Kleinig TJ, et al. EXTEND-IA Investigators. Endovascular therapy for ischemic stroke with perfusion-imaging selection. N Engl J Med. 2015; 372(11):1009–1018

[3] Goyal M, Demchuk AM, Menon BK, et al. ESCAPE Trial Investigators. Randomized assessment of rapid endovascular treatment of ischemic stroke. N Engl J Med. 2015; 372(11):1019–1030

[4] Saver JL, Goyal M, Bonafe A, et al. SWIFT PRIME Investigators. Stent-retriever thrombectomy after intravenous t-PA vs. t-PA alone in stroke. N Engl J Med. 2015; 372(24):2285–2295

[5] Jovin TG, Chamorro A, Cobo E, et al. REVASCAT Trial Investigators. Thrombectomy within 8 hours after symptom onset in ischemic stroke. N Engl J Med. 2015; 372(24):2296–2306

[6] Ribo M, Flores A, Rubiera M, et al. Difficult catheter access to the occluded vessel during endovascular treatment of acute ischemic stroke is associated with worse clinical outcome. J Neurointerv Surg. 2013; 5 Suppl 1:i70–i73

[7] Jadhav AP, Ribo M, Grandhi R, et al. Transcervical access in acute ischemic stroke. J Neurointerv Surg. 2014; 6(9):652–657

[8] Mokin M, Snyder KV, Levy EI, Hopkins LN, Siddiqui AH. Direct carotid artery puncture access for endovascular treatment of acute ischemic stroke: technical aspects, advantages, and limitations. J Neurointerv Surg. 2015; 7 (2):108–113

[9] Kaesmacher J, Gralla J, Mosimann PJ, et al. Reasons for reperfusion failures in stent-retriever-based thrombectomy: registry analysis and proposal of a classification system. AJNR Am J Neuroradiol. 2018; 39(10):1848–1853

[10] Liebeskind DS, Jahan R, Nogueira RG, Zaidat OO, Saver JL, SWIFT Investigators. Impact of collaterals on successful revascularization in Solitaire FR with the intention for thrombectomy. Stroke. 2014; 45(7):2036–2040

[11] Brinjikji W, Duffy S, Burrows A, et al. Correlation of imaging and histopathology of thrombi in acute ischemic stroke with etiology and outcome: a systematic review. J Neurointerv Surg. 2017; 9(6):529–534

[12] Gunning GM, McArdle K, Mirza M, Duffy S, Gilvarry M, Brouwer PA. Clot friction variation with fibrin content; implications for resistance to thrombectomy. J Neurointerv Surg. 2018; 10(1):34–38

[13] Leischner H, Flottmann F, Hanning U, et al. Reasons for failed endovascular recanalization attempts in stroke patients. J Neurointerv Surg. 2019; 11 (5):439–442

[14] van der Marel K, Chueh JY, Brooks OW, et al. Quantitative assessment of device-clot interaction for stent retriever thrombectomy. J Neurointerv Surg. 2016; 8(12):1278–1282

[15] Haussen DC, Rebello LC, Nogueira RG. Optimizing clot retrieval in acute stroke: the push and fluff technique for closed-cell stentrievers. Stroke. 2015; 46(10):2838–2842

[16] Lapergue B, Blanc R, Gory B, et al. ASTER Trial Investigators. Effect of endovascular contact aspiration vs stent retriever on revascularization in patients with acute ischemic stroke and large vessel occlusion: the ASTER randomized clinical trial. JAMA. 2017; 318(5):443–452

[17] Chueh JY, Puri AS, Wakhloo AK, Gounis MJ. Risk of distal embolization with stent retriever thrombectomy and ADAPT. J Neurointerv Surg. 2016; 8 (2):197–202

[18] Chueh JY, Kühn AL, Puri AS, Wilson SD, Wakhloo AK, Gounis MJ. Reduction in distal emboli with proximal flow control during mechanical thrombectomy: a quantitative in vitro study. Stroke. 2013; 44(5):1396–1401

[19] Brinjikji W, Starke RM, Murad MH, et al. Impact of balloon guide catheter on technical and clinical outcomes: a systematic review and meta-analysis. J Neurointerv Surg. 2018; 10(4):335–339

[20] Yoo AJ, Andersson T. Thrombectomy in acute ischemic stroke: challenges to procedural success. J Stroke. 2017; 19(2):121–130

[21] Mokin M, Ionita CN, Nagesh SV, Rudin S, Levy EI, Siddiqui AH. Primary stentriever versus combined stentriever plus aspiration thrombectomy approaches: in vitro stroke model comparison. J Neurointerv Surg. 2015; 7 (6):453–457

[22] Stampfl S, Pfaff J, Herweh C, et al. Combined proximal balloon occlusion and distal aspiration: a new approach to prevent distal embolization during neurothrombectomy. J Neurointerv Surg. 2017; 9(4):346–351

[23] Adeeb N, Griessenauer CJ, Moore JM, et al. Ischemic stroke after treatment of intraprocedural thrombosis during stent-assisted coiling and flow diversion. Stroke. 2017; 48(4):1098–1100

[24] Goh DH, Jin SC, Jeong HW, Ha SY. Mechanical Solitaire thrombectomy with low-dose booster tirofiban injection. Neurointervention. 2016; 11(2):114–119

[25] Seker F, Pfaff J, Wolf M, et al. Correlation of thrombectomy maneuver count with recanalization success and clinical outcome in patients with ischemic stroke. AJNR Am J Neuroradiol. 2017; 38(7):1368–1371

[26] Aydin K, Barburoglu M, Oztop Cakmak O, et al. Crossing Y-Solitaire thrombectomy as a rescue treatment for refractory acute occlusions of the middle cerebral artery. J Neurointerv Surg. 2018

[27] Baek JH, Kim BM, Kim DJ, Heo JH, Nam HS, Yoo J. Stenting as a rescue treatment after failure of mechanical thrombectomy for anterior circulation large artery occlusion. Stroke. 2016; 47(9):2360–2363

[28] Ahmed SU, Mann J, Houde J, Barber E, Kelly ME, Peeling L. Permanent implantation of the Solitaire device as a bailout technique for large vessel intracranial occlusions. J Neurointerv Surg. 2019; 11(2):133–136

[29] Forbrig R, Lockau H, Flottmann F, et al. Intracranial rescue stent angioplasty after stent-retriever thrombectomy: multicenter experience. Clin Neuroradiol. 2019; 29(3):445–457

30 Rescue Permanent Stenting

30.1 Case Description

30.1.1 Clinical Presentation

A 57-year-old male presents to the emergency department (ED) 180 minutes after sudden onset of left arm and leg weakness as well as facial droop. Clinical examination confirms a right middle cerebral artery (MCA) syndrome, with a National Institutes of Health Stroke Scale (NIHSS) score of 17.

30.1.2 Imaging Workup and Investigations

- Noncontrast computed tomography (NCCT) performed shortly after presentation to the emergency department (200 minutes after symptoms onset) showed no early infarction, with an ASPECTS score of 10.
- CT angiography (CTA) showed occlusion of the M1 segment of the right MCA and moderate collateral circulation.
- CT perfusion (CTP) showed increased mean transit time (MTT) in the right MCA cortical branch territories, with mildly reduced cerebral blood flow (CBF) and normal cerebral blood volume (CBV), indicating tissue at risk of infarction, but potentially salvageable with reperfusion.

30.1.3 Diagnosis

Right M1 occlusion without early infarction in the MCA territory and large ischemic penumbra (mismatch on CTP).

30.1.4 Management

- The patient had no contraindication to intravenous thrombolysis based on clinical history, clinical assessment, and CT findings.
- He received an initial bolus and infusion of a full dose of intravenous tissue plasminogen activator (IV-tPA), commencing 220 minutes after symptom onset. Endovascular therapy was considered appropriate, based on time from onset of symptoms, location of the arterial occlusion and CT findings, suggesting potentially salvageable tissue. He patient was brought to the angiography suite and groin puncture was performed 235 minutes after onset of symptoms.

30.1.5 Endovascular Treatment

Materials

- 8 Fr × 11 cm AVANTI Vascular Access Sheath (Cordis).
- 8 Fr × 95 cm FlowGate Balloon Guide Catheter (Stryker Neurovascular).
- 6 Fr × 130 cm Berenstein tip Diagnostic Catheter (Stryker Neurovascular).
- 6 Fr × 132 cm ACE 68 Reperfusion Catheter (Penumbra).
- 2.95-Fr × 160 cm Velocity Microcatheter (Penumbra).
- 4 × 20 mm Solitaire 2 Stentriever Device (Medtronic).
- 6 × 30 mm Solitaire 2 Stentriever Device (Medtronic).
- 4.5 × 20 mm Separator 3D Stentriever (Penumbra).
- 3 × 15 mm Solitaire AB Device (Medtronic).
- 0.035 in × 145 cm J-wire (Cook Medical).
- 0.035 in × 180 cm Glidewire Advantage (Terumo).
- 0.014 in × 200 cm Synchro-14 Microwire (Stryker Neurovascular).

Technique

- The patient was brought to the neuroangiography suite and both groins were prepped and draped in the typical sterile fashion.
- Right common femoral artery (CFA) puncture was performed, and a 0.035 inch x 145 cm J-wire was inserted into the descending thoracic aorta under real-time fluoroscopy.
- An 8 Fr × 11 cm femoral sheath was inserted into the right iliac artery over the J-wire and was connected with continuous heparinized flush.
- An 8 Fr × 95 cm FlowGate balloon guide catheter (BCG) was prepped and introduced through the femoral sheath.
- A 6 Fr × 130 cm Berenstein tip Catheter was then introduced into the BCG over a 0.035 in × 180 cm Glidewire Advantage ultimately to catheterize the right common carotid artery (CCA) under fluoroscopy.
- A roadmap was then obtained to characterize the bifurcation and used to gain access into the right internal carotid artery (ICA).
- An angiography was obtained. This demonstrated persistent occlusion of the right M1. The diagnostic catheter was then removed (▶ Fig. 30.1).
- A 6 Fr × 132 cm ACE 68 Reperfusion Catheter and a 2.95 Fr × 160 cm Velocity Microcatheter were prepped and introduced through the BCG over a 0.014 in × 200 cm Synchro-14 microwire, and we were able to cross the thrombus into the superior M2 division.
- The Synchro-14 microwire was then navigated to the right MCA and across the occlusive clot. The Velocity Microcatheter was then positioned distal to the clot in the M2 segment, and the ACE 68 Reperfusion Catheter at the origin of the MCA.
- A 4 × 20 mm Solitaire 2 Stentriever Device was then deployed from the proximal M2 to the mid M1 segment, resulting in restoration of flow to the remainder of the MCA. The stent remained in place for about 5 minutes after which it was retrieved under flow arrest with the BCG inflated and continuous aspiration. Manual suction was continued after the aspiration catheter was removed through the BCG. This demonstrated some clot that was within the Solitaire 2 Stentriever and the ACE 68. The patient remained hemodynamically stable during this maneuver (▶ Fig. 30.2).
- Angiography via the BCG demonstrated persistent clot within the right M1 and with partial distal recanalization.
- We decided to perform a second pass with 4 × 20 mm Solitaire 2 Stentriever using the same technique (▶ Fig. 30.3).
- A second angiography via the BCG demonstrated partial flow restoration.

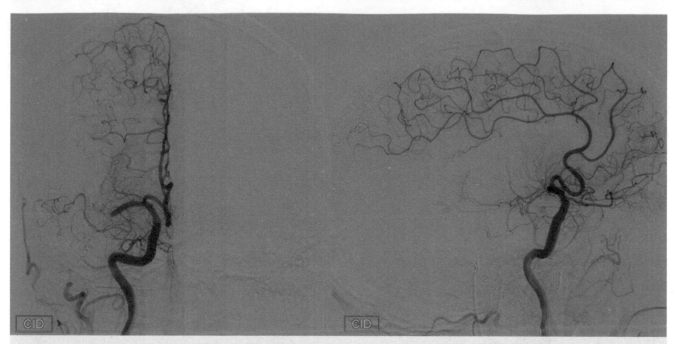

Fig. 30.1 Diagnostic cerebral angiography. Right internal carotid artery injection via diagnostic catheter. Imaging demonstrated persistent occlusion of the right M1.

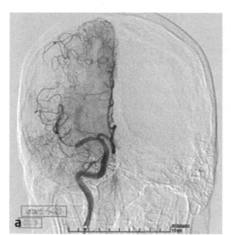
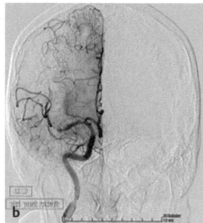

Fig. 30.2 (a) Mechanical thrombectomy using an ACE 68 Reperfusion Catheter and a 4 mm × 20 mm Solitaire 2 Stentriever Device. The device was deployed from the proximal M2 to the mid M1 segment, resulting in restoration of flow to the remainder of the middle cerebral artery. The stent remained in place for about 5 minutes, after which it was retrieved under flow arrest with the Balloon Guide Catheter inflated and continuous aspiration. (b) Angiography via the Balloon Guide Catheter demonstrated persistent clot within the right M1 and with partial distal recanalization.

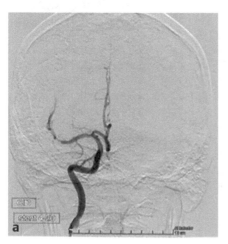
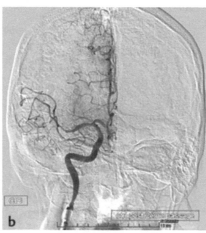

Fig. 30.3 (a) Mechanical thrombectomy using an ACE 68 Reperfusion Catheter and a 4 × 20 mm Solitaire 2 Stentriever Device. Second pass using the same technique. (b) A second angiography via the Balloon Guide Catheter demonstrated partial flow restoration.

- We decided to perform a third pass with a bigger stent. A 6 × 30 mm Solitaire Stentriever was then deployed from the proximal M2 to the mid M1 segment (▶ Fig. 30.4).
- A third angiography via the BCG demonstrated persistent occlusion of the right M1, same as described in the beginning.
- We decided to perform a fourth pass with a different stentriever. A 4.5 × 20 mm Separator 3D Stentriever was then deployed from the proximal M2 to the mid M1 segment (▶ Fig. 30.5).
- A fourth angiography via the BCG demonstrated partial flow restoration.
- After four passes with three different devices, we attempted a direct aspiration technique. Therefore, the ACE 68 Reperfusion Catheter was advanced into the proximal end of the thrombus and suction was initiated. Unfortunately, this maneuver was also unsuccessful (▶ Fig. 30.5).
- We decide to deploy a permanent self-expandable stent. A 3 × 15 mm Solitaire AB Device was deployed from the proximal M2 to the mid M1 segment, resulting in restoration of flow to the remainder of the MCA (▶ Fig. 30.6).
- Final angiographic runs demonstrated satisfactory distal perfusion (thrombolysis in cerebral infarction [TICI]: 3) (▶ Fig. 30.7).

30.1.6 Postprocedure Care

- The patient was transferred to the intensive care unit (ICU).

- After the thrombectomy procedure, a NCCT was performed to rule out intracranial hemorrhage. The NCCT did not show hemorrhagic transformation (▶ Fig. 30.8).
- The patient was loaded with clopidogrel 600 mg plus aspirin 325 mg for the first 24 hours immediately after the procedure.
- The patient was closely monitored with subsequent improvement in neurological status over 24 hours. Repeat NCCT 24 hours later showed small infarct in the posterior MCA cortex territory.
- After 24 hours, the patient was loaded with a second loading dose consisting of clopidogrel 300 mg plus aspirin 325 mg. After 48 hours, clopidogrel 75 mg plus aspirin 325 mg for 6 weeks. Then, clopidogrel 75 mg plus aspirin 81 mg for 6 months. Finally, aspirin 81 mg lifelong.
- A repeat of NCCT 48 hours later showed no further infarct extension or hemorrhagic conversion.

30.1.7 Outcome

- Right MCA occlusive stroke.
- Reperfusion therapy with IV-tPA and rescue permanent self-expanding stent placement, following failed mechanical thrombectomy.
- Final infarct volume based on day 4 NCCT remained largely similar to the initial 24 hours of NCCT, and significantly smaller than the predicted infarct on CTP.

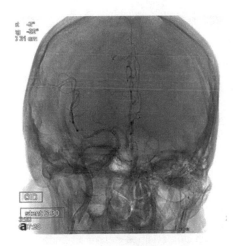
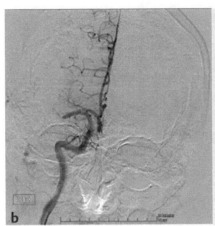

Fig. 30.4 (a) Third pass with a bigger stent. A 6 × 30 mm Solitaire 2 Stentriever was then deployed from the proximal M2 to the mid M1 segment. (b) A third angiography via the Balloon Guide Catheter demonstrated persistent occlusion of the right M1.

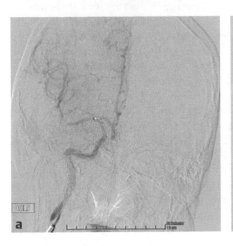
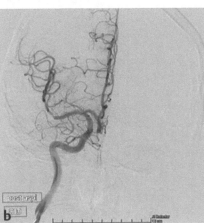

Fig. 30.5 (a) Fourth pass with a different stent. A 4.5 × 20 mm Separator 3D Stentriever was then deployed from the proximal M2 to the mid M1 segment. (b) A fourth angiography via the Balloon Guide Catheter demonstrated partial flow restoration.

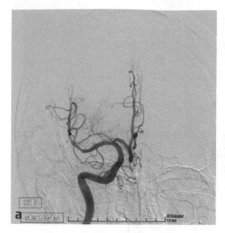
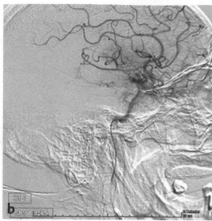

Fig. 30.6 (a) Permanent self-expandable stent placement. A 3 × 15 mm Solitaire AB Device was deployed from the proximal M2 to the mid M1 segment, resulting in restoration of flow to the remainder of the middle cerebral artery. (b) Final angiographic runs demonstrated satisfactory distal perfusion (TICI: 3).

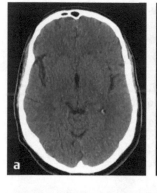
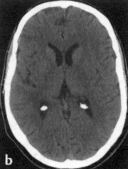
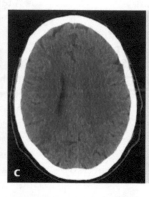

Fig. 30.7 Repeat NCCT 24 hours later showed small infarct in the posterior right MCA cortex territory. No hemorrhagic transformation.

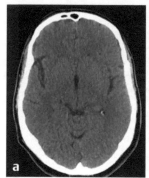
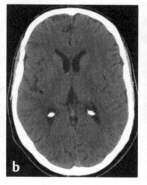
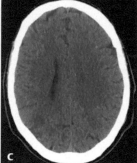

Fig. 30.8 Repeat NCCT 24 hours later showed small infarct in the posterior MCA cortex territory. No hemorrhagic transformation.

- The patient was discharged 4 days after admission to a rehabilitation hospital, with a modified Rankin scale (mRS) score of 2.
- Follow-up CTA at 6 weeks showed stent patency.

30.1.8 Background

Mechanical thrombectomy using a stentriever device has become the standard of care for acute large-vessel occlusions in the anterior circulation.[1,2,3,4,5,6,7,8] Successful reperfusion (modified TICI [mTICI], 2b–3) is the most powerful predictor of a favorable clinical outcome (mRS score of ≤ 2 at 3 months).[1,2,3,4,5,6,7,8] Nevertheless, thrombectomy may not accomplish recanalization in all patients. Arterial reocclusion rate in those five successful trials was 28.9%.[1,2,3,4,5] New scientific evidence suggests that there is a technical failure rate of 14 to 41% whether using a stentriever with a BGC, distal aspiration catheter, or a combination of devices and techniques.[2,3,4,5,6,7,9,10,11,12,13,14,15]

Mechanical thrombectomy may fail due to technical and/or patient factors (see Chapter 29). A failed stentriever technique may be due to a fibrin-rich clot, calcified clot, or an underlying arterial atherosclerotic stenosis.[21,22,23] Procedural time, number of stentriever passes, tandem occlusions of cervical artery and intracranial artery, severe arterial tortuosity, physical properties of the clot,[16] and pathomechanism of the artery occlusion[17] are crucial for the success of the mechanical thrombectomy. Longer procedural times, extending beyond 90 minutes, and multiple device passes are associated with worse outcomes.[18,19] A recent study showed that more than three passes of stentriever is an independent predictor of parenchymal hematoma in acute ischemic stroke and a trend toward a worse clinical outcome.[20] Furthermore, recanalization failure postthrombectomy is well described in cases of intracranial atherosclerotic disease.[23] Although this is relatively rare in Caucasian populations, it may account for a third of proximal intracranial occlusions among Asians.[24,25] The presence of a thrombus on presentation

CTA can mask an underlying atherosclerotic plaque and/or stenosis. Moreover, use of a stent-retriever in these cases can cause endothelial damage to an underlying atherosclerotic plaque or dissection, leading to thrombus formation and reocclusion.

The natural history of arterial reocclusion in acute ischemic stroke patients is poor. In the REVASCAT trial, 54% of patients with successful reperfusion assessed at 24 hours achieved functional independence compared with only 29% without successful reperfusion.[1] Comparably, in the SWIFT PRIME trial, 70% of patients with arterial patency, assessed at 27 hours, had achieved functional independence compared with only 18% in those with lesser degrees of patency.[4] A number of studies have assessed the outcome in cohorts of patients with arterial reocclusion, whose favorable outcome rate is 16.6 to 22%.[26,27]

Successful recanalization in large vessel occlusive stroke is associated with a favorable outcome. In cases of mechanical thrombectomy failure due to device–clot interaction, or underlying arterial stenosis, alternative strategies are necessary. One possible technique is the intra-arterial infusion of thrombolytics or glycoprotein IIb/IIIa inhibitors. The catheter delivery of thrombolytics, such as tPA or urokinase and/or antiplatelets as glycoprotein IIb/IIIa inhibitors, can promote successful recanalization in some refractory stroke cases.[27,28,29,30,31,32] Other rescue techniques have also been described, such as angioplasty,[33] crossing Y stentriever thrombectomy, or a combination of techniques like stent retriever and aspiration catheter thrombectomy ("Solumbra").[34] Data regarding the efficacy of these approaches is, however, limited to a small series.[35,36]

Placement of a permanent, self-expanding stent has been suggested both as a primary approach and a rescue tool for the recanalization of an acute large vessel occlusion.[27,37,38] As mentioned above, the refractoriness of a large artery occlusion might occur in different scenarios. In the case of an intracranial atherosclerotic stenosis occlusion, the problem is mainly due to arterial reocclusion.[29,38,39] A glycoprotein IIb/IIIa inhibitor may help prevent such repeated arterial occlusion.

Intracranial atherosclerotic steno-occlusions are often refractory to glycoprotein IIb/IIIa inhibitors, which may be due to endothelial damage, plaque rupture, and/or dissection during stent-retriever mechanical thrombectomy. In these cases, permanent stenting combined with a glycoprotein IIb/IIIa inhibitor has been shown to achieve recanalization and reperfusion in some series.[27,29,30,37,38,39,40,41,42,43,44,45] Baek et al[27] demonstrated that permanent stenting following a failed stentriever thrombectomy may be safe and effective. They retrospectively evaluated 208 patients who underwent stentriever thrombectomy for anterior circulation large artery occlusion between September 2010 and September 2015. Unsuccessful mechanical thrombectomy occurred in 45 of 208 patients (21.6%), with 17 undergoing permanent stent placement and 28 without stent placement. Although it is unclear how the authors determined which patients were stented, 83.3% of stented patients had mTICI 2b–3. In addition, stented patients had significantly more favorable outcomes (mRS of 0–2, 35.5%) and less cerebral herniation (11.8%) than the nonstented patients (mRS of 0–2, 7.1%; cerebral herniation, 42.9%). Symptomatic intracranial hemorrhage (SICH) and mortality rates did not differ between groups (symptomatic hemorrhage and mortality, 11.8 and 23.9%, respectively, in the stented group vs. 14.3 and 39.4%, respectively, in the nonstented group). Solitaire AB was used in 10 patients, and Wingspan stent was used in seven patients. Among 17 stented cases, only 40% underwent balloon angioplasty. A retrospective analysis of the cohorts of 16 comprehensive stroke centers between September 2010 and December 2015 by Chang et al[46] concluded that rescue stenting was independently associated with good outcomes without increasing SICH or mortality. In a meta-analysis of seven retrospective studies and one prospective study of rescue stenting for failed mechanical thrombectomy in 160 patients by Wareham et al,[11] the authors found that permanent self-expanding stent placement as a rescue procedure is associated with mTICI 2b–3 in 71% and 90-day mRS of 0 to 2 in 43%.[11] The Solitaire stent (Medtronic) was the most commonly deployed stent following failed thrombectomy attempts (66%; 95% confidence interval [CI]: 31–89%). Pre- or poststent angioplasty was performed in 39% of patients (95% CI: 29–48%).

The advantage of using a self-expandable stent is that it adapts itself to the shape and diameter of the injured artery and minimizes the trauma inflicted on the vessel wall. The Solitaire AB (Medtronic) has been the most frequently used stent in published studies to date.[26,27,46,47,48,49,50,51] The Solitaire AB (Medtronic) is a nitinol closed cell stent, which is easy to deploy and can be re-sheathed if necessary. The radial force of this stent is often enough to keep a vessel open; however, angioplasty may be necessary in some cases. Recrossing the stent and performing an angioplasty can be challenging, especially in the setting of intracranial atherosclerotic stenoocclusion, as suboptimal angioplasty has been shown to be associated with acute in-stent thrombosis.[23] Krischek et al[52] compared in vitro physical features and functional properties of different self-expanding intracranial stents. They showed variable results dependent on the test method used. However, irrespective of method, the open cell Wingspan stent (Stryker Neurovascular) showed greater radial force compared to the closed cell Enterprise stent (Johnson and Johnson), Solitaire AB, and open cell Neuroform Atlas (Stryker Neurovascular) stents.[52] The Solitaire AB showed greater radial force at higher oversizing, whereas the Neuroform Atlas showed greater radial force at lower oversizing.[52] No comparative study exists on the safety and efficacy of different self-expanding intracranial stents available. Stent selection may depend on physical and anatomical factors of each individual patient. Knowledge of the stent characteristics, procedural experience, and proper technical skills are mandatory for safe and successful endovascular treatment on the basis of individualized decision making.

A key consideration in choosing between permanent stent deployment and aborting a failed mechanical thrombectomy is the need for platelet inactivation.[29] Heparinization and long-term dual-antiplatelet therapy are necessary during and after stent placement. In addition, platelet inactivation is necessary during the procedure, with some authors starting a GPIIb/IIIa infusion just prior to stent placement, while others prefer loading doses of aspirin and clopidogrel. Regardless of the regimen, the additional blood thinners and degree of anticoagulation needed increases the risk of intracranial bleeding in an acute stroke setting.

Although recent studies affirm that the benefit of achieving a complete recanalization with intracranial stenting compared to failed stentriever thrombectomy with nonrecanalization,[27,30] there is a vast majority of retrospective studies with selection biases likely present. In the meta-analysis by Wareham et al,[11] the SICH rate was 12%. This rate is similar to recent real-world published rates of SICH in stentriever registries,[53] but higher than those seen in the mechanical thrombectomy randomized trials (0–8%).[1,2,3,4,5,6,7,8] Many of the patients included in the meta-analysis were treated with thrombolytics prior to stent deployment, which may have increased the bleeding rate (89% of patients were treated with glycoprotein IIb/IIIa inhibitors and 95% had antiplatelet therapy with postprocedure). The data regarding the safety of glycoprotein IIb/IIIa inhibitors are controversial. Recent registry data suggest that postprocedural dual-antiplatelet treatment is safe in the context of large vessel occlusion and cervical ICA stenting[54] with no significant increase in SICH but with more favorable recanalization rates. The use of NCCT to assess for contrast staining in areas of core infarct postprocedure might guide the use of antiplatelet therapy after stent placement.

Long-term stent patency is also a concern and necessitates close follow-up. Data governing this cannot be gleaned from big prospective studies. However, mid-term angiographic follow-up was obtained following the small, prospective SARIS trial.[37] Among all the survivors, none developed an in-stent stenosis of greater than 50%.

In conclusion, recanalization failure is not uncommon during mechanical endovascular procedures. The natural history of patients with large vessel occlusion acute ischemic stroke and failed thrombectomy is poor. Permanent self-expanding stent placement appears to be a promising and reasonable approach following the failure of a stentriever and aspiration thrombectomy, if the procedural time is extending beyond 90 minutes or over three passes with no progress; however, the size of core infarct and time from stroke onset should be considered in light of the need for anticoagulation during and after stent placement. Optimal stent device and antiplatelet regimen remain to be elucidated. A prospective registry of patients undergoing rescue stenting would be a useful project to obtain further evidence in order to guide future recommendations.

30.1.9 Pearls and Pitfalls

1. Failed mechanical thrombectomy is not uncommon and the natural history of these patients is poor.
2. Permanent self-expanding stent placement following the failure of mechanical thrombectomy may be a safe and effective modality if the procedural time is extending beyond 90 minutes or over multiple passes with no progress.
3. The major concern with permanent stenting is that it requires intraprocedural and postprocedural platelet inactivation, which increases the risk of intracranial hemorrhage in an acute stroke setting. Based on limited studies to date, the benefit of recanalization may outweigh the increased risk of intracranial hemorrhage; however, larger prospective studies are needed.
4. The advantage of using a self-expandable stent is that it adapts itself to the shape and diameter of the injured artery and minimizes the trauma inflicted on the vessel wall. Most series have reported use of Solitaire AB and/or Wingspan stent; however, no stent is currently considered ideal.

References

[1] Jovin TG, Chamorro A, Cobo E, et al. REVASCAT Trial Investigators. Thrombectomy within 8 hours after symptom onset in ischemic stroke. N Engl J Med. 2015; 372(24):2296–2306

[2] Goyal M, Demchuk AM, Menon BK, et al. ESCAPE Trial Investigators. Randomized assessment of rapid endovascular treatment of ischemic stroke. N Engl J Med. 2015; 372(11):1019–1030

[3] Campbell BCV, Mitchell PJ, Kleinig TJ, et al. EXTEND-IA Investigators. Endovascular therapy for ischemic stroke with perfusion-imaging selection. N Engl J Med. 2015; 372(11):1009–1018

[4] Saver JL, Goyal M, Bonafe A, et al. SWIFT PRIME Investigators. Stent-retriever thrombectomy after intravenous t-PA vs. t-PA alone in stroke. N Engl J Med. 2015; 372(24):2285–2295

[5] Berkhemer OA, Fransen PSS, Beumer D, et al. MR CLEAN Investigators. A randomized trial of intraarterial treatment for acute ischemic stroke. N Engl J Med. 2015; 372(1):11–20

[6] Albers GW, Marks MP, Kemp S, et al. DEFUSE 3 Investigators. Thrombectomy for stroke at 6 to 16 hours with selection by perfusion imaging. N Engl J Med. 2018; 378(8):708–718

[7] Nogueira RG, Jadhav AP, Haussen DC, et al. DAWN Trial Investigators. Thrombectomy 6 to 24 hours after stroke with a mismatch between deficit and infarct. N Engl J Med. 2018; 378(1):11–21

[8] Goyal M, Menon BK, van Zwam WH, et al. HERMES Collaborators. Endovascular thrombectomy after large-vessel ischaemic stroke: a meta-analysis of individual patient data from five randomised trials. Lancet. 2016; 387(10029):1723–1731

[9] Bracard S, Ducrocq X, Mas JL, et al. THRACE Investigators. Mechanical thrombectomy after intravenous alteplase versus alteplase alone after stroke (THRACE): a randomised controlled trial. Lancet Neurol. 2016; 15(11):1138–1147

[10] Mocco J, Zaidat OO, von Kummer R, et al. THERAPY Trial Investigators*. Aspiration thrombectomy after intravenous alteplase versus intravenous alteplase alone. Stroke. 2016; 47(9):2331–2338

[11] Wareham J, Flood R, Phan K, Crossley R, Mortimer A. A systematic review and meta-analysis of observational evidence for the use of bailout self-expandable stents following failed anterior circulation stroke thrombectomy. J Neurointerv Surg. 201 9; 11(7):675–682

[12] Muir KW, Ford GA, Messow C-M, et al. PISTE Investigators. Endovascular therapy for acute ischaemic stroke: the pragmatic ischaemic stroke thrombectomy evaluation (PISTE) randomised, controlled trial. J Neurol Neurosurg Psychiatry. 2017; 88(1):38–44

[13] Saver JL, Goyal M, Bonafe A, et al. Aspiration thrombectomy after intravenous alteplase versus intravenous alteplase alone. N Engl J Med. 2017; 378(1):11–21

[14] Hesse AC, Behme D, Kemmling A, et al. Comparing different thrombectomy techniques in five large-volume centers: a 'real world' observational study. J Neurointerv Surg. 2018; 10(6):525–529

[15] Lapergue B, Blanc R, Gory B, et al. ASTER Trial Investigators. Effect of endovascular contact aspiration vs stent retriever on revascularization in patients with acute ischemic stroke and large vessel occlusion: the ASTER randomized clinical trial. JAMA. 2017; 318(5):443–452

[16] Singh P, Kaur R, Kaur A. Clot composition and treatment approach to acute ischemic stroke: The road so far. Ann Indian Acad Neurol. 2013; 16(4):494–497

[17] Kim BM. Causes and solutions of endovascular treatment failure. J Stroke. 2017; 19(2):131–142

[18] Kass-Hout T, Kass-Hout O, Sun CJ, Kass-Hout TA, Nogueira R, Gupta R. Longer procedural times are independently associated with symptomatic intracranial hemorrhage in patients with large vessel occlusion stroke undergoing thrombectomy. J Neurointerv Surg. 2016; 8(12):1217–1220

[19] Linfante I, Starosciak AK, Walker GR, et al. Predictors of poor outcome despite recanalization: a multiple regression analysis of the NASA registry. J Neurointerv Surg. 2016; 8(3):224–229

[20] Bourcier R, Saleme S, Labreuche J, et al. More than three passes of stent retriever is an independent predictor of parenchymal hematoma in acute ischemic stroke. J Neurointerv Surg. 201 9; 11(7):625–629

[21] Fennell VS, Setlur Nagesh SV, Meess KM, et al. What to do about fibrin rich 'tough clots'? Comparing the Solitaire stent retriever with a novel geometric clot extractor in an in vitro stroke model. J Neurointerv Surg. 2018; 10 (9):907–910

[22] Dobrocky T, Piechowiak E, Cianfoni A, et al. Thrombectomy of calcified emboli in stroke. Does histology of thrombi influence the effectiveness of thrombectomy? J Neurointerv Surg. 2018; 10(4):345–350

[23] Kim GE, Yoon W, Kim SK, et al. Incidence and clinical significance of acute reocclusion after emergent angioplasty or stenting for underlying intracranial stenosis in patients with acute stroke. AJNR Am J Neuroradiol. 2016; 37 (9):1690–1695

[24] Al Kasab S, Almadidy Z, Spiotta AM, et al. Endovascular treatment for AIS with underlying ICAD. J Neurointerv Surg. 2017; 9(10):948–951

[25] Jia B, Feng L, Liebeskind DS, et al. EAST Study Group. Mechanical thrombectomy and rescue therapy for intracranial large artery occlusion with underlying atherosclerosis. J Neurointerv Surg. 2018; 10(8):746–750

[26] Baracchini C, Farina F, Soso M, et al. Stentriever thrombectomy failure: a challenge in stroke management. World Neurosurg. 2017; 103:57–64

[27] Baek J-H, Kim BM, Kim DJ, Heo JH, Nam HS. Stenting as a rescue treatment after failure of mechanical thrombectomy for anterior circulation large artery occlusion. Stroke. 2016; 47(9):2360–2363

[28] Kang D-H, Kim Y-W, Hwang Y-H, Park S-P, Kim Y-S, Baik SK. Instant reocclusion following mechanical thrombectomy of in situ thromboocclusion and the role of low-dose intra-arterial tirofiban. Cerebrovasc Dis. 2014; 37 (5):350–355

[29] Moon Kim B. Refractory occlusion to stentriever thrombectomy: etiological considerations and suggested solutions. Acute Ischemic Stroke. 2017:213–226

[30] Baek J-H, Kim BM, Kim DJ, et al. Importance of truncal-type occlusion in stentriever-based thrombectomy for acute stroke. Neurology. 2016; 87 (15):1542–1550

[31] Seo JH, Jeong HW, Kim ST, Kim E-G. Adjuvant tirofiban injection through deployed Solitaire stent as a rescue technique after failed mechanical thrombectomy in acute stroke. Neurointervention. 2015; 10(1):22–27

[32] Goh D-H, Jin S-C, Jeong HW, Ha SY. Mechanical Solitaire thrombectomy with low-dose booster tirofiban injection. Neurointervention. 2016; 11(2):114–119

[33] Yoo AJ, Andersson T. Thrombectomy in acute ischemic stroke: challenges to procedural success. J Stroke. 2017; 19(2):121–130

[34] Aydin K, Barburoglu M, Oztop Cakmak O, Yesilot N, Vanli ENY, Akpek S. Crossing Y-Solitaire thrombectomy as a rescue treatment for refractory acute occlusions of the middle cerebral artery. J Neurointerv Surg. 2019; 11 (3):246–250

[35] IMS II Trial Investigators. The interventional management of stroke (IMS) II study. stroke. 2007; 38(7):2127–2135

[36] IMS Study Investigators. Combined intravenous and intra-arterial recanalization for acute ischemic stroke: the interventional management of stroke study. Stroke. 2004; 35(4):904–911

[37] Levy EI, Siddiqui AH, Crumlish A, et al. First Food and Drug Administration-approved prospective trial of primary intracranial stenting for acute stroke: SARIS (stent-assisted recanalization in acute ischemic stroke). Stroke. 2009; 40(11):3552–3556

[38] Mocco J, Hanel RA, Sharma J, et al. Use of a vascular reconstruction device to salvage acute ischemic occlusions refractory to traditional endovascular recanalization methods. J Neurosurg. 2010; 112(3):557–562

[39] Qureshi AI, Siddiqui AM, Kim SH, et al. Reocclusion of recanalized arteries during intra-arterial thrombolysis for acute ischemic stroke. AJNR Am J Neuroradiol. 2004; 25(2):322–328

[40] Brekenfeld C, Schroth G, Mattle HP, et al. Stent placement in acute cerebral artery occlusion: use of a self-expandable intracranial stent for acute stroke treatment. Stroke. 2009; 40(3):847–852

[41] Suh SH, Kim BM, Roh HG, et al. Self-expanding stent for recanalization of acute embolic or dissecting intracranial artery occlusion. AJNR Am J Neuroradiol. 2010; 31(3):459–463

[42] Yoon W, Seo JJ, Kim JK, Cho KH, Park JG, Kang HK. Contrast enhancement and contrast extravasation on computed tomography after intra-arterial thrombolysis in patients with acute ischemic stroke. Stroke. 2004; 35 (4):876–881

[43] Yoon W, Kim SK, Park MS, Kim BC, Kang HK. Endovascular treatment and the outcomes of atherosclerotic intracranial stenosis in patients with hyperacute stroke. Neurosurgery. 2015; 76(6):680–686, discussion 686

[44] Levy EI, Mehta R, Gupta R, et al. Self-expanding stents for recanalization of acute cerebrovascular occlusions. AJNR Am J Neuroradiol. 2007; 28(5):816–822

[45] Zaidat OO, Wolfe T, Hussain SI, et al. Interventional acute ischemic stroke therapy with intracranial self-expanding stent. Stroke. 2008; 39(8):2392–2395

[46] Chang Y, Kim BM, Bang OY, et al. Rescue stenting for failed mechanical thrombectomy in acute ischemic stroke: a multicenter experience. Stroke. 2018; 49(4):958–964

[47] Sauvageau E, Samuelson RM, Levy EI, Jeziorski AM, Mehta RA, Hopkins LN. Middle cerebral artery stenting for acute ischemic stroke after unsuccessful MERCI retrieval. Neurosurgery. 2007; 60(4):701–706, discussion 706

[48] Delgado Acosta F, Jiménez Gómez E, Bravo Rey I, Bravo Rodríguez FA, Ochoa Sepúlveda JJ, Oteros Fernández R. Intracranial stents in the endovascular treatment of acute ischemic stroke. Radiologia (Madr). 2017; 59(3):218–225

[49] Nappini S, Limbucci N, Leone G, et al. Bail-out intracranial stenting with Solitaire AB device after unsuccessful thrombectomy in acute ischemic stroke of anterior circulation. J Neuroradiol. 2019; 46(2):141–147

[50] Zhou T, Li T, Zhu L, et al. Intracranial stenting as a rescue therapy for acute ischemic stroke after stentriever thrombectomy failure. World Neurosurg. 2018; 120:e181–e187

[51] Ahmed SU, Mann J, Houde J, Barber E, Kelly ME, Peeling L. Permanent implantation of the Solitaire device as a bailout technique for large vessel intracranial occlusions. J Neurointerv Surg. 2019; 11(2):133–136

[52] Krischek O, Miloslavski E, Fischer S, Shrivastava S, Henkes H. A comparison of functional and physical properties of self-expanding intracranial stents [Neuroform3, Wingspan, Solitaire, Leo+, Enterprise]. Minim Invasive Neurosurg. 2011; 54(1):21–28

[53] Mokin M, Abou-Chebl A, Castonguay AC, et al. Real-world stent retriever thrombectomy for acute ischemic stroke beyond 6 hours of onset: analysis of the NASA and TRACK registries. J Neurointerv Surg. 2019; 11(4):334–337

[54] Papanagiotou P, Haussen DC, Turjman F, et al. TITAN Investigators. carotid stenting with antithrombotic agents and intracranial thrombectomy leads to the highest recanalization rate in patients with acute stroke with tandem lesions. JACC Cardiovasc Interv. 2018; 11(13):1290–1299

31 Acute Dissection with Hemodynamic Infarctions

31.1 Case Description

31.1.1 Clinical Presentation

A 49-year-old woman presented initially with a history of blurred vision for 1 hour. Three days later, she again presented with sudden onset of blurred vision in her left eye and right-sided weakness. On examination, she had left mydriasis and a right-sided pronator drift. A CTA of the carotids and circle of Willis was performed, which demonstrated a left internal carotid artery (ICA) dissection. MRI demonstrated no evidence of acute infarct on diffusion-weighted imaging. She was initially managed with anticoagulation in the form of a heparin infusion; however, over the next 24 hours, she deteriorated neurologically with development of aphasia, worsening right arm weakness, and a right-sided facial droop, and thus MRI was repeated.

31.1.2 Imaging Studies

- Sagittal reconstruction of the CT angiography (CTA) of the carotids performed at the time of presentation demonstrates abrupt narrowing, leading to occlusion of the proximal left ICA just above the carotid bulb (▶ Fig. 31.1).
- Diffusion-weighted MRI of the brain demonstrated classical deep border-zone infarctions in keeping with global left hemispheric hypoperfusion (▶ Fig. 31.2).

31.1.3 Diagnosis

Left internal carotid dissection with hemodynamic infarction affecting the left centrum semiovale.

31.1.4 Treatment

- Once the patient developed hemodynamic infarcts while on heparin infusion, intervention was deemed necessary.

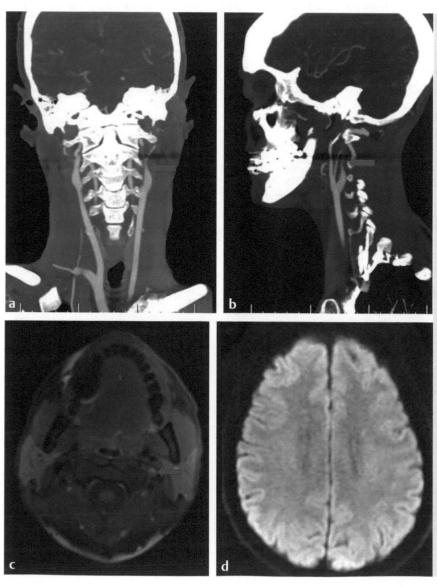

Fig. 31.1 Investigations performed on re-presentation to the hospital included CTA of the carotids and MRI of the head and neck. CTAs of the carotids in the coronal (a) and sagittal (b) demonstrate the transition between the normal caliber ICA to the string-like ICA just beyond the carotid bulb, as indicated by the *arrow*. Fat-saturated T1-weighted MRI (c) demonstrates increased T1 signal within the left ICA wall in keeping with intramural hematoma from a dissection. The diffusion-weighted imaging (d) demonstrates no evidence of infarct.

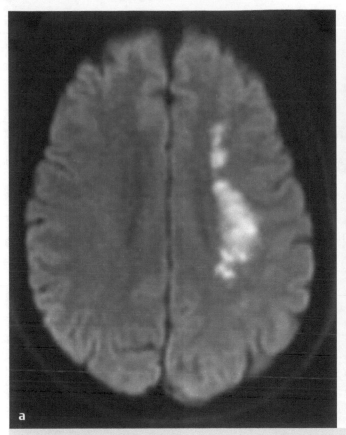
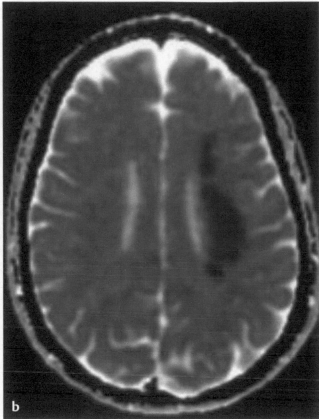

Fig. 31.2 Repeat MRI scan performed at the time of the patients' deterioration demonstrates acute infarcts in the centrum semiovale in a watershed distribution on diffusion-weighted imaging (**a**), and ADC maps (**b**).

- Digital subtraction angiography following injection into the left common carotid artery (CCA) demonstrated the classical appearance of an ICA dissection with a focal narrowing just above the carotid bulb with the "string sign" indicating severely compromised arterial lumen.
- Immediate postprocedural final angiography demonstrated successful reconstruction of the acutely dissected left ICA using stents. The ICA was reconstructed from proximal (carotid bifurcation with two carotid Wallstents) to distal (skull base with an overlapping Pipeline stent).

Endovascular Treatment: Left Carotid Stenting

Material

- 8-Fr short vascular sheath.
- 5 Fr × 100 cm Berenstein catheter.
- 8-Fr MERCI balloon guide.
- 5-Fr VTK Slip catheter.
- 0.035 in × 150 cm Glide wire.
- 0.014 in × 200 cm Synchro-2 guidewire.
- 0.014 in Traxcess hydrophilic guidewire.
- 0.014 in × 115 cm Traxcess Docking wire.
- 7 × 40 mm to 6 × 48 mm carotid wall stent.
- 5 × 30 mm to 4 × 36 mm Carotid wall stent.

- 4 × 20 mm Scepter C Balloon Catheter.
- 4 mm × 2 cm 142 cm shaft Aviator Plus PTA Balloon.
- 5.0 × 25 mm Pipeline Flex Embolization Device.

Technique

The procedure was performed with general anesthesia and full systemic heparinization. The right common femoral artery was punctured and an 8-Fr short vascular sheath inserted. The 5-Fr Berenstein catheter was used to perform diagnostic angiography from the left CCA. This demonstrated the long-segment left ICA dissection with filling of the distal ICA via the left ophthalmic artery, which fills retrogradely from the external carotid artery (▶ Fig. 31.3).

An 8-Fr MERCI balloon guide was then advanced into the distal left CCA over a 5-Fr VTK slip catheter with the aid of an angled Terumo Glide wire. A Marksman catheter, over a Synchro-2 microwire shaped with a "J" tip, was then used to cross the dissected segment into the petrous ICA. Intraluminal positioning was confirmed by microcatheter injection (▶ Fig. 31.4).

A Traxcess microwire with the docking exchange wire was inserted via the Marksmen catheter to the level of the cavernous ICA, and used as an exchange wire to maintain access through the dissected segment, during the stenting procedure. A 7 × 40 mm carotid wall stent was then advanced over the Traxcess exchange

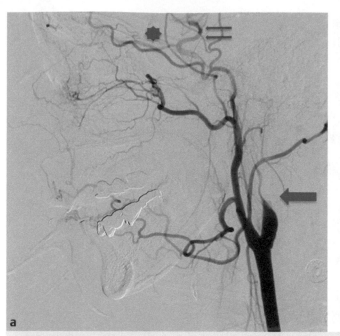
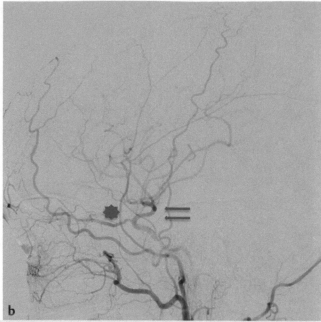

Fig. 31.3 (a) CCA injection in the arterial phase (b) demonstrates the abrupt transition in caliber of the internal carotid artery (*arrow*) with the distal internal carotid artery (*double arrow*) seen to fill via the ophthalmic artery (*) which fills retrogradely from the ECA.

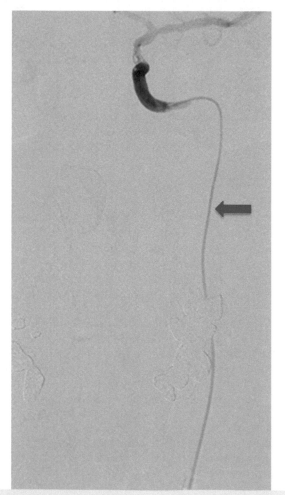

Fig. 31.4 Microcatheter (*arrow*) injection confirms and intraluminal position after crossing the dissection.

wire and deployed in the distal ICA from the lower border of C1 to the level of the carotid bulb (▶ Fig. 31.5, ▶ Fig. 31.6). At this point, Integrilin was commenced intravenously.

A rapid exchange maneuver was then used to deploy a second telescoped 5 × 30 mm carotid wall stent from just below the skull base. Following this, the Marksman catheter was again inserted over the Traxcess wire; through this, a 5 × 25 mm Pipeline flex device was then deployed from the petrous ICA back to telescope with the already delivered carotid wall stents (▶ Fig. 31.7).

Although delivery of these stents resulted in improved antegrade flow through the left ICA, there was an area of narrowing in the region of the pipeline stent from the level of the skull base back to the carotid wall stent. This was in the region where the MRI demonstrated thrombus within the false lumen of the ICA and as such was thought to be secondary to compression. A 4 × 20 mm Scepter balloon was then advanced over the Traxcess wire left in place for access through the stents.

Angioplasty was performed with some improvement in caliber; however, there was persistent narrowing. Three mg of intra-arterial verapamil was administered to assess if some of the narrowing may be due to vasospasm; however, control angiography following this demonstrated increased intraluminal narrowing with associated reduced flow in the ICA. A 4 × 20 mm Aviator Plus angioplasty Balloon was then inserted and angioplasty performed with two inflations. Resolution of the stenosis and complete stent opening with good wall opposition and improved left ICA flow was achieved. Normal antegrade flow and good cerebral perfusion was also observed. (▶ Fig. 31.8).

Hemostasis at the puncture site was achieved with an 8-Fr Angio-Seal closure device. The Integrilin was continued as an infusion for 24 hours postprocedure, and the patient was given a 600-mg loading dose of clopidogrel and 325 mg of aspirin. Clopidogrel and aspirin were continued for 6 weeks.

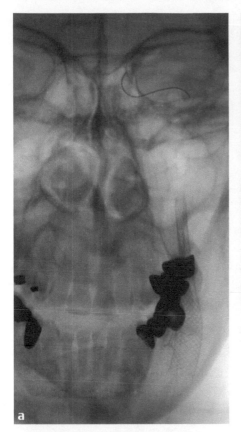
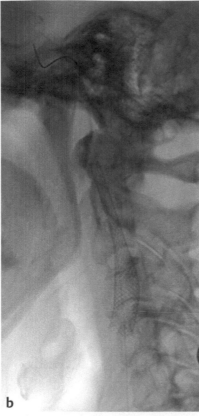

Fig. 31.5 AP (**a**) and lateral (**b**) deployment of a 7 × 40 mm carotid wall stent from the lower border of C1 back to the carotid bulb, with Traxcess wire seen in situ maintaining access across the dissection.

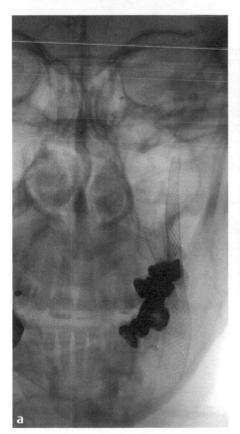
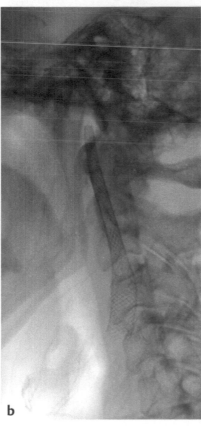

Fig. 31.6 AP (**a**) and lateral (**b**) radiographs demonstrating the position of the second 5 × 30 mm carotid wall stent. The Marksmen catheter is seen in position for the delivery of the Pipeline stent.

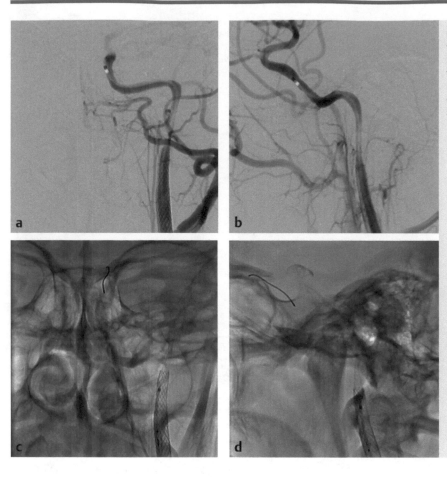

Fig. 31.7 AP (**a**) and lateral (**b**) angiographic run following deployment of the two carotid wall stents and with the Marksman catheter in situ for the deployment of the Pipeline stent. AP (**c**) and lateral (**d**) radiographs demonstrated the pipeline deployed and telescoped through the carotid wall stents.

31.2 Outcome

The Integrilin was continued as an infusion for 24 hours post-procedure, and the patient was given a 600-mg loading dose of clopidogrel and 325 mg of aspirin. Clopidogrel and aspirin were continued for 6 weeks. The patient made an uneventful recovery.

Follow-up CTA (▶ Fig. 31.9) performed at 2 years demonstrated complete patency of the stent construct with flow in the left ICA and no evidence of in-stent stenosis.

31.3 Discussion

Carotid dissection is responsible for approximately 2% of all strokes; however, it accounts for up to a quarter of strokes in patients younger than 45 years.[1,2] Dissections result from a tear in the intima that leads to separation of the arterial wall layers due to hematoma formation. The dissection may lead to stenosis or formation of a dissecting aneurysm, depending on where the bleeding occurs. If the bleeding is subintimal, the result will be ICA stenosis, and if the bleeding is subadventitial, a dissecting aneurysm will form.[3] Both stenotic lesions and dissecting aneurysms can result in ischemic complications. In addition, the disruption to the endothelium can lead to thrombus formation with subsequent embolization.

Pain in the face, head, or neck; partial Horner syndrome; and subsequent cerebral or retinal ischemia are the classic clinical triad seen with ICA dissection. It is rare for patients to present with all three; however, the presence of any two strongly suggests the diagnosis.[3]

Traditionally, digital subtraction catheter angiography has been considered the gold standard radiological test for the diagnosis of carotid artery dissection; however, with improvements in the resolution of MRI, this noninvasive modality is rapidly replacing traditional angiography as the gold standard for diagnosis.[3] Findings on catheter angiography include a long, irregular stenosis sparing the carotid bulb. The intimal flap or false lumen may be visualized.[4] In the presence of carotid occlusion, a flame-like appearance may be observed, and in cases involving the adventitia, a pseudoaneurysm may be demonstrated.[4] The diagnosis on MRI is made by identification of an intramural hematoma. T1-weighted sequences with fat saturation permit the visualization of the crescentic high T1 intramural hematoma.[4] Fat saturation allows differentiation from the surrounding soft tissues.[3] However, it is important to note that the sensitivity of MRI is limited in the first 72 hours, as the oxyhemoglobin in the hyperacute stage and the deoxyhemoglobin in the acute stage make the hematoma isointense on T1-weighted imaging.[4]

The mainstay of treatment is currently anticoagulation or antiplatelet therapy with the aim of preventing recurrent stroke.[5,6] There is no evidence demonstrating superiority of anticoagulation over antiplatelet therapy.[7] However, it has been suggested that antiplatelets are preferable in patients with a National Institutes of Health Stroke Scale (NIHSS) score of 15 or greater, accompanying intracranial dissection, local

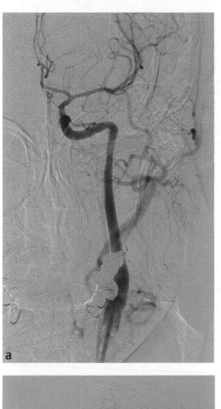
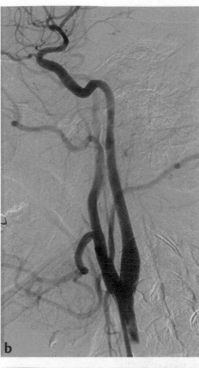
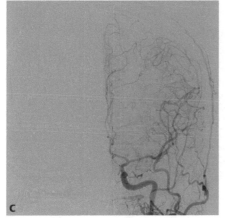
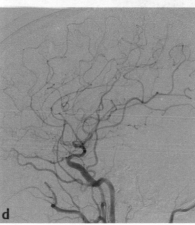

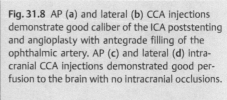

Fig. 31.8 AP (**a**) and lateral (**b**) CCA injections demonstrate good caliber of the ICA poststenting and angioplasty with antegrade filling of the ophthalmic artery. AP (**c**) and lateral (**d**) intracranial CCA injections demonstrated good perfusion to the brain with no intracranial occlusions.

compression syndromes without ischemic events, or concomitant diseases with increased bleeding risk. On the contrary, anticoagulation is preferred in patients with pseudo-occlusion of the dissected artery, high-intensity transient signals in transcranial ultrasound studies despite dual antiplatelets, multiple ischemic events in the same circulation, or with free floating thrombus.[8] It is known that by using this medical therapy, up to 90% of dissections will heal and stenotic lesions will resolve within 3 months.[1] In the remaining, further management including endovascular therapies need to be considered. Indications for endovascular treatment include recurring ischemic events despite antithrombotic therapy, severe stenosis (> 70%) failing to heal 3 months after initial presentation with prior cerebral ischemia or persistence of nonischemic symptoms attributable to that lesion, worsening stenosis on follow-up imaging with a history of ischemic or flow-related symptoms, hemodynamically significant stenosis with completely occluded contralateral carotid, tandem ICA and MCA occlusion due to carotid dissection in the setting of acute stroke within 8 hours of onset, and clinical evidence of hemodynamic insufficiency or hypoperfusion on imaging in a symptomatically unstable patient.[6]

Carotid stenting has been shown to be a safe and viable treatment option for carotid dissections.[6] When done electively, the patient should be premedicated with clopidogrel and aspirin for at least 10 days.

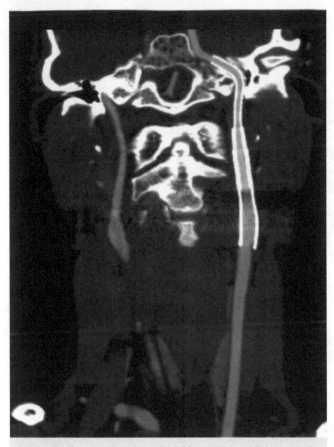

Fig. 31.9 Follow-up CT angiography (oblique MIP reconstruction in the coronal plane) performed at 2 years demonstrates complete patency of the stent construct, with flow in the left ICA and no evidence of in-stent stenosis.

References

[1] Lee VH, Brown RD, Jr, Mandrekar JN, Mokri B. Incidence and outcome of cervical artery dissection: a population-based study. Neurology. 2006; 67 (10):1809–1812

[2] Giroud M, Fayolle H, André N, et al. Incidence of internal carotid artery dissection in the community of Dijon. J Neurol Neurosurg Psychiatry. 1994; 57(11):1443

[3] Schievink WI. Spontaneous dissection of the carotid and vertebral arteries. N Engl J Med. 2001; 344(12):898–906

[4] Ben Hassen W, Machet A, Edjlali-Goujon M, et al. Imaging of cervical artery dissection. Diagn Interv Imaging. 2014; 95(12):1151–1161

[5] Debette S. Pathophysiology and risk factors of cervical artery dissection: what have we learnt from large hospital-based cohorts? Curr Opin Neurol. 2014; 27(1):20–28

[6] Asif KS, Lazzaro MA, Teleb MS, Fitzsimmons BF, Lynch J, Zaidat O. Endovascular reconstruction for progressively worsening carotid artery dissection. J Neurointerv Surg. 2015; 7(1):32–39

[7] Kennedy F, Lanfranconi S, Hicks C, et al. CADISS Investigators. Antiplatelets vs anticoagulation for dissection: CADISS nonrandomized arm and meta-analysis. Neurology. 2012; 79(7):686–689

[8] Engelter ST, Brandt T, Debette S, et al. Cervical Artery Dissection in Ischemic Stroke Patients (CADISP) Study Group. Antiplatelets versus anticoagulation in cervical artery dissection. Stroke. 2007; 38(9):2605–2611

32 The SAVE Technique

32.1 Case Description

32.1.1 Clinical Presentation

An 85-year-old, high functioning, male patient was last seen well at 14:00 hours. He woke up at 16:00 hours and was found to be aphasic and weak on the right. He was taken by emergency medical services (EMS) to the hospital and reached at 16:45 hours. The National Institutes of Health Stroke Scale (NIHSS) score was 21 upon arrival. The patient was alert but globally aphasic. His pupils were equal and reactive. There was forced gaze deviation to the left, and mild right upper motor neuron facial asymmetry. Also, there was right hemiplegia, and extensor plantar response on the right. Asymmetric response to sensory stimuli on the right compared to left was observed. He was unable to test for visual fields and was afflicted with ataxia.

32.1.2 Imaging Workup and Investigations

- Noncontrast CT (**NCCT**): Showed ASPECTS score of 7 with loss of gray-white differentiation over left insula, caudate, and lentiform nucleus (▶ Fig. 32.1).
- CTA: Revealed left proximal M1 occlusion.
- CT perfusion (**CTP**): Demonstrated perfusion mismatch 4 mL core, and 181 mL penumbra with 45.3 mismatch ratio.

32.1.3 Diagnosis

Acute stroke due to left M1 occlusion.

32.1.4 Management

- 6 mg tissue plasminogen activator (tPA) bolus was given at 17:04 hours, as no contradiction was identified, followed by 56 mg of tPA infusion.
- Was taken to angiography suite for endovascular thrombectomy (EVT) promptly, while tPA infusion was run after obtaining consent.

32.1.5 Endovascular Treatment

Materials

- 8-Fr short vascular access sheath.
- 8-Fr FlowGate balloon guide catheter (BGC).
- 6-Fr Berenstein tip guide assist FlowGate Slip-Cath.
- Terumo guidewire.
- AXS Catalyst 6 Distal Access Catheter (aspiration catheter).
- Synchro-14 guidewire.
- Trevo XP ProVue microcatheter and 4 mm × 30 mm stentriever.

Technique

- The procedure was performed under conscious sedation while anesthesia present in the room.

- Right common femoral artery (CFA) puncture with placement of an 8-Fr short vascular access sheath into the CFA.
- An 8-Fr FlowGate BGC placed in the left common carotid artery (CCA) coaxially over a slip-cath with the aid of Terumo guidewire.
- Control anteroposterior and lateral angiographic runs confirmed persistent M1 occlusion (▶ Fig. 32.2a).
- The Trevo XP ProVue microcatheter and the AXS Catalyst 6 Distal Access Catheter were prepped and connected to the continuous flushing system.
- The Trevo XP ProVue microcatheter was navigated into the left middle cerebral artery (MCA) with the aid of Synchro-14 guidewire bypassing the clot.
- Microinjection confirmed the location of the Trevo microcatheter with no perforation (▶ Fig. 32.2b).
- A Trevo 4 mm × 30 mm stentriever was deployed into the left M2 superior division, with the proximal third of the stent engaging the thrombus.
- The FlowGate BGC was inflated.
- The AXS Catalyst 6 Distal Access Catheter was advanced to wedge the clot, while being connected to the Stryker aspiration pump with the suction turned on (▶ Fig. 32.2c).
- A penumbra aspiration tubing was primed and connected to the pump and the guide catheter
- After 90 seconds of flow arrest, both the Trevo stent and the AXS Catalyst 6 were pulled gradually with both aspiration pumps turned on.
- Final angiographic runs demonstrated optimal distal perfusion (thrombolysis in cerebral infarction [TICI]: 3; ▶ Fig. 32.2d).

32.1.6 Postprocedure Care

The patient was transferred to the ICU for 24 hours, following which he was transferred to the stroke unit and to the rehabilitation center.

32.1.7 Outcome

NIHSS score dipped below 21. Follow-up imaging showed evolution of the left MCA core infarction with no infarction of the penumbral tissue (▶ Fig. 32.3).

Unfortunately, the patient developed depression, requiring psychiatric assessment, which led to weight loss and poor compliance with the rehabilitation.

32.1.8 Background

Stent-retriever assisted vacuum-locked extraction (SAVE) is a novel technique first described by Manus et al for EVT.[1] The technique utilizes both stent retrievers and direct aspiration devices, along with a vacuum pressure syringe. It is well established through several randomized control trials that EVT for stroke secondary to large vessel occlusion is effective; however, there is no consensus regarding which EVT technique works best.[2] The principal idea that differentiates the SAVE technique from the so-called Solumbra technique is that continuous

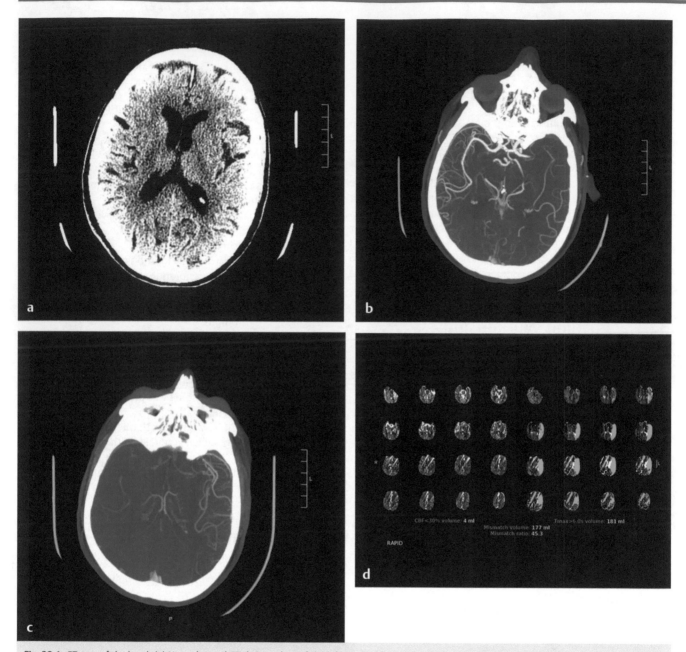

Fig. 32.1 CT scan of the head. (**a**) Nonenhanced CT showing loss of the left insult ribbon and indistinct left caudate and lentiform nucleus (ASPECTS 7). (**b**) CTA demonstrates left M1 occlusion. (**c**) Late-phase CTA demonstrates good collaterals. (**d**) RAPID perfusion images depicting small core and large penumbra.

aspiration is provided through the guide catheter in the internal carotid artery (ICA) to prevent clot fragments from migrating into the anterior cerebral artery (ACA) and MCA during retrieval of the stent under vacuum pressure via a 60-mL syringe. The authors report fast, safe, and effective results in a retrospective review of 32 patients undergoing this novel technique. The original study using the SAVE technique was followed up by a multicenter study of 200 patients undergoing EVT using the SAVE technique across four German stroke centers.[3] They confirmed complete/near-complete reperfusion of 77% with an overall successful reperfusion rate of 95%. They report first-pass rates of complete/near-complete reperfusion of 57%. These rates are

much higher than their self-reported complete reperfusion rate, utilizing direct aspiration first-pass technique (ADAPT) of 26%. Overall, the technique appears promising; however, one must exercise caution, as there are limited data on the effectiveness of the technique, with only one multicenter study reported.

32.1.9 Discussion

The SAVE technique is a unique combination of previously described thrombectomy technique in addition to some extra steps. The key steps of SAVE technique as described by Manus et al are as follows:

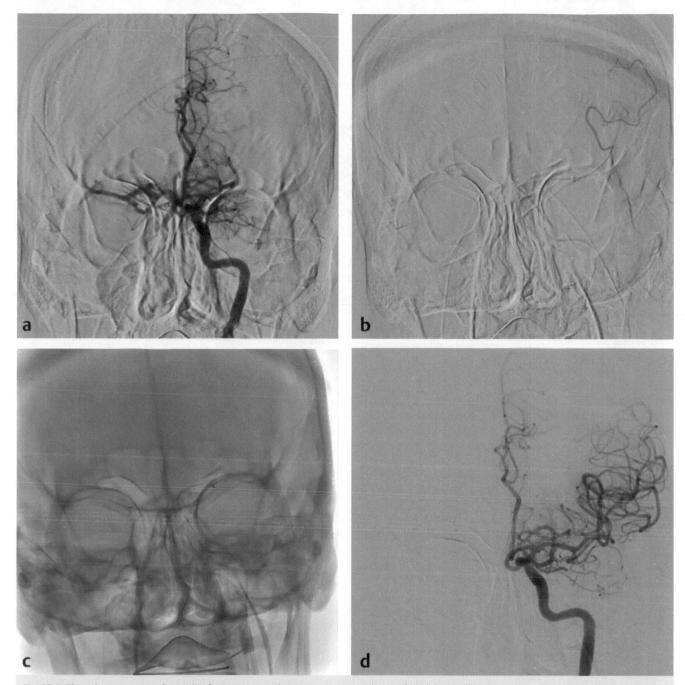

Fig. 32.2 Thrombectomy procedure. (**a**) Left ICA injection showing persistent occlusion of the left M1. (**b**) Microinjection through the Trevo XP ProVue microcatheter confirming position distal to the occlusion with no perforation. (**c**) The Trevo 4 mm × 30 mm stentriever was deployed distally into the M2 with the proximal third over the occlusion, and the AXS Catalyst 6 aspiration catheter was advanced while the aspiration pump is active to wedge the clot. (**d**) TICI 3 reperfusion of the left MCA territory.

- Triaxial approach to gain access of the brain vasculature.
- An 8-Fr guide catheter (8-Fr Cordis Vista, Johnson & Johnson, New Brunswick, NY) or long sheath (8-Fr Destination, Terumo Medical, Somerset, NJ) is advanced distally into the ICA; an 8-Fr BGC (FlowGate,[2] Stryker Neurovascular, Fremont, CA) could also be used. A 7-Fr guide (Mach 1, Boston Scientific, Marlborough, MA) for posterior circulation is advanced into the distal vertebral artery.
- A stent retriever microcatheter is advanced through a 5/6-Fr aspiration catheter (AXS Catalyst, Stryker Neurovascular;

Sofia/ Sofia Plus, MicroVention, Tustin, CA) past the occlusion site in an M2/A2/P1 vessel under continuous aspiration or with the help of a 0.014-in microwire.
- The stent retriever (Trevo variants, Stryker Neurovascular; Solitaire AB/FR; Covidien, Irvine, CA; EmboTrap, Neuravi, Galway, Ireland) is placed and advanced primarily distally, with the proximal third across the occlusion using active push deployment technique (push and fluff technique).[4] The distal part of the stent serves as a distal embolization protection device, capturing dislodge clot fragments to

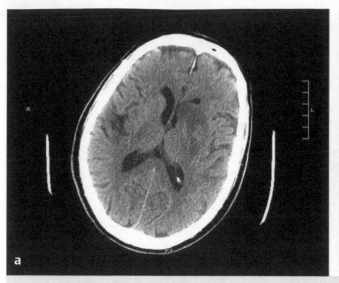 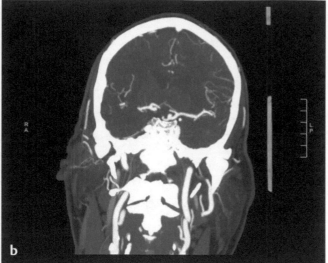

Fig. 32.3 Postthrombectomy CT. (**a**) Evolution of the known infarction with no new infarct. (**b**) CTA showing recanalized left MCA.

prevent distal emboli or embolization into another territory.

- The stent retriever is kept open for 2 to 8 minutes according to operator preference.
- The stent retriever microcatheter is then slowly removed (bare wire technique) to improve aspiration flow rate.[5]
- The aspiration catheter is connected to the aspiration pump and primed and activated. It is then advanced to the proximal part of the thrombus.
- Thereafter, the stent retriever is pulled slowly and gently, while advancing the aspiration catheter to wedge the clot.
- A 60-mL vacuum syringe (VacLok, Merit Medical, South Jordan, UT) is used to keep the negative pressure in the aspiration catheter after disconnecting the pump aspiration tubing.
- The aspiration tubing and the aspiration pump are connected to the guide catheter; if two pumps are available, dual aspiration can be performed from the guide catheter and the aspiration catheter.
- Both the stent retriever and the aspiration catheter are pulled as a unit into the guide catheter.
- If no back flow is noted through the guide catheter, it will be retrieved under permanent aspiration.

32.1.10 Pearls and Pitfalls

- Distal stent deployment with the occlusion at the proximal third helps in preventing clot fragments from embolization

distally, as the distal part of the stent serves as a distal protection device.

- Dual aspiration from the aspiration catheter and the guide catheter also maximizes the prevention of clot dislodgment and distal embolization at different stages of thrombus retrieval.
- Wedging the clot between the aspiration catheter and the stent retriever is a key step in the SAVE technique.

References

[1] Maus V, Behme D, Kabbasch C, et al. Maximizing first-pass complete reperfusion with SAVE. Clin Neuroradiol. 2018; 28(3):327–338

[2] Goyal M, Menon BK, van Zwam WH, et al. HERMES Collaborators. Endovascular thrombectomy after large-vessel ischaemic stroke: a meta-analysis of individual patient data from five randomised trials. Lancet. 2016; 387(10029):1723–1731

[3] Maus V, Henkel S, Riabikin A, et al. The SAVE technique: large-scale experience for treatment of intracranial large vessel occlusions. Clin Neuroradiol. 2018:[Epub ahead of print]

[4] Haussen DC, Rebello LC, Nogueira RG. Optimizing clot retrieval in acute stroke: the push and fluff technique for closed-cell stentrievers. Stroke. 2015; 46(10):2838–2842

[5] Nikoubashman O, Alt JP, Nikoubashman A, et al. Optimizing endovascular stroke treatment: removing the microcatheter before clot retrieval with stent-retrievers increases aspiration flow. J Neurointerv Surg. 2017; 9 (5):459–462

33 Aspiration-Retriever Technique for Stroke (ARTS)

33.1 Case Description

33.1.1 Clinical Presentation

An 85-year-old male presented with sudden onset of confusion, speech difficulties, and right-sided weakness, predominantly in the face and arm. He was last seen well 1 hour prior by his wife. Neurological examination revealed he was disoriented and aphasic. He had left gaze preference associated with right hemianopsia. There was a right, upper motor neuron facial palsy with absent movement in the right arm and mild weakness in the right leg (able to sustain suspended against gravity). His National Institutes of Health Stroke Scale (NIHSS) score was 20.

33.1.2 Imaging

Noncontrast computed tomography (CT) of the head showed only subtle loss of grey-white differentiation in the anterior frontal region (M1) consistent with an Alberta Stroke Program Early CT (ASPECTS) score of 9. CT angiography demonstrated a left M1 segment occlusion with corresponding nonmatched perfusion defect on CT perfusion (▶ Fig. 33.1).

33.1.3 Management

- He was not a candidate for tissue plasminogen activator, as his current medications included low-dose apixaban and aspirin for deep venous thrombosis prophylaxis in the setting of malignancy and cardiac disease. Mechanical thrombectomy was pursued (▶ Fig. 33.2).
- Pretreatment left internal carotid artery (ICA) injection showed persistent occlusion.

- Lateral view of the microcatheter injection demonstrated distal access beyond the M1 thrombus. The microcatheter was supported by a balloon guide catheter (BGC) within the distal cervical ICA and a distal aspiration catheter whose tip was positioned in the mid-M1 segment (▶ Fig. 33.3).
- Unsubtracted oblique view following deployment of the stentriever device (Trevo XP ProVue 4 × 30 mm) and removal of the microcatheter. The distal aspiration catheter (ACE68, Penumbra) remained in the proximal M1 segment, at the proximal end of the stent, to engage the thrombus (▶ Fig. 33.4).
- Postmechanical thrombectomy anteroposterior (left) and lateral (right) views demonstrated complete reperfusion (▶ Fig. 33.5).

33.1.4 Endovascular Devices

9-Fr 80-cm Teleflex Arrow-Flex sheath.
  9-Fr 92-cm Medtronic Cello BGC.
  Penumbra 5-Fr 130-cm Berenstein Select catheter.
  Terumo Advantage Glidewire 180 cm.
  Penumbra ACE 68 reperfusion catheter 132 cm.
  Penumbra Velocity Delivery microcatheter 170 cm.
  Boston Scientific Fathom 16 180 cm microwire.
  Stryker Trevo XP ProVue 4 mm × 30 mm stent.

33.1.5 Outcome

Thrombolysis in cerebral infarction (TICI) 3 reperfusion was achieved after a single stentriever pass. Clinically, his right arm improved to 4 + /5 in strength with a minor pronator drift and right leg to 5/5 strength. He had persisting partial aphasia and a

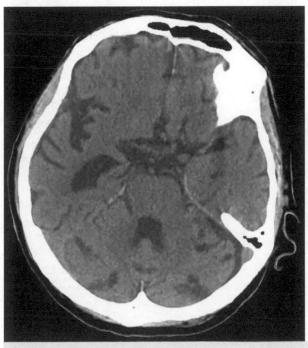
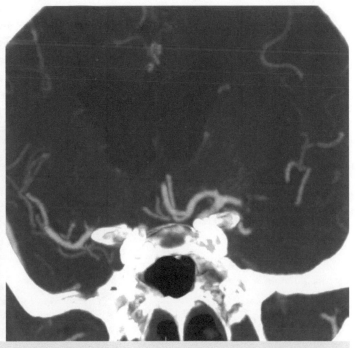

Fig. 33.1 Noncontrast CT of the head (left) demonstrating a hyperdense vessel involving the left M1 segment. Coronal reformatted image of CT angiography (right), with corresponding left M1 occlusion and distal reconstitution.

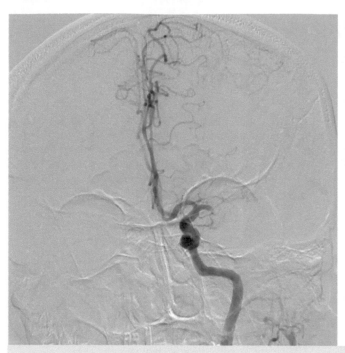

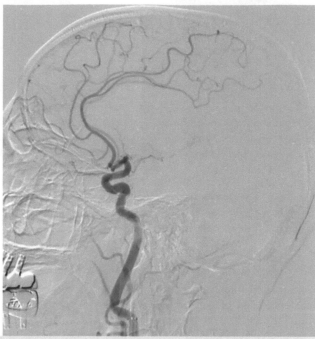

Fig. 33.2 Pretreatment left internal carotid artery (ICA) injection, anteroposterior (left) and lateral views (right).

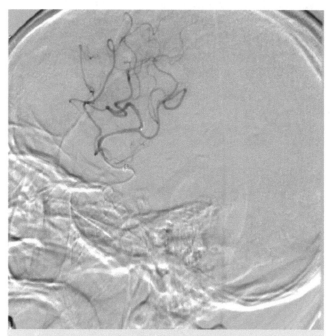

Fig. 33.3 Lateral view of a microcatheter injection demonstrating distal access beyond the M1 thrombus. The microcatheter is supported by a balloon guide catheter within the distal cervical ICA and by a distal aspiration catheter whose tip is positioned in the mid-M1 segment.

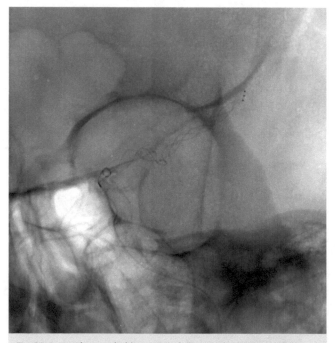

Fig. 33.4 Unsubtracted oblique view following deployment of the stentriever device (Trevo XP ProVue 4 × 30 mm) and removal of the microcatheter. The distal aspiration catheter (ACE68, Penumbra) remains in the proximal M1 segment at the proximal end of the stent to engage the thrombus.

right facial droop. He was transferred to a peripheral hospital for rehabilitation.

33.2 Background

The advent of stent retrievers and their utilization in acute ischemic stroke has revolutionized endovascular treatment of proximal intracranial large vessel occlusions. These in combination with large bore, distal access aspiration catheters have led to the development of a variety of techniques to promote mechanical thrombectomy success by increasing recanalization rates, decreasing the number of passes required, and shortening time to reperfusion while reducing thrombus fragmentation

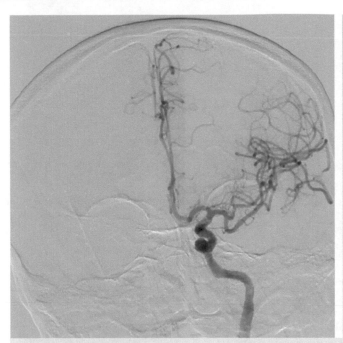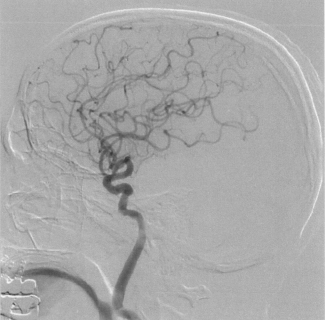

Fig. 33.5 Postmechanical thrombectomy anteroposterior (left) and lateral (right) views demonstrating complete reperfusion.

with subsequent distal embolization. The aspiration (catheter)-(stent) retriever technique for stroke (ARTS) was created to achieve these criteria.[1]

For access, an 8- to 9-Fr BGC is used and positioned within the distal cervical ICA. A triaxial assembly is then established with a distal access aspiration catheter navigated over a 0.021- to 0.027-in microcatheter and 0.014- to 0.016-in microwire, which are navigated through the clot. The aspiration catheter is then brought close to the proximal end of the clot (either over the microcatheter or, if it does not track, later "railed" over the deployed stentriever). The microwire is removed; after a microcatheter injection to confirm suitable position, a stent retriever is unsheathed across the clot and given several minutes to incorporate. The microcatheter is then removed. Retrieval of the stent is initiated with inflation of the BGC, followed by continuous aspiration through the distal access catheter by means of a mechanical pump. The stent is then pulled; simultaneously, the aspiration catheter advances slightly until there is resistance or reduction in flow through the aspiration tubing at which point, the entire system is locked. One may then wait a few minutes to promote "corking" of the clot. Thereafter, the stent retriever and microcatheter are withdrawn simultaneously through the BGC. The principle of this treatment revolves around "corking" the aspiration catheter with the stent-ensnared clot followed by retrieval under continuous aspiration and flow arrest.

Using ARTS, Massari et al[1] were able to achieve TICI ≥ 2b/3 recanalization in 97.6% of 42 consecutive patients, a majority of which were anterior circulation and M1 occlusions. Of these recanalizations, 43% were successful on the first pass. Distal emboli occurred in 4.7% of patients downstream into a M3 or M4 branch, and 2.4% (1 patient) into a nontarget territory. The procedure was associated with four cases (9.5%) of symptomatic intracerebral hemorrhage (two subarachnoid hemorrhages secondary to stent retrieval and two intraparenchymal

hemorrhages), which is comparable to the hemorrhagic complication rate observed in the multicenter randomized clinical trial of endovascular treatment for acute ischemic stroke in the Netherlands trial (MR CLEAN; 7.7%). At the 90-day follow-up, 65.7% of patients had a modified Rankin scale (mRS) score of ≤ 2, falling in the higher range of what was observed in the major stent-retriever trials from 2015 (32.6% in MR CLEAN to 71% in Extending the Time for Thrombolysis in Emergency Neurological Deficits—Intra-Arterial [EXTEND-IA] trial).

33.2.1 Discussion

ARTS utilizes the advantages of stent retrieval and direct catheter aspiration by combining them in a synergistic manner. A key component of this technique is the partial recapturing of the stent into the distal aspiration catheter until the clot is "corked," and simultaneous removal into the BGC, while maintaining this relationship rather than complete retrieval of the stent through the distal aspiration catheter as performed in SOLUMBRA and first described by Deshaies et al.[2] This minimizes the "apple-coring" effect that can occur as a large, ensnared clot/stent complex is forcefully withdrawn into the aspiration catheter. It is theorized that this action contributes to fragmentation of the clot and iatrogenic distal embolization. This is supported by a higher rate of new territory embolus in the series by Humphries et al[3] using SOLUMBRA (5.7%) compared to the series by Massari et al[2] using ARTS (2.4%).

The continuous aspiration prior to intracranial vascular embolectomy (CAPTIVE) technique of McTaggart et al[4] employs a similar method of stent retrieval; however, ARTS has the advantage of using a BGC. Inflation of the BGC initiates flow arrest which has been shown, in vitro, to reduce distal embolization during thrombectomy.[5] In practice, this has been observed to improve clinical and angiographic outcomes in patients with acute large vessel occlusion strokes. A recent systematic review compared stroke patients treated using mechanical thrombectomy with (1,083 patients) and without (939 patients) a BGC.[6] Use of BGC was associated with a higher first-pass recanalization rate (63.1 vs. 45.2%), greater chance of achieving TICI 2b/3 reperfusion (78.9 vs. 67%), less distal embolization evidenced by a higher TICI 3 rate (57.9 vs. 38.2%), and fewer number of passes (mean: 1.7 vs. 2.0). These patients also experienced improved clinical outcomes with a greater number achieving a 90-day mRS score of ≤ 2 (59.7 vs. 43.8%).

Both ARTS and CAPTIVE attempt to maximize the suction capabilities of the distal aspiration catheter through removal of the microcatheter after deployment of the stent retriever. The absence of a microcatheter not only increases the surface area for aspiration but also augments flow by increasing the volume accessible to fluid and reducing contact surfaces which contribute to drag forces. In vitro, Nikoubashman et al[7] were able to demonstrate that microcatheter absence (termed the "bare wire technique") significantly increased the volume aspirated over time. This, in turn, enables improved blood flow control toward reversal (particularly in the setting of an inflated balloon guide), thereby reducing the clot disruption and distal embolization. Together, these maneuvers that comprise the ARTS technique build upon the fundamentals of stentriever use, as described in the original thrombectomy trials coupled with aspiration via an intermediate catheter close to the clot and flow arrest, hopefully translating to more effective large vessel recanalization therapy while minimizing the risks of nontarget embolization or clot release. However, a limitation to the earlier discussion is the lack of randomized trials comparing these techniques and hence the lack of comparisons based on retrospective data.

33.3 References

[1] Massari F, Henninger N, Lozano JD, et al. ARTS (aspiration-retriever technique for stroke): initial clinical experience. Interv Neuroradiol. 2016; 22(3):325–332

[2] Deshaies EM. Tri-axial system using the Solitaire-FR and penumbra aspiration microcatheter for acute mechanical thrombectomy. J Clin Neurosci. 2013; 20(9):1303–1305

[3] Humphries W, Hoit D, Doss VT, et al. Distal aspiration with retrievable stent assisted thrombectomy for the treatment of acute ischemic stroke. J Neurointerv Surg. 2015; 7(2):90–94

[4] McTaggart RA, Tung EL, Yaghi S, et al. Continuous aspiration prior to intracranial vascular embolectomy (CAPTIVE): a technique which improves outcomes. J Neurointerv Surg. 2017; 9(12):1154–1159

[5] Chueh JY, Kühn AL, Puri AS, Wilson SD, Wakhloo AK, Gounis MJ. Reduction in distal emboli with proximal flow control during mechanical thrombectomy: a quantitative in vitro study. Stroke. 2013; 44(5):1396–1401

[6] Brinjikji W, Starke RM, Murad MH, et al. Impact of balloon guide catheter on technical and clinical outcomes: a systematic review and meta-analysis. J Neurointerv Surg. 2018; 10(4):335–339

[7] Nikoubashman O, Alt JP, Nikoubashman A, et al. Optimizing endovascular stroke treatment: removing the microcatheter before clot retrieval with stent-retrievers increases aspiration flow. J Neurointerv Surg. 2017; 9 (5):459–462

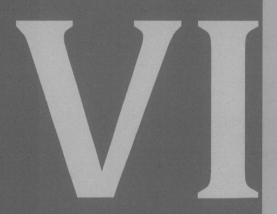

Part VI

Complications

VI

34 Clot Migration with Emboli to Distal Territories

34.1 Case Description

34.1.1 Clinical Presentation

An 86-year-old woman presented with left-sided hemiplegia and aphasia 2 hours before hospital admission. Clinically, she displayed a full right middle cerebral artery (MCA) occlusion syndrome with hemineglect, hemiplegia, and gaze preference to the left. The National Institutes of Health Stroke Scale (NIHSS) score at presentation was 24. Intravenous thrombolysis was administered after initial noncontrast CT (NCCT) of the brain confirmed no intracranial hemorrhage.

34.1.2 Imaging Workup and Investigations

CT angiography of the brain confirmed a complete right M1 MCA occlusion with moderate pial collateral vessels. The thrombus measured 8 mm in length. CT perfusion demonstrated a clear ischemic penumbra in the entire right hemisphere, with no established infarct core as defined by regional cerebral blood flow less than 30% (▶ Fig. 34.1).

Endovascular Treatment

The patient was brought to the angio suite and transfemoral endovascular thrombectomy with conscious sedation was performed. A balloon guiding catheter (BGC; FlowGate, Stryker) was navigated to the right cervical internal carotid artery (ICA) over a 5-Fr diagnostic catheter and Terumo Glidewire. Digital subtraction angiography again demonstrated the complete right M1 occlusion just distal to the origin of the medial lenticulostriate vessels. (▶ Fig. 34.2a) Stent-retriever thrombectomy was performed by first navigating a microcatheter (Trevo Pro 18, Stryker) to the superior M2 trunk over a microguidewire, followed by deployment of the Trevo ProVue 6 × 25 mm stent retriever across the occluding thrombus. The first pass with proximal flow reversal yielded a piece of thrombus, but control angiography demonstrated fragmentation and distal migration of the clot, resulting in occlusion of the inferior M2 trunk as well as more distal occlusion of the opercular M3 branch (▶ Fig. 34.2b, c).

Using a similar setup, the inferior M2 trunk was recanalized by a second pass of stent retriever with proximal flow reversal at the level of the BGC. Another couple of attempts to revascularize the opercular branch was unsuccessful due to the distality of the clot and tortuous vascular anatomy. Finally, modified treatment in cerebral infarction 2a revascularization was achieved with the right opercular branch of the MCA remaining occluded (▶ Fig. 34.2d, e). Follow-up CT scan of the brain demonstrated infarction of the right insula and the basal ganglia, correlating to the area supplied by the opercular branch (▶ Fig. 34.2f). Patients' neurological symptoms improved to NIHSS 15, but remained disabled with left hemiparesis and a modified Rankin scale score of 3 at discharge.

34.1.3 Discussion

Mechanical thrombectomy with newer generation devices have consistently demonstrated better rates of reperfusion; however, this has not resulted in equally high rates of good clinical outcome.[1,2,3]

The aim of mechanical thrombectomy is to reperfuse the affected territory in order to reduce, if not prevent, ischemic injury to the brain; however, when removing the clot from the affected vessel, one of the risks is the formation of emboli in a new vascular territory (ENT) and the consequent development of an infarct in a previously unaffected part of the brain. This may contribute to the discrepancy between the rates of reperfusion and good clinical outcome. In the major trials, the rate of ENT has been reported to be between 0 and 11.4% (▶ Table 34.1).[1,2,3,4,5,6,7,8,9] In addition to ENT, there is also risk of emboli downstream from the originally occluded vessel; for example, Gascou et al reported this phenomenon in 3.5% of their patient cohort.[9] The clinical impact of these downstream emboli is not fully known; however, Kurre et al reported clinical worsening by more than 4 points on the NIHSS scale in 3 of the six patients who experienced ENT. Gascou et al reported clinical worsening among 13 of 18 patients who had ENT or emboli downstream for the occluded vessel within the same vascular territory, and Davalos et al reported that 2 of 9 patients experienced a clinically significant stroke following ENT.[8,9,10] In contrast, the two patients in EXTEND IA who experienced ENT had no clinical symptoms attributable to these distal emboli.[5] Rescue therapy can be performed to revascularize the newly occluded vessel as performed in six of the patients from the Kurre series; this proved to be successful in five patients, and in three out of those five patients, there was no evidence of new infarcts.[8] Attempts at rescue, however, mean additional instrumentation, which is associated with increased risk, as illustrated in the present case. Given that not all of these emboli are eloquent territory or clinically symptomatic, it may be that in some instances, there is no need to chase ENT. When patients are under conscious sedation, on-table examination can be performed to determine if there is a need to perform rescue therapy.

Both clot and treatment strategy factors may be considered to be related to the risk of ENT. These factors include clot composition, administration of intravenous tissue plasminogen activator (IV-tPA), location and length of the clot, thrombectomy device, and choice of access/ guiding catheter. Conceptually, longer clots that are soft, lodged across bifurcations, or angulated segments of a vessel would be more prone to fragmentation and ENT. This risk may be aggravated by the use of IV-tPA. Nevertheless, the two patients in the STAR trial who experienced ENT did not receive IV-tPA, and other studies have not shown any difference in the rate of ENT with the administration of fibrinolystics.[9,10]

More importantly, the thrombectomy strategy may be crucial in preventing ENT. Although a recent meta-analysis of 2,893 patients comparing aspiration-first and stent-retriever-first

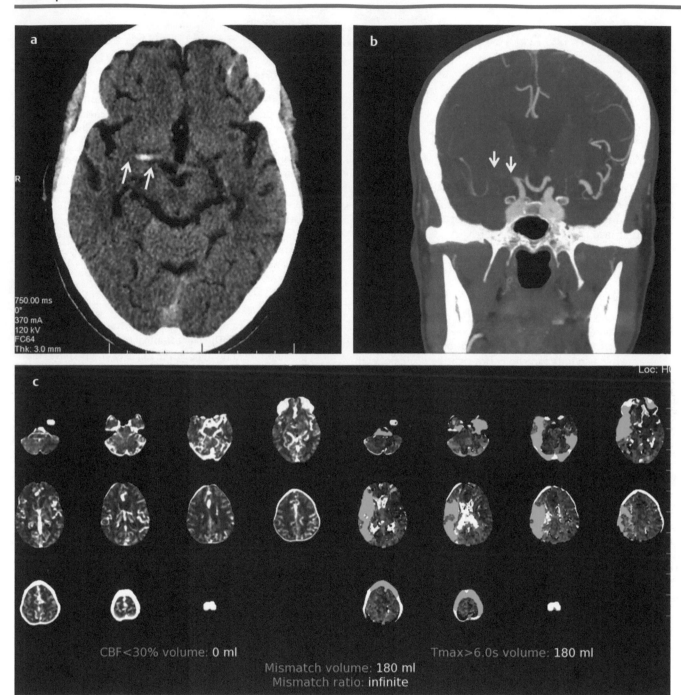

Fig. 34.1 (a) Noncontrast CT of the brain of the patient showing a dense right MCA sign (*arrow*). (b) CT angiography coronal reconstruction showing the filling defect of the M1 segment of the right MCA, correlating to the acute MCA occlusion. (c) CT perfusion and RAPID software summary demonstrating the penumbra.

thrombectomy did not demonstrate a difference in the rate of ENT,[11] Chueh et al found the use of proximal flow reversal with a BGC to be most effective in preventing soft elastic clot fragmentation in in vitro studies.[12] Kurre et al likewise observed a trend toward fewer ENT when distal aspiration was performed with distal emboli seen in 3.3% of those who underwent distal aspiration versus 14.6% who did not.[8] It is therefore advisable to adopt BGC or distal aspiration in conjunction with stent-retriever thrombectomy when the risk of ENT or distal emboli is high, such as in cases with embolic, long thrombus across bifurcations.

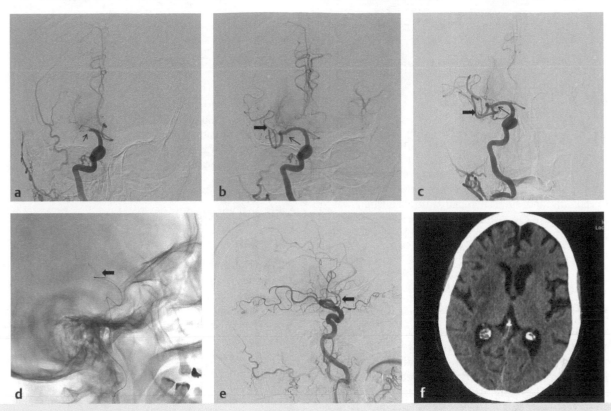

Fig. 34.2 (a) Anteroposterior view of right ICA angiography from the balloon guiding catheter at the proximal cervical ICA, confirming the right M1 occlusion. (b,c) After first pass of stent retriever, the M1 and superior M2 trunk were recanalized. There were distal emboli to the opercular branch (*thick arrow*), and the inferior M2 trunk (*thin arrow*), which required further passes of stent retriever. The inferior M2 trunk was revascularized after the second pass thrombectomy. (d,e) Further attempts to reopen the occluded opercular branch was unsuccessful (*thick arrow*). (f) Follow-up CT of the brain demonstrating infarction of the right insula and basal ganglia.

Table 34.1 Reported rates of emboli to new vascular territory in the literature

Trial	Rate of emboli to new vascular territory n/N (%)
SWIFT (solitaire arm)[2]	0/89 (0)
Dávalos et al[10]	9/141 (6.4)
NASA registry (BGC + no BGC group)[6]	18/338 (5.3)
STAR[1]	2/202[1]
Kurre et al[8]	12/105 (11.4)
Gascou et al[9]	14/144 (9.7)
Behme et al[7]	4/176[2]
MR CLEAN[4]	20/233 (8.6)
EXTEND-IA[5]	2/35 (5.7)

References

[1] Pereira VM, Gralla J, Davalos A, et al. Prospective, multicenter, single-arm study of mechanical thrombectomy using Solitaire Flow Restoration in acute ischemic stroke. Stroke. 2013; 44(10):2802–2807

[2] Saver JL, Jahan R, Levy EI, et al. SWIFT Trialists. Solitaire flow restoration device versus the MERCI Retriever in patients with acute ischaemic stroke (SWIFT): a randomised, parallel-group, non-inferiority trial. Lancet. 2012; 380(9849):1241–1249

[3] Nogueira RG, Lutsep HL, Gupta R, et al. TREVO 2 Trialists. Trevo versus MERCI retrievers for thrombectomy revascularisation of large vessel occlusions in acute ischaemic stroke (TREVO 2): a randomised trial. Lancet. 2012; 380 (9849):1231–1240

[4] Berkhemer OA, Fransen PS, Beumer D, et al. MR CLEAN Investigators. A randomized trial of intraarterial treatment for acute ischemic stroke. N Engl J Med. 2015; 372(1):11–20

[5] Campbell BC, Mitchell PJ, Kleinig TJ, et al. EXTEND-IA Investigators. Endovascular therapy for ischemic stroke with perfusion-imaging selection. N Engl J Med. 2015; 372(11):1009–1018

[6] Nguyen TN, Malisch T, Castonguay AC, et al. Balloon guide catheter improves revascularization and clinical outcomes with the Solitaire device: analysis of the North American Solitaire acute stroke registry. Stroke. 2014; 45 (1):141–145

[7] Behme D, Gondecki L, Fiethen S, Kowoll A, Mpotsaris A, Weber W. Complications of mechanical thrombectomy for acute ischemic stroke-a retrospective single-center study of 176 consecutive cases. Neuroradiology. 2014; 56(6):467–476

[8] Kurre W, Aguilar-Pérez M, Niehaus L, et al. Predictors of outcome after mechanical thrombectomy for anterior circulation large vessel occlusion in patients aged ≥ 80 years. Cerebrovasc Dis. 2013; 36(5–6):430–436

[9] Gascou G, Lobotesis K, Machi P, et al. Stent retrievers in acute ischemic stroke: complications and failures during the perioperative period. AJNR Am J Neuroradiol. 2014; 35(4):734–740

[10] Dávalos A, Pereira VM, Chapot R, Bonafé A, Andersson T, Gralla J, Solitaire Group. Retrospective multicenter study of Solitaire FR for revascularization in the treatment of acute ischemic stroke. Stroke. 2012; 43(10):2699–2705

[11] Tsang COA, Cheung IHW, Lau KK, Brinjikji W, Kallmes DF, Krings T. Outcomes of stent retriever versus aspiration-first thrombectomy in ischemic stroke: a systematic review and meta-analysis. AJNR Am J Neuroradiol. 2018; 39 (11):2070–2076

[12] Chueh JY, Puri AS, Wakhloo AK, et al. Risk of distal embolization with stent retriever thrombectomy and ADAPT. J Neurointerv Surg. 2016; 8(2):197–202

35 Endothelial Damage

35.1 Case Description

35.1.1 Clinical Presentation

A 59-year-old female inpatient under the care of cardiology developed a sudden-onset aphasia, right hemiplegia, and neglect. Her National Institutes of Health Stroke Scale (NIHSS) score was 28. Three days previously, the patient had undergone ablation procedure for atrial fibrillation, complicated by left atrial perforation and pericardial tamponade, and followed by ministernotomy and surgical repair. Anticoagulation was on hold. In addition to the history of atrial fibrillation, comorbidities included hypertension, which was well controlled. There were no other cardiovascular risk factors.

35.1.2 Imaging Workup and Investigations

Noncontrast computed tomography (NCCT) of the brain obtained 90 minutes from symptom onset (▶ Fig. 35.1a–c) demonstrated already loss of gray-white matter differentiation in the left insular region and lentiform nucleus in keeping with early infarction. Elsewhere, gray-white matter differentiation was preserved. There was hyperdensity consistent with thrombus in the left carotid termination and proximal middle cerebral artery (MCA; ▶ Fig. 35.1a).

CT angiography (CTA) demonstrated absence of contrast opacification of the left supraclinoid internal carotid artery (ICA), carotid terminus, M1 segment of left MCA, and proximal M2 branches (▶ Fig. 35.1d, e). Left MCA branches in the sylvian fissure filled through leptomeningeal collaterals. The left A1 segment (▶ Fig. 35.1e, *arrow*) and more distal anterior cerebral artery (ACA) was patent, opacified by contrast from the contralateral side through the anterior communicating artery.

35.1.3 Diagnosis

Cardioembolic occlusion of the left carotid terminus in the setting of atrial fibrillation off anticoagulation.

35.1.4 Treatment

In view of the high NIHSS score, presentation clearly within the time window, relative lack of early change on CT (other than left lentiform and insular region infarction), and the presence of large artery occlusion on CTA, a decision was made to proceed with intervention.

Initial Management

Intravenous tissue plasminogen activator (IV-tPA) was contraindicated in view of the recent surgery and therefore not administered. The patient was transferred directly to the neurointerventional suite.

Endovascular Treatment

Materials

- 8-Fr short angiographic sheath.
- 8-Fr MERCI balloon guide catheter.
- 5-Fr VTK slip catheter.
- 0.035 angled hydrophilic wire.
- Trevo 18 microcatheter.
- Synchro-14 microguidewire.
- Trevo ProVue 4 × 20 mm stent retriever.
- 8-Fr Angio-Seal closure device.

Technique

Intervention was performed with conscious sedation and local anesthetic. A single-wall, left common femoral artery (CFA) puncture was performed, and the 8-Fr short vascular access sheath inserted. The right femoral artery had been recently accessed for cardiac intervention. The 8-Fr balloon guide catheter was advanced to the midcervical level of the left ICA over a 5-Fr VTK slip catheter with the aid of an angled Terumo guidewire using roadmap guidance. Left ICA angiography in frontal (▶ Fig. 35.2a) and lateral (▶ Fig. 35.2b) views showed slow filling of the left carotid artery to the level of the supraclinoid segment, where there was distal sharp cutoff with meniscus sign at the proximal clot face. There was no anterograde flow and no opacification of the MCA or ACA. Contrast stagnation and layering was noted in the cervical and supraclinoid ICA. A Trevo 18 microcatheter was navigated across the occluded carotid terminus and left M1 segment of MCA, and into an opercular branch of the superior division of MCA. Microcatheter injection (not shown) confirmed position distal to thrombus in a good caliber M2 branch. A Trevo ProVue 4 × 20 mm stent-retriever device was then deployed from the proximal M2 segment back to the supraclinoid segment of the ICA.

Control angiography with the stent in situ (▶ Fig. 35.2c, d) showed some antegrade flow through the deployed stent, with filling defect consistent with thrombus in the supraclinoid ICA and carotid terminus region. The stent was left in situ for 5 minutes to allow incorporation of thrombus and then retrieved with flow arrest and suction. Some small clot fragments were retrieved in the stent; however, there was no back bleeding through the guide catheter, even with aspiration. The guide catheter was removed and flushed on the angiography table. Three large pieces of thrombus were flushed from the guide catheter. Total retrieved thrombus length was approximately 2 cm. The catheter was cleaned thoroughly and flushed. Using the same coaxial approach as before, the guide catheter was again placed in the left ICA. Control angiography showed complete recanalization of the left ICA, MCA, and now filling of left ACA from the carotid injection (▶ Fig. 35.2d, e). There was complete reperfusion of the distal territory, with no evidence of distal clot migration or distal emboli, and no evidence of narrowing or spasm at site of thrombectomy.

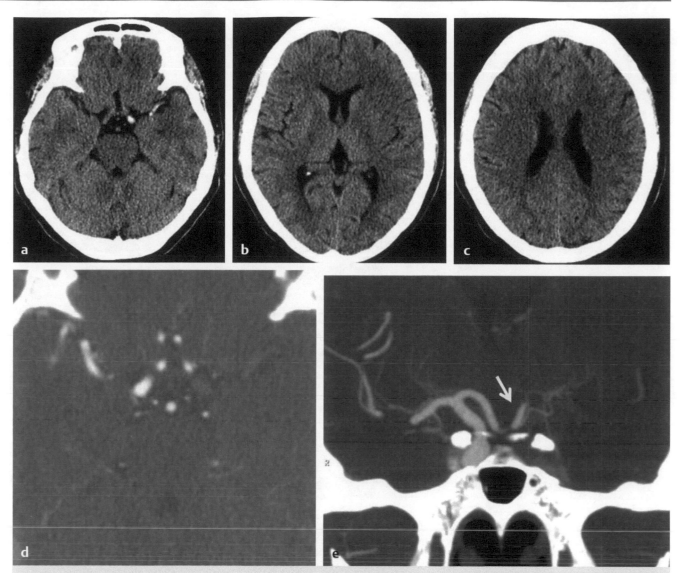

Fig. 35.1 Noncontrast enhanced CT of the brain obtained 90 minutes from symptom onset (**a–c**) demonstrated already loss of gray-white matter differentiation in the left insular region and lentiform nucleus in keeping with early infarction. Elsewhere, gray-white matter differentiation was preserved. There was hyperdensity consistent with thrombus in the left carotid termination and proximal MCA (**a**). CT angiography demonstrated absence of contrast opacification of the left supraclinoid ICA, carotid terminus, M1 segment of left MCA, and proximal M2 branches (**d, e**). Left MCA branches in the sylvian fissure filled through leptomeningeal collaterals. The left A1 segment (**e**, arrow) and more distal ACA was patent, opacified by contrast from the contralateral side through the anterior communicating artery.

All devices were removed. Hemostasis of the femoral artery puncture site was achieved by insertion of an 8-Fr Angio-Seal.

Postprocedure Care/Outcome

The patient demonstrated on-table improvement following recanalization and reperfusion, with improved power in the right arm and leg, along with improvement of aphasia and neglect. She was transferred to the neuro high-dependency unit (HDU) in stable condition for further monitoring and care. NCCT of the head performed 24 hours postprocedure demonstrated infarction in the left lentiform nucleus, caudate, insula, and small-volume patchy left frontal lobe infarction, with no evidence of hemorrhage. Following CT, the patient was

commenced on IV heparin infusion for anticoagulation. Subsequently, anticoagulation with apixaban was commenced.

MRI with time of flight (TOF) MRA and vessel wall imaging were performed at 3 Tesla 5 days postthrombectomy. Diffusion-weighted imaging showed diffusion restriction in a pattern similar to previous postprocedural CT (► Fig. 35.3a, b), involving left lentiform nucleus posteriorly, caudate, insular region, and small-volume infarction in the left frontal lobe, with sparing otherwise of basal ganglia, internal capsule, and most of the left MCA territory. MRA (► Fig. 35.3c) showed normal appearance to the left ICA, carotid terminus, MCA, and ACA with no evidence of luminal irregularity or narrowing. Vessel-wall imaging was performed (► Fig. 35.4a–f) with the following protocol: pre- and postcontrast T1 FLAIR and T2-weighted images in

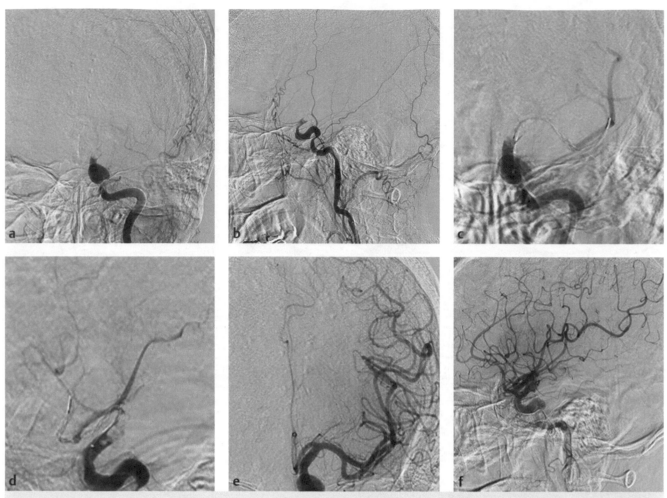

Fig. 35.2 Left ICA angiography in frontal (**a**) and lateral (**b**) views showed slow filling of the left carotid artery to the level of the supraclinoid segment, where there was distal sharp cut off with meniscus sign at the proximal clot face. There was no anterograde flow and no opacification of the MCA or ACA. Contrast stagnation and layering was noted in the cervical and supraclinoid ICA. Control angiogram with the stent in situ (**c,d**) showed some antegrade flow through the deployed stent with filling defect consistent with thrombus in the supraclinoid ICA and carotid terminus region. Control angiogram showed complete recanalization of the left ICA, MCA, and now filling of left ACA from the carotid injection (**d,e**).

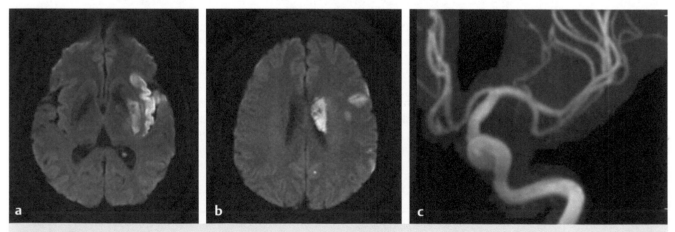

Fig. 35.3 Diffusion-weighted imaging showed diffusion restriction in a similar pattern to previous postprocedural CT (**a,b**), involving left lentiform nucleus posteriorly, caudate, insular region, and small volume infarction in the left frontal lobe, with sparing otherwise of basal ganglia, internal capsule, and most of the left MCA territory. MR angiography (**c**) showed normal appearance to the left ICA, carotid terminus, MCA, and ACA, with no evidence of luminal irregularity or narrowing.

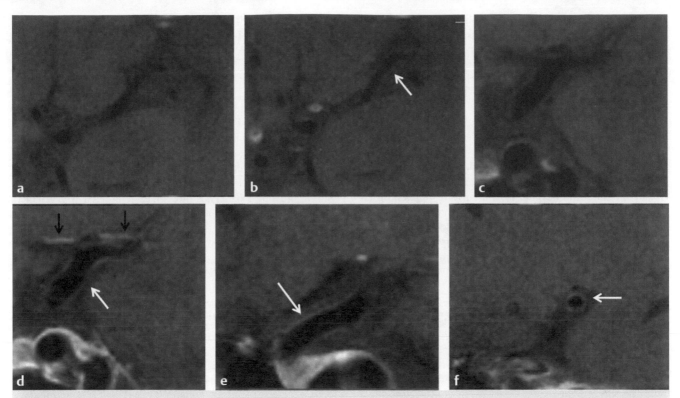

Fig. 35.4 Vessel wall imaging was performed (**a–f**) with the following protocol: pre- and postcontrast T1 FLAIR and T2-weighted images in axial, coronal, and sagittal oblique planes with slice thickness of 2 to 3 mm and matrix size 512 × 512. There was no evidence of intrinsic T1 hyperintensity to suggest intramural thrombus on the precontrast imaging (**a,c**). Gadolinium-enhanced T1 FLAIR showed concentric wall thickening and enhancement of the left M1 and proximal M2 segment of MCA (**b,f**) and enhancement of the left supraclinoid ICA and ICA termination (**d,e**). This corresponded to location of deployment of the stent retriever.

axial, coronal, and sagittal oblique planes with slice thickness of 2 to 3 mm and matrix size 512 × 512. There was no evidence of intrinsic T1 hyperintensity to suggest intramural thrombus on precontrast imaging (▶ Fig. 35.4a, c). Gadolinium-enhanced T1 FLAIR showed concentric wall thickening and enhancement of the left M1 and proximal M2 segment of MCA (▶ Fig. 35.4b, f), and enhancement of the left supraclinoid ICA and ICA termination (▶ Fig. 35.4d, e). This corresponded to the location of deployment of the stent retriever.

There was continued clinical improvement throughout her in-patient stay, and she was discharged to rehabilitation 7 days following the thrombectomy procedure; 2 weeks later, she was discharged home. On the 3-month follow-up in the clinic, the patient was well, with no residual motor or sensory deficits, and complete resolution of language difficulties (modified Rankin scale score of 0).

35.2 Discussion

35.2.1 Background

Acute ischemic stroke due to intracranial large artery occlusion is independently associated with poor functional outcomes and high-mortality rates. Broadly speaking, the underlying cause for intracranial arterial occlusion can be either embolic, or, less commonly, related to diseases of the occluded vessel itself such as atherosclerosis. IV thrombolysis is an established treatment for acute ischemic stroke presenting within the 4.5 hour

thrombolysis window. However, intracranial large arterial occlusion has been shown to be relatively resistant to treatment with IV thrombolytic therapy, and recent randomized controlled trials such as MR CLEAN, ESCAPE, EXTEND-IA, and SWIFT-PRIME have proven beneficial for mechanical thrombectomy over IV thrombolytic therapy alone in patients with large artery occlusive stroke. Mechanical thrombectomy is now the standard of care for such patients.

Little is currently known regarding the aftereffects of mechanical thrombectomy on the arterial wall in human subjects, as this has not been extensively studied to date. There is, however, some evidence from animal studies with regard to histopathological correlation that mechanical thrombectomy can result in arterial wall damage. In addition, there are some emerging studies in human subjects on angiographic follow-up postthrombectomy, showing delayed development of luminal narrowing/stenosis at the site of previous intracranial thrombectomy.

High-resolution 3-Tesla MRI can be used to study the wall of intracranial arteries, and can give valuable information regarding underlying abnormality. The MRI appearance of the arterial wall in disease states such as atherosclerosis and vasculitis is now well reported. Recently, this imaging technique has also been used to study the wall of intracranial arteries following stent retriever thrombectomy.

In this illustrative case, the patient presented with cardioembolic occlusion of the left carotid terminus in the setting of atrial fibrillation off anticoagulation. Mechanical thrombectomy was performed. MRI of the vessel wall subsequently showed abnormality of the intracranial arterial wall at the site of the deployed stent retriever.

35.2.2 Workup and Diagnosis

Patient History

In the acute setting, when a patient presents with large artery occlusive stroke, it may be difficult to gather information regarding relevant medical history quickly, particularly if the patient is aphasic, as it was in this case. If the patient has previously attended the hospital or is a current inpatient, then a review of the patients' medical records or collateral from the physicians caring for the patient could yield helpful information, particularly regarding possible cardiovascular risk factors and any contraindications to treatment. In this case, for example, given the recent surgical history, IV-tPA was contraindicated, and the patient was brought directly to the neurointerventional suite for thrombectomy. Collateral history from witnesses, family, friends, or staff could help determine time of symptom onset, which is also an important consideration for treatment.

In the follow-up, in the context of potential endothelial damage to the arterial wall, or development of a de-novo stenosis at the site of prior thrombectomy, it is conceivable that the patient may report a history of new onset stroke or transient ischemic attack–like symptoms related to either embolic disease or, if there is stenosis, hypoperfusion of watershed territories. It should, however, be noted that the limited literature available in this area of discussion shows that the patients generally remain asymptomatic.

Examination and Investigations

Findings from physical examination in patients presenting with acute stroke, or symptomatic sequelae of endothelial damage, will manifest depending on the ischemic or hypoperfused territory and/or neurologic deficits from previously infarcted territory.

There are currently no formal recommendations regarding imaging follow-up of patients post–mechanical thrombectomy in terms of assessing the arterial wall, or assessing for luminal stenosis. Generally, patients will have, at least, a NCCT of the brain at 24 hours postprocedure to assess extent of infarction, and look for any evidence of hemorrhagic conversion and mass effect. This will, however, not assess the arterial wall. Some centers perform CTA at 24 hours poststroke treatment to confirm continued patency of the artery, although generally this is most applicable to cases treated with IV thrombolysis alone, or in cases where patient develops new or progressive symptoms to suggest reocclusion or a new arterial occlusion. CTA follow-up in this subacute stage will generally not demonstrate a de novo stenosis, as, based on the limited available literature, this is seen more in the delayed setting and therefore develops over time.

High-resolution contrast-enhanced vessel wall MRI (MRI) can not only be used to study the wall of intracranial arteries, but also provide valuable information regarding underlying abnormality. This is usually performed at 3 Tesla, and various protocols exist in the literature. The protocol used in our institution is as follows: Signa HD × 3.0-T scanner with an 8-channel

head coil (GE Healthcare, Milwaukee, WI). TOF MRA of the circle of Willis and T1-weighted black blood vessel wall sequences (single inversion recovery-prepared, two-dimensional fast spin echo acquisition with field of view = 22 × 22 cm, acquired matrix = 512 × 512; slice thickness = 2 mm; total slab thickness = 3 cm, TR/TI/TE = 2263/860/13 ms) before and after IV administration of gadolinium. The same scan parameters are used for the nonenhanced and enhanced sequences. High-resolution T2 FRFSE, 2-mm slice thickness, for 3-cm slab thickness can also be obtained. Imaging can be targeted to the vessel which was occluded on the initial CTA at the time of stroke presentation. It would be ideal if the vessel wall sequences are obtained in both short- and long-axis planes through each targeted artery, which can be planned in the TOF MRA.

Using this approach, the TOF MRA can be used to not only assess the arterial lumen for confirmation of recanalization but also identify any stenosis. Nonenhanced T1-weighted vessel wall sequence will demonstrate if there is any hyperintensity within the arterial wall, that is, evidence of intramural blood product, as might be seen in dissection. Using the nonenhanced and contrast-enhanced vessel wall sequences, arterial wall thickening and arterial wall enhancement can be identified and categorized.

A cross-sectional study of consecutive patients with acute ischemic stroke secondary to large intracranial arterial occlusion who underwent contrast-enhanced vessel wall MRI within days of stroke presentation and stent-retriever mechanical thrombectomy was published by Power et al in Stroke 2014. MRA showed no evidence of luminal narrowing in the group of patients post–mechanical thrombectomy. There was also no evidence of T1 hyperintensity within the arterial wall on the pre-contrast imaging to suggest blood products in the wall or dissection. On the postgadolinium T1 imaging, the arterial wall at site of stent-retriever deployment and thrombectomy showed varying degrees of thickening and concentric smooth enhancement. Arterial wall edema may account for the arterial wall thickening observed in these patients. Endothelial damage and denudation may result in increased endothelial permeability to IV gadolinium, accounting for the arterial wall enhancement observed in patients who had undergone mechanical thrombectomy. Duration of persistence of wall imaging abnormality is not yet known. Based on limited local experience, there does seem to be some improvement of wall imaging appearances over the first 6 to 12 months following thrombectomy, although in some cases, residual mild thickening and enhancement remains.

Postthrombectomy, digital subtraction angiography (DSA), CTA, or MRA will assess the arterial lumen for evidence of narrowing/stenosis. While DSA remains the definitive, gold standard technique for assessing the lumen, and measuring degree of stenosis, it does not image the arterial wall. CTA and MRA have the advantage of being noninvasive imaging modalities, with MRA having the added benefit of lack of radiation and can even be performed without contrast. Our experience, to date, with TOF intracranial MRA at 3 Tesla suggests it is a sufficient screening tool to assess the development of a de novo stenosis. The technique is, however, prone to motion artifact, and degree of stenosis can be overestimated on MRA, particularly if it is severe. Kurre et al in 2013 reported an angiographic follow-up study in patients following mechanical thrombectomy, performing DSA follow-up at a median of 107 days postprocedure.

De novo stenosis was found in 3.4% of treated segments. Patients were all asymptomatic. Eugène et al in 2015 reported MRA follow-up in patients treated with stent-retriever mechanical thrombectomy at 1 year postprocedure. In total, 10 of the 39 patients imaged had luminal abnormality on MRI; however, only 4 of these (4/39 patients, 10.3%) represented delayed de novo arterial stenosis. Again, all four of these patients were asymptomatic.

35.2.3 Decision-Making Process

The presence of an intracranial large artery occlusion calls for immediate treatment in an effort to prevent or reduce the clinical implications of disabling stroke. The benefits of mechanical thrombectomy in intracranial large artery occlusive stroke have been proven in several randomized controlled clinical trials and is now the standard of care. IV thrombolysis is considered an established treatment for acute ischemic stroke presenting within the 4.5-hour thrombolysis window, and should be administered unless contraindicated, as most of the trials to date were placed in the context of mechanical thrombectomy being performed as adjunct to IV-tPA, if administrable. The potential risk of endothelial damage and development of a delayed de novo stenosis at the site of thrombectomy should not factor into the decision as to whether thrombectomy should be performed, particularly as the clinical implications are as yet unknown; also, from the limited data available, patients seem to remain largely asymptomatic. Decision making, instead, should still hinge on the usual considerations of patient's premorbid state, time from symptom onset, severity of stroke symptoms/NIHSS score, absence or presence and extent of early change on CT at presentation, location of arterial occlusion, and degree of collateralization to the territory if any.

35.2.4 Management

Medication

In terms of management of large artery occlusive stroke, IV-tPA can be administered if the patient presents within 4.5 hours of last seen normal and no contraindications are present.

Treatment

Intracranial mechanical thrombectomy can be performed with stent retriever, as in this case using the earlier-described technique. Aspiration thrombectomy, using a distal access catheter and either manual or pump aspiration (such as the penumbra aspiration system), is also an option, particularly if the clot is proximal, for example, in the ICA, carotid terminus, or M1 segment of MCA. The recently published randomized controlled trial evidence, it should be noted, is largely relevant to stent-retriever thrombectomy. The two techniques, that is, stent-retriever thrombectomy and penumbra system aspiration, can also be combined, and may be particularly effective for more distal occlusions, for example, M2 occlusion where flow arrest in the ICA and aspiration from the level of the carotid can potentially be ineffective.

Histopathological studies in swine and canine models have shown that mechanical thrombectomy can result in injury to the arterial wall. Gory et al in 2013 studied a variety of thrombectomy devices in a swine model, including the Solitaire stent retriever and an aspiration device known as the Penumbra System 0.32. All of the mechanical thrombectomy devices studied resulted in damage to the arterial wall, with histopathological examination revealing varying degrees of endothelial denudation, disruption of the internal elastic lamina, and edema in the intimal and medial layers of the arterial wall. There were no statistically significant differences between the device groups. While the aspiration device created less endothelial denudation and mural thrombus than the wall-contact devices, there was more intimal and medial layer edema in the aspiration group, although the differences were not significant. Nogueira et al reported similar findings with the Trevo stent retriever. Therefore, it seems that since devices seem to have similar effects on the arterial wall, they should not be factored into the decision-making process of which device to use.

35.2.5 Postprocedure Care

Following mechanical thrombectomy, stroke patients should be managed in a dedicated stoke unit, HDU, or ICU depending on the level of care needed.

If possible, a closure device should be used to achieve hemostasis at the puncture site. An external compression device may be helpful in maintaining hemostasis if closure device fails or cannot be inserted. If a closure device is not used, then consideration can be given to leaving the sheath in situ until tPA/heparin is no longer in the system, and then obtaining hemostasis with manual pressure.

In terms of specific treatment targeted at the intracranial wall at the site of thrombectomy, there is no proposed treatment to reduce arterial inflammation or edema as yet. Aspirin or other antiplatelet agents are frequently administered following large artery occlusive stroke in the context of secondary prevention strategies. Antiplatelet agents are not, however, always administered, as was the case here where stroke etiology was cardioembolic due to atrial fibrillation, and the patient was discharged on anticoagulation only. Consideration could be given, in view of the arterial wall abnormalities seen on imaging, to administering aspirin in all cases postthrombectomy; however, there is currently no evidence for this. Outcome effects of such empiric treatment would likely have to be based on imaging appearances alone, as patients seem largely asymptomatic, unless clinical effects are seen in the future when longer term follow-up is available for thrombectomy patients.

35.2.6 Literature Synopsis

After effects of mechanical thrombectomy on the arterial wall have not been studied well. There is limited histological data from humans postthrombectomy. There is, however, as outlined in earlier sections, some evidence from animal studies that mechanical thrombectomy causes arterial wall damage.

High-resolution MRI can be used to image the wall of intracranial arteries, providing important information regarding underlying abnormality. Wall imaging findings in diseases such as intracranial atherosclerotic plaque and vasculitis are now well reported. Until recently, the effects of embolus on the arterial wall and the after effects of mechanical thrombectomy on the arterial wall on wall imaging were not known. Power et al in 2014 reported the results of a cross-sectional study on consecutive patients with large artery stroke treated with either medical therapy alone or appropriate medical therapy and mechanical thrombectomy with stent retriever. Among the six patients treated with stent-retriever mechanical thrombectomy, wall imaging demonstrated definite arterial wall thickening in five (83%) and possible thickening in one (17%) of the cases, with definite wall enhancement in four (67%) and possible enhancement in two (33%). Among the 10 patients treated with medical therapy alone, wall imaging demonstrated definite arterial wall thickening in three (30%) and possible thickening in two (20%) of the cases, while there was definite wall enhancement in two (20%) and possible enhancement in two (20%). Arterial wall thickening and enhancement were both significantly more common in patients treated with mechanical thrombectomy than with medical therapy alone ($p = 0.037$ and $p = 0.016$, respectively). Therefore, while it appears that thrombus itself may have some inflammatory effect on the wall, it is mild overall. Arterial wall edema may account for the arterial wall thickening. Endothelial denudation may result in increased endothelial permeability to IV gadolinium, accounting for the arterial wall enhancement in thrombectomy patients. A potential alternative mechanism of arterial wall enhancement is leakage of gadolinium from vasa vasorum; however, intracranial arteries normally lack vasa vasorum. Histopathological studies have demonstrated intramural thrombus after stent-retriever use; however, there is no evidence of hyperintensity in the arterial wall on the nonenhanced T1-weighted vessel wall images to suggest presence of intramural blood products.

There are now reports of delayed luminal stenosis on follow-up at the site of mechanical thrombectomy on DSA and MRA. These data are at present limited to small case series and single-case reports. Kurre et al reported that vasospasm following mechanical thrombectomy was seen more frequently in patients who subsequently went onto develop de novo stenosis. It is pos-sible that development of delayed stenosis is related to arterial wall damage at the time of thrombectomy, and later development of intimal hyperplasia. Evidence for development of delayed stenosis is, however, as yet limited, and so far, despite development of stenosis, reports suggest patients are largely asymptomatic.

Suggested Readings

Swartz RH, Bhuta SS, Farb RI, et al. Intracranial arterial wall imaging using high-resolution 3-tesla contrast-enhanced MRI. Neurology. 2009; 72(7):627–634

Skarpathiotakis M, Mandell DM, Swartz RH, Tomlinson G, Mikulis DJ. Intracranial atherosclerotic plaque enhancement in patients with ischemic stroke. AJNR Am J Neuroradiol. 2013; 34(2):299–304

Küker W, Gaertner S, Nagele T, et al. Vessel wall contrast enhancement: a diagnostic sign of cerebral vasculitis. Cerebrovasc Dis. 2008; 26(1):23–29

Mandell DM, Matouk CC, Farb RI, et al. Vessel wall MRI to differentiate between reversible cerebral vasoconstriction syndrome and central nervous system vasculitis: preliminary results. Stroke. 2012; 43(3):860–862

Power S, Matouk C, Casaubon LK, et al. Vessel wall magnetic resonance imaging in acute ischemic stroke: effects of embolism and mechanical thrombectomy on the arterial wall. Stroke. 2014; 45(8):2330–2334

Vergouwen MD, Silver FL, Mandell DM, Mikulis DJ, Swartz RH. Eccentric narrowing and enhancement of symptomatic middle cerebral artery stenoses in patients with recent ischemic stroke. Arch Neurol. 2011; 68(3):338–342

Gory B, Bresson D, Kessler I, et al. Histopathologic evaluation of arterial wall response to 5 neurovascular mechanical thrombectomy devices in a swine model. AJNR Am J Neuroradiol. 2013; 34(11):2192–2198

Nogueira RG, Levy EI, Gounis M, Siddiqui AH. The Trevo device: preclinical data of a novel stroke thrombectomy device in two different animal models of arterial thrombo-occlusive disease. J Neurointerv Surg. 2012; 4(4):295–300

Yin NS, Benavides S, Starkman S, et al. Autopsy findings after intracranial thrombectomy for acute ischemic stroke: a clinicopathologic study of 5 patients. Stroke. 2010; 41(5):938–947

Kurre W, Pérez MA, Horvath D, Schmid E, Bäzner H, Henkes H. Does mechanical thrombectomy in acute embolic stroke have long-term side effects on intracranial vessels? An angiographic follow-up study. Cardiovasc Intervent Radiol. 2013; 36(3):629–636

Eugène F, Gauvrit JY, Ferré JC, et al. One-year MR angiographic and clinical follow-up after intracranial mechanical thrombectomy using a stent retriever device. AJNR Am J Neuroradiol. 2015; 36(1):126–132

Akpınar S, Yılmaz G. Early middle cerebral artery stenosis following stent-assisted thrombectomy. Interv Neuroradiol. 2015; 21(3):337–340

36 Management of Vessel Perforation during Stroke Intervention

36.1 Case Description:

36.1.1 Clinical Presentation

A 55-year-old male presented to the emergency department (ED) at 3 p.m. with onset of left-sided hemiparesis and mild left sensory loss which began at 10 a.m. He was awake, although moderately drowsy, and able to follow basic commands. The patient's National Institutes of Health Stroke Scale (NIHSS) score was 16.

Past medical history is significant for coronary artery disease, hypertension, hyperlipidemia, and sleep apnea. He has known intracranial atherosclerosis with a prior MRI demonstrating mild right M1 stenosis.

36.1.2 Imaging Workup and Investigations

- Noncontrast CT (NCCT) of the head demonstrated mild hyperdensity in the right middle cerebral artery (MCA). His ASPECTS score was 10.
- CTA demonstrated an occlusive clot in the right M1 (▶ Fig. 36.1).

36.1.3 Diagnosis

Acute ischemic stroke secondary to right MCA M1 occlusion, possibly secondary to intracranial atherosclerosis.

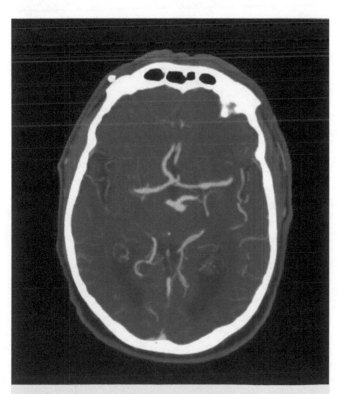

Fig. 36.1 CTA MIP image demonstrates occlusion of the right M1.

36.1.4 Treatment

Initial Management

- Patient is not a tissue plasminogen activator (tPA) candidate due to time of onset.
- The patient was immediately transferred to the angio suite for endovascular intervention. Anesthesia was administered using conscious sedation.

Endovascular Treatment

Material

- Micropuncture set.
- 8-Fr sheath.
- 5-Fr Simmons 2 catheter.
- 8-Fr balloon guide catheter (BGC).
- Avigo guidewire (0.014 in).
- Rebar 18 (0.021 microcatheter).
- Solitaire 4 × 20 device.

Technique

- Micropuncture was set to access the right common femoral artery and a 5-Fr sheath was placed in it.
- 5-Fr Simmons 2 catheter was then placed in the right common carotid artery where digital subtraction angiography (DSA) was performed. The Simmons catheter was used due to the patient's tortuous aortic arch.
- Angiography demonstrated a patent right internal carotid artery (ICA) and occlusion of the proximal right M1 (▶ Fig. 36.2).
- Using exchange technique, the Simmons catheter was exchanged for an 8-Fr BGC. The catheter tip was placed in the distal cervical ICA.
- The Rebar 18 microcatheter was advanced over an Avigo guidewire to the location of the occlusion in the M1. Multiple attempts were made to cross the lesion but were unsuccessful. A microcatheter injection demonstrated extravasation of contrast into the subarachnoid space and into the sylvian fissure. The findings were consistent with a vessel perforation (▶ Fig. 36.3).
- Anticoagulation was reversed with 25 mg of protamine. Following this, the BGC was inflated for approximately 1 minute. Repeat angiography demonstrated no more extravasation of contrast (▶ Fig. 36.4). The procedure was ended at this time due to risk of further perforation.

Outcomes

- Iodine subtracted dual energy CT demonstrated a small amount of subarachnoid hemorrhage (▶ Fig. 36.5); no acute infarct was present immediately after the procedure.
- At 24 hours, the patient's NIHSS score was 2. The improvement in NIHSS was likely due to spontaneous recanalization of the M1 occlusion. The patient had no

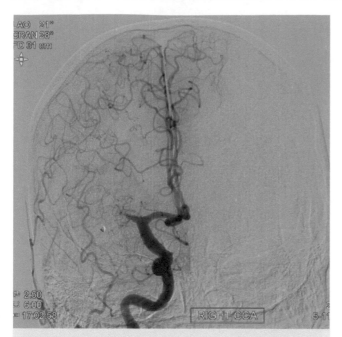

Fig. 36.2 Right ICA cerebral angiography demonstrates occlusion of the right M1 with a large amount of collaterals coming from the right ACA.

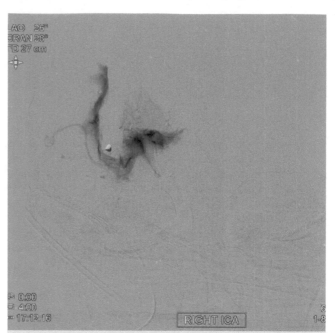

Fig. 36.3 Right M1 cerebral angiography demonstrates active extravasation of contrast into the subarachnoid space. The contrast lines the sylvian fissure.

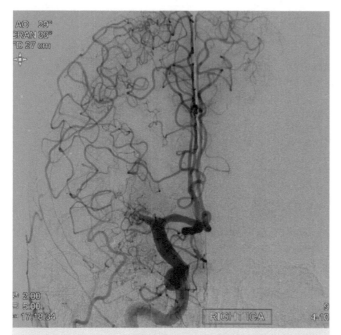

Fig. 36.4 Right ICA cerebral angiography following reversal of anticoagulation and inflation of the balloon guide catheter demonstrates no evidence of residual contrast extravasation. In addition, there are substantial collaterals arising from the right ACA filling the right MCA territory.

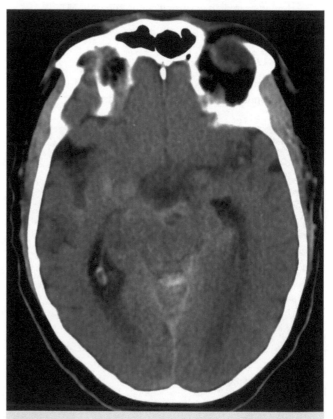

Fig. 36.5 Iodine subtracted noncontrast of the head demonstrates a small to moderate amount of subarachnoid blood secondary to the vessel perforation.

evidence of infarct on follow-up imaging. This is likely secondary to the fact that the patient had robust collaterals due to a long-standing M1 stenotic lesion.

36.2 Companion Case

36.2.1 Clinical Presentation

A 59-year-old woman from home presented with right temporal headache and collapse. Her husband noted a left hemiparesis. She was transferred to the ED by ambulance, arriving 3 hours following symptom onset.

Her past history included Meniere's disease and migraine. Examination at presentation revealed a left gaze palsy, left hemianopia, left facial weakness, and a dense left hemiparesis. Dysarthria and neglect were also present. New atrial fibrillation was noted. Initial NIHSS score was 14.

36.2.2 Imaging Workup and Investigations

- NCCT, performed at 3 hours 50 minutes, demonstrated a subtle low density in the right lentiform nucleus, with an ASPECTS score of 9 (▶ Fig. 36.6a).
- CTA showed a right M1 occlusion with reduced arborization of the right MCA cortical vessels and left M3 occlusion (▶ Fig. 36.6b).
- Perfusion imaging revealed a large region of increased mean transit time (MTT) and decreased cerebral blood flow involving the right lentiform nucleus, insular cortex, and right posterior frontoparietal region. Cerebral blood volume suggested a small area of core infarct in the right lentiform nucleus (▶ Fig. 36.6c, d).

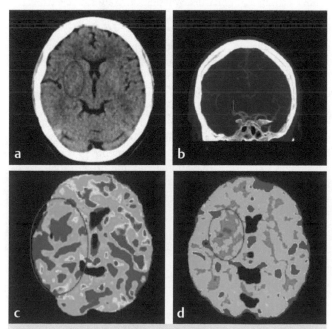

Fig. 36.6 (a) NCCT at the level of the basal ganglia and (b, top right) coronal CT angiography maximum intensity projection demonstrating corresponding occlusion. Same-session CTP shows (c) MTT at the level of the basal ganglia and (d) CBV at similar level.

36.2.3 Diagnosis

Right M1 occlusion in the setting of new atrial fibrillation.

36.2.4 Treatment

Initial Management

- Alteplase was administered 4 hours 50 minutes following symptom onset.

Endovascular Management

- The patient was randomized to the intravenous:intra-arterial arm of the EXTEND-IA trial.
- A Neuron Max catheter was placed in the right ICA and target vessel occlusion in the right MCA was confirmed. Prowler select plus catheter was placed over the Fathom microwire into the right MCA.
- Initial microcatheter injection demonstrated an intravascular location. Repeat screening demonstrated layering of contrast in the right sylvian fissure, likely from the right MCA (▶ Fig. 36.7).
- This was presumed to be from the microwire or microcatheter perforation. No active bleeding was detected. The thrombus had migrated down the dominant inferior division.
- Right ICA DSA demonstrated recanalization of the target M1 occlusion, with reperfusion of the superior division territory and persistent occlusion inferiorly.
- Overall, TICI 2a reperfusion was demonstrated.

36.2.5 Progress

- Repeat NIHSS score on the table following angiography was 4.
- Postprocedure dual-energy CT, with water and iodine maps, demonstrated a small amount of subarachnoid blood and a large amount of contrast due to vessel perforation (▶ Fig. 36.8a, b).
- Repeat CT perfusion demonstrated a reduced volume of ischemia on MTT and time to peak maps compared with initial imaging.
- NCCT 5 hours following showed a large right sylvian fissure hematoma and subarachnoid blood from persistent hemorrhage (▶ Fig. 36.8c).
- MRI confirmed the hematoma, measuring 5.8 × 5.2 × 5 cm and causing subfalcine herniation and sulcal effacement (▶ Fig. 36.8d).

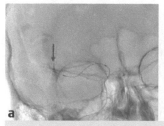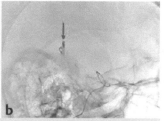

Fig. 36.7 (a) Initial injections showed intravascular position of the microcatheter; however, repeat injection demonstrated (b) layering of contrast in the right sylvian fissure.

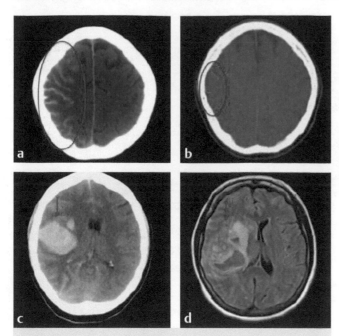

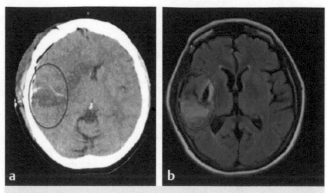

Fig. 36.9 Postevacuation (a) NCCT and (b) FLAIR MRI.

Fig. 36.8 Dual-energy CT (a) iodine map demonstrating extravasated contrast, less conspicuous on (b) water map. Five hours postprocedure (c) showed a rapidly expanding hematoma later characterized on (d) FLAIR MRI.

- Concurrent clinical deterioration was noted, with dense left hemiparesis and decreased conscious state.

36.2.6 Further Treatment

- The patient underwent right pterional craniotomy and evacuation of sylvian fissure hematoma without complication (▶ Fig. 36.9).

36.2.7 Progress

- Following surgery, there was a slow, steady neurological recovery.
- On discharge, her NIHSS score was 9.
- With extensive rehabilitation, mild residual hemiparesis was present, with NIHSS score 5.

36.2.8 Case Discussion

Vessel perforation during mechanical thrombectomy for acute ischemic stroke is a rare but potentially devastating complication.[1] Overall, the rate of vessel perforation is thought to be between 1 and 3%, with similar rates when comparing thrombectomy with aspiration or stent retriever, and up to 10% with older devices such as the MERCI device.[2,3,4] The primary clinical risk factors contributing to vessel perforation include catheterization of small vessels (i.e., distal MCA branches) and atheromatous disease.

Vessel perforations during stroke intervention are generally secondary to perforation by the microguidewire or stent-retriever device. Perforations as a result of stent-retriever devices can occur either during deployment of the device or during device withdrawal. The distal end of many stent-retriever devices has many tines. If the device is pushed out during delivery rather than unsheathed, these tines can potentially engage the vessel wall, resulting in perforation. Unsheathing of the stent retriever is the preferred technique of device deployment, as it is a smoother process and minimizes the risk of vessel perforation. Vessel perforation during device withdrawal can occur secondary to tearing of an atheromatous plaque or injury to a small branch artery such as a lenticulostriate.[5] Vessel perforation with microguidewires can generally be avoided through the use of roadmap guidance. This is especially important when the microguidewire is crossing the thrombus.

In general, vessel perforation during stroke intervention is a devastating complication resulting in significant morbidity and mortality. One review of outcomes of vessel perforation during neuroendovascular procedures found a mortality rate of 72%.[6] The first clinical clue to vessel perforation is sometimes an acute rise in blood pressure immediately following recanalization. Follow-up angiographic runs will demonstrate active extravasation of contrast into the subarachnoid space.

There are several different management options for vessel perforation during a stroke intervention. The conservative approach involves reversal of anticoagulation with protamine sulfate followed by rapid reduction of blood pressure.[5] One can attempt to temporarily inflate a balloon proximal to the perforation in the hope that the perforation will spontaneously thrombose due to stasis. More aggressive strategies include vessel sacrifice with coils, liquid embolic agents, detachable balloons, or stent/flow diverter placement.[6,7] The obvious advantages to conservative approaches and/or stent placement is the fact that flow through the parent vessel can be preserved.[6] However, in many cases, especially in cases of M2 or M3 branch perforations, sacrifice of the vessel may result in the lowest degree of morbidity.

Pearls and Pitfalls

- Vessel perforations can be avoided in most cases by using careful technique.
- Conservative treatment of vessel perforation includes reversal of anticoagulation and reduction in blood pressure.
- Potential treatments for vessel perforation include vessel sacrifice, balloon inflation, and stenting.

References

[1] Carneiro AA, Rodrigues JT, Pereira JP, Alves JV, Xavier JA. Mechanical thrombectomy in patients with acute basilar occlusion using stent retrievers. Interv Neuroradiol. 2015; 21(6):710–714

[2] Penumbra Pivotal Stroke Trial Investigators. The penumbra pivotal stroke trial: safety and effectiveness of a new generation of mechanical devices for clot removal in intracranial large vessel occlusive disease. Stroke. 2009; 40 (8):2761–2768

[3] Jovin TG, Chamorro A, Cobo E, et al. REVASCAT Trial Investigators. Thrombectomy within 8 hours after symptom onset in ischemic stroke. N Engl J Med. 2015; 372(24):2296–2306

[4] Nogueira RG, Lutsep HL, Gupta R, et al. TREVO 2 Trialists. Trevo versus MERCI retrievers for thrombectomy revascularisation of large vessel occlusions in acute ischaemic stroke (TREVO 2): a randomised trial. Lancet. 2012; 380 (9849):1231–1240

[5] Leishangthem L, Satti SR. Vessel perforation during withdrawal of Trevo ProVue stent retriever during mechanical thrombectomy for acute ischemic stroke. J Neurosurg. 2014; 121(4):995–998

[6] Gulati D, et al. Abstract T P18: incidence and management of intracranial wire perforation during acute stroke endovascular therapy. Stroke. 2015; 46: ATP18–ATP18

[7] Velioglu M, Ozturk E, Sonmez G, Kendirli T, Mutlu H, Basekim C. Flow diverter as a rescue therapy for a complicated basilar angioplasty. Diagn Interv Radiol. 2013; 19(4):345–348

37 Arterial Access Complications

37.1 Case Description

37.1.1 Clinical Presentation

Traditionally, the common femoral artery (CFA) has been used for arterial access in interventional neuroradiology, both for diagnostic and therapeutic procedures. However, particularly for acute stroke treatment (AIS) treatment, where patients are elderly, vasculopaths, or both, femoral artery access may present challenges. Aortic arch anatomy may influence the approach strategy, since a femoral approach may be not favorable and other routes of access such as the radial or brachial artery may be required. Regardless of the site of access, complications can occur related to the puncture as well as the methods used to obtain hemostasis following completion of the procedure. Hemorrhagic complications are the most common, and in cardiac catheterization patients, the risk has been shown to be increased with the administration of antithrombotic agents, clopidogrel, and postprocedural heparin. It stands to reason that hemorrhagic complications are also likely to be more common in patients receiving tissue plasminogen activator (tPA) in combination with intra-arterial therapy. Other complications include arterial dissection, and thrombotic and embolic complications. These complications can be a source of significant morbidity and mortality despite successful neurointerventional therapy; therefore, it is imperative that the interventionalist is capable of recognizing and managing these complications should they occur.

The following cases present a range of complications that can occur at the arterial puncture site.

37.1.2 Mini-Case A: Active Extravasation Round the Vascular Sheath

The CFA was punctured and a 6-Fr sheath was inserted. Active bleeding was noted around the sheath, so the sheath was upsized to 8 Fr. The amount of bleeding slowed but did not abate. The patient received a therapeutic dose of tPA which was thought to contribute to the bleeding. At the conclusion of the procedure, an 8-Fr Angio-Seal was inserted. This resulted in complete hemostasis.

Contrast was seen surrounding the sheath adjacent to the entry point into the CFA (▶ Fig. 37.1), demonstrating active extravasation.

37.1.3 Mini-Case B: Femoral Artery Pseudoaneurysm

Arterial access was obtained with a right femoral artery puncture and insertion of a 6-Fr sheath. Following the procedure, hemostasis was achieved with manual compression. Later that day, the patient was noticed to have a palpable lump in the right groin in the region of the puncture. Arterial vascular ultrasound (US) was performed and demonstrated a large pseudoaneurysm. Initial attempts were made to treat this with US-guided compression; however, this was not successful due to the large size of the pseudoaneurysm. US-guided thrombin injection procedure was performed with resultant thrombosis of the pseudoaneurysm.

Duplex US demonstrated an arterialized jet (▶ Fig. 37.2) projecting away from the CFA. Immediately superior to the visualized jet, a bilobed pseudoaneurysm was identified with the classic yin-yang appearance.

37.1.4 Mini-Case C: Hematomas in Anticoagulated Patients

Patient 1

A patient underwent bilateral CFA punctures with insertion of bilateral 6-Fr sheaths earlier in the day. The patient was entirely anticoagulated with a heparin infusion and was taking clopidogrel and aspirin. He felt unwell in the evening after the procedure and was found to experience a sudden drop in blood pressure. Hemoglobin had dropped from 100 g/L pre procedure to 70 g/L. CTA demonstrated bilateral hematomas at the puncture sites (▶ Fig. 37.3) as well as a retroperitoneal hematoma involving the right iliopsoas muscle (▶ Fig. 37.3b).

The heparin infusion was discontinued and the patient was managed with supportive measures including fluid resuscitation as well as blood transfusion. The patient had a prolonged admission because of the hematomas; however, he ultimately made a full recovery.

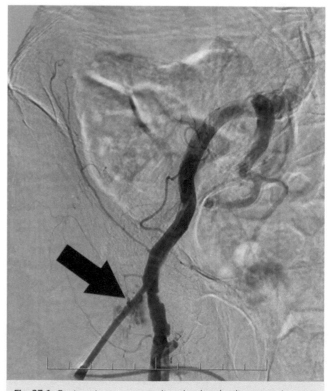

Fig. 37.1 Contrast is seen surrounding the sheath adjacent to the entry point into the CFA (*arrow*) demonstrating active extravasation.

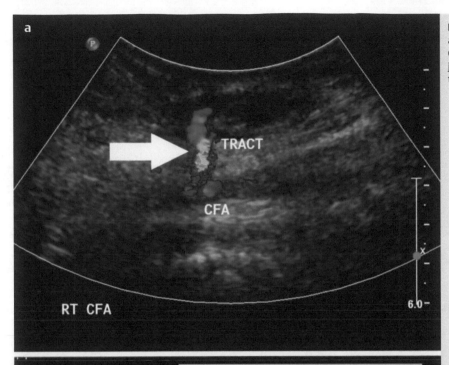

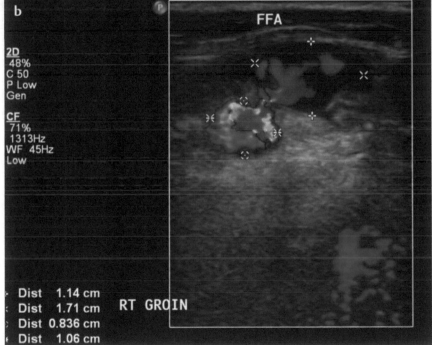

Fig. 37.2 (a) Duplex ultrasound demonstrates an arterialized jet (*arrow*) projecting away from the CFA. (b) Immediately superior to the visualized jet, a bilobed pseudoaneurysm is identified with the classic yin-yang appearance.

Patient 2

A patient underwent a brachial artery puncture followed by insertion of a 6-Fr sheath. The patient was on aspirin and clopidogrel and was administered systemic heparinization during the procedure. At the conclusion of the procedure, manual compression was applied for a total of 45 minutes at which time hemostasis was achieved. Two hours after hemostasis was achieved, the patient's arm was noticed to be swollen and a firm hematoma was palpable. Neurovascular examination revealed brachial and radial pulses. The hand was warm with good capillary return. There was no increased pain on extension of the wrist to suggest compartment syndrome. US confirmed the presence of a large hematoma and excluded a pseudoaneurysm. The patient was managed conservatively with prolonged half-hourly neurovascular vitals to ensure any signs of compartment syndrome were recognized early.

Color Doppler US of the brachial artery demonstrated no pseudoaneurysm of arterialized tract extending from the artery (▶ Fig. 37.3). Color Doppler of the hematoma demonstrated no vascularity.

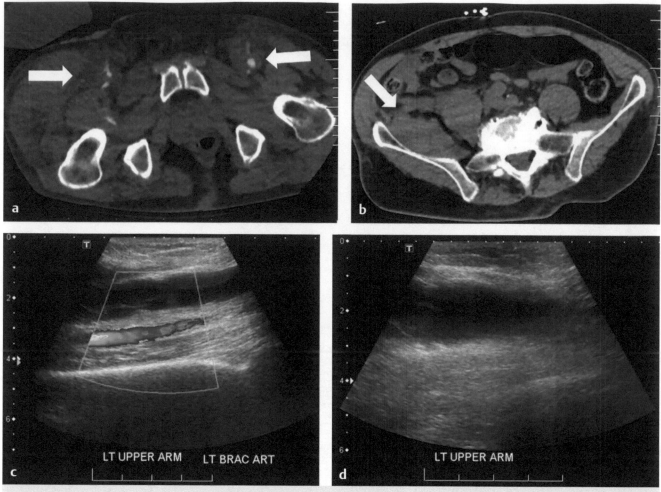

Fig. 37.3 (a) CTA demonstrates bilateral hematomas at the puncture sites (*arrows*) as well as (b) a retroperitoneal hematoma involving the right iliopsoas muscle (*arrow*). (c) Color Doppler ultrasound of the brachial artery demonstrates no pseudoaneurysm or arterialized tract extending from the artery. (d) Color Doppler of the hematoma demonstrates no vascularity.

37.1.5 Mini-Case D: Distal Embolic Occlusion

A patient underwent a right CFA puncture and insertion of a 6-Fr sheath. At the conclusion of the procedure, the patient complained of severe pain over the lower lateral aspect of the right leg. CTA run off was performed on the lower limbs and this demonstrated a distal segmental occlusion of the anterior tibial artery. The patient had a good posterior tibial artery and peroneal artery and was taking aspirin and clopidogrel. Given that the patient was on dual-antiplatelet therapy, no additional anticoagulation was given. One week later, the patient presented with increasing pain and repeat CTA confirmed persistent occlusion of the anterior tibial artery. Given change in clinical symptoms, anticoagulation with Coumadin was given for 2 weeks. The aspirin was withheld during this period.

Reconstructed coronal CTA image of the legs demonstrated an abrupt cutoff of the mid anterior tibial artery (▶ Fig. 37.4), with no gross evidence of peripheral vascular evidence.

37.1.6 Mini-Case E: Vessel Dissection

Puncture of the right CFA was performed; initially, the wire advanced normally, but then resistance was encountered. As a sufficient length of wire had been advanced to safely insert the vascular access sheath, the sheath was inserted and angiography performed. Angiography demonstrated a dissection at the level of a loop of the wire within the common iliac artery. As this was an uphill dissection and not flow limiting, it was expected that the antegrade blood flow would compress the dissection flap and no active management would be required. The contralateral CFA was punctured and once access was obtained, the right vascular access sheath was removed and the groin puncture sealed with an 8-Fr Angio-Seal device. The procedure was continued through the left CFA and the patient suffered no further clinical consequences from the dissection.

After the CFA was accessed, contrast was injected, demonstrating abrupt smooth occlusion of the CIA consistent with arterial dissection. Antegrade angiography performed demonstrated a non–flow-limiting dissection flap of the CFA (▶ Fig. 37.5).

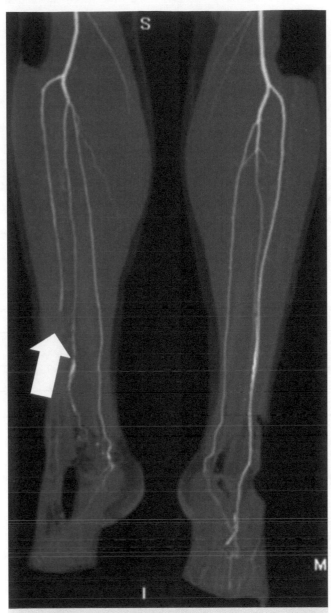

Fig. 37.4 Reconstructed coronal CTA image of the legs demonstrates an abrupt cutoff of the midanterior tibial artery (*arrow*) with no gross evidence of peripheral vascular disease.

37.1.7 Mini-Case F: Delayed Thrombus Formation on the Angio-Seal Foot Plate

Hemostasis of the CFA was achieved with a 6-Fr Angio-Seal (St. Jude Medical, St. Paul, MN), following removal of a 6-Fr sheath, and there were no noted immediate complications. One week later, the patient presented complaint of linear firmness in the region of the puncture site. US demonstrated nonocclusive thrombus that had formed on the Angio-Seal footplate. The patient was referred for a vascular surgery opinion. As the thrombus was nonocclusive, the patient was given the option of anticoagulation and observation or surgical excision of the Angio-Seal with embolectomy. The patient opted for surgical intervention.

The string of the Angio-Seal device within CFA (▶ Fig. 37.6). Within the CFA, the hemostatic plug was identified with surrounding thrombus.

37.1.8 Mini-Case G: Acute Loss of Pulse

Arterial access was obtained via the CFA for the purpose of neurointervention. The access was difficult due to a heavily calcified femoral artery that was noted based on tactile sensation. After completion of the intervention, a 6-Fr Angio-Seal was used to obtain hemostasis. The patient immediately complained of thigh and leg pain with loss of a palpable femoral pulse. Acute thrombosis related to the Angio-Seal at the puncture site was suspected. The patient was taken to the operating room emergently. Femoral cutdown revealed that the footplate and plug were both within the artery, with the string sticking out of the arterial puncture site.

Intraoperative cutdown demonstrated the Angio-Seal string extending through the arterial puncture site (▶ Fig. 37.6), with no hemostatic plug visible on the artery surface.

37.1.9 Pearls and Pitfalls

- Preprocedure identification of distal arterial pulses is very important for postoperative monitoring and assessment.
- Any suspicion of femoral arterial complication during the procedure should be evaluated with a femoral angiographic run for the purposes of identification, management, and documentation.
- Extravasations around the sheath can be stopped by changing it for a larger sheath.
- Pseudoaneurysms can be conservatively managed with US-guided compression in most of the cases. Occasionally, interventional measures may be required. US-guided percutaneous thrombin injection, endovascular embolization of the arterial tear or, in rare cases, a covered stent can be used as alternative techniques.
- Percutaneous closure devices are well tolerated in the context of AIS treatment and are highly recommended in patients who have received recombinant tPA, who will require immediate anticoagulation, anti-aggregation therapy, or 2B/3A inhibitors to counter the increased risk of hemorrhagic complications. Experience and/or training minimizes technical complications.
- Distal occlusion/thrombosis should be monitored by assessing distal pulses. The features of acute limb ischemia are the six Ps: painful, pulseless, pale, perishing cold, paresthesia, and paralysis.
- If small emboli to distal well-perfused territories occur, then typically only supportive measures such as analgesia are required. Patients with loss of motor function and sensation require emergent treatment with open or endovascular approaches.
- If vessel dissection is uphill, following CFA puncture, removing the sheath and allowing antegrade blood flow to compress the dissection flap is typically considered sufficient management.
- Iatrogenic femoral arteriovenous fistulas (AVFs) have been reported to occur in approximately 1% of cardiac

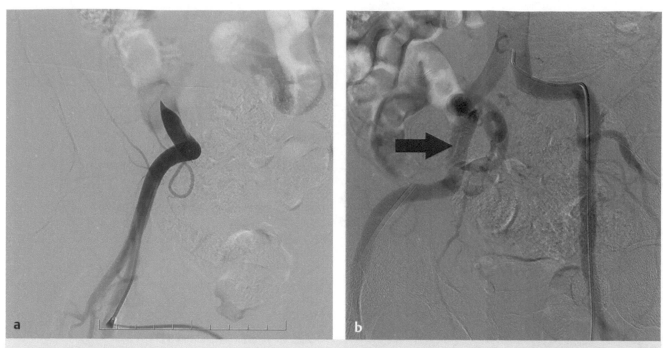

Fig. 37.5 (a) After access of the CFA, contrast was injected, demonstrating abrupt smooth occlusion of the CIA, consistent with arterial dissection. (b) Antegrade angiogram performed demonstrates a nonflow limiting dissection flap of the CFA (*arrow*).

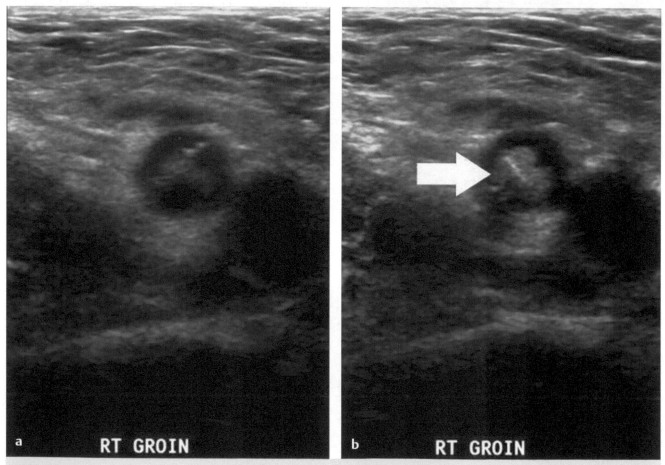

Fig. 37.6 (a) String of Angio-Seal device seen within CFA (*arrow*). (b) Within the CFA, the hemostatic plug is identified with surrounding thrombus (*arrow*).

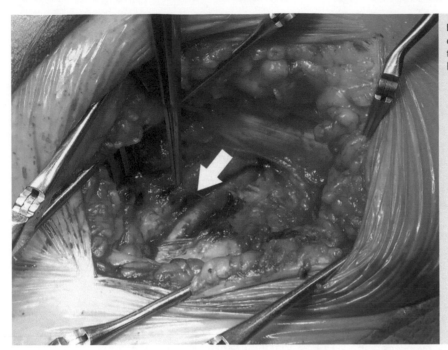

Fig. 37.7 Image of intraoperative cutdown demonstrating Angio-Seal string and extending through the arterial puncture site (*arrow*) with no hemostatic plug visible on the artery surface.

catheterization patients, of which one third will occlude spontaneously in one year. Treatment of AVF should begin with US-guided compression, as this is least invasive and then progress should be made toward placement of covered stents or surgical repair as required.

• US-guided puncture of the CFA allows for identification of atheromatous plaques. Avoiding these with arterial puncture avoids complications with use of closure devices.

38 Intraprocedural Vasospasm during Thrombectomy

38.1 Case Description

38.1.1 Clinical Presentation

A 45-year-old African American female with past medical history of hypertension and diabetes mellitus type II was brought to the hospital after her husband found her shaking in bed with right lower facial droop and left-sided weakness.

At presentation, the patient's Glasgow Coma Scale (GCS) was 6, withdrawing bilaterally to pain, less on the right side, and not opening eyes to voice stimulus. The National Institutes of Health Stroke Scale (NIHSS) score could not be accurately assessed due to intubation. She was intubated in the emergency department. Alteplase was not given due to unknown time of onset.

38.1.2 Imaging Workup and Investigations

- Noncontrast CT (NCCT) demonstrated subtle hypodensity in the right frontotemporal region with poor gray-white differentiation (▶ Fig. 38.1a).
- CT angiography showed right M2 artery occlusion and left M1 artery occlusion (▶ Fig. 38.1b).
- Perfusion imaging showed a mismatch volume of 33 mL and a ratio of 5.7, bilateral penumbra with core on the right only.

38.1.3 Diagnosis

Left M1 artery occlusion and right M2 artery occlusion.

38.1.4 Treatment

Initial Management

- Alteplase was not given due to unknown time of onset of symptoms.

Endovascular Management

- The right groin was prepped and draped in the usual sterile manner. An 8-Fr sheath was placed in the right femoral artery.
- A JB 1 catheter was advanced over a 0.035 Glidewire and selective catheterization of the following vessels was obtained: bilateral common carotid arteries and bilateral internal carotid arteries (ICA).
- Initial diagnostic angiogram showed a complete occlusion of the right M2 (▶ Fig. 38.2).
- A Neuron Max catheter was placed into the distal cervical segment of the right ICA.
- A microcatheter was advanced over a 0.014-in microwire.
- Jet 7 aspiration catheter was advanced over the microcatheter and placed at the M1 segment proximal to the occlusion and proceeded to aspirate using the aspiration pump.
- TICI 3 was achieved in the right M2 (▶ Fig. 38.3).
- Same procedure was performed on the left M1 occlusion along with a Trevo stent retriever deployment.
- This was followed by vasospasm of the left M1 and distal clot migration (▶ Fig. 38.4, ▶ Fig. 38.5).
- After a total of seven stent passes combined with aspiration, the vasospasm was resolved, and the clot was retrieved (▶ Fig. 38.6).
- Overall, TICI 2a reperfusion was achieve on left M1.

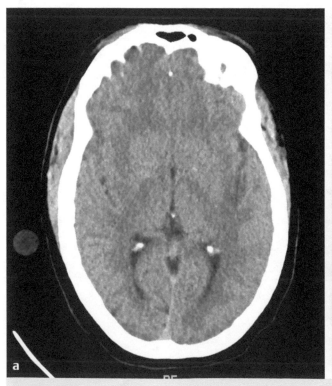
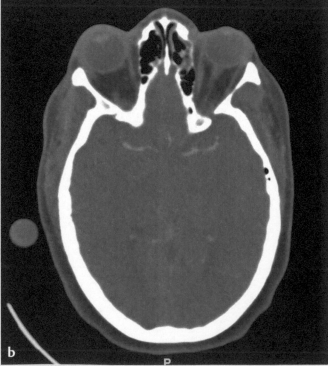

Fig. 38.1 Noncontrast CT showed no gross ischemic stroke (a), while CT angiography showed signs of bilateral MCA occlusion (b).

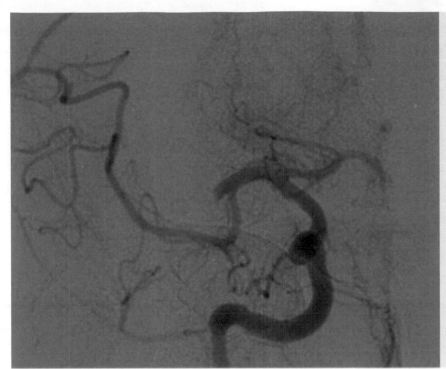

Fig. 38.2 Prethrombectomy digital subtracted angiography confirmed the presence of complete right M2 occlusion.

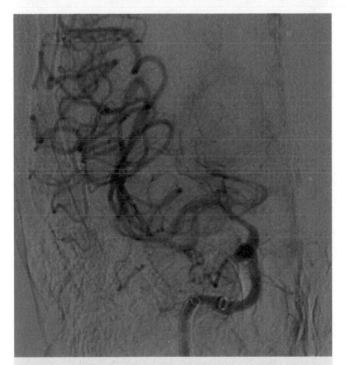

Fig. 38.3 Postthrombectomy digital subtracted angiography showed complete reperfusion of the previously occluded right M2.

38.1.5 Progress

• Postprocedure, the patient continued to have poor neurological condition with right-sided hemiplegia and a GCS score of 6.
• NCCT at 24 hours showed evolved left MCA and right basal ganglia stroke.
• The patient was started on aspirin 81 mg.

• The family elected not to proceed with further treatment and the patient was placed on comfort measures.

38.2 Discussion

The future potential and role of mechanical thrombectomy in the treatment of acute ischemic stroke (AIS) may be jeopardized by a lack of profound knowledge regarding the inherent risks of the procedure.[1] Vasospasm of the target vessel or the access vessel (e.g., ICA or vertebral artery) is one such complication, which if detected in time can be resolved without any clinical sequelae.[2] Vasospasm usually results from "irritation" of the vessels by catheter manipulation during a neurointervention procedure.[3] Specifically, during a mechanical thrombectomy, application of negative pressure (suction) to the catheter tip, or the shear stress from the stentriever, can result in vasospasm of the target cerebral vessel.[4] Vasospasm and the ensuing compromised blood flow through the target vessel can adversely influence the course of the AIS by hampering reperfusion of the "at-risk tissue."

38.2.1 Incidence and Clinical Sequelae

Theoretically, vasospasm after mechanical thrombectomy may represent a potential etiology for poor recanalization, particularly if it is severe enough to cause complete occlusion.[1,4] A review of literature revealed that vasospasm was a common intraprocedural event but was usually without any adverse neurological outcome. In one of the earlier reports on vasospasm in mechanical thrombectomy, Gupta described two patients who developed arterial vasospasm at the site of deployment of the L5 MERCI retrieval device.[4] The vasospasm was significant in nature and occlusive to one division of the MCA. Both patients were treated with infusion of calcium channel antagonists with resolution of the narrowing.[4] In a

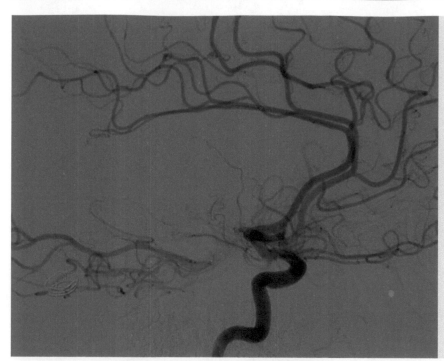

Fig. 38.4 Prethrombectomy digital subtracted angiography confirmed the presence of complete left M1 occlusion.

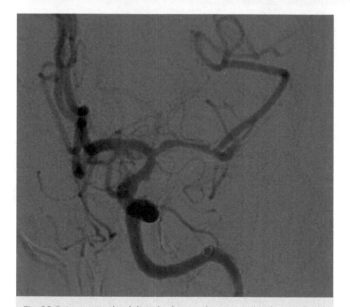

Fig. 38.5 Intraprocedural digital subtracted angiography shows left M1 vasospasm.

complications for 30 patients of either primary or, following mechanical thrombectomy, secondary occlusion of the anterior cerebral artery (ACA).[7] In this specific cohort of distal cerebral vessel occlusion, they reported on three cases [3/30 (10%)] of vasospasms in the distal ACA following a retrieval maneuver in the superior A3 segment ($n = 2$) and the callosomarginal artery ($n = 1$). Arterial vasospasm resolved completely after intra-arterial administration of nimodipine into the affected segment via a microcatheter in two cases. The third case of vasospasm was self-limiting without any intervention and resolved within 5 minutes. Dorn et al, in their single-center experience with 108 recanalization procedures, reported vasospasm in 14 of 108 (13%) of the target vessels.[8] In their study as well, vasospasm did not have any negative clinical influence.

38.2.2 Intraprocedural Management

For catheter or guidewire-induced vasospasm, the device should be immediately retracted to minimize irritation of the vessel wall and control imaging performed to ensure flow is not occluded.[3] In most cases, vasospasm will diminish within minutes without further treatment. If vasospasm persists, blood pressure (BP) may be increased and intra-arterial nimodipine can be injected slowly—typically 0.5 to 1 mg—over several minutes (NB: Nimodipine is not licensed for this use). While calcium channel blockers are effective, their propensity for lowering BP necessitates close monitoring of mechanical thrombectomy stroke patients. Prophylaxis against vasospasm in neurointerventional procedures may be affected by the use of glyceryl trinitrate patch or addition of nimodipine to catheter flush bags. However, in AIS, neither maneuver can be recommended due to the risks posed by hypotension in large vessel occlusion stroke patients. The use of pharmacological agents to treat suspected vasospasm should be considered during endovascular revascularization procedures for AIS, but care must be taken in monitoring decreases in BP.[4]

retrospective analysis of 176 consecutive AIS cases that were treated with mechanical thrombectomy, Behme et al, noted vasospasm of the access vessel in five (3%) cases.[1] The vasospasm in all five cases could be treated successfully with intra-arterial nimodipine, and the authors could proceed with mechanical thrombectomy without any clinically sequelae. Arterial vasospasm was the most common procedural complication in THRACE trial, reported in 33 of 200 patients (23%).[5] Akins et al in their review of the SWIFT database for procedural complications noted that angiographic vasospasm was a common finding and was observed in 29 of 144 patients (20%), but none had any resulting adverse effects or clinical deterioration.[6] Pfaff et al studied the clinical outcomes and procedural

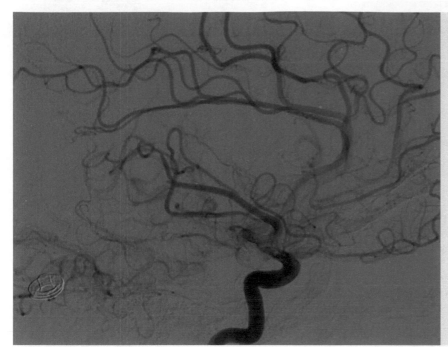

Fig. 38.6 Postthrombectomy digital subtracted angiography showed resolution of the left M1 vasospasm and partial reperfusion of the previously occluded left M1.

References

[1] Behme D, Gondecki L, Fiethen S, Kowoll A, Mpotsaris A, Weber W. Complications of mechanical thrombectomy for acute ischemic stroke a retrospective single-center study of 176 consecutive cases. Neuroradiology. 2014; 56(6):467–476

[2] Emprechtinger R, Piso B, Ringleb PA. Thrombectomy for ischemic stroke: meta-analyses of recurrent strokes, vasospasms, and subarachnoid hemorrhages. J Neurol. 2017; 264(3):432–436

[3] Balami JS, White PM, McMeekin PJ, Ford GA, Buchan AM. Complications of endovascular treatment for acute ischemic stroke: Prevention and management. Int J Stroke. 2018; 13(4):348–361

[4] Gupta R. Arterial vasospasm during mechanical thrombectomy for acute stroke. J Neuroimaging. 2009; 19(1):61–64

[5] Bracard S, Ducrocq X, Mas JL, et al. THRACE investigators. Mechanical thrombectomy after intravenous alteplase versus alteplase alone after stroke (THRACE): a randomised controlled trial. Lancet Neurol. 2016; 15(11):1138–1147

[6] Akins PT, Amar AP, Pakbaz RS, Fields JD, SWIFT Investigators. Complications of endovascular treatment for acute stroke in the SWIFT trial with solitaire and MERCI devices. AJNR Am J Neuroradiol. 2014; 35(3):524–528

[7] Pfaff J, Herweh C, Pham M, et al. mechanical thrombectomy of distal occlusions in the anterior cerebral artery: recanalization rates, periprocedural complications, and clinical outcome. AJNR Am J Neuroradiol. 2016; 37(4):673–678

[8] Dorn F, Stehle S, Lockau H, Zimmer C, Liebig T. Endovascular treatment of acute intracerebral artery occlusions with the solitaire stent: single-centre experience with 108 recanalization procedures. Cerebrovasc Dis. 2012; 34 (1):70–77

39 Hemorrhagic Transformation after Endovascular Stroke Therapy

39.1 Case Description

39.1.1 Clinical Presentation

A 79-year-old male presented with acute onset of language disturbance and right hemiparesis 75 minutes post–stroke onset. His past medical history revealed hypertension and hyperlipidemia, with a baseline modified Rankin scale (mRS) score of 1. Examination in the emergency department confirmed complete left middle cerebral artery (MCA) syndrome with a National Institutes of Health Stroke Scale (NIHSS) score of 23. Emergent noncontrast CT (NCCT) at 90 minutes post–stroke onset revealed hyperattenuating left M1 MCA and ASPECTS score of 8. Following bolus intravenous thrombolysis at 94 minutes post onset of symptoms, endovascular treatment is contemplated.

39.1.2 Imaging Workup and Investigations

- NCCT at 90 minutes post–stroke onset reveals hyperattenuating left M1 MCA (▶ Fig. 39.1a) and ASPECTS score of 8.
- CTA of the head confirms proximal left M1 MCA occlusion with good collaterals (▶ Fig. 39.1b).
- CTA of the neck reveals focal noncalcified thrombus at the left internal carotid artery (ICA) origin (Fig▶ Fig. 39.1c).

39.1.3 Diagnosis

- Acute proximal left MCA occlusion, presumed large artery-to-artery embolism from thrombus at the left ICA origin.

39.1.4 Treatment

Initial Management

- Intravenous thrombolysis was administered after initial NCCT, 94 minutes after stroke onset.
- A decision is made to proceed to emergent endovascular treatment, based on time from onset, presence of large vessel occlusion, and favorable ASPECTS score.
- For collateral augmentation, a 500-mL normal saline fluid bolus is administered, and systolic blood pressure (SBP) maintained at 150 to 180 mm Hg en route to the neuroangiography suite.

39.1.5 Endovascular Treatment

Material

- 7-Fr-long (90-cm) sheath for access (micropuncture kit; 6F dilator; 7F KSAW-7.0–38–90-RB-SHTL-FLEX- HC sheath).
- 125-cm Davis catheter (Cook Medical Inc) and 0.038 Glidewire (Terumo).
- Abbott Vascular XACT stent 9–7 mm × 40 mm.
- Penumbra 5 Max ACE catheter.
- Velocity 0.025 microcatheter.
- Synchro-2 standard microwire 200 cm.
- Synchro-2 standard microwire 300 cm.
- Solitaire 4 mm × 40 mm stentriever.

Technique

- The endovascular procedure was carried out under local anesthesia and conscious sedation administered by the anesthesia team.

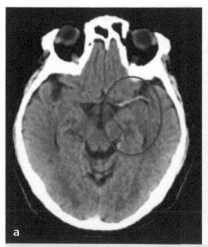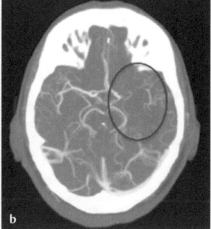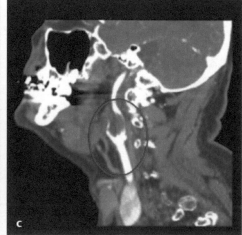

Fig. 39.1 NCCT (a) and subsequent CTA axial and sagittal maximum intensity projection (b,c) demonstrate a dense left MCA, M1 occlusion, and noncalcified thrombus at the ICA origin.

- SBP was maintained at 150 to 180 mm Hg to maximize collateral support, while the intracranial occlusion remained present, but not exceeding the recommended upper limit post–intravenous tissue plasminogen activator (IV-tPA) administration.
- The 7-Fr-long sheath was advanced into the left common carotid artery (CCA) over the 125-cm Davis catheter.
- Since the appearances on the CTA of the neck suggested soft thrombus, a decision was made to trap the cervical ICA thrombus with a stent. In light of the documented intracranial occlusion, a distal protection device was not used.
- A Velocity microcatheter was used to carefully navigate an exchange length Synchro 2 standard microwire across the narrowed left ICA origin, aiming to avoid displacing the thrombus.
- The microcatheter was removed, and the 9 to 7 mm × 40 mm XACT stent was navigated across the thrombus site over the exchange length 0.014 microwire. The XACT stent was successfully deployed with full expansion. However, postdeployment angiography demonstrated that a portion of the cervical ICA thrombus had migrated distally to cause a complete ICA terminus occlusion.
- The stent system was removed, and a Penumbra 5 Max ACE catheter was used to attempt primary aspiration of the ICA terminus thrombus, but without success.
- Subsequently, a triaxial system of the Penumbra 5 Max ACE, the Velocity microcatheter, and 200 cm Synchro 2 standard microwire were navigated across the thrombus into the M2 left MCA, microwire was removed, and a 4 × 40 mm Solitaire stentriever used to recanalize both the left MCA and ICA. Two passes were required, and TICI 2b reperfusion was achieved (▶ Fig. 39.2a).
- Subsequent angiogram revealed active contrast pooling in the lenticulostriate territory (▶ Fig. 39.2b). Since active bleeding was suspected, the procedure was immediately terminated and SBP reduced to less than 140 mm Hg.
- Time from groin puncture to TICI 2b reperfusion was 51 minutes; time from initial stentriever deployment to TICI 2b reperfusion was 21 minutes.

39.1.6 Postprocedure Care

- There was no immediate intra- or postprocedural neurological deterioration; emergent intubation was not required.
- Emergent repeat NCCT confirmed large basal ganglia hemorrhage (▶ Fig. 39.2c), with denser contrast pooling in the posterior margin of the hematoma, which was compatible with the angiographic findings.
- A meeting with the family was held and the options of intubation, external ventricular drainage, and aggressive medical management were balanced against the option of transitioning to hospice care. Given the patient's age, significant clinical deficit, and imaging findings, a high disability and mortality rate was expected. Based on the patient's previously stated wishes, a decision was made for supportive hospice care.

39.1.7 Outcome

- Comfort care measures were instituted, and the patient died 24 hours later.

39.2 Companion Case

39.2.1 Case

Hemorrhagic transformation 27 hours after mechanical thrombectomy.

39.2.2 Clinical Presentation

A 58-year-old female presents with a left MCA occlusion and a NIHSS score of 14 3 hours after the beginning of stroke symptoms. Emergent NCCT reveals early ischemic changes in the left lentiform nucleus with an ASPECTS score of 9. The patient received IV-rtPA and was taken to the angiography suite for endovascular treatment.

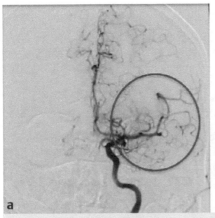
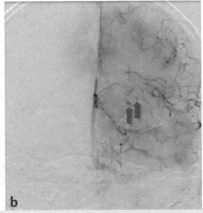
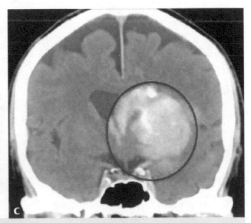

Fig. 39.2 Catheter angiographic images (**a,b**) demonstrate active contrast extravasation in the lenticulostriate territory after recanalization. Subsequent NCCT (**c**) demonstrates a large left basal ganglia hematoma with intraventricular extension. Note the denser areas within the hematoma on CT reflecting extravasated contrast.

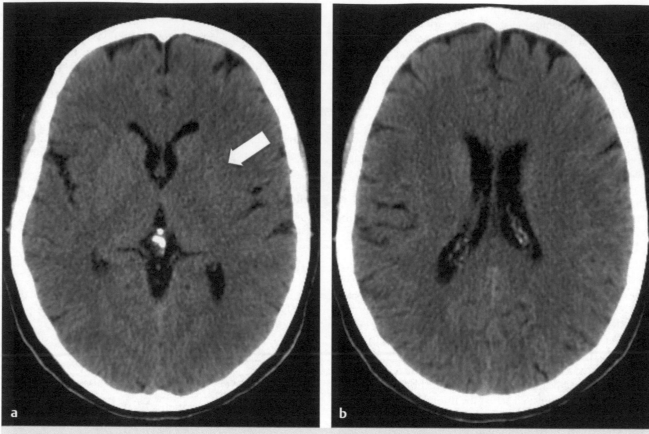

Fig. 39.3 NCCT demonstrates hypoattenuation/early infarction of the left lentiform nucleus (ASPECTS score of 9).

39.2.3 Imaging Workup and Investigations

NCCT (▶ Fig. 39.3) and CTA demonstrate hypoattenuation of the left lentiform nucleus, an ASPECTS score of 9, and a left M1 occlusion.

39.2.4 Diagnosis

- Acute proximal left MCA occlusion.

39.2.5 Treatment

Initial Management

- Intravenous thrombolysis.
- Patient is transferred to the angiography suite for mechanical thrombectomy.

39.2.6 Endovascular Treatment

Material

- Solitaire 4 mm × 40 mm stentriever.

Technique

- The endovascular procedure was carried out under local anesthesia and conscious sedation administered by the anesthesia team.

- No intraprocedural heparin was administered.
- Initial catheter angiogram confirmed the left proximal M1 occlusion (▶ Fig. 39.4a).
- The Solitaire device was deployed across the M1 thrombus with immediate reperfusion.
- 3 passes performed with final TICI 2B reperfusion (▶ Fig. 39.4b).
- Time from groin puncture to TICI 2B reperfusion: 40 minutes.
- On table NIHSS score following reperfusion: 4.
- Xper CT demonstrated hyperattenuation in the caudate head and the lentiform nucleus, keeping with contrast staining, but there was no evidence of hemorrhage (▶ Fig. 39.4c).

39.2.7 Postprocedure Care

- Prophylactic heparin and aspirin commenced the next day.
- 27 hours after the end of the procedure, the patient experienced sudden clinical deterioration. Emergent repeat NCCT demonstrated large basal ganglia hemorrhage (▶ Fig. 39.5) with intraventricular extension.

39.2.8 Outcome

- Patient was managed conservatively; mRS score was 4 at 90 days.

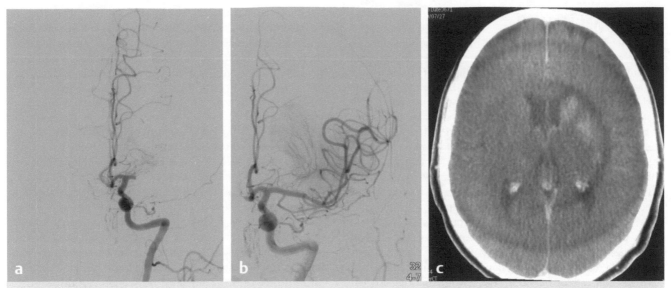

Fig. 39.4 Catheter angiogram demonstrates left proximal M1 occlusion (**a**) with TICI 2B reperfusion postthrombectomy (**b**). Xper CT (**c**) demonstrates hyperattenuation in the caudate head and the lentiform nucleus in keeping with contrast staining, but no evidence of hemorrhage. Note that the staining in the lentiform nucleus corresponds to the area of infarction seen on the pretreatment NCCT (▶ Fig. 39.3).

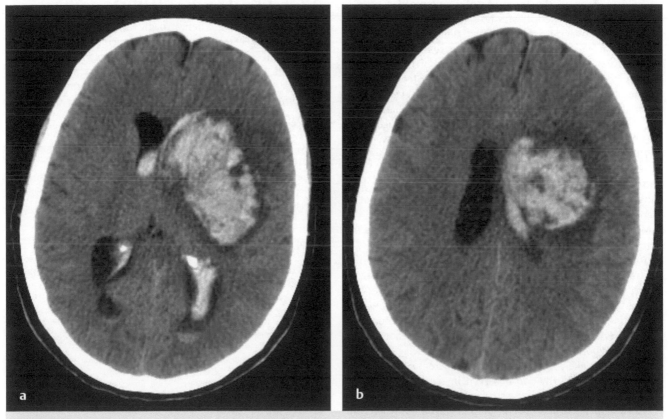

Fig. 39.5 NCCT demonstrates a large left basal ganglia hematoma with intraventricular extension.

39.3 Discussion

Minor hemorrhagic transformation may be the natural consequence of some forms of ischemic stroke. The unifying pathophysiological process is that of reperfusion of infarcted brain tissue with a compromised blood–brain barrier.[1] In an attempt to classify hemorrhagic transformation for the purposes of stroke trial research, the ECASS trials defined hemorrhagic events on CT as hemorrhagic infarction (HI) types I and II and parenchymal hematoma (PH) types I and II.[2,3] HI I was defined as small petechiae along the infarct margins; HI II was confluent petechiae within the infarct, but without mass effect; PH I was a focal blood clot occupying < 30% of the infarct area with mild mass effect, and PH II was a focal blood clot occupying > 30% the infarct volume with significant mass effect. In the trials, CT was used to assess posttreatment hemorrhagic events. However, new MRI techniques such as susceptibility-weighted imaging (SWI) increase the detection of intracranial hemorrhage, and increase the detection rate of minor HI that is common after ischemic stroke, particularly after reperfusion therapy.[4] HI has little impact on clinical outcome, in contrast to PH II,[5] and is often considered as an imaging biomarker of symptomatic intracranial hemorrhage, given the impact on patient's 90-day outcomes.

The risk of symptomatic intracranial hemorrhage after endovascular therapy in the three recent randomized controlled trials ranged from 0 to 8%, with no significant difference compared to intravenous thrombolysis alone.[6,7,8] Symptomatic hemorrhage is usually defined as an increase of 4 points on the NIHSS at the baseline stroke scale. Acute hemorrhagic transformation with contrast extravasation from the lenticulostriate arteries, as distinct to contrast extravasation from vessel perforation during endovascular stroke treatment, is rare and generally limited to case reports.[9,10,11] In the 300 endovascular stroke treatments at the Massachusetts General hospital between July 2010 and December 2014, there have been two instances of active contrast extravasation from lenticulostriate arteries. In both cases, the procedures were terminated, and large basal ganglia hemorrhages (PH 2) were evident on subsequent CT scans; both patients died.

More commonly, hemorrhagic transformation manifests in a delayed fashion after endovascular treatment. Regardless of infarct mechanism, the common pathophysiology of hemorrhagic transformation is that of reperfusion of infarcted tissue, in which there is abnormally increased blood-brain barrier permeability and dysfunction of the vascular basal lamina.[1] Direct interaction of fibrinolytic agents such as tPA with various proteinases, which exacerbate damage to vascular endothelium, has been hypothesized to contribute to hemorrhagic transformation, and is likely to contribute to the increased incidence of hemorrhagic transformation observed in the setting of intra-arterial thrombolysis for acute stroke. Intra-arterial thrombolysis has a higher risk of hemorrhagic transformation when compared to the intravenous route, probably, in part, due to increased localized effects of the thrombolytic agent on the vascular endothelium. Lending weight to this theory is the animal model observation of increased rates of hemorrhagic transformation with intra-arterial tPA compared with intravenous therapy utilizing the same total.[12]

Risk factors contributing to hemorrhagic transformation of ischemic stroke include age, cardioembolic mechanism of stroke, atrial fibrillation, oral anticoagulation, hypertension, elevated body temperature, hyperglycemia, low serum cholesterol, higher dose of thrombolytic agent, and intra-arterial route of thrombolytic administration.[1] Risk factors contributing to hemorrhagic transformation in ischemic stroke patients treated with intra-arterial thrombolysis include higher NIHSS scores, longer time to recanalization, low platelet count, and hyperglycemia.[13,14]

One potential pitfall of identifying postprocedure hemorrhagic transformation is the presence of parenchymal contrast staining, a frequently observed phenomenon after intra-arterial therapy for acute stroke.[15,16,17,18,19] Identifying hemorrhage and distinguishing it from contrast staining may have treatment implications by influencing the decision to anticoagulate, reversal of IV-tPA effect, blood pressure parameters, and identification of patients who may require early or closer imaging surveillance. Distinguishing between contrast staining and hemorrhage may be achieved with serial CT imaging, MRI with the use of blood-sensitive sequences, or dual-energy CT. Our practice is to obtain a dual-energy CT for any postoperative CT scan obtained within 12 hours of the procedure (see Chapter 49).

39.4 Pearls and Pitfalls

- Asymptomatic minor hemorrhagic transformation after ischemic stroke is common. PH II hemorrhagic conversion is important to identify because this negatively impacts patients 90-day outcomes; symptomatic intracranial hemorrhage after endovascular stroke treatment occurs in less than 10% of cases.
- Acute hemorrhage with active contrast extravasation from the lenticulostriate arteries during endovascular stroke treatment is extremely rare, but is typically fatal.
- Parenchymal contrast staining after endovascular stroke therapy may mimic hemorrhagic transformation, and may be distinguished from hemorrhage using advanced imaging techniques including dual energy CT.

References

[1] Álvarez-Sabín J, Maisterra O, Santamarina E, Kase CS. Factors influencing haemorrhagic transformation in ischaemic stroke. Lancet Neurol. 2013; 12 (7):689–705

[2] Hacke W, Kaste M, Fieschi C, et al. The European Cooperative Acute Stroke Study (ECASS). Intravenous thrombolysis with recombinant tissue plasminogen activator for acute hemispheric stroke. JAMA. 1995; 274 (13):1017–1025

[3] Hacke W, Kaste M, Fieschi C, et al. Randomised double-blind placebo-controlled trial of thrombolytic therapy with intravenous alteplase in acute ischaemic stroke (ECASS II). Second European-Australasian Acute Stroke Study Investigators. Lancet. 1998; 352:1245–1251

[4] Zhang J, Yang Y, Sun H, Xing Y. Hemorrhagic transformation after cerebral infarction: current concepts and challenges. Ann Transl Med. 2014; 2(8):81

[5] Fiorelli M, Bastianello S, von Kummer R, et al. Hemorrhagic transformation within 36 hours of a cerebral infarct: relationships with early clinical deterioration and 3-month outcome in the European Cooperative Acute Stroke Study I (ECASS I) cohort. Stroke. 1999; 30(11):2280–2284

[6] Goyal M, Demchuk AM, Menon BK, et al. ESCAPE Trial Investigators. Randomized assessment of rapid endovascular treatment of ischemic stroke. N Engl J Med. 2015; 372(11):1019–1030

[7] Campbell BCV, Mitchell PJ, Kleinig TJ, et al. EXTEND-IA Investigators. Endovascular therapy for ischemic stroke with perfusion-imaging selection. N Engl J Med. 2015; 372(11):1009–1018

[8] Berkhemer OA, Fransen PS, Beumer D, et al. MR CLEAN Investigators. A randomized trial of intraarterial treatment for acute ischemic stroke. N Engl J Med. 2015; 372(1):11–20

[9] Komiyama M, Nishijima Y, Nishio A, Khosla VK. Extravasation of contrast medium from the lenticulostriate artery following local intracarotid fibrinolysis. Surg Neurol. 1993; 39(4):315–319

[10] Prince EA, Jayaraman MV, Schirmang T, Haas R. Angiographically documented hemorrhagic conversion of a left middle cerebral artery embolic stroke during intra-arterial thrombolysis. J Neurointerv Surg. 2011; 3 (3):246–248

[11] Urbach H, Bendszus M, Brechtelsbauer D, Solymosi L. [Extravasation of contrast medium in local intra-arterial fibrinolysis of the carotid territory]. Nervenarzt. 1998; 69(6):490–494

[12] Crumrine RC, Marder VJ, Taylor GM, et al. Intra-arterial administration of recombinant tissue-type plasminogen activator (rt-PA) causes more intracranial bleeding than does intravenous rt-PA in a transient rat middle cerebral artery occlusion model. Exp Transl Stroke Med. 2011; 3(1):10

[13] Kidwell CS, Saver JL, Carneado J, et al. Predictors of hemorrhagic transformation in patients receiving intra-arterial thrombolysis. Stroke. 2002; 33(3):717–724

[14] Kase CS, Furlan AJ, Wechsler LR, et al. Cerebral hemorrhage after intra-arterial thrombolysis for ischemic stroke: the PROACT II trial. Neurology. 2001; 57(9):1603–1610

[15] Lummel N, Schulte-Altedorneburg G, Bernau C, et al. Hyperattenuated intracerebral lesions after mechanical recanalization in acute stroke. AJNR Am J Neuroradiol. 2014; 35(2):345–351

[16] Nakano S, Iseda T, Kawano H, Yoneyama T, Ikeda T, Wakisaka S. Parenchymal hyperdensity on computed tomography after intra-arterial reperfusion therapy for acute middle cerebral artery occlusion: incidence and clinical significance. Stroke. 2001; 32(9):2042–2048

[17] Parrilla G, García-Villalba B, Espinosa de Rueda M, et al. Hemorrhage/contrast staining areas after mechanical intra-arterial thrombectomy in acute ischemic stroke: imaging findings and clinical significance. AJNR Am J Neuroradiol. 2012; 33(9):1791–1796

[18] Wildenhain SL, Jungreis CA, Barr J, Mathis J, Wechsler L, Horton JA. CT after intracranial intraarterial thrombolysis for acute stroke. AJNR Am J Neuroradiol. 1994; 15(3):487–492

[19] Yoon W, Seo JJ, Kim JK, Cho KH, Park JG, Kang HK. Contrast enhancement and contrast extravasation on computed tomography after intra-arterial thrombolysis in patients with acute ischemic stroke. Stroke. 2004; 35 (4):876–881

40 Endovascular Treatment of Cerebral Venous Thrombosis

40.1 Case Description

40.1.1 Clinical Presentation

A 23-year old woman presented to the emergency room of a community hospital with confusion and a 2-day history of severe headache. At examination, she had a score of 12 on the Glasgow Coma Scale (GCS) and mild left-sided weakness. Shortly after admission, she developed epileptic seizures, became comatose, and developed a fixed and dilated right pupil. She was then sedated, intubated, and transferred to our hospital.

40.1.2 Baseline Imaging

- Noncontrast CT (NCCT) showed bilateral areas of edema in the frontal lobes, mostly subcortical and more pronounced in the right hemisphere. Within the lesions were patchy areas of hemorrhage. There was mass effect and a midline shift of 6 mm. The right transverse and sigmoid sinus demonstrated a region of hyperdensity, and a cord sign was visible in one of the cortical veins (▶ Fig. 40.1).
- MRI confirmed the presence of bilateral hemorrhagic infarctions. Contrast-enhanced MR venography showed thrombosis of the anterior part of the superior sagittal sinus, and nonocclusive thrombi in the posterior part of the superior sagittal sinus, right transverse sinus, and right sigmoid sinus. The cortical veins overlaying the frontal lobes were also thrombosed. The left internal jugular vein was hypoplastic (▶ Fig. 40.2).

40.2 Diagnosis

Cerebral venous thrombosis with bilateral hemorrhagic infarctions.

40.3 Treatment

- Because of clinical and radiological signs of impending transtentorial and subfalcine herniation, the patient underwent emergency bilateral decompressive hemicraniectomy and placement of an external ventricular drain. Prior to surgery, she had a GCS score of 4 and bilateral fixed and dilated pupils.
- Immediately after the operation, she was transferred to the angio suite for mechanical thrombectomy (▶ Fig. 40.3). Balloon angioplasty was performed using a 7 × 20 mm Amiia balloon. Successful recanalization of the right transverse sigmoid and sigmoid sinus was achieved, and flow was improved in the posterior third of the superior sagittal sinus. Recanalization of the anterior part of the superior sagittal sinus was attempted with a 3.5 × 10 mm balloon, but was unsuccessful.
- NCCT after the bilateral hemicraniectomy and thrombectomy demonstrated a decrease in mass effect. The hemorrhagic component of the venous infarcts had increased, most likely

as a result of the decrease in intracranial pressure (▶ Fig. 40.4).
- After the surgical and endovascular procedure, the patient was started on unfractionated heparin in the therapeutic dose.

40.3.1 Outcome

- Initially, after the interventions, the clinical condition of the patient was unchanged, but after an extended stay in the intensive care unit (ICU), she began to improve.
- Two months after admission, she was discharged to a rehabilitation clinic on warfarin and antiseizure medication. She continued to improve and was discharged home several weeks later. Cranioplasty was performed approximately 1 year after initial admission.
- The patient continued to improve clinically and at her last follow-up visit, 5 years after admission, she had no focal neurological deficits. She followed a part-time education for a legal profession. She did develop epilepsy over time, which was controlled with levetiracetam, carbamazepine and clobazam. Apart from oral contraceptive use, no cause for the thrombosis was identified.
- CT scan at follow-up showed encephalomalacia in both frontal lobes, predominantly in the white matter (▶ Fig. 40.5). Contrast-enhanced MR venography performed about 18 months after admission showed that the anterior part of the superior sagittal sinus had recanalized (▶ Fig. 40.6).

40.4 Discussion

Cerebral venous thrombosis (CVT) is a rare cause of stroke that mainly affects young adults and children.[1,2] In adults, women are affected three times more often than men, which is the result of hormonal risk factors (oral contraceptives and pregnancy).[3] The most common clinical manifestations of CVT are headache (90%), focal neurological deficits (50%), and epileptic seizures (40%). Approximately 40 to 60% of patients have a brain parenchymal lesion on imaging, usually in the form of a venous hemorrhagic infarct.[4,5] Coma at admission, as was the case in our patient, occurs in less than 5% of patients and is usually caused by mass effect from large venous infarcts, bilateral edema of the thalami and basal ganglia, or recurrent seizures.

The standard treatment of CVT is anticoagulation with heparin, either with unfractionated or low-molecular weight heparin, and this therapy should be initiated as soon as possible after the diagnosis is established.[6,7,8,9] In our patient, heparin was not started immediately because emergency neurosurgical intervention was required. Transtentorial herniation is the most important cause of early death in patients with CVT, and recent data suggest that decompressive hemicraniectomy can be life-saving and result in good functional outcomes in these patients.[10,11,12] Our patient was in a very severe condition prior to surgery, with bilateral fixed and dilated pupils, but even in these patients, good recovery has been reported.[13]

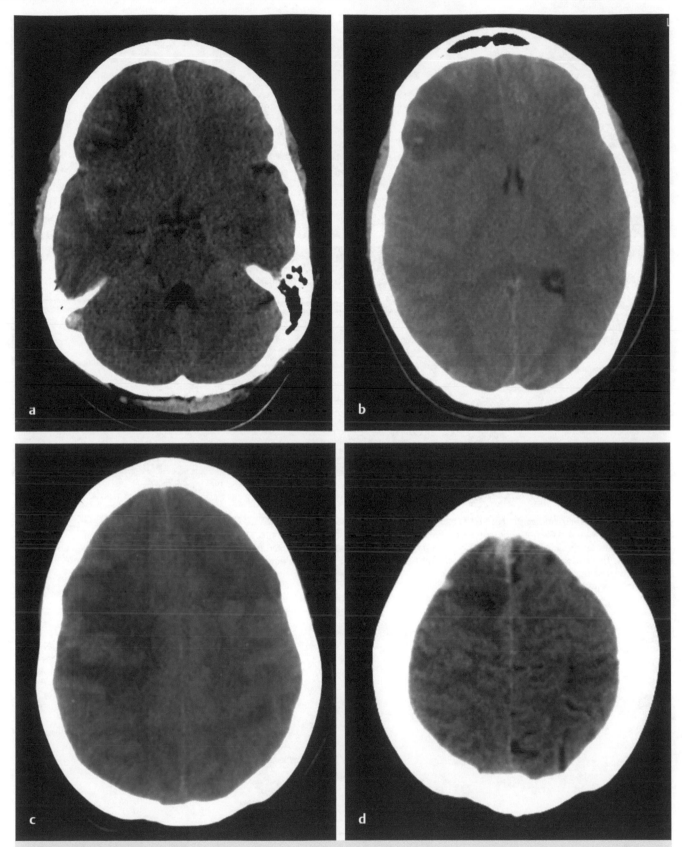

Fig. 40.1 Baseline CT. (a–d) Pretreatment axial noncontrast CT scan. There are bilateral areas of edema visible in the frontal lobes, more pronounced in the right hemisphere. Within these lesions are small, patchy areas of hemorrhage. There is mass effect, with a midline shift of approximately 6 mm. The right sigmoid sinus has a hyperdense aspect **(a)**, and there is cord sign visible in one of the cortical veins overlying the right hemisphere **(d)**.

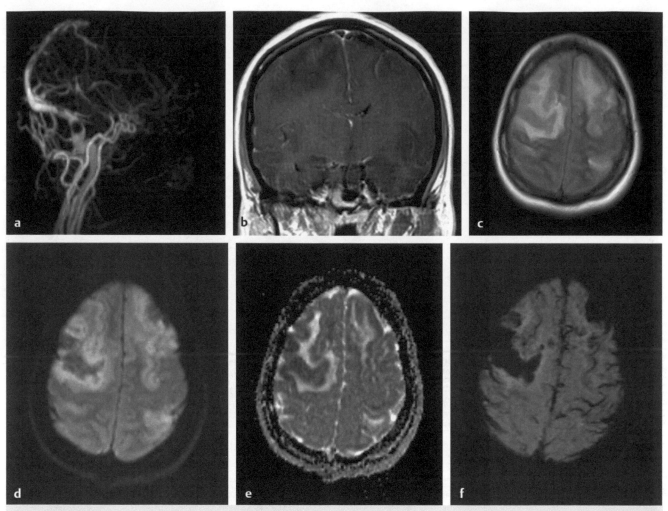

Fig. 40.2 Baseline MRI. (a) Sagittal contrast enhanced MR venography shows thrombosis of the anterior part of the superior sagittal sinus and nonocclusive thrombi in the posterior part of the superior sagittal sinus, right transverse sinus, and right sigmoid sinus.**(b)** Coronal contrast enhanced MRI demonstrates septation of the superior sagittal sinus with absent flow in both channels.**(c)** Aligned axial FLAIR (**c**), DWI (**d**), ADC (**e**), and SWI (**f**) sequences. There are bilateral lesions visible, with a mixture of edema and blood. The edema consists mostly of vasogenic edema, but at the outer parts of the lesions, there are also areas of cytotoxic edema, most likely due to leptomeningeal compression. The SWI also shows venous congestion in the cortical veins.

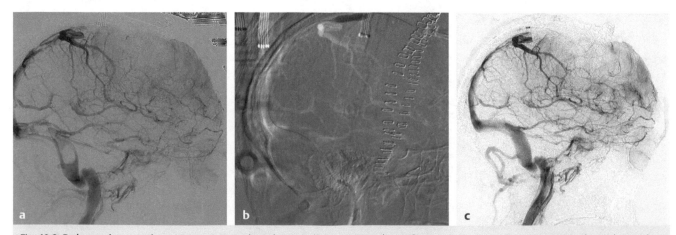

Fig. 40.3 Endovascular procedure. (a) Pretreatment lateral view catheter angiography confirming the findings of the MR venography, with complete occlusion of the anterior part of the superior sagittal sinus, and nonocclusive thrombi in the posterior part of the superior sagittal sinus, right sigmoid and transverse sinus.**(b)** Balloon angioplasty with a 7 × 20 mm Amiia balloon in the superior sagittal sinus **(c)** Postintervention lateral view catheter angiography, showing improved filling of the right sigmoid and transverse sinus, and the posterior part of the superior sagittal sinus. The speed of the venous outflow was also improved compared to before treatment. Persistent thrombosis of the anterior part of the superior sagittal sinus.

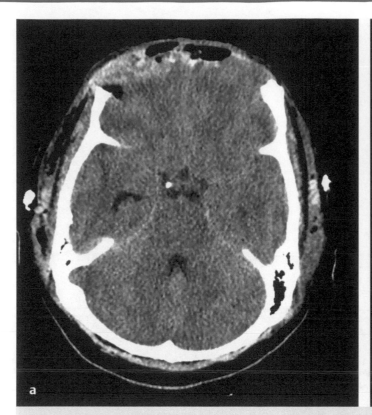
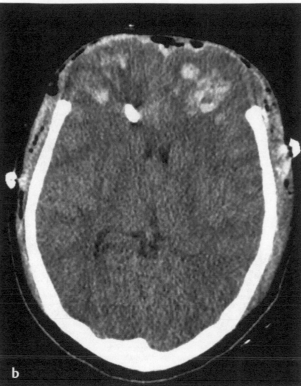

Fig. 40.4 Postoperative CT scan. (a,b) Status after bilateral frontal decompressive hemicraniectomy. There is a decrease in mass effect and midline shift. The hemorrhagic component in the venous infarctions has increased, most likely as a result of the decrease in intracranial pressure. External ventricular drain through the right frontal lobe in the lateral ventricle (b). Hyperdensity is no longer visible in the right sigmoid sinus (a).

The use of endovascular treatment (ET) in patients with CVT is increasingly reported in the literature. Most of these studies report good outcomes; however, almost all of them are case reports or small case series.[14,15,16] It is difficult to draw any conclusions on the basis of these data, because of the high risk of publication bias and the fact that the prognosis of CVT is also favorable in many patients who do not undergo ET.[3,17] Thus far, no controlled studies have been performed, although there is one ongoing randomized trial, the TO-ACT trial.[18] In this study, patients with CVT and a high risk of poor outcome are randomized to standard therapy or standard therapy in combination with ET. The trial has a pragmatic design and does not prescribe a specific endovascular method. Instead, the interventionalist can use the strategy that he/she thinks is best suited for that particular case. Intrasinus thrombolysis (using recombinant tissue plasminogen activator [rtPA] or urokinase), mechanical thrombectomy, or a combination of both can be used. The results of the TO-ACT trial were presented at the European Stroke Conference. Among 67 randomized patients, ET did not improve clinical outcome over standard therapy. The full results of the study are expected to be published this year.

In the absence of trial data on its efficacy and safety in CVT, the decision to use ET must be weighed in each separate case. The guideline of the American Heart Association advises to reserve ET for patients who deteriorate despite heparin treatment, or if patients who develop mass effect from a venous infarction that causes intracranial hypertension are resistant to standard therapies.[6] If ET is done in a patient with impending herniation, it is important that it is preceded by decompressive surgery. ET alone is insufficient to reverse the process of herniation and in the absence of decompressive surgery, there is a high risk of fatal herniation while the patient is under anesthesia for the intervention.[19,20]

Judging from the number of publications in recent years, mechanical thrombectomy is currently favored over intrasinus thrombolysis, despite the fact that there is no evidence that one technique is superior over the other.[21] Theoretically, the risk of hemorrhagic complications is lower with mechanical thrombectomy, because of the obvious risk of using a thrombolytic drug in a condition where most patients already have an intracerebral hemorrhage prior to the intervention. On the other hand, devices that are used for mechanical thrombectomy are generally more bulky, which could increase the risk of perforating a sinus. The Angiojet device, for example, is frequently used in ET for CVT, but a recent systematic review suggested that it is associated with a higher risk of complications and a lower chance of successful recanalization.[22]

In our case, ET was partially successful. We managed to recanalize the posterior part of the superior sagittal sinus and the dominant transverse and sigmoid sinus. The venous outflow was also substantially improved after the procedure; however, we did not succeed in recanalizing the anterior part of the superior sagittal sinus. After two attempts, we decided not to pursue this any further for the following reasons: (1) risk of hemorrhagic complications and (2) the cortical veins in that region were all thrombosed, and even if we would managed to open the sinus, the flow in the cortical veins could not be restored with ET.

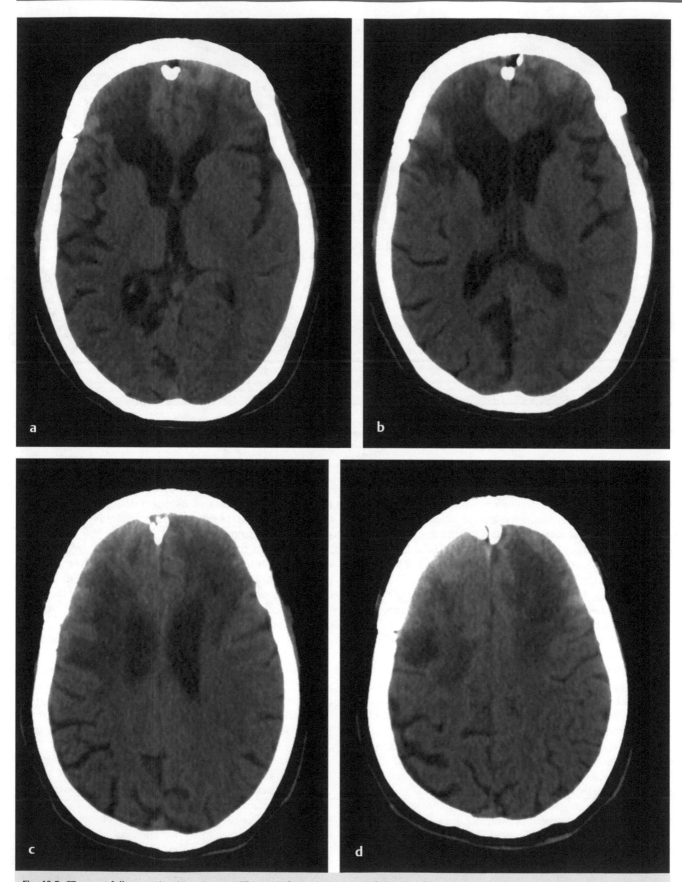

Fig. 40.5 CT scan at follow-up. (a–c) Noncontrast CT scan performed approximately 5 years after admission showed encephalomalacia bilateral in the frontal lobes, which was located predominantly in the white matter.

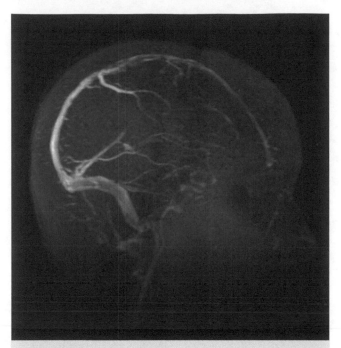

Fig. 40.6 MR venography at follow-up. Lateral contrast enhanced MR venography showing that the anterior part of the superior sagittal sinus has recanalized partially over time.

In summary, ET can be considered in patients with a severe form of CVT, but currently there is insufficient evidence on its efficacy and safety from controlled studies. Analysis of the full results of the TO-ACT trial may help in delineating the role of ET in the treatment of CVT.

References

[1] Stam J. Thrombosis of the cerebral veins and sinuses. N Engl J Med. 2005; 352 (17):1791–1798

[2] Coutinho JM, Zuurbier SM, Aramideh M, Stam J. The incidence of cerebral venous thrombosis: a cross-sectional study. Stroke. 2012; 43(12):3375–3377

[3] Ferro JM, Canhão P, Stam J, Bousser MG, Barinagarrementeria F, Investigators I, ISCVT Investigators. Prognosis of cerebral vein and dural sinus thrombosis: results of the International Study on Cerebral Vein and Dural Sinus Thrombosis (ISCVT). Stroke. 2004; 35(3):664–670

[4] Leach JL, Fortuna RB, Jones BV, Gaskill-Shipley MF. Imaging of cerebral venous thrombosis: current techniques, spectrum of findings, and diagnostic pitfalls. Radiographics. 2006; 26 Suppl 1:S19–S41, discussion S42–S43

[5] Coutinho JM, van den Berg R, Zuurbier SM, et al. Small juxtacortical hemorrhages in cerebral venous thrombosis. Ann Neurol. 2014; 75(6):908–916

[6] Saposnik G, Barinagarrementeria F, Brown RD, Jr, et al. American Heart Association Stroke Council and the Council on Epidemiology and Prevention. Diagnosis and management of cerebral venous thrombosis: a statement for healthcare professionals from the American Heart Association/American Stroke Association. Stroke. 2011; 42(4):1158–1192

[7] Einhäupl K, Stam J, Bousser MG, et al. European Federation of Neurological Societies. EFNS guideline on the treatment of cerebral venous and sinus thrombosis in adult patients. Eur J Neurol. 2010; 17(10):1229–1235

[8] Coutinho J, de Bruijn SF, Deveber G, Stam J. Anticoagulation for cerebral venous sinus thrombosis. Cochrane Database Syst Rev. 2011(8):CD002005

[9] Coutinho JM, Stam J. How to treat cerebral venous and sinus thrombosis. J Thromb Haemost. 2010; 8(5):877–883

[10] Ferro JM. Causes, predictors of death, and antithrombotic treatment in cerebral venous thrombosis. Clin Adv Hematol Oncol. 2006; 4(10):732–733

[11] Ferro JM, Crassard I, Coutinho JM, et al. Second International Study on Cerebral Vein and Dural Sinus Thrombosis (ISCVT 2) Investigators. Decompressive surgery in cerebrovenous thrombosis: a multicenter registry and a systematic review of individual patient data. Stroke. 2011; 42 (10):2825–2831

[12] Coutinho JM, Majoie CB, Coert BA, Stam J. Decompressive hemicraniectomy in cerebral sinus thrombosis: consecutive case series and review of the literature. Stroke. 2009; 40(6):2233–2235

[13] Stefini R, Latronico N, Cornali C, Rasulo F, Bollati A. Emergent decompressive craniectomy in patients with fixed dilated pupils due to cerebral venous and dural sinus thrombosis: report of three cases. Neurosurgery. 1999; 45 (3):626–629, discussion 629–630

[14] Rahman M, Velat GJ, Hoh BL, Mocco J. Direct thrombolysis for cerebral venous sinus thrombosis. Neurosurg Focus. 2009; 27(5):E7

[15] Newman CB, Pakbaz RS, Nguyen AD, Kerber CW. Endovascular treatment of extensive cerebral sinus thrombosis. J Neurosurg. 2009; 110(3):442–445

[16] Zhang A, Collinson RL, Hurst RW, Weigele JB. Rheolytic thrombectomy for cerebral sinus thrombosis. Neurocrit Care. 2008; 9(1):17–26

[17] Coutinho JM, Zuurbier SM, Stam J. Declining mortality in cerebral venous thrombosis: a systematic review. Stroke. 2014; 45(5):1338–1341

[18] Coutinho JM, Ferro JM, Zuurbier SM, et al. Thrombolysis or anticoagulation for cerebral venous thrombosis: rationale and design of the TO-ACT trial. Int J Stroke. 2013; 8(2):135–140

[19] Stam J, Majoie CB, van Delden OM, van Lienden KP, Reekers JA. Endovascular thrombectomy and thrombolysis for severe cerebral sinus thrombosis: a prospective study. Stroke. 2008; 39(5):1487–1490

[20] Coutinho JM, Hama-Amin AD, Vleggeert Lankamp C, Reekers JA, Stam J, Wermer MJ. Decompressive hemicraniectomy followed by endovascular thrombosuction in a patient with cerebral venous thrombosis. J Neurol. 2012; 259(3):562–564

[21] Siddiqui FM, Banerjee C, Zuurbier SM, et al. Mechanical thrombectomy versus intrasinus thrombolysis for cerebral venous sinus thrombosis: a non-randomized comparison. Interv Neuroradiol. 2014; 20(3):336–344

[22] Siddiqui FM, Dandapat S, Banerjee C, et al. Mechanical thrombectomy in cerebral venous thrombosis: systematic review of 185 cases. Stroke. 2015; 46 (5):1263–1268

41 Endovascular Thrombectomy for Pediatric Acute Ischemic Stroke

41.1 Case Description

41.1.1 Clinical Presentation

A 14-year-old female patient presented to the pediatric emergency department with quadriparesis, obtundation, and dysconjugate eye movements.

41.1.2 Imaging Workup and Investigations

- Noncontrast CT (NCCT) of the head (▸ Fig. 41.1a) demonstrated a "hyperdense" basilar artery sign, representing an acute thromboembolic occlusion of the basilar artery. Low-attenuation changes, representing evolving perforator infarcts, were seen in the pons (▸ Fig. 41.1b), with no abnormalities in the remaining posterior fossa parenchyma, thalami, or the occipital lobes bilaterally.
- CT angiography arch to vertex demonstrated a right cervical rib and associated thrombosed pseudoaneurysm of the right subclavian artery (▸ Fig. 41.2a), with digital subtraction angiography confirming the basilar artery thrombosis, as predicted by unenhanced CT (▸ Fig. 41.2b).

41.2 Diagnosis

Acute basilar artery thromboembolic occlusion due to a right subclavian thrombosed pseudoaneurysm that was believed to be a result of repetitive traumatic injuries due to an adjacent right cervical rib.

41.2.1 Treatment

As the pediatric hospital had no expertise in pediatric stroke intervention, the patient was transferred to an adult tertiary care hospital where emergency mechanical thrombectomy was performed by the adult interventional neuroradiology service.

Materials

- 5-Fr Micropuncture kit.
- 6-Fr 90-cm Neuron Max 0.088-in guide sheath (Penumbra, Alameda, CA).
- Berenstein Select catheter (Penumbra).
- Rotating Tuohy Borst Hemostatic valve (Merit Medical, South Jordan, UT).
- ACE 60 aspiration catheter (Penumbra).
- Velocity microcatheter (Penumbra).
- Fathom 16 microwire (Boston Scientific, Fremont, CA).

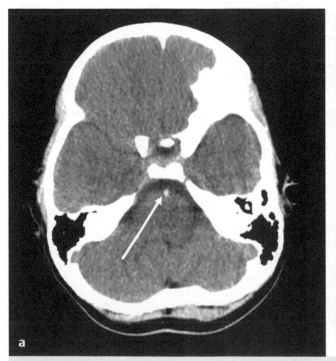 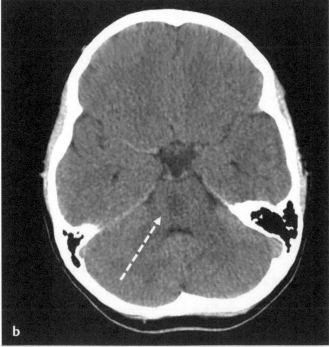

Fig. 41.1 Noncontrast CT of the head (a) demonstrated a "hyperdense" basilar artery sign, representing an acute thromboembolic occlusion of the basilar artery. Low-attenuation changes, representing evolving perforator infarcts, were seen in the pons (b), with no abnormalities in the remaining posterior fossa parenchyma, thalami, or the occipital lobes bilaterally.

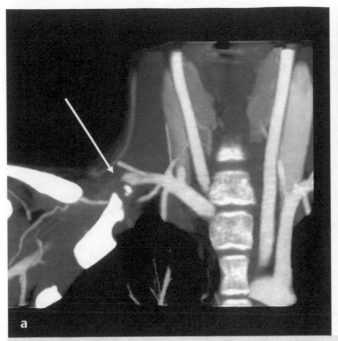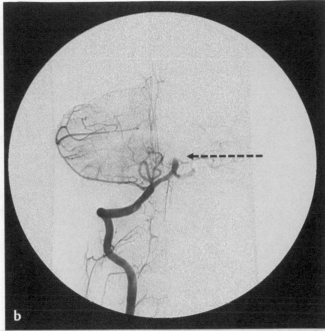

Fig. 41.2 CT angiography arch to vertex demonstrated a right cervical rib and associated thrombosed pseudoaneurysm of the right subclavian artery (a), with digital subtraction angiography confirming the basilar artery thrombosis, as predicted by unenhanced CT (b).

- Vascular closure device (6-Fr Angio-Seal, Terumo Medical, Somerset, NJ).

Technique

- Endotracheal intubation and general anesthesia support of the patient was provided on an emergent basis by the adult anesthesia department due to the impaired level of consciousness of the patient.
- Percutaneous ultrasound (US)-guided access to the right common femoral artery (CFA) was achieved using a 5-Fr micropuncture kit, with placement of a 5-Fr vascular sheath.
- After placement of an Amplatz Extra Stiff guidewire in the abdominal aorta, the 5-Fr sheath was removed, with subsequent advancement of a 6-Fr Neuro Max guide sheath (over its dilator), with the guide sheath serving as the primary access sheath.
- As the right vertebral artery was the dominant vessel of the posterior circulation, using a Berenstein Select catheter and Terumo guidewire, the Neuron Max guide sheath was positioned in the right subclavian artery, proximal to the right vertebral artery origin.
- With the Select catheter removed, the detachable sheath valve was replaced with a Tuohy Borst rotating hemostatic valve, with the guide sheath placed on continuous flush, and side-arm access provided for performing angiography.
- Control angiography confirmed the proximal basilar artery occlusion (▶ Fig. 41.3a). A coaxial system of an ACE 60 aspiration catheter and a Velocity microcatheter was advanced over a Fathom 16 guidewire to the level of the basilar artery occlusion.
- After one pass of aspiration, there was complete recanalization of the basilar artery (thrombolysis in cerebral artery 3) with no distal emboli (▶ Fig. 41.3b).

41.2.2 Postprocedure Care

- A 6-Fr vascular closure device (Angio-Seal, Terumo Medical) was deployed for hemostasis.
- CT of the head was performed immediately following the intervention, as well as 24 hours later.

41.2.3 Outcome

- The patient was extubated shortly after completion of the procedure, with her being able to move all extremities better than the preprocedural phase. She was significantly better 24 hours postprocedure, with marked improvement in her strength, wakefulness, alertness, and orientation. At 3 months, she had no residual deficits (modified Rankin scale [mRS] score of 0).

41.2.4 Background

Although the role of intravenous thrombolysis (IVT) and endovascular therapy (EVT) is now well established in adults presenting with acute ischemic stroke (AIS) due to a large cerebral artery occlusion, randomized controlled trials demonstrating the same benefit in pediatric AIS patients is lacking. Despite this paucity of data, there are increasing reports in the literature of EVT in the setting of pediatric AIS, with techniques used being similar to adult therapy for certain AIS pathologies.

41.3 Discussion

Many publications on pediatric AIS exist in the literature, describing its incidence, prevalence, as well as mechanisms and etiologies, including the differences in comparison to adults

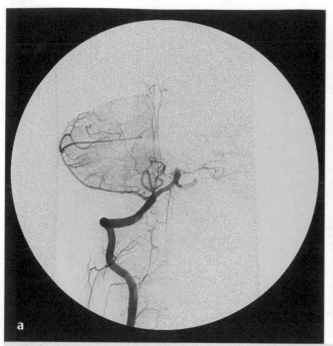
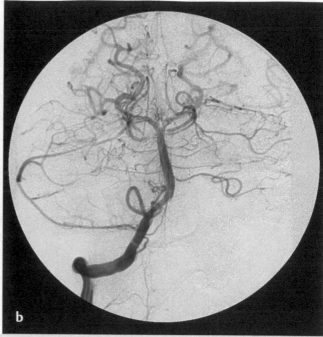

Fig. 41.3 Control angiography confirmed the proximal basilar artery occlusion (**a**). After one passage of aspiration, there was complete recanalization of the basilar artery (TICI 3) with no distal emboli (**b**).

presenting with the same syndromes.[1,2] Advances in medicine, including genetics, have been able to provide a better understanding of the many different factors playing a role in pediatric AIS. However, in most instances, rapid diagnosis and initiation of therapy able to improve patient outcome remain challenging due to the relative rarity of AIS in children compared to adults, its variable presentation, and the resultant lack of development of clinical and imaging protocols meant to recognize those able to receive IVT/EVT.

Despite the commonly held belief that pediatric patients suffering from AIS have better outcomes than adults with the same strokes, more recent literature shows that the long-term impact of stroke in children cannot simply be assessed through motor, sensory, or language deficits. Even though stroke-specific mortality is roughly 5%, persisting neurological deficits can be seen in up to 70% of older children.[1] Deotto et al have demonstrated an association with a reduction in intellectual functioning.[3] Children with AIS demonstrated poorer functioning in math, spelling, metacognition, and behavioral regulation. Williams et al not only confirmed these learning and intellectual disabilities but also demonstrated the psychological impact of AIS, especially the development of attention-deficit hyperactivity disorder.[4] Westmacott et al examined the impact of AIS on children with respect to intellectual ability, academics, attention, executive function, and psychological disorders, and reached many of the same conclusions already described. However, they demonstrated the impact of lesion location, size, and age at time of AIS with respect to the intellectual and psychological challenges these children faced afterward.[5]

As in adult AIS, imaging plays a vital role in determining the type, location, and possibly the etiology of pediatric AIS.[6] Given the different etiologies that exist for pediatric AIS (compared to adult AIS), the decision to offer medical or EVT rests on correct identification of the pathology causing flow impairment to brain tissue. While adult AIS amenable to EVT is most commonly a result of cardioembolic or artery-to-artery embolism, these diagnoses are rare in children. However, congenital heart disease and other cardiac disorders, arteriopathies, infections, traumatic head and neck disorders, as well as acute and chronic systemic conditions and prothrombotic states may give rise to large vessel occlusion in the pediatric setting.[1,2] Imaging paradigms should focus on rapid diagnosis of those AIS that are related to mechanisms amenable to emergency therapy, especially in extended time windows validated in adult EVT through DAWN) and DEFUSE 3 trials.

Several authors have published case reports, case series, as well as meta-analyses on EVT in pediatric AIS.[7,8,9,10,11,12,13,14,15,16,17,18] All have demonstrated high rates of revascularization, with excellent clinical outcomes. Although long-term outcomes, as well as prospective randomized controlled data, are lacking, techniques currently applied for adult EVT can be adapted to the pediatric setting, with the time taken to reach the target vessel occlusion likely faster in children due to the lack of arterial tortuosity. The specific technique used (stent retrievers, aspiration systems, or both) is dependent on patient-specific factors, including size and weight of the child, location of the thromboembolic occlusion, and considerations such as arterial access and target vessel diameter. Savastano et al have reported successful endovascular management of a basilar artery thrombosis in a 22-month-old patient.[19] Although significant work remains to be done in finding the true place of EVT in pediatric AIS, the ultimate goal remains the same as in adults: rapid clinical and imaging diagnosis of AIS amenable to EVT, with emergency mobilization of appropriately trained teams to perform this procedure in as short a time as possible.

41.3.1 Pearls and Pitfalls

- Pediatric AIS has many far-reaching negative impacts on the affected child, including learning and intellectual difficulties, as well as a range of psychological disorders. These can occur (and persist) despite potential rapid improvements in initial motor, sensory, and speech deficits.
- Pediatric AIS amenable to EVT is much less common than that seen in adults.
- Rapid clinical and imaging evaluation is necessary to identify those children in whom EVT may be appropriate.
- Current techniques used for performing adult EVT can be used in the pediatric setting, and may, in fact, be easier, given the relative lack of arterial tortuosity seen in children.
- The procedure likely requires general anesthetic with endotracheal intubation to ensure patient cooperation.
- Specific techniques (i.e., choice of stent retriever and/or aspiration catheter) will depend on various factors, including the weight, age, and size of the child; location of the culprit lesion; groin sheath considerations; and other medically relevant issues.

References

[1] deVeber GA, Kirton A, Booth FA, et al. Epidemiology and outcomes of arterial ischemic stroke in children: the Canadian Pediatric Ischemic Stroke Registry. Pediatr Neurol. 2017; 69:58–70

[2] Mackay MT, Wiznitzer M, Benedict SL, Lee KJ, Deveber GA, Ganesan V, International Pediatric Stroke Study Group. Arterial ischemic stroke risk factors: the International Pediatric Stroke Study. Ann Neurol. 2011; 69 (1):130–140

[3] Deotto A, Westmacott R, Fuentes A, deVeber G, Desrocher M. Does stroke impair academic achievement in children? The role of metacognition in math and spelling outcomes following pediatric stroke. J Clin Exp Neuropsychol. 2018; 413. :1–13

[4] Williams TS, McDonald KP, Roberts SD, Dlamini N, deVeber G, Westmacott R. Prevalence and predictors of learning and psychological diagnoses following pediatric arterial ischemic stroke. Dev Neuropsychol. 2017; 42(5):309–322

[5] Westmacott R, McDonald KP, Roberts SD, et al. Predictors of cognitive and academic outcome following childhood subcortical stroke. Dev Neuropsychol. 2018; 43(8):708–728

[6] Khalaf A, Iv M, Fullerton H, Wintermark M. Pediatric stroke imaging. Pediatr Neurol. 2018; 86:5–18

[7] Pacheco JT, Siepmann T, Barlinn J, et al. Safety and efficacy of recanalization therapy in pediatric stroke: a systematic review and meta-analysis. Eur J Paediatr Neurol. 2018; 22(6):1035–1041

[8] Stowe RC, Kan P, Breen DB, Agarwal S. Mechanical thrombectomy for pediatric acute stroke and ventricular assist device. Brain Dev. 2018; 40 (1):81–84

[9] Kim ES, Mason EK, Koons A, Quinn SM, Williams RL. Successful utilization of mechanical thrombectomy in a presentation of pediatric acute ischemic stroke. Case Rep Pediatr. 2018; 2018:5378247

[10] Cappellari M, Moretto G, Grazioli A, Ricciardi GK, Bovi P, Ciceri EFM. Primary versus secondary mechanical thrombectomy for anterior circulation stroke in children: An update. J Neuroradiol. 2018; 45(2):102–107

[11] Bigi S, Dulcey A, Gralla J, et al. Feasibility, safety, and outcome of recanalization treatment in childhood stroke. Ann Neurol. 2018; 83(6):1125–1132

[12] Wilson JL, Eriksson CO, Williams CN. Endovascular therapy in pediatric stroke: utilization, patient characteristics, and outcomes. Pediatr Neurol. 2017; 69:87–92.e2

[13] Satti S, Chen J, Sivapatham T, Jayaraman M, Orbach D. Mechanical thrombectomy for pediatric acute ischemic stroke: review of the literature. J Neurointerv Surg. 2017; 9(8):732–737

[14] Kulhari A, Dorn E, Pace J, et al. Acute ischemic pediatric stroke management: an extended window for mechanical thrombectomy? Front Neurol. 2017; 8:634

[15] Buompadre MC, Andres K, Slater LA, et al. Thrombectomy for acute stroke in childhood: a case report, literature review, and recommendations. Pediatr Neurol. 2017; 66:21–27

[16] Madaelil TP, Kansagra AP, Cross DT, Moran CJ, Derdeyn CP. Mechanical thrombectomy in pediatric acute ischemic stroke: clinical outcomes and literature review. Interv Neuroradiol. 2016; 22(4):426–431

[17] Lena J, Eskandari R, Infinger L, et al. Basilar artery occlusion in a child treated successfully with mechanical thrombectomy using ADAPT. BMJ Case Rep. 2016. DOI: 10.1136/bcr-2015-012195

[18] Huded V, Kamath V, Chauhan B, et al. Mechanical thrombectomy using Solitaire in a 6-year-old child. J Vasc Interv Neurol. 2015; 8(2):13–16

[19] Savastano L, Gemmete JJ, Pandey AS, Roark C, Chaudhary N. Acute ischemic stroke in a child due to basilar artery occlusion treated successfully with a stent retriever. BMJ. 2015. DOI: 10.1136/bcr-2015-011821

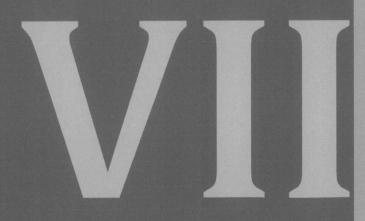

42 Hemiplegic Migraine

42.1 Case Description

42.1.1 Clinical Presentation

A 36-year-old male patient presented with 3-hour history of neurological deficit. Initial presenting symptoms were diplopia and dizziness, followed by nausea and left hemiparesthesia, with progression of symptoms to include left-sided weakness. Subsequently, during the course of his assessment in the emergency department, a right-sided headache developed with pain behind the right eye. An examination revealed normal vital signs, left facial droop, inability to visually track toward the left, left visual and sensory neglect, impaired proprioception in the left arm, and reduced power in the left upper and lower extremity. On questioning, a past medical history of migraine with aura was revealed. Otherwise there were no relevant comorbidities and cardiovascular risk factors, and family history was noncontributory.

42.1.2 Imaging Workup and Investigations

Noncontrast computed tomography (NCCT) of brain was normal, with no evidence of infarction, hyperdense vessel sign, or hemorrhage (▶ Fig. 42.1). No intracranial proximal large artery occlusion was seen on computed tomography angiography (CTA). Note was, however, made of generalized paucity of distal middle cerebral artery (MCA) branches over the right hemisphere compared to the contralateral left side (▶ Fig. 42.1). Computed tomography perfusion (CTP; ▶ Fig. 42.2) demonstrated prolonged time to peak (TTP) within the right cerebral hemisphere compared to the left, indicating delayed flow and hypoperfusion of the right hemisphere; relative cerebral blood volume was preserved.

Magnetic resonance imaging (MRI) was performed to further investigate (▶ Fig. 42.3). No abnormality was seen on T2 fluid-attenuated inversion recovery (FLAIR), or diffusion-

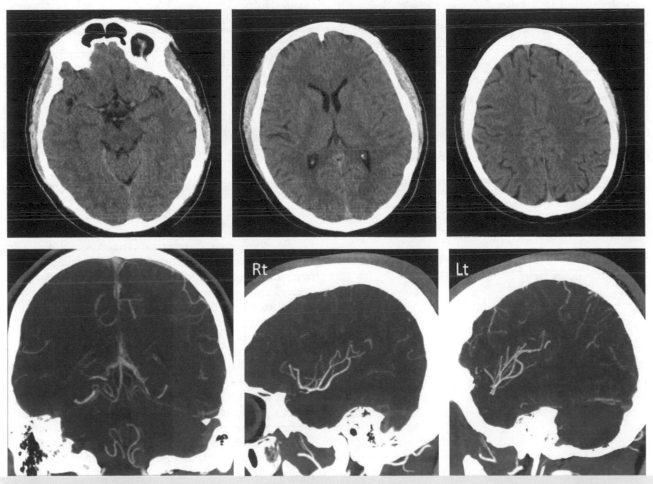

Fig. 42.1 NCCT of brain was normal, with no evidence of infarction, hyperdense vessel sign, and hemorrhage. No intracranial proximal large artery occlusion was seen on CTA. Note was however made of generalized paucity of distal MCA branches over the right hemisphere compared to the contralateral left side.

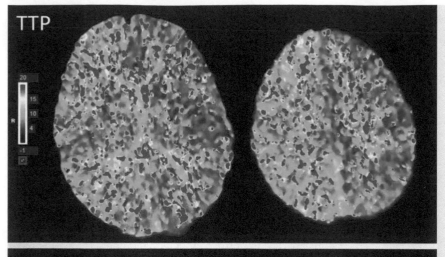

TTP

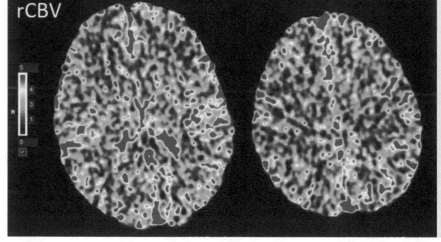

rCBV

Fig. 42.2 CTP demonstrated prolonged TTP within the right cerebral hemisphere compared to the left, indicating delayed flow and hypoperfusion of the right hemisphere.

weighted imaging (DWI). Contrast-enhanced MR angiography of the extracranial arterial system was normal, with no evidence of proximal disease or stenosis of the right common or internal carotid artery (ICA). MR venogram was also normal.

42.1.3 Diagnosis

Sporadic hemiplegic migraine (SHM).

42.1.4 Treatment

Aspirin 325 mg was administered orally at the time of initial presentation when etiology was unclear. Supportive management was instigated with intravenous fluids (500 mL normal saline), intravenous antiemetic for nausea (10 mg metoclopramide), and simple analgesia (500 mg acetaminophen). The patient's symptoms gradually improved. He was discharged from hospital 10 hours following initial onset of symptoms, at which time the left weakness and sensory disturbance were fully resolved, with residual mild headache and nausea remaining. Follow-up CTP study performed 2 days later showed reversal of previously noted prolonged right hemispheric TTP with no residual perfusion defect remaining (▶ Fig. 42.4).

42.2 Discussion

42.2.1 Background

Hemiplegic migraine is a rare form of migraine with aura, where aura includes motor weakness.[1] Typical hemiplegic migraine starts in the first or second decade of life. Patients who have an affected first- or second-degree relative are diagnosed as having familial hemiplegic migraine (FHM), whereas patients without an affected relative are considered to have SHM. FHM has an autosomal dominant mode of inheritance. Genetic studies have shown mutations in genes that encode proteins involved in ion transportation, with three genetic subtypes identified: in FHM 1, the mutation is in the CACNA1A gene on chromosome 19 which encodes for calcium channels; in FHM 2, the mutation is in the ATP1A2 gene on chromosome 1 which encodes for a subunit of the sodium–potassium ATPase pump; in FHM 3, the mutation is in the SCN1A gene on chromosome 2 which encodes for a sodium channel. Sporadic cases can be caused by a de novo mutation in a gene that causes the familial form or by inheritance of a gene mutation from an asymptomatic parent.[2] However, at least a quarter of familial and most sporadic cases do not have a mutation in these three genes, suggesting there are other involved genes still to be identified.

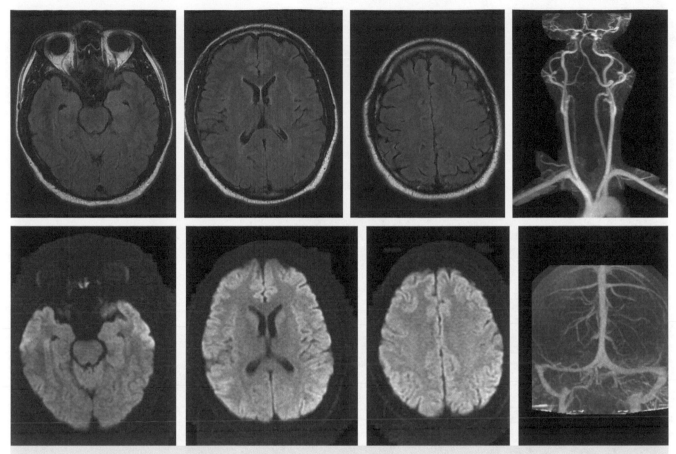

Fig. 42.3 No abnormality was seen on T2 FLAIR or DWI. Contrast-enhanced MRA of the extracranial arterial system was normal, with no evidence of proximal disease or stenosis of the right common or ICA. MR venogram was also normal.

Migraine aura pathophysiology is most probably that of cortical spreading depression, where a brief neuronal excitation initiates a depolarization wave that moves across the cortex and is followed by prolonged inhibition of neuronal activity. Dysfunction of the ion transporters coded by the gene mutations in FHM not only results in abnormal glutamate metabolism and neuronal hyperexcitability, but also reduces the threshold for cortical spreading depression.[2]

42.2.2 Workup and Diagnosis

Patient History

Diagnosis of hemiplegic migraine relies on meticulous description of the aura as well as the exclusion of symptomatic causes. The International Classification of Headache Disorders, 3rd edition (ICHD-3) lists the following diagnostic criteria for hemiplegic migraine. There must be at least two attacks which fulfill both of the following criteria: First is an aura which consists of a fully reversible motor weakness as well as fully reversible visual, sensory, and/or speech/language symptoms. Second, there must be at least two of the following four characteristics: (1) at least one aura symptom spreads gradually over 5 minutes or more and/or two or more symptoms that occur in succession; (2) each individual nonmotor aura symptom lasts 5 to 60 minutes and motor symptoms last less than 72 hours; (3) at least one aura symptom is unilateral; and (4) the aura is

accompanied or followed within 60 minutes by a headache. Finally, the symptoms should not be better accounted for by another ICHD-3 diagnosis and transient ischemic attack and stroke should have been excluded.

As seen from the diagnostic criteria, motor weakness is always associated with at least one other aura symptom, the most frequent being sensory symptoms (98%), followed by visual aura (89–90%), aphasia (72–81%), and brainstem aura (69–72%).[2,3,4]

Examination and Investigations

Motor weakness typically involves the areas affected by sensory symptoms and can vary from profound weakness to mild clumsiness.[2] Symptoms usually start in the hand, gradually spreading to involve the arm and face, and can be restricted to one limb or involve the whole hemibody. Symptoms and findings can be bilateral, or unilateral, and can switch side from attack to attack or always involve the same side. It can be difficult to distinguish weakness from sensory loss if depending solely on patient history without examination. The motor aura should be a clear deficit, that is, weakness with difficulty moving the hand, arm, or leg.[2]

A first episode of motor deficit with or without headache requires urgent and exhaustive investigations to rule out causes such as stroke, transient ischemic attack, intraparenchymal hemorrhage, and mass lesion, among others. Urgent imaging with NCCT and CTA is indicated to assess any evidence of

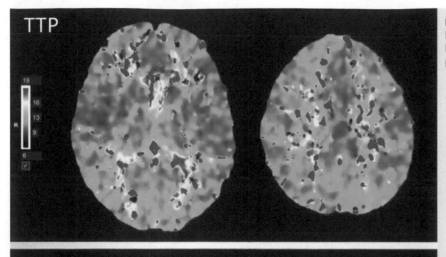

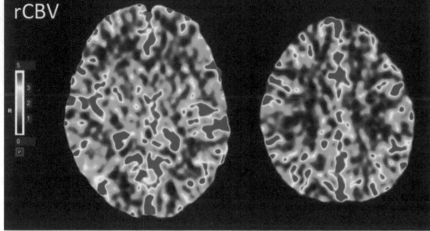

Fig. 42.4 Follow-up CTP study performed 2 days later showed reversal of previously noted prolonged right hemispheric TTP with no residual perfusion defect remaining.

hemorrhage, early or established infarction, and rule out large vessel occlusive stroke or dissection. CTP can also be performed as part of the acute stroke workup. MRI is more sensitive than CT for identifying early or small volume infarcts and should be performed if no causative abnormality is seen on CT.

Catheter angiography should be avoided as it might trigger and worsen hemiplegic migraine attacks.[2]

Cerebrospinal fluid (CSF) analysis can show an aseptic meningitis picture with elevated white blood cells (usually 12–290 white cells per mm^3) and elevated protein (up to 1 g/L), with normal glucose concentrations. CSF profile is normal between attacks. Electroencephalography can show diffuse slow wave activity contralateral to the motor deficit which may persist for several weeks.[2]

Imaging Findings

Imaging studies performed during an attack of hemiplegic migraine usually have a normal appearance; however, substantial abnormalities have been described, in particular when the attack is severe.

Perfusion abnormalities have been described in hemiplegic migraine patients investigated by MR, CT, and nuclear medicine perfusion studies during an attack. While there are some reports of patients demonstrating hyperperfusion or finding dilated vessels on angiographic imaging, patients with vasoconstriction and hypoperfusion abnormalities have also been reported, as in the

case described here. These differing findings may be related to timing of the imaging study relative to the onset of the attack, as some suggest that migraine aura is initially associated with transient hypoperfusion followed by hyperperfusion.[5]

In a study describing MR perfusion findings in acute-onset migrainous aura mimicking stroke, a clear relationship between the perfusion abnormality and aura symptoms of the patients was documented.[6] Perfusion abnormality (hypoperfusion) was evident in 14 of 20 patients in this study (70%). Patients with motor deficits, paraesthesia, or aphasia, mostly demonstrated hypoperfusion in the area of the MCA. In patients with posterior predominance of hypoperfusion, visual deterioration and nausea and/or vertigo were seen.

Other reported findings on CT or MRI include cortical edema contralateral to the hemiparesis, sometimes involving the whole hemisphere. Cortical or meningeal contrast enhancement contralateral to the hemiparesis has also been described. Imaging between attacks is usually normal with complete resolution of abnormalities seen during the attack. Cerebellar atrophy is, however, frequently observed in patients with FHM 1.[2] In severe cases of hemiplegic migraine, cortical hemispheric atrophy and cortical laminar necrosis may be seen on MRI.

42.2.3 Decision-Making Process

Once patency of the intracranial arterial system has been demonstrated, a possible differential for this pattern of hypoperfusion would be severe stenosis or dissection of the extracranial carotid artery; however, this can be ruled out by performing MRA/CTA of the neck vessels. In our acute stroke protocol, we perform CTA from the level of aortic arch to vertex in order to allow assessment of the extracranial arterial system.

Extensive unilateral cortical venous thrombosis might also show a similar pattern of hypoperfusion; however, absence of hyperdensity within cortical veins on NCCT, and absence of findings suggestive of venous thrombosis on MRI, together with patency of veins on late-phase CTA or CT/MR venography, can rule out this pathology.

42.2.4 Management

Management mainly relies on supportive treatment and use of abortive and preventative medications. Patients with prolonged symptoms or severe attacks often require hospitalization due to fever, decreased level of consciousness, or seizures.

Use of triptans in hemiplegic migraine remains controversial as there is concern that the vasoconstrictor properties of triptans may worsen the aura.[2] In a retrospective series of 76 patients with hemiplegic migraine, use of triptans appeared safe and effective for treating the headache in attacks, although one patient had a prolonged attack of hemiplegic migraine that persisted for several months following treatment.[7]

Prophylactic treatment is given in patients with frequent, long-lasting, or severe attacks. There is no randomized controlled trial evidence for therapies, specifically in hemiplegic migraine. Some limited evidence is available from case reports and small series. Prophylactic medications which can be given include oral verapamil, acetazolamide, and lamotrigine.[2]

42.2.5 Literature Synopsis

Migraine is a common disorder, affecting 15% of the population. Among one third of patients, migraine is accompanied by aura. The rare cases where there is motor weakness during the aura qualify for hemiplegic migraine. Approximately 100 to 200 families affected by FHM and approximately 200 patients affected by SHM have been published.[2] From limited epidemiological studies, prevalence of the sporadic form is approximately 0.002%[4] and prevalence of the familial form is at least 0.003%.[3]

The diagnosis of hemiplegic migraine remains a clinical one. Mean frequency of attacks is approximately three per year, but is highly variable. Frequency and severity often decrease with age. Long intervals without an attack are possible.

Some patients experience severe attacks, accompanied by encephalopathy or coma. Seizures, fever, meningism, and cerebral edema can occur with severe attacks. Aura symptoms in a severe attack may be prolonged and last from days to months before resolving. Rarely, a severe attack can result in permanent brain injury, cerebral infarction, or cerebral atrophy.

42.2.6 Pearls and Pitfalls

- Ischemic abnormalities on imaging are not typically found during hemiplegic migraine, presumably because the reduced regional cerebral blood flow after cortical spreading depression remains above the threshold for ischemia.
- In contrast to the typical pattern in stroke, the perfusion abnormality in hemiplegic migraine is usually not limited to a single vascular territory.
- Headache may not be present at presentation, but in most cases will develop at some point during the attack, mostly during the aura or after onset of visual symptoms. In rare cases, patients with hemiplegic migraine may experience no headache at all.

References

[1] et al. The international classification of headache disorders, 3rd edition (beta version). Cephalgia. 2013; 33(9):629–808

[2] Russell MB, Ducros A. Sporadic and familial hemiplegic migraine: pathophysiological mechanisms, clinical characteristics, diagnosis, and management. Lancet Neurol. 2011; 10(5):457–470

[3] Thomsen LL, Eriksen MK, Roemer SF, Andersen I, Olesen J, Russell MB. A population-based study of familial hemiplegic migraine suggests revised diagnostic criteria. Brain. 2002; 125(Pt 6):1379–1391

[4] Thomsen LL, Ostergaard E, Olesen J, Russell MB. Evidence for a separate type of migraine with aura: sporadic hemiplegic migraine. Neurology. 2003; 60(4):595–601

[5] Iizuka T, Tominaga N, Kaneko J, et al. Biphasic neurovascular changes in prolonged migraine aura in familial hemiplegic migraine type 2. J Neurol Neurosurg Psychiatry. 2015; 86(3):344–353

[6] Floery D, Vosko MR, Fellner FA, et al. Acute-onset migrainous aura mimicking acute stroke: MR perfusion imaging features. AJNR Am J Neuroradiol. 2012; 33(8):1546–1552

[7] Artto V, Nissilä M, Wessman M, Palotie A, Färkkilä M, Kallela M. Treatment of hemiplegic migraine with triptans. Eur J Neurol. 2007; 14(9):1053–1056

43 Intra-arterial Contrast Injection during Computed Tomography Angiography

43.1 Case Description

43.1.1 Clinical Presentation

A 79-year-old female patient presented with right-sided facial weakness. Medical history included metastatic breast carcinoma, hypertension, and previous surgical management of a giant anterior communicating artery (AComm) aneurysm over 30 years previously. She was a nonsmoker, with no other relevant comorbidities and cardiovascular risk factors. Family history was noncontributory.

43.1.2 Imaging Workup and Investigations

Noncontrast computed (NCCT) of the brain showed evidence of previous surgery, and a complex, multilobulated, hyperdense, partly calcified mass in the region of the inferior anterior interhemispheric fissure, in keeping with the known history of previously treated giant AComm aneurysm. There was no evidence of acute infarction (▶ Fig. 43.1a, b).

CT angiography (CTA) was also performed (▶ Fig. 43.2a–g). Iodinated contrast material was administered through peripheral vascular access in the right antecubital fossa. A total of 60 mL of contrast material was administered at an injection rate of 4 mL per second. On the CTA, only the right carotid and vertebral arteries were seen filling in the neck (▶ Fig. 43.2a). Intracranially, there was contrast opacification of the right middle cerebral artery (MCA), and bilateral anterior cerebral artery (ACA) territories, but no filling of the left internal carotid artery (ICA), left MCA or left posterior cerebral artery (PCA) territory (▶ Fig. 43.2b–g). In the posterior circulation, the right vertebral artery, basilar artery, and right cerebellar and right PCA branches were filling. There was opacification of the left anterior inferior cerebellar artery and left superior cerebellar artery territories, but no filling of the left vertebral artery or left

posterior inferior cerebellar artery territory (▶ Fig. 43.2b, c, g). The visualized intracranial arteries were densely opacified with contrast, avid enhancement of leptomeningeal vessels, and greater than expected brain parenchymal enhancement, giving an appearance which could be referred to as a "superscan."

The previously treated aneurysm did not fill on CTA. An incidental note was also made of dense sclerosis and thickening of the bones of the cranial vault, and a destructive process involving the left occipital condyle (arrow), in keeping with boney metastatic disease.

43.1.3 Diagnosis

Stroke mimic: inadvertent intra-arterial administration of iodinated contrast material for CTA.

43.1.4 Treatment

The referring physicians were immediately notified that an inadvertent intra-arterial contrast administration had occurred, the vascular access in the right antecubital fossa, which was believed to be venous had instead been inadvertently placed in the right brachial artery. The cannula was immediately removed, and hemostasis achieved with local pressure. The patient was observed, and had no adverse effects after the injection or on the next day, and required no further management. There was no recurrence of the right transient facial weakness, examination showed no focal neurological deficit, and further management was not instigated.

43.2 Discussion

43.2.1 Background

Inadvertent intra-arterial injection of contrast for CT studies is rare, but is of potential significance when it does occur. There

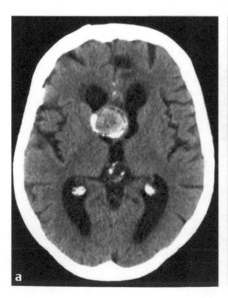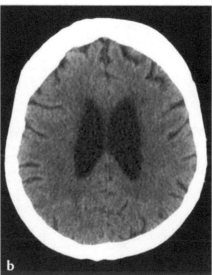

Fig. 43.1 Noncontrast enhanced CT of the brain showed evidence of previous surgery, and a complex multilobulated, hyperdense, partly calcified mass in the region of the inferior anterior interhemispheric fissure, in keeping with the known history of previously treated giant anterior communicating artery aneurysm. There was no evidence of acute infarction.

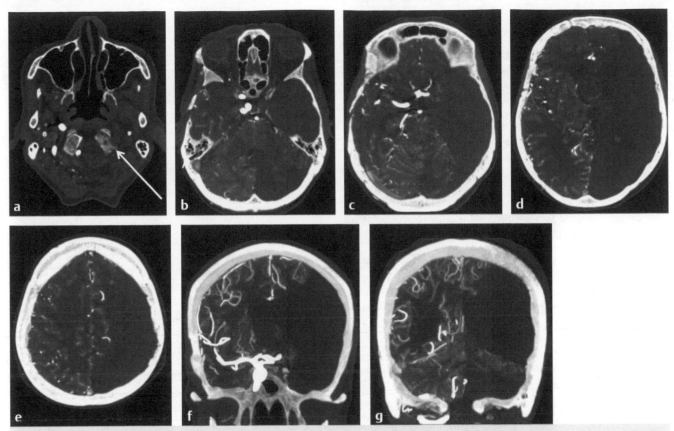

Fig. 43.2 On the CTA, only the right carotid and vertebral arteries were seen filling in the neck (**a**). Intracranially, there was contrast opacification of the right MCA, and bilateral ACA territories, but no filling of the left ICA, left MCA, or left PCA territory (**b–g**). In the posterior circulation, the right vertebral artery, basilar artery, and right cerebellar and right PCA branches were filling. There was opacification of the left anterior inferior cerebellar artery and left superior cerebellar artery territories, but no filling of the left vertebral artery or left posterior inferior cerebellar artery territory (**b, c, g**). The visualized intracranial arteries were densely opacified with contrast, avid enhancement of leptomeningeal vessels, and greater than expected brain parenchymal enhancement.

are two main concerns: first, regarding the potential adverse clinical effects of an intra-arterial injection; second, regarding the potential for either a nondiagnostic study or misinterpretation of the appearances on subsequent CT.

43.2.2 Workup and Diagnosis

Patient History

Correlation with the provided patient history can prove to be not only invaluable for the interpreting radiologist but also help avoid misinterpretation. For example, in this case, it would be extremely unlikely that a patient with nonfilling of almost the entire left hemisphere on CTA would have symptoms only of a transient right facial weakness. While it is possible that a patient with large artery occlusion could present in such a way, if there was excellent collateralization to the occluded territory, for example, through the circle of Willis or leptomeningeal collaterals, no such "collateralization" was evident on CTA in this case. This discrepancy between imaging appearance and history can alert the radiologist to the fact that something is amiss.

From an inadvertent intra-arterial access point of view, indicators in the patient history suggestive of an intra-arterial

rather than venous injection would include a report of intense pain on administration of the administered drug, pulsatile return of blood from the access cannula, vascular access in a site such as the antecubital fossa where there is proximity of an artery to vein, and possibly later symptoms of complicating distal limb ischemia.[1]

Examination and Investigations

When obtaining peripheral vascular access, distinguishing a superficial vessel as an artery rather than vein is not always straightforward. Absence of sensation of pulsation is not always reliable, and partial occlusion of arterial flow by an applied tourniquet may be one reason for this.[1] Awareness of the common patterns of arterial variation in the upper limb can facilitate early detection of inadvertent intra-arterial cannulation, and the possibility of this occurring should be kept in mind whenever cannulation is performed in the antecubital fossa or ventromedial aspect of the forearm.

In situations where cannulation has been performed, and there is uncertainty as to whether artery or vein has been accessed, blood gas analysis can be performed to help distinguish arterial from venous access.[2]

Imaging Findings

In the case described here, the CTA appearances were a result of intra-arterial injection into the right brachial artery, with resultant retrograde filling of the right vertebral, innominate, and right carotid arteries. The appearance of avid enhancement of leptomeningeal vessels and greater than expected brain parenchymal enhancement was due to the large volume of contrast reaching the cerebral circulation on the right without dilution in the systemic circulation. The absence of filling of the left PCA territory can be explained by a left fetal type PCA, which is a normal anatomical variant. A further clue on imaging in this case was the absence of filling of the left vertebral artery and left posterior inferior cerebellar artery (PICA) territory, as contrast was not injected with sufficient pressure to reflux from the right vertebral artery to retrogradely fill the left side.

If the inadvertent intra-arterial access had been in the left upper limb, then retrograde filling of only the left vertebral artery and distal territory would be seen on intracranial CTA, unless there was contribution to the anterior circulation through a posterior communicating (PComm) artery or other normal variant anatomy.

43.2.3 Decision-Making Process

The appearance of avid enhancement of leptomeningeal vessels and greater than expected brain parenchymal enhancement on the CTA study alerts the radiologist that something is amiss. With no evidence of established infarction, the combination of nonfilling of the left vertebral artery and PICA territory, as well as nonfilling of the left ICA, PCA and MCA territories would require concomitant occlusion of at least the left ICA and left vertebral artery. Multifocal arterial occlusion can occur, with some literature reporting up to 20% of cases showing arterial occlusion in different territories[3,4]; however, this usually refers to the intracranial circulation, and the likelihood of simultaneous acute occlusion of a vertebral and carotid artery would be relatively low.

Correlation with NCCT for absence of early or established ischemic change, correlation with patient history and examination, and a knowledge of intracranial arterial anatomy and normal variants allows the correct diagnosis to be reached.

Performing CTA from the level of the aortic arch, rather than from the upper neck or base of skull level, adds additional information, showing contrast in the ipsilateral subclavian artery with nonopacification of the contralateral subclavian artery and other great vessels from the aortic arch, thus simplifying the decision-making process and diagnosis.

43.2.4 Management

Management mainly relies on removal of the inadvertently placed cannula, supportive treatment, and observation of limb complications such as distal ischemia. Anecdotally from this case, and other described cases in the literature,[2,5] permanent adverse effects of inadvertent intra-arterial iodinated contrast administrations were not seen. There is, however, extensive literature describing complications such as distal ischemia and gangrene following inadvertent intra-arterial administration of medications, including antibiotics, narcotics, and anesthetic agents.[6]

43.2.5 Literature Synopsis

There are some published case reports of inadvertent intra-arterial administration of iodinated contrast material during CT.[2,5] Morhard et al[2] have described a case of inadvertent intra-arterial contrast administration mimicking bilateral ICA occlusion in a suspected stroke patient on CT perfusion (CTP) imaging. In this case, CTP maps demonstrated substantially delayed and decreased perfusion of the entire bilateral anterior circulation, with normal filling of all intracranial arteries on subsequently acquired CTA. Once significant stenosis of the supraaortic arteries had been ruled out, the discrepant CTA and CTP findings were presumed to be due to erroneous analysis of the CTP data. However, review of the raw data which showed isolated contrast enhancement of the posterior circulation only in the early phase, and subsequent delayed enhancement of intracranial circulation together with blood gas analysis from the antecubital fossa, allowed the correct conclusions of inadvertent intra-arterial administration of contrast to be drawn.

Gupta et al[5] have described a case of inadvertent intra-arterial cannulation and iodinated contrast administration in a patient undergoing coronary CTA. In this case, the study was performed with bolus-tracking technique, and an unexpected delay was noted in the triggering of the scan. Review of the images showed no contrast in the coronary arteries and minimal contrast in the aortic arch; however, there was contrast opacification of the right subclavian and common carotid arteries, allowing the correct diagnosis of inadvertent intra-arterial contrast administration to be made.

In both of these cases from the literature, no adverse sequelae occurred following the intra-arterial contrast administration.

An awareness of arterial anatomical variation of the upper limb is important, potentially facilitating early recognition of inadvertent intra-arterial cannulation. Patterns of arterial variations of the upper limb have been described by Rodriguez-Niedenfuhr et al.[7,8] A superficial ulnar artery is the most commonly seen superficial artery in the forearm, seen in almost 4% of subjects, which is closely related to the course of the basilic vein. A superficial radial artery is a less commonly encountered aberrant superficial artery, seen in less than 0.2% of subjects, which is also at risk of puncture due to its proximity to the cephalic vein. As a result, the possibility of inadvertent intra-arterial cannulation should be borne in mind when attempting venous cannulation in the antecubital fossa and ventromedial forearm.

43.2.6 Pearls and Pitfalls

- On CTA, the presence of intense enhancement and absence of filling in an entire hemisphere, or filling of only a single vascular territory (e.g., filling of only the left vertebral artery territory in a patient with left-sided intra-arterial access), should alert the radiologist to the possibility that inadvertent intra-arterial contrast administration has occurred.
- Early recognition of this constellation of imaging findings is essential to avoid misinterpretation of CTA and erroneous diagnosis of large territory stroke.

- Correlation with NCCT for absence of early or established ischemic change, correlation with patient history and examination, and a knowledge of intracranial arterial anatomy and normal variants allows the correct diagnosis to be reached.
- Early recognition of inadvertent intra-arterial cannulation is crucial to avoid potential repetition of further nondiagnostic, contrast-enhanced studies, as well as potential intra-arterial injection of drugs associated with high incidence of limb complications. If there is doubt during cannulation, blood gas analysis can help distinguish arterial from venous access.

References

[1] Chin KJ, Singh K. The superficial ulnar artery–a potential hazard in patients with difficult venous access. Br J Anaesth. 2005; 94(5):692–693

[2] Morhard D, Pellkofer H, Reiser MF, Ertl-Wagner B. Inadvertent intra-arterial contrast agent injection mimicking bilateral occlusion of the internal carotid arteries in a patient with suspected stroke on maximum-slope, nondeconvolution perfusion computed tomography. Stroke. 2009; 40(3): e46–e49

[3] Galimanis A, Jung S, Mono ML, et al. Endovascular therapy of 623 patients with anterior circulation stroke. Stroke. 2012; 43(4):1052–1057

[4] Power S, McEvoy SH, Cunningham J, et al. Value of CT angiography in anterior circulation large vessel occlusive stroke: imaging findings, pearls, and pitfalls. Eur J Radiol. 2015; 84(7):1333–1344

[5] Gupta P, Gulati GS, Guleria M. Contrast injected, scan triggered, but where has contrast gone? Indian J Radiol Imaging. 2012; 22(3):186–187

[6] Sen S, Chini EN, Brown MJ. Complications after unintentional intra-arterial injection of drugs: risks, outcomes, and management strategies. Mayo Clin Proc. 2005; 80(6):783–795

[7] Rodríguez-Niedenführ M, Vázquez T, Nearn L, Ferreira B, Parkin I, Sañudo JR. Variations of the arterial pattern in the upper limb revisited: a morphological and statistical study, with a review of the literature. J Anat. 2001; 199(Pt 5):547–566

[8] Rodriguez-Niedenfuhr M, Vazquez T, Parkin IG, et al. Arterial patterns of the human upper limb: update of anatomical variations and embryological development. Eur J Anat. 2003; 7 Suppl 1:21–28

44 Mitochondrial Encephalomyopathy, Lactic Acidosis, and Stroke-Like Episodes (MELAS)

44.1 Case Description

44.1.1 Clinical Presentation

A 26-year-old Chinese male patient was brought to the emergency department with a history of transient nausea and vomiting 3 weeks prior to presentation, which was followed by gradual progressive confusion with a sudden inability to express himself on the day of his arrival to the hospital. On examination, he was somnolent and was found to have dysphasia, dysarthria, and a right homonymous hemianopia.

His past medical history was remarkable for insulin-dependent diabetes mellitus and for the development of gradual hearing loss over the last few months prior to presentation. He had a strikingly short stature, a poor physical tolerance since childhood, and learning difficulties. His family history was noncontributory.

He was admitted for further investigations. During admission, he developed focal occipital seizures with secondary generalization treated with carbamazepine.

44.1.2 Imaging Workup and Investigations

The initial noncontrast enhanced CT of the brain showed multiple hypodense areas within the left occipital, parietal, and temporal lobes (▶ Fig. 44.1).

Subsequent MRI of the brain performed on the same day revealed hyperintensity on T2 fluid-attenuated inversion recovery (FLAIR) imaging in the left parietal, occipital, and temporal lobe (▶ Fig. 44.2a) as well as in the left thalamus with a high signal on diffusion-weighted imaging (DWI; ▶ Fig. 44.2b) but without decreased signal on apparent diffusion coefficient (ADC; ▶ Fig. 44.2c). Abnormality mainly affected the cortical gray matter with gyral swelling and some subcortical white

matter involvement. Contrast-enhanced T1-weighted images showed mild leptomeningeal enhancement in the affected areas (▶ Fig. 44.2d). MR angiography including MR venography was unremarkable (not shown). Note was also made of mild generalized atrophy for age.

MR spectroscopy was obtained. In the region of abnormal signal in the left hemisphere, a double peak was found between 1.2 and 1.4 ppm, in the expected location of lactate (resonates at 1.3 ppm), and inversion of the doublet was seen at a longer echo time (▶ Fig. 44.3). Also in the contralateral nonaffected brain tissue, a lactate peak was found, although less pronounced.

On serum and cerebrospinal fluid (CSF) analysis, lactate was elevated, while infectious workup was negative and electroencephalography (EEG) did not demonstrate ongoing epileptic discharges.

Electrocardiography showed sinus rhythm with Wolff–Parkinson–White conduction abnormality.

On molecular investigations, an A3243G transition was found, which confirmed the diagnosis of mitochondrial encephalomyopathy with lactic acidosis and stroke-like episodes (MELAS).

44.1.3 Diagnosis

MELAS.

44.1.4 Treatment

This patient received a metabolic cocktail consisting of idebenone, L-arginine, riboflavin, creatine, and ascorbic acid. He gradually recovered from his strokes and did not develop new stroke-like episodes over a 5-year period. His seizures were well controlled with carbamazepine and he remained stable from a cardiac standpoint.

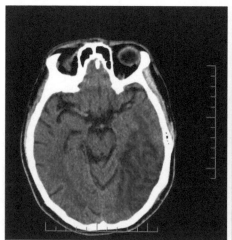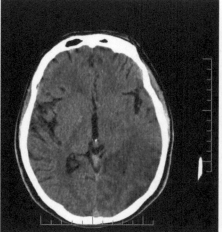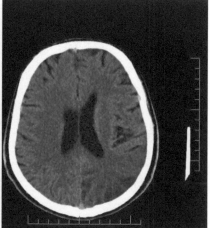

Fig. 44.1 Noncontrast CT of the head, axial images, demonstrated low-attenuation in the left occipital, parietal, and temporal lobe involving cortex and subcortical white matter with sulcal effacement.

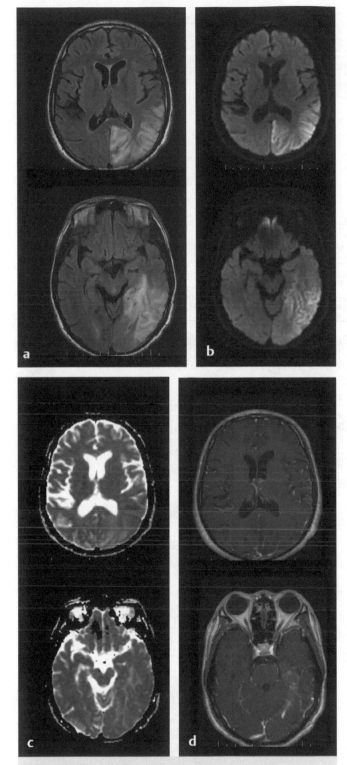

Fig. 44.2 MRI brain, performed on same day as CT in ▶ Fig. 44.1, revealed hyperintensity on T2 FLAIR imaging in the left parietal, occipital, and temporal lobe (a) as well as in the left posterior thalamus. There was high signal on DWI in the occipital, temporal and parietal region (b) but without decreased signal on ADC (c). Signal abnormality on imaging affected mainly the cortical gray matter with gyral swelling. To a lesser extent there was some subcortical white matter involvement (a). Contrast-enhanced T1-weighted images showed mild leptomeningeal enhancement in the affected areas (d).

44.2 Discussion

44.2.1 Background

Mutations in the mitochondrial DNA (mDNA), or in nuclear genes coding for proteins involved in the respiratory chain, may result in mitochondrial dysfunction, which typically affects organs with high-energy requirements such as the brain and skeletal muscles. In mitochondrial diseases, the mutation is not present in all cells and tissues, the so-called heteroplasmy, and the number of mutated cells needs to exceed a certain threshold to become clinically manifest (threshold effect). Even if clinically manifest, the amount of mutant mDNA does not correlate with the severity of the disease. This together with the heteroplasmy and threshold effect makes the diagnosis of mitochondrial diseases challenging. Diagnosis usually relies on a combination of clinical features, biochemical test results, and structural findings on imaging.

The prevalence of mitochondrial disease is higher than previously thought; clinical studies have found a frequency of 9.2/100,000 adults younger than 65 years with clinically manifested mitochondrial disease caused by a mutation in mDNA, making this one of the most common inherited neuromuscular disorders. MELAS is one of the most frequent maternally inherited mitochondrial diseases. In 80% of patients, it is caused by an A to G point mutation at position 3243 in the mDNA in the MT-TL1 gene. There are also other mitochondrial and nuclear DNA mutations associated with MELAS, such as mutations in the POLG (polymerase gamma 1) gene. The A3243G point mutation has a frequency up to 1 in 400 in the general population. The prevalence of manifest disease was found to be 0.2:100,000 in a study from Japan.

44.2.2 Workup and Diagnosis

Patient History

Symptoms typically manifest before the age of 20 years, and only 1 to 6% of patients present after the age of 40. The disease is progressive and clinical manifestations are diverse, as several organ systems are involved. Patients can present with stroke-like episodes, dementia, epilepsy, lactic acidemia, myopathy, migrainous headaches, sensorineural hearing loss, diabetes mellitus, and short stature caused by growth hormone deficiency. In addition, cardiac diseases such as hypertrophic cardiomyopathy or conduction abnormalities, psychiatric manifestations, cyclic vomiting, peripheral neuropathy, and progressive encephalopathy can be part of this syndrome. The most recent diagnostic criteria for a definitive diagnosis of MELAS require the presence of two category A and two category B criteria. Category A criteria include clinical stroke-like episodes, headache with vomiting, seizures, hemiplegia, cortical blindness/hemianopsia, or an acute focal lesion observed via brain imaging. Category B criteria comprise evidence of mitochondrial dysfunction, high-lactate levels in plasma/CSF or deficiency of mitochondrial-related enzyme activities, mitochondrial abnormalities in muscle biopsy, or definitive gene mutation related to MELAS.

Stroke-like episodes are a hallmark of MELAS; however, the mechanism of these episodes is not well understood. Patients

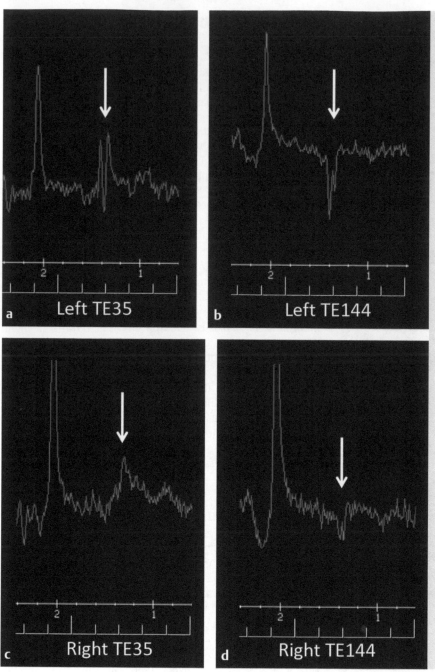

Fig. 44.3 MR spectroscopy was obtained. In the region of abnormal signal in the left hemisphere, a double peak was found at 1.3 ppm (**a**), with inversion of the doublet seen at a longer echo time (**b**), features in keeping with a lactate peak. Also in the contralateral nonaffected brain tissue, a lactate peak was found, though less pronounced (**c,d**).

present with acute or subacute focal neurological deficits, typically hemiparesis and visual field defects, which can improve over time. There are three hypotheses to explain the pathophysiology of stroke-like episodes. The first theory is an ischemic vascular mechanism, presumably caused by mitochondrial angiopathy, where cerebral infarcts occur as a result of impaired autoregulation and segmental impairment of vasodilation of the small arteries induced by mitochondrial dysfunction. It remains unknown whether ischemic processes trigger the onset of the stroke-like episodes. The ischemic vascular theory cannot explain some of the features of MELAS, such as continuous spread of the stroke-like lesions and the predominant nature of vasogenic edema. The second hypothesis is the generalized cytopathic theory, wherein a defect in the oxidative phosphorylation pathway causes generalized cytopathy. This

would explain why a lactate peak is also found in normal-appearing brain tissue on imaging and the cerebrovascular reserve capacity is spared in MELAS patients. The third hypothesis concerns a nonischemic neurovascular cellular underlying mechanism where neuronal hyperexcitability (i.e., epileptic activity) increases the energy demand, which cannot be delivered due to the oxidative phosphorylation defect.

Examination and Investigations

Findings on examination of patients presenting with stroke-like episodes are dependent on the region of brain involvement, and clinical findings typically correlate with location of abnormality on imaging. Classically, the occipital lobe is affected with or without the involvement of the parietal lobe.

Wolff–Parkinson–White syndrome and conduction block are often identified on an electrocardiogram, and cardiac ultrasound may demonstrate hypertrophic cardiomyopathy that can remain asymptomatic until an advanced stage.

Serum and CSF lactate are increased due to impaired oxidative phosphorylation.

A muscle biopsy can demonstrate ragged red fibers and succinate dehydrogenase reactive vessels. This is not a specific finding for MELAS but indicative of mitochondrial disease.

Imaging Findings

In patients with MELAS, imaging can be normal even in the case of a high mutation load.

Noncontrast CT can demonstrate hypodensities, often in the parietooccipital and parietotemporal regions. Bilateral calcifications in the basal ganglia may be found as well as generalized atrophy, findings which are more prominent features in older patients.

MRI can also demonstrate stroke-like lesions, most often involving the parietooccipital and parietotemporal regions. Lesions do not follow arterial vascular territories and predominantly involve cortex which has a high-energy demand. This suggests that the underlying mechanism is not disruption of arterial blood supply but rather metabolic failure. Acute lesions will show cortical swelling and may demonstrate enhancement. Subcortical white matter can also be involved. Lesions are hyperintense on T2-weighted images, and also show high signal on DWI. ADC is reportedly variable; ADC may be increased, normal, or decreased. Apart from focal lesions, MRI in MELAS may show diffuse white matter changes and generalized atrophy.

The diverse ADC changes in MELAS are poorly understood. It has been suggested that the diverse ADC changes reflect the gradual evolution of cytotoxic edema in this condition in contrast to the more acute evolution of cytotoxic edema seen with arterial strokes. Patients may be scanned at different points in time, which would explain the differing ADC reports in the literature. There still exist conflicting reports of lesions with differing ADC values even when imaging is performed in the early stage of presentation. It is possible, since the symptoms in MELAS are nonspecific, that even in "early presentation," findings of normal or increased ADC may reflect an already evolving lesion and pseudonormalization of cytotoxic edema. Alternatively, based on the hyperexcitability theory, the mismatch between energy demand and availability may cause vasogenic and cytotoxic edema. This is supported by the finding that 80% of patients who present with stroke-like episodes have epileptic activity on EEG. Several reports have demonstrated a slowly progressive and spreading pattern of the infarct-like lesions in MELAS; therefore, as lesions evolve and new areas become involved, this could lead to a temporal overlap of the processes of vasogenic and cytotoxic edema.

Although there are some reversible lesions, the edematous swelling can evolve to cortical laminar necrosis and eventually to irreversible encephalomalacia indicating irreversible damage, regardless of the initial ADC changes.

Angiographic techniques (CT angiography, MR angiography, and digital subtraction angiography) are usually normal.

Perfusion studies may show hyperperfusion in the acute stage (< 1 month) and hypoperfusion in the chronic stage several months later. A common finding is hypoperfusion in the posterior cingulate cortex, which is also a finding in Alzheimer disease.

Positron emission tomography during symptomatic presentations may reveal normal or increased cerebral blood flow in cortical regions, reduced cerebral metabolic rate for oxygen, and preservation/increase of the cerebral metabolic rate for glucose, further evidence that pathophysiology is that of metabolic failure.

In MELAS, MR spectroscopy demonstrates a lactate peak in areas of parenchymal abnormality on brain imaging as well as in normal appearing brain parenchyma. N-acetylaspartate/creatine ratio is reduced.

When the clinical picture and imaging findings are suggestive of MELAS, testing for mDNA mutations and sequencing of the POLG gene are indicated.

44.2.3 Decision-Making Process

In the acute setting of a stroke-like episode, one may not immediately search for diagnostic clues toward mitochondrial disease. The pattern on CT or MRI will likely trigger this rare differential diagnosis of ischemic stroke. Especially when a stroke-like lesion is predominantly located in the cortex, does not follow an arterial territory, involves the occipital with or without the parietal lobe, with a normal arterial and venous angiography, one should include MELAS in the differential diagnosis. An EEG should be performed to rule out status epilepticus. For further diagnosis of the disease, one should search for involvement of other organ systems, assess lactate levels in serum and CSF, consider MR spectroscopy, and proceed with testing for mDNA mutations.

44.2.4 Management

There is currently no definite effective treatment for MELAS. Various supportive measures are available, although no controlled trial has proven efficacy. Long-term benefits of dietary manipulations are not known. There are reports on the positive effect of coenzyme Q10 and its analogue idebenone. Also, riboflavin may be effective in specific cases. Studies in Japan reported on the positive effect of L-arginine in the acute treatment as well as in the prevention of stroke-like episodes. L-arginine is a nitric oxide precursor and may compensate for the impaired vasodilation in intracerebral arteries caused by mitochondrial dysfunction and thereby reduce ischemic damage. There is growing evidence that treatment with arginine is beneficial in MELAS patients to prevent stroke and to decrease stroke severity.

When patients have recurrent symptomatic tachyarrhythmia caused by Wolff–Parkinson–White syndrome, radiofrequency ablation should be considered.

Certain medications should be avoided in patients with mitochondrial disease, such as sodium valproate, since it has been associated with significant liver disease. Carbamazepine should be used with caution as it increases the risk of developing hyponatremia. Alternatives are levetiracetam, lamotrigine, and clonazepam. Other medications that should be avoided are aspirin, metformin, aminoglycosides, halothane, barbiturates, Ringer lactate, and statins.

44.2.5 Literature Synopsis

MELAS is a progressive neurodegenerative mitochondrial disorder with a wide range of clinical manifestations including stroke-like episodes, a hallmark of the disease. The pathophysiology of these episodes is unclear and the stroke-like lesions on MRI seem to be a combination of vasogenic and cytotoxic edema. The diagnosis is based on the combination of clinical presentation, imaging patterns, and molecular testing. There is currently no effective treatment for this condition.

44.2.6 Pearls and Pitfalls

- In 80% of patients, MELAS is caused by an A3245G mutation in mitochondrial DNA.
- MRI demonstrates stroke-like lesions that are predominantly located in the cortex, can have subcortical white matter involvement, and do not follow an arterial territory.
- Predominantly affected areas on imaging are the parietooccipital and parietotemporal regions.
- MR spectroscopy demonstrates a lactate peak in areas of parenchymal abnormality on brain imaging as well as in normal-appearing brain parenchyma.
- On MRI, ADC changes of lesions in MELAS can be diverse.
- Venous angiography should be considered to rule out venous infarction and EEG should rule out status epilepticus.

Further Readings

Schaefer AM, McFarland R, Blakely EL, et al. Prevalence of mitochondrial DNA disease in adults. Ann Neurol. 2008; 63(1):35–39

El-Hattab AW, Adesina AM, Jones J, Scaglia F. MELAS syndrome: clinical manifestations, pathogenesis, and treatment options. Mol Genet Metab. 2015; 116(1–2):4–12

Yatsuga S, Povalko N, Nishioka J, et al. Taro Matsuoka for MELAS Study Group in Japan. MELAS: a nationwide prospective cohort study of 96 patients in Japan. Biochim Biophys Acta. 2012; 1820(5):619–624

Iizuka T, Sakai F. Pathogenesis of stroke-like episodes in MELAS: analysis of neurovascular cellular mechanisms. Curr Neurovasc Res. 2005; 2(1):29–45

Ito H, Mori K, Harada M, et al. Serial brain imaging analysis of stroke-like episodes in MELAS. Brain Dev. 2008; 30(7):483–488

McFarland R, Taylor RW, Turnbull DM. A neurological perspective on mitochondrial disease. Lancet Neurol. 2010; 9(8):829–840

Oppenheim C, Galanaud D, Samson Y, et al. Can diffusion weighted magnetic resonance imaging help differentiate stroke from stroke-like events in MELAS? J Neurol Neurosurg Psychiatry. 2000; 69(2):248–250

Ito H, Mori K, Kagami S. Neuroimaging of stroke-like episodes in MELAS. Brain Dev. 2011; 33(4):283–288

Manwaring N, Jones MM, Wang JJ, et al. Population prevalence of the MELAS A3243G mutation. Mitochondrion. 2007; 7(3):230–233

Sproule DM, Kaufmann P, Engelstad K, Starc TJ, Hordof AJ, De Vivo DC. Wolff-Parkinson-White syndrome in patients with MELAS. Arch Neurol. 2007; 64 (11):1625–1627

Koga Y, Povalko N, Nishioka J, Katayama K, Kakimoto N, Matsuishi T. MELAS and L-arginine therapy: pathophysiology of stroke-like episodes. Ann N Y Acad Sci. 2010; 1201:104–110

Tzoulis C, Bindoff LA. Serial diffusion imaging in a case of mitochondrial encephalomyopathy, lactic acidosis, and stroke-like episodes. Stroke. 2009; 40 (2):e15–e17

Pfeffer G, Majamaa K, Turnbull DM, Thorburn D, Chinnery PF. Treatment for mitochondrial disorders. Cochrane Database Syst Rev. 2012; 18(4):CD004426

Wilichowski E, Pouwels PJ, Frahm J, Hanefeld F. Quantitative proton magnetic resonance spectroscopy of cerebral metabolic disturbances in patients with MELAS. Neuropediatrics. 1999; 30(5):256–263

Castillo M, Kwock L, Green C. MELAS syndrome: imaging and proton MR spectroscopic findings. AJNR Am J Neuroradiol. 1995; 16(2):233–239

Koenig MK, Emrick L, Karaa A, et al. Recommendations for the management of strokelike episodes in patients with mitochiondrial encephalomyopathy lactic acidosis, and strokelike episodes. JAMA Neurol. 2016; 73(5):591–594

45 Reversible Cerebral Vasoconstriction Syndrome

45.1 Case Description

45.1.1 Clinical Presentation

A 65-year-old female patient of Filipina-Canadian descent presented with acute-onset headache with a 10 out of 10 severity. Headache had begun acutely 4 days prior to visiting the hospital. It was characterized as diffuse and bilateral, centered at the vertex of her skull. The headache was described as different in character from the patients' normal migraines. There were no associated symptoms such as visual symptoms, nausea or vomiting, photophobia, phonophobia, meningismus, or focal neurological deficits. The patient's headache improved 30 to 45 minutes after taking ibuprofen, although it did not resolve completely. She continued to take ibuprofen every 4 to 6 hours over the next 4 days; however, the headache worsened. The patient went to her local hospital where a noncontrast CT of the head was performed, which showed subarachnoid hemorrhage over the left frontal convexity (▶ Fig. 45.1). She was then transferred to a tertiary hospital and was assessed by neurology and neurosurgery; thereafter, she was admitted for treatment and further investigations. On physical examination, no focal neurological deficits were found. Laboratory investigations showed the patient to be a chronic hepatitis B carrier. Her hepatitis was not active during the course of admission. Rheumatology was consulted with working diagnosis of cerebral vasculitis versus reversible cerebral vasoconstriction syndrome (RCVS). Rheumatology blood panel was negative.

45.1.2 Imaging Workup and Investigations

- Initial noncontrast CT of the head demonstrated a focal area of hyperdensity, compatible with subarachnoid hemorrhage,

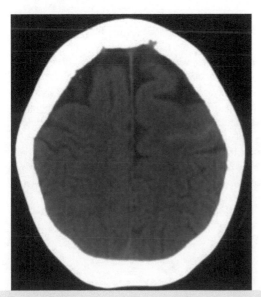

Fig. 45.1 Noncontrast CT of the head, axial image, demonstrated subarachnoid hemorrhage involving high left cerebral convexity sulci.

within a left frontal convexity sulcus. Subsequent CTA did not demonstrate a vascular cause for subarachnoid hemorrhage.
- MRI of the brain exhibited sulcal hyperintensity on the fluid-attenuated inversion recovery (FLAIR) sequence and gradient echo T2 hyperintensity overlying the left frontal and parietal lobes adjacent to the central sulcus, in keeping with subarachnoid hemorrhage.
- Catheter angiography was performed which exhibited multiple focal segmental areas of mild arterial narrowing, involving the pericallosal artery and distal cortical anterior cerebral artery branches, as well as the mid and distal middle cerebral artery branches. There were also similar findings in the distal posterior cerebral arteries more prominent on the left (▶ Fig. 45.2).
- Follow-up angiogram was performed four weeks after the initial catheter angiography, and there was interval resolution of the previously noted areas of arterial narrowings.

45.1.3 Diagnosis

Reversible cerebral vasoconstriction syndrome.

45.1.4 Treatment and Follow-up

The patient was treated with Solu-Medrol and prednisone for the working diagnosis of vasculitis, with a tapering dose over 3 months following discharge. She was also initially treated with Nimodipine and then Verapamil for possible RCVS. Acute pain service provided supportive management for pain control. She was discharged with satisfactory resolution of her headaches and returned for follow-up catheter angiogram 4 weeks following discharge.

45.1.5 Outcome

The patient remained asymptomatic on her last follow-up visit, 7 months after initial presentation.

45.2 Discussion

45.2.1 Background

RCVS is a clinicoangiographic syndrome characterized angiographically by reversible diffuse-multifocal narrowing of the cerebral arteries, and typically associated with single or recurrent episodes of sudden and severe thunderclap headaches. This may be complicated by ischemic or hemorrhagic strokes and a variety of other neurological complications.[1,2,3,4,5,6]

It was also previously known as Call–Fleming syndrome among other names such as thunderclap headache with reversible vasospasm, postpartum cerebral angiitis, central nervous system pseudovasculitis, and benign angiopathy of the central nervous system.[5,7,8,9,10]

The syndrome is considered relatively rare and its exact incidence is unknown.[5] It appears to be more common in women than in men with a ratio of 2.4:1 and the mean age of presentation is 42 years (range: 10–76 years) with no clear ethnicity group specification.[2,3,4,5,11]

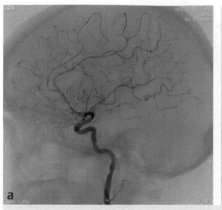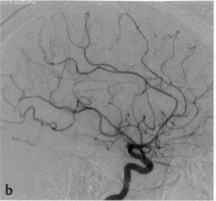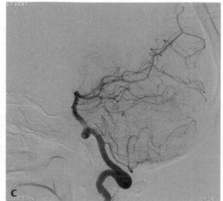

Fig. 45.2 Catheter angiography anteroposterior (a) and 3D spin (b) images show multiple focal segmental areas of mild arterial narrowing involving the pericallosal artery and distal cortical ACA branches, as well as the mid and distal MCA branches. Similar findings were evident in the distal PCAs (c).

45.2.2 Pathology

The pathophysiology of RCVS is poorly understood. Many theories have been postulated, including sympathetic overactivity, dysregulation of vascular tone of intracranial arteries, and blood–brain barrier (BBB) breakdown. The latter was demonstrated in a study conducted by Lee et al.[12] It was based on the idea that the contrast-enhancing FLAIR MRI sequence will show gadolinium leakage into the cerebrospinal fluid (CSF) spaces and brain parenchyma secondary to a disturbed BBB. This finding was showed in two-thirds of patients with RCVS. This would suggest that the cerebral capillaries are also affected. Further studies are needed to better understand the relationship between BBB breakdown and vasoconstrictions in RCVS.[12]

Dysregulation of intracranial vascular tone leading to vasoconstriction is believed to be the key pathophysiologic mechanism. It occurs secondary to spontaneous or evoked sympathetic overactivity by a release of exogenous or endogenous factors like vasoconstrictive drugs and female hormones among other immunologic and biochemical factors. This is supported by the absence of histologic changes in brain biopsy such as active inflammation or vasculitis.[1,2,3,8,13,14,15,16]

Serotonin-producing tumors and serotonin-enhancing medication have been found to be associated with RCVS, which suggests that serotonin plays an important role in the pathophysiology of RCVS.[9]

Several triggers for RCVS have been identified, including early puerperium, late pregnancy, preeclampsia, vasoactive drugs (phenylpropanolamine, pseudoephedrine, ergotamine, tartrate, methysergide, bromocriptine, lisuride, selective serotonin reuptake inhibitors, sumatriptan, and isometheptene), recreational drugs (cocaine, ecstasy, marijuana, and amphetamines), tacrolimus, cyclophosphamide, pheochromocytoma, and carcinoid.[5,17,18,19,20,21]

45.2.3 Presentation

RCVS is most commonly a monophasic self-limiting condition. The most prominent symptom is a severe thunderclap headache reaching its peak intensity within seconds. Up to 80% of the patients have a thunderclap headache; thus, less severe, subacute, or even absent headache is rare. In 70 to 80% of the patients, it is the only presenting symptom. The thunderclap

headaches can recur up to three weeks and may occur spontaneously or be triggered by coughing, orgasm, physical exertion, acute stressful or emotional situations, straining, sneezing, bathing, or swimming.[1,5,8,9,10,18]

Other focal neurological symptoms can be associated with RCVS. Most commonly, these are visual symptoms; however, aphasia and sensory symptoms have also been reported. They can mimic transient ischemic attacks or migraine auras.[1,5]

45.2.4 Diagnosis

The diagnostic criteria in Box 1 were proposed by Calabrese et al.[2] The new International Classification of Headache Disorders, 3rd edition (ICHD-3; beta version) has proposed the diagnostic criteria shown in Box 2 for headaches attributed to RCVS and headache probably attributed to RCVS.[6,14]

Box 1: Diagnostic criteria of RCVS by Calabrese et al[2]:

- Acute and severe headache (often thunderclap) with or without focal deficits or seizures.
- Uniphasic course without new symptoms more than 1 month after clinical onset.
- Segmental vasoconstriction of cerebral arteries shown by indirect (e.g., MR or CT) or direct catheter angiography.
- No evidence of aneurysmal subarachnoid hemorrhage.
- Normal or near-normal CSF (protein concentrations < 100 mg/dL, < 15 white blood cells per μL).
- Complete or substantial normalization of arteries shown by follow-up indirect or direct angiography within 12 weeks of clinical onset.

Box 2: Diagnostic criteria of RCVS in the ICHD-3b[6]:

a) Any new headache fulfilling criterion C.
b) RCVS has been diagnosed
c) Evidence of causation demonstrated by either or both of the following:

---

1. Headache, with or without focal deficits and/or seizures, has led to angiography (with "string of beads" appearance) and diagnosis of RCVS.
2. Headache has one or more of the following characteristics:
   a) Thunderclap onset.
   b) Triggered by sexual activity, exertion, Valsalva maneuvers, emotion, bathing and/or showering.
   c) Present or recurrent during ≤ 1 month after onset, with no new significant headache after > 1 month.
d) Either of the following:
   1. Headache has resolved within 3 months of onset.
   2. Headache has not yet been resolved, but 3 months from onset have not yet passed.
e) Not better accounted for by another ICHD-3 diagnosis.

Acute headache *probably* attributed to RCVS:
a) Any new headache fulfilling criterion C.
b) RCVS is suspected but cerebral angiography is normal.
c) Probability of causation demonstrated by all of the following:
   1. At least two headaches within 1 month, with all three of the following characteristics:
      a) Thunderclap onset, and peaking in < 1 minute.
      b) Severe intensity.
      c) Lasting ≥ 5 minutes.
   2. At least one thunderclap headache has been triggered by one of the following:
      a) Sexual activity (just before or at orgasm).
      b) Exertion.
      c) Valsalva-like maneuver.
      d) Emotion.
      e) Bathing and/or showering.

Investigations and Imaging Findings

Imaging features together with the clinical presentation are crucial in making an early diagnosis. The initial angiography (CT, MR, or conventional) can be normal, especially in the first 3 to 5 days after symptom onset. Moreover, the detection of narrowed cerebral arteries has substantial interobserver variations, especially when using noninvasive imaging modalities. Cerebral angiographic studies typically show diffuse segmental multifocal narrowing and dilatation "string of beads" appearance of multiple cerebral arteries which usually reverse within weeks. It can involve both the anterior and the posterior circulation, and are mostly bilateral and diffuse. Maximum vasoconstriction occurs at approximately 2 weeks post-onset and the constricted vessel segments are not necessarily in the area of the intracerebral or subarachnoid hemorrhage. Centripetal propagation of vasoconstriction in RCVS has been postulated in many studies with limited evidence and unclear mechanism. It showed an initial distal vasoconstriction followed by more proximal vessels' involvement in time interval follow-up imaging. By diagnostic criteria, image evidence of vasoconstriction should be resolved by 12 weeks.[1,2,7,10,22,23,24,25]

Vessel wall MRI: It may be used as an adjunct to differentiate between RCVS, vasculitis, and atherosclerotic plaques. It will show wall thickening with no or very mild contrast enhancement of the affected arterial wall. In case of vasculitis, it will show intense concentric contrast enhancement, and a focal contrast enhancement in case of an active atherosclerotic processes.[26,27]

Initial CT or MR brain scans may show normal finding or spectrum of parenchymal abnormalities, including nonaneurysmal convexity subarachnoid hemorrhage, intracerebral hemorrhage, ischemic stroke, and brain edema. Contrast-enhancing FLAIR MRI assessment of BBB breakdown can be used as an adjuvant finding or a clue to support the diagnosis, as explained earlier.[1,12,23,24,28,29,30,31]

Routine blood tests are usually normal, but other tests are useful in ruling out systemic diseases that have been associated with RCVS: rheumatoid factor, antinuclear and antinuclear cytoplasmic antibodies, Lyme disease antibodies, urine vanillylmandelic acid and 5-hydroxyindoleacetic acid, and serum and urine toxicology screens. CSF examination findings are benign in more than 85% of patients. Other than to rule out cerebral vasculitis, there is no role for brain biopsy or temporal artery biopsy.[3,4,17,23,32]

45.2.5 Differential Diagnosis

The diversity of the RCVS clinical and imaging features carries a wide range of differential diagnoses. Thunderclap headaches can also indicate a variety of serious threatening conditions such as aneurysmal subarachnoid hemorrhage, parenchymal hemorrhage, cerebral artery dissection, and cerebral venous sinus thrombosis. Typical precipitants of RCVS can also trigger headache in primary (such as primary thunderclap headache, primary exertional headache, and orgasmic and migraine headache) or secondary headache disorders other than RCVS.[3,5,7,9,11]

Migraine should be cautiously considered in the sitting of severe headache and migraine-related stroke, because treating it inappropriately with agents such as sumatriptan may exacerbate vasoconstriction and stroke.[4,13,18]

The most challenging and difficult to exclude differential diagnosis is the primary angiitis of the central nervous system (PACNS), given the close sharing and common overlapping of the clinical and radiological features in both conditions. RCVS has the favor of stable or improving clinical course early on in comparison with continuous deterioration in PACNS. The presenting features of explosive recurrent thunderclap headaches with normal CSF findings and normal brain imaging suggest a diagnosis of RCVS. Also, the presence of history of common triggers and associated cofactors may provide clues to the diagnosis. Other characteristic radiological features that may guide the RCVS diagnosis in the appropriate clinical setting are the absence of brain lesions on initial imaging and the presence of cortical convexal subarachnoid hemorrhages as well as the angiographic findings "string of beads" appearance.[13,33,34,35,36]

45.2.6 Clinical Course

RCVS is considered self-limited and one of the defining features of it is transient cerebral vasoconstriction, which resolves within 1 to 3 months. The prognosis is generally considered very good.[5,11] However, complications can occur and include: ischemic or hemorrhagic stroke, cortical subarachnoid hemorrhage, cervical artery dissection, posterior reversible encephalopathy syndrome, and seizures. Brain hemorrhage and brain edema are usually early phase complications, during the first week, while ischemic complications occur at a delayed phase, at the end of or after the second week. Ischemic complications may thus occur when the headaches have improved or even resolved.[1,10,11,23,24,30,31]

Unfortunately, no known clinical or imaging features to reliably predict disease progression; however, evidence of BBB breakdown existence is suggested to be an independent risk factor for hemorrhagic neurological complications.[12]

45.2.7 Management and Prognosis

There is no proven treatment currently and no placebo-controlled trials carried out yet, hence the management is based on observational data and real-world evidence from an expert opinion and consensus.

Oral calcium–channel blockers (nimodipine, nifedipine, and verapamil) have been generally used but there is no strong evidence on their effectiveness in improving vasospasm or preventing disease progression, as they mainly work as supportive treatment for symptomatic relieve of the headache.[5,11] Triptans should be avoided, as they have been associated with RCVS.[37] Intra-arterial vasodilator therapy (papaverine, milrinone, nicardipine, and nimodipine) has been attempted in fulminant cases with variable success.[38,39,40]

Glucocorticoids are showed to contribute to disease progression with clinical worsening and poor outcome.[41]

Seizures should be looked at and treated accordingly. Routine stroke preventive medications, such as antiplatelets, anticoagulants, and cholesterol-lowering agents, are probably not indicated. Blood pressure control is an important part of the management since high pressure may worsen the vasoconstriction and increase the risk of hemorrhagic complications, and mild hypotension in a vasoconstricted brain may increase the risk of the ischemic stroke.

Although RCVS is mostly a self-remitting syndrome (95%)[18]; however, it is not necessarily an absolute benign condition and it may be fatal in extreme rare cases due to progressive vasoconstriction process in less than 5%. Recurrence of RCVS is extremely rare.

45.2.8 Pearls and Pitfalls

- RCVS is characterized by:
  - Severe acute headaches (recurrent) (thunderclap) with or without focal neurological deficits.
  - Reversible, diffuse segmental centripetal propagation of cerebral artery vasoconstrictions.
  - Biphasic course of early hemorrhagic complications followed by ischemic phase.
- Etiology remains unknown. Potential triggers: vasoactive medications, illicit drugs, sexual intercourse, pregnancy, and postpartum.
- Angiographic imaging:
  - Diffuse, multifocal, segmental narrowing and dilatation, and "string of beads."
  - High-resolution MRI with vessel wall imaging may avoid the need for further invasive investigations.

- The final diagnosis is confirmed only when the reversibility of previously identified vasoconstriction is identified.
- Treatment:
  - To discontinue and avoid any vasoactive medications and precipitating and triggering factors.
  - Vasodilators (calcium-channel blockers) are usually used with no strong evidence or proof. It is more effective for symptomatic headache control rather than treating the vasoconstriction.
  - Glucocorticoid has been associated with poor outcome.
- RCVS is not necessarily benign. Although vasoconstriction is typically reversible, it might rarely result in fatal ischemic and or hemorrhagic stroke.

References

[1] Ducros A, Boukobza M, Porcher R, Sarov M, Valade D, Bousser MG. The clinical and radiological spectrum of reversible cerebral vasoconstriction syndrome. A prospective series of 67 patients. Brain. 2007; 130(Pt 12):3091–3101

[2] Calabrese LH, Dodick DW, Schwedt TJ, Singhal AB. Narrative review: reversible cerebral vasoconstriction syndromes. Ann Intern Med. 2007; 146 (1):34–44

[3] Ducros A, Bousser MG. Reversible cerebral vasoconstriction syndrome. Pract Neurol. 2009; 9(5):256–267

[4] Sheikh HU, Mathew PG. Reversible cerebral vasoconstriction syndrome: updates and new perspectives. Curr Pain Headache Rep. 2014; 18(5):414

[5] Ducros A. Reversible cerebral vasoconstriction syndrome. Lancet Neurol. 2012; 11(10):906–917

[6] et al. The international classification of headache disorders, 3rd edition (beta version). Cephalalgia. 2013; 33:629–808

[7] Dodick DW, Brown RD, Jr, Britton JW, Huston J, III. Nonaneurysmal thunderclap headache with diffuse, multifocal, segmental, and reversible vasospasm. Cephalalgia. 1999; 19(2):118–123

[8] Call GK, Fleming MC, Sealfon S, Levine H, Kistler JP, Fisher CM. Reversible cerebral segmental vasoconstriction. Stroke. 1988; 19(9):1159–1170

[9] Singhal AB, Caviness VS, Begleiter AF, Mark EJ, Rordorf G, Koroshetz WJ. Cerebral vasoconstriction and stroke after use of serotonergic drugs. Neurology. 2002; 58(1):130–133

[10] Marder CP, Donohue MM, Weinstein JR, Fink KR. Multimodal imaging of reversible cerebral vasoconstriction syndrome: a series of 6 cases. AJNR Am J Neuroradiol. 2012; 33(7):1403–1410

[11] Miller TR, Shivashankar R, Mossa-Basha M, Gandhi D. Reversible cerebral vasoconstriction syndrome, part 1: epidemiology, pathogenesis, and clinical course. AJNR Am J Neuroradiol. 2015; 36(8):1392–1399

[12] Lee MJ, Cha J, Choi HA, et al. Blood-brain barrier breakdown in reversible cerebral vasoconstriction syndrome: Implications for pathophysiology and diagnosis. Ann Neurol. 2017; 81(3):454–466

[13] Ducros A. L37. Reversible cerebral vasoconstriction syndrome: distinction from CNS vasculitis. Presse Med. 2013; 42(4, Pt 2):602–604

[14] Arrigan MT, Heran MKS, Shewchuk JR. Reversible cerebral vasoconstriction syndrome: an important and common cause of thunderclap and recurrent headaches. Clin Radiol. 2018; 73(5):417–427

[15] Kunchok A, Castley HC, Aldous L, et al. Fatal reversible cerebral vasoconstriction syndrome. J Neurol Sci. 2018; 385:146–150

[16] Robert T, Kawkabani Marchini A, Oumarou G, Uské A. Reversible cerebral vasoconstriction syndrome identification of prognostic factors. Clin Neurol Neurosurg. 2013; 115(11):2351–2357

[17] Chen SP, Fuh JL, Wang SJ. Reversible cerebral vasoconstriction syndrome: current and future perspectives. Expert Rev Neurother. 2011; 11(9):1265–1276

[18] Singhal AB, Hajj-Ali RA, Topcuoglu MA, et al. Reversible cerebral vasoconstriction syndromes: analysis of 139 cases. Arch Neurol. 2011; 68 (8):1005–1012

[19] Garcin B, Clouston J, Saines N. Reversible cerebral vasoconstriction syndrome. J Clin Neurosci. 2009; 16(1):147–150

[20] Katz BS, Fugate JE, Ameriso SF, et al. Clinical worsening in reversible cerebral vasoconstriction syndrome. JAMA Neurol. 2014; 71(1):68–73

[21] Mawet J, Boukobza M, Franc J, et al. Reversible cerebral vasoconstriction syndrome and cervical artery dissection in 20 patients. Neurology. 2013; 81 (9):821–824

[22] Slivka A, Philbrook B. Clinical and angiographic features of thunderclap headache. Headache. 1995; 35(1):1–6

[23] Miller TR, Shivashankar R, Mossa-Basha M, Gandhi D. Reversible cerebral vasoconstriction syndrome, Part 2: diagnostic work-up, imaging evaluation, and differential diagnosis. AJNR Am J Neuroradiol. 2015; 36(9):1580–1588

[24] Topcuoglu MA, Singhal AB. Hemorrhagic reversible cerebral vasoconstriction syndrome. Features and mechanisms. Stroke. 2016; 47(7):1742–1747

[25] Shimoda M, Oda S, Shigematsu H, et al. Clinical significance of centripetal propagation of vasoconstriction in patients with reversible cerebral vasoconstriction syndrome: A retrospective case-control study. Cephalalgia. 2018; 38(12):1864–1875

[26] Mandell DM, Mossa-Basha M, Qiao Y, et al. Vessel Wall Imaging Study Group of the American Society of Neuroradiology. Intracranial vessel wall MRI: principles and expert consensus recommendations of the American Society of Neuroradiology. AJNR Am J Neuroradiol. 2017; 38(2):218–229

[27] Obusez EC, Hui F, Hajj-Ali RA, et al. High-resolution MRI vessel wall imaging: spatial and temporal patterns of reversible cerebral vasoconstriction syndrome and central nervous system vasculitis. AJNR Am J Neuroradiol. 2014; 35(8):1527–1532

[28] Ansari SA, Rath TJ, Gandhi D. Reversible cerebral vasoconstriction syndromes presenting with subarachnoid hemorrhage: a case series. J Neurointerv Surg. 2011; 3(3):272–278

[29] Xing B, Lenck S, Krings T, Hengwei J, Jaigobin CS, Schaafsma JD. Angiographic characteristics of hemorrhagic and ischemic phases of reversible cerebral vasoconstriction syndrome. Clin Neuroradiol. 2018:[Epub ahead of print]

[30] Chen SP, Fuh JL, Wang SJ, et al. Magnetic resonance angiography in reversible cerebral vasoconstriction syndromes. Ann Neurol. 2010; 67(5):648–656

[31] Ducros A, Fiedler U, Porcher R, Boukobza M, Stapf C, Bousser M-G. Hemorrhagic manifestations of reversible cerebral vasoconstriction syndrome: frequency, features, and risk factors. Stroke. 2010; 41(11):2505–2511

[32] Sattar A, Manousakis G, Jensen MB. Systematic review of reversible cerebral vasoconstriction syndrome. Expert Rev Cardiovasc Ther. 2010; 8(10):1417–1421

[33] Singhal AB, Topcuoglu MA, Fok JW, et al. Reversible cerebral vasoconstriction syndromes and primary angiitis of the central nervous system: clinical, imaging, and angiographic comparison. Ann Neurol. 2016; 79(6):882–894

[34] de Boysson H, Parienti JJ, Mawet J, et al. Primary angiitis of the CNS and reversible cerebral vasoconstriction syndrome: a comparative study. Neurology. 2018; 91(16):e1468–e1478

[35] Kraayvanger L, Berlit P, Albrecht P, Hartung HP, Kraemer M. Cerebrospinal fluid findings in reversible cerebral vasoconstriction syndrome: a way to differentiate from cerebral vasculitis? Clin Exp Immunol. 2018; 193(3):341–345

[36] Hajj-Ali RA, Singhal AB, Benseler S, Molloy E, Calabrese LH. Primary angiitis of the CNS. Lancet Neurol. 2011; 10(6):561–572

[37] Kato Y, Hayashi T, Mizuno S, et al. Triptan induced reversible cerebral vasoconstriction syndrome: two case reports with a literature review. Intern Med. 2016; 55(23):3525–3528

[38] Ioannidis I, Nasis N, Agianniotaki A, Katsouda E, Andreou A. Reversible cerebral vasoconstriction syndrome: treatment with multiple sessions of intra-arterial nimodipine and angioplasty. Interv Neuroradiol. 2012; 18 (3):297–302

[39] Zuber M, Touzé E, Domigo V, Trystram D, Lamy C, Mas JL. Reversible cerebral angiopathy: efficacy of nimodipine. J Neurol. 2006; 253(12):1585–1588

[40] Bouchard M, Verreault S, Gariépy JL, Dupré N. Intra-arterial milrinone for reversible cerebral vasoconstriction syndrome. Headache. 2009; 49(1):142–145

[41] Singhal AB, Topcuoglu MA. Glucocorticoid-associated worsening in reversible cerebral vasoconstriction syndrome. Neurology. 2017; 88(3):228–236

46 Acute Ischemic Stroke Secondary to Cardiac Myxoma Embolus

46.1 Case Description

46.1.1 Clinical Presentation

A 28-year-old female initially presented to the emergency department as a code stroke with left-sided deficits. She underwent successful thrombectomy, but sustained residual loss of vision in the left eye. Poststroke workup with echocardiography revealed a left atrial mass, and CT of the abdomen revealed emboli to the liver and spleen. She underwent minimally invasive cardiac surgery 2 days after her initial presentation with pathology, demonstrating a left atrial myxoma. Four years after her initial episode, she presented with headaches, which prompted MRI evaluation.

46.1.2 Imaging Workup and Investigations

- MRI at the time of the second presentation revealed a fusiform aneurysm of the distal right M1 and proximal right M2 branches.

46.1.3 Diagnosis

Acute ischemic stroke secondary to cardiac myxoma and subsequent development of myxomatous aneurysm.

46.1.4 Treatment

Acute Management

- On the initial presentation, the patient underwent successful thrombectomy.
- Subsequent discovery of the fusiform right middle cerebral artery (MCA) aneurysm prompted initiation of acetylsalicylic acid (ASA) to prevent potential future ischemia.

Surgical Treatment

- Resection of the cardiac myxoma

Outcomes

- From her initial presentation, the patient sustained minimal deficits after a successful thrombectomy and resection of the cardiac myxoma.
- Subsequent discovery of the right MCA fusiform aneurysm prompted initiation of ASA treatment. Surveillance MRI imaging over the next three years demonstrated no complications (▶ Fig. 46.1).

46.2 Companion Case

46.2.1 Clinical Presentation

A 25-year-old female presented to the emergency department 5 hours post onset of sudden weakness of the right face and arm. Since initial CT was normal but symptoms persisted, the patient underwent emergency MRI for evaluation of acute ischemic stroke. MR demonstrated acute ischemic infarcts in the left occipital lobe, left midbrain/cerebral peduncle, and left thalamocapsular region (▶ Fig. 46.2). Past medical history was significant for migraines and Crohn disease.

46.2.2 Imaging Workup and Investigations

- Intracranial and cervical MRA are normal without any findings for vasculitis or atherosclerosis.
- Serum antinuclear antibody is positive. Antiphospholipid antibody is borderline. Coagulation studies are normal.
- Transesophageal echocardiogram demonstrates a left atrial mass (▶ Fig. 46.3). This mass went on to be resected, and pathology was consistent with a cardiac myxoma.

46.2.3 Diagnosis

Acute ischemic stroke secondary to cardiac myxoma.

46.2.4 Treatment

Acute Management

- The patient was not considered to be a tissue plasminogen activator candidate, as she presented outside the therapeutic window. Additionally, the absence of a large vessel occlusion and the low National Institutes of Health Stroke Scale (NIHSS) score meant she was not a candidate for endovascular treatment.

Surgical Treatment

- Resection of the cardiac myxoma.

Outcomes

- Two years following treatment, the patient presented with flashing lights in her right eye. MRI was performed, which revealed three hemorrhagic foci in the left occipital lobe (▶ Fig. 46.4). These were thought to possibly represent metastatic lesions.
- Diagnostic cerebral angiography was performed which demonstrated distal fusiform aneurysms in the region of these hemorrhagic lesions. These findings were suggestive of oncotic aneurysms secondary to myxomatous emboli (▶ Fig. 46.5). These were treated conservatively with close imaging follow-up.

46.3 Discussion

46.3.1 Background

Cardiac myxomas are reported to be the cause of 0.5% of acute ischemic strokes.[1] Furthermore, approximately 30% of myxoma

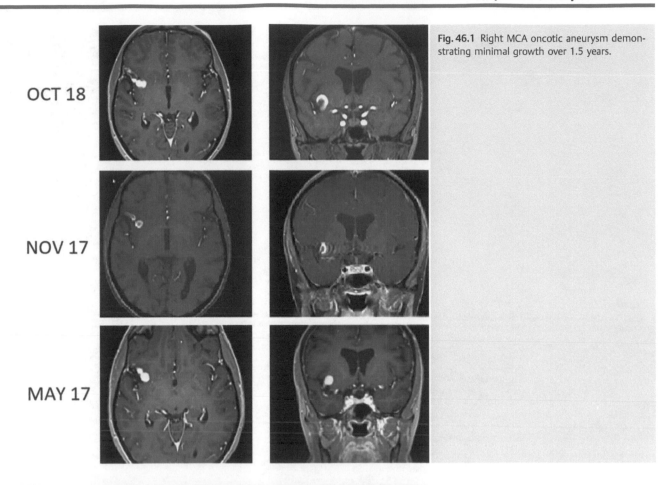

OCT 18

NOV 17

MAY 17

Fig. 46.1 Right MCA oncotic aneurysm demonstrating minimal growth over 1.5 years.

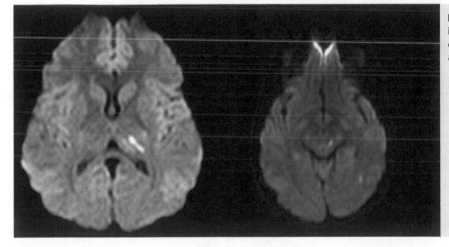

Fig. 46.2 DWI MRI for evaluation of acute ischemic stroke demonstrates infarcts in the left occipital lobe, left midbrain/cerebral peduncle, and left thalamocapsular region.

patients present with systemic or cerebral emboli.[2] Cerebral infarction in myxoma patients is secondary to embolization of tumor particles or thrombotic material covered with tumor cells.[3] In fact, several case reports on mechanical thrombectomy for treatment of acute ischemic stroke in myxoma patients have demonstrated myxomatous tissue in the retrieved emboli.[4,5]

Stroke Secondary to Cardiac Myxoma

Infarction due a cardiac myxoma commonly manifests as multiple infarcts in more than one vascular territory due to its cardioembolic nature.[3] Case series on the prognosis of myxomatous

emboli have found that nearly 50% of patients have severe neurological deficits and 20% of patients die related to complications of cerebral infarction. The multivessel territory of the infarcts are thought to contribute to a poorer prognosis in these patients.[6] Reported complications following ischemic stroke secondary to cardiac myxoma include herniation and hemorrhagic transformation.[7]

While there are several cases describing the use of intravenous thrombolysis in the treatment of ischemic strokes secondary to myxoma, the results have been mixed.[5,8,9,10,11] This is thought to be secondary to the fact that emboli are primarily

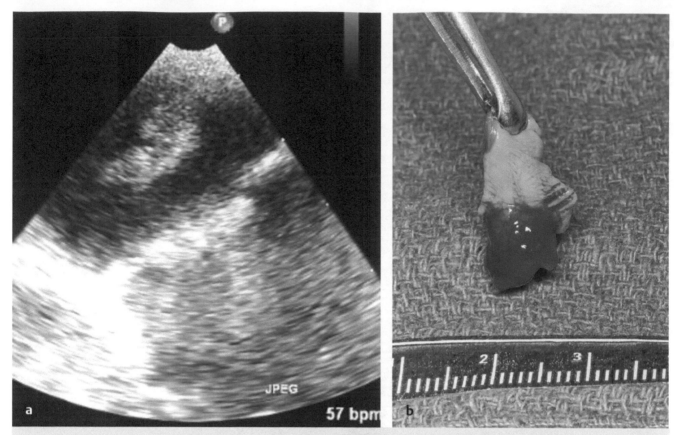

Fig. 46.3 (a) Echocardiographic image demonstrates a large pedunculated mass in the left atrium. (b) surgical specimen of the pedunculated soft tissue mass, which was a pathologically proven cardiac myxoma.

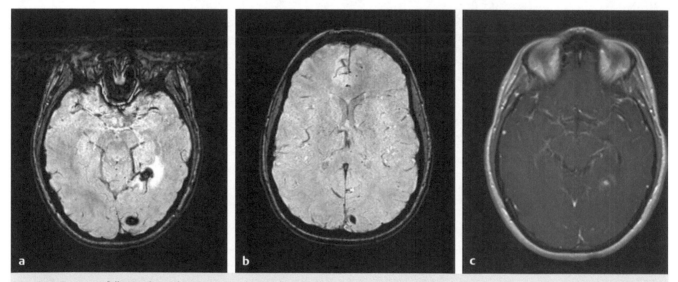

Fig. 46.4 Two years following her ischemic events, she developed a flashing sensation in her right eye. (a–c) MRI demonstrated three hemorrhagic foci, the largest of which demonstrated marked contrast enhancement on post-gadolinium T1-weighted images.

composed of tumor cells rather than thrombus. Case reports of endovascular recanalization in the setting of large vessel occlusion have yielded promising results. Overall, most authors favor the use of thrombolysis or endovascular recanalization when no contraindications exist.[4,5]

Aneurysms

Oncotic cerebral aneurysms are late manifestations of cardiac myxoma metastatic disease and are seen in up to 25% of patients.[6,12,13] These aneurysms are usually fusiform, multiple,

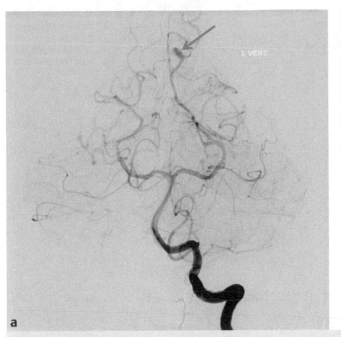
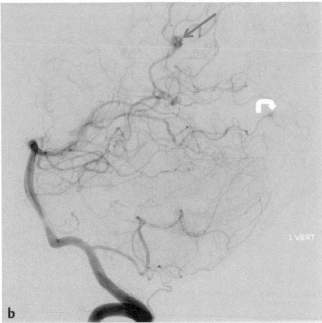

Fig. 46.5 (a) Digital subtraction angiography following left vertebral artery injection demonstrates scattered areas of irregular caliber in several mid through distal branches in the left PCA territory. (b) Smaller fusiform aneurysm distal left calcarine branch above tentorium near the calvarium, corresponding to the hemorrhage focus seen in the left occipital lobe (*curved arrow*). (c) There is a large serpiginous, fusiform aneurysm in the distal left parietooccipital artery at a bifurcation which appears to correlate with the enhancing lesion (*straight arrow*).

and located in peripheral cerebrovascular territories. They are thought to result from implantation of metastatic emboli which infiltrate and subsequently weaken the vessel wall. The myxomatous tissue proliferates into the vessel wall, resulting in weakening of the subintimal tissue and subsequent aneurysm formation. This hypothesis is supported by clinical studies which have demonstrated that a high proportion of cardiac myxoma aneurysm patients had embolic events prior to discovery of their aneurysms, with pathologic studies demonstrating penetration of vessel walls by myxomatous cells.[14,15] Because of the slow growth of myxomatous tissue, there is often a long delay between the diagnosis of cardiac myxoma and the diagnosis of a myxomatous aneurysm. Optimal treatment of myxomatous oncotic aneurysms has not been established. Prophylactic treatment with ASA to prevent distal emboli can be considered. Prior studies examining the role of endovascular embolization, chemotherapy, and radiation in decreasing the growth of these aneurysms have yielded equivocal results.[16,17] These treatments fail as they do not address the underlying pathological process which is centered within the vessel wall with growth of embedded myxomatous tissue.

46.3.2 Pearls and Pitfalls

- Cardiac myxoma is a rare cause of acute ischemic stroke but should be considered as a possible stroke etiology among younger patients.
- No consensus exists regarding the best treatment modality for stroke in myxoma patients; however, most authors favor the use of thrombolysis or endovascular recanalization when no contraindications exist.

- Oncotic aneurysm formation in distal cerebrovascular territories is thought to be a late manifestation of myxomatous emboli.

References

[1] Koeltgen D, Kidwell CS. Neurologic complications of cardiac tumors. Handb Clin Neurol. 2014; 119:209–222

[2] Mattle HP, Maurer D, Sturzenegger M, Ozdoba C, Baumgartner RW, Schroth G. Cardiac myxomas: a long term study. J Neurol. 1995; 242(10):689–694

[3] Long Y, Gao C. Brain embolism secondary to cardiac myxoma in fifteen Chinese patients. ScientificWorldJournal. 2014; 2014:718246

[4] Vega RA, Chan JL, Anene-Maidoh TI, Grimes MM, Reavey-Cantwell JF. Mechanical thrombectomy for pediatric stroke arising from an atrial myxoma: case report. J Neurosurg Pediatr. 2015; 15(3):301–305

[5] Baek SH, Park S, Lee NJ, Kang Y, Cho KH. Effective mechanical thrombectomy in a patient with hyperacute ischemic stroke associated with cardiac myxoma. J Stroke Cerebrovasc Dis. 2014; 23(9):e417–e419

[6] Lee SJ, Kim JH, Na CY, Oh SS. Eleven years' experience with Korean cardiac myxoma patients: focus on embolic complications. Cerebrovasc Dis. 2012; 33 (5):471–479

[7] Lee VH, Connolly HM, Brown RD, Jr. Central nervous system manifestations of cardiac myxoma. Arch Neurol. 2007; 64(8):1115–1120

[8] Abe M, Kohama A, Takeda T, et al. Effective intravenous thrombolytic therapy in a patient with cerebral infarction associated with left atrial myxoma. Intern Med. 2011; 50(20):2401–2405

[9] Gassanov N, Nia AM, Dahlem KM, et al. Local thrombolysis for successful treatment of acute stroke in an adolescent with cardiac myxoma. ScientificWorldJournal. 2011; 11:891–893

[10] Kamiya Y, Ichikawa H, Mizuma K, Itaya K, Shimizu Y, Kawamura M. [Case of acute ischemic stroke due to cardiac myxoma treated by intravenous thrombolysis and endovascular therapy]. Rinsho Shinkeigaku. 2014; 54 (6):502–506

[11] Kohno N, Kawakami Y, Hamada C, Toyoda G, Bokura H, Yamaguchi S. Cerebral embolism associated with left atrial myxoma that was treated with thrombolytic therapy. Case Rep Neurol. 2012; 4(1):38–42

[12] Ekinci EI, Donnan GA. Neurological manifestations of cardiac myxoma: a review of the literature and report of cases. Intern Med J. 2004; 34(5):243–249

[13] Viganò S, Papini GD, Cotticelli B, et al. Prevalence of cerebral aneurysms in patients treated for left cardiac myxoma: a prospective study. Clin Radiol. 2013; 68(11):e624–e628

[14] Budzilovich G, Aleksic S, Greco A, Fernandez J, Harris J, Finegold M. Malignant cardiac myxoma with cerebral metastases. Surg Neurol. 1979; 11(6):461–469

[15] Sabolek M, Bachus-Banaschak K, Bachus R, Arnold G, Storch A. Multiple cerebral aneurysms as delayed complication of left cardiac myxoma: a case report and review. Acta Neurol Scand. 2005; 111(6):345–350

[16] Branscheidt M, Frontzek K, Bozinov O, et al. Etoposide/carboplatin chemotherapy for the treatment of metastatic myxomatous cerebral aneurysms. J Neurol. 2014; 261(4):828–830

[17] Altundag MB, Ertas G, Ucer AR, et al. Brain metastasis of cardiac myxoma: case report and review of the literature. J Neurooncol. 2005; 75(2):181–184

47 Seizure

47.1 Case Description

47.1.1 Clinical Presentation

A 67-year-old man was brought to the emergency department (ED) by ambulance after being found at home with new onset of left hemiparesis and dysarthria. He was last seen well 30 minutes earlier by his wife.

On further history, there was a prior episode of left hemiparesis and dysarthria 2 years ago. The patient's wife was told it was a stroke, and at the time, he had received tissue plasminogen activator (tPA) with resolution of deficits. No stroke etiology was found. His only home medication was aspirin 81 mg daily.

In the ED, his National Institutes of Health Stroke Scale (NIHSS) score was 5 for mild left hemiparesis (drift in left upper and lower extremity—1 point each), mild dysarthria (1 point), drowsiness (1 point), and left visual extinction (1 point).

47.1.2 Investigations

His routine stroke laboratory panel was normal, including cell counts, glucose, electrolytes, and coagulation studies.

A noncontrast CT of the head showed old right frontal infarction (▶ Fig. 47.1a). CT angiography (CTA) was normal (▶ Fig. 47.1b). CT perfusion demonstrated a large area of hyperperfusion of the right hemisphere—increased cerebral blood flow (CBF) and cerebral blood volume (CBV) with decreased mean transit time (MTT)—extending beyond the expected middle cerebral artery territory (▶ Fig. 47.1c). Electroencephalography (EEG) later showed a nonspecific area of focal slowing over the right frontal lobe and no active seizure.

Follow-up MRI did not reveal any new infarction corresponding to the perfusion abnormality (▶ Fig. 47.2).

47.1.3 Clinical Reassessment

Ten minutes later, he was found to experience twitching of the left lower face and left thumb, which evolved into a clonic activity of the left arm. His head and gaze deviated to the left. He was given 2 mg of lorazepam intravenously and the movements quickly abated. He then became drowsier. Postictally, the tone in the left hemibody was flaccid, while the tone and power in the right hemibody appeared normal.

One hour later, his deficits resolved entirely.

47.1.4 Diagnosis

Seizure secondary to remote right frontal stroke, causing mild postictal paralysis and dysarthria. No evidence of new cerebral infarct.

47.1.5 Treatment

Lorazepam 2 mg IV aborted the initial seizure. He received phenytoin 20 mg/kg IV (rate < 50 mg/min) loading dose in the ED to prevent seizure recurrence acutely.

He was eventually discharged from hospital with a diagnosis of poststroke epilepsy. The following day, he started levetiracetam 500 mg PO BID for long-term seizure prevention. Counselling was provided regarding potential side effects, including mood or behavior changes. Follow-up was booked in the epilepsy clinic in 3 months' time.

Secondary stroke prevention strategies were reassessed in the light of his remote stroke, and recommendations for ongoing management of this issue were shared with the family doctor.

47.2 Discussion

47.2.1 Background

Cerebrovascular clinicians must become familiar with the bidirectional relationship between strokes and seizures. Seizures can mimic strokes, and strokes can mimic seizures; alternatively, both can coexist in the same patient, either because strokes precipitate seizures or due to a common underlying mechanism.

Seizure as a Stroke Mimic

Among stroke mimics, seizures have been consistently ranked as one of the most common—accounting for 21 to 41% of mimics.[1,2,3] The International League Against Epilepsy (ILAE) defines seizure as "a transient occurrence of signs and/or symptoms due to abnormal excessive or synchronous neuronal activity in the brain."[4] Seizures may be considered in four phases: prodrome, aura, ictus, and postictus. Classically, it is the postictal phase that mimics strokes, but other phases may do so less commonly. These will be reviewed in sequence.

Prodrome

The first phase, prodrome, is only recognized in about 20% of patients.[5] Its onset may precede seizures by up to several days. The most common prodromal symptoms are "funny feeling," "confusion," "anxiety," "irritability," "speech disturbance," and "headache" in decreasing frequency. Seizure prodrome does not usually mimic cerebral ischemia.

Aura

An aura is defined as "a subjective *ictal* phenomenon that comprises all experienced sensations in a patient and may precede an observable seizure."[6] The aura often precedes other manifestations of the ictus, but occasionally it is isolated; in other words, a focal seizure may produce only subjective symptoms without evolving into an observable seizure.[7] Typically, an aura lasts seconds to minutes; rarely, it is prolonged— a phenomenon called "aura-continua," a form of focal status epilepticus.[8] The incidence of auras among patients with epilepsy has ranged from 20 to 94%.[8] The most common specific manifestations of an aura are sensory (visual hallucinations, paresthesias, numbness, pain, and stiffness) and autonomic (gastrointestinal discomfort and palpitations).[6] An epileptic aura is most apt to

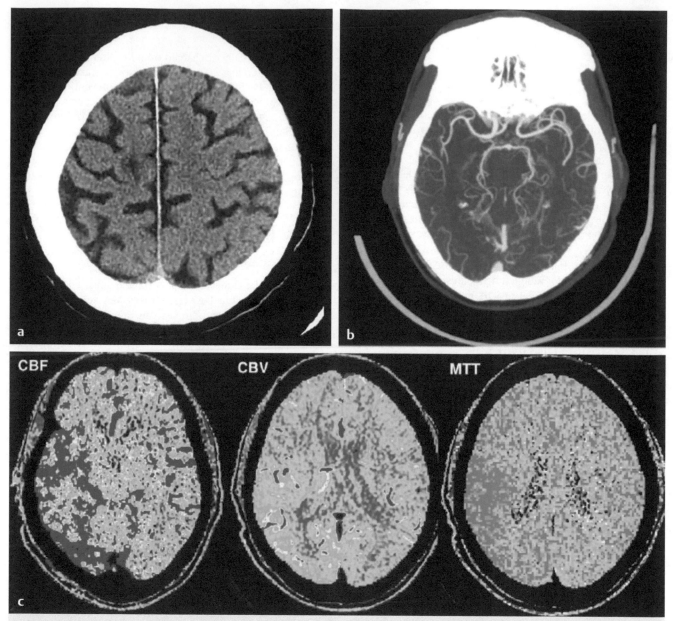

Fig. 47.1 (a) Noncontrast CT showing right old frontal infarction. (b) CTA showing patent MCA bilaterally. (c) CT perfusion cross-section of the brain, demonstrating increased CBF and CBV, with decreased MTT in a large area of the right hemisphere, suggesting hyperperfusion.

be confused with an ischemic event when it is prolonged, and/or when it is manifested by purely negative (loss of function) symptoms such as numbness, speech disturbance, or vertigo.

Ictus

Observable seizures (ictus) may occur with or without preceding epileptic auras. Occasionally, this portion of seizures may mimic cerebral ischemia. The most striking example is when seizures manifest as acute unilateral weakness.[7,9,10,11] Purported responsible cortical regions include the primary sensorimotor area, primary negative motor area, and supplementary negative motor area.[12] Ictal hemiparesis can also be a feature of temporal lobe epilepsy and may be accompanied by ipsilateral automatisms.[11] Speech arrest, aphasia, or other speech changes may be

seen with seizures involving the anterior or posterior language areas of the dominant frontal or temporal lobes.[7,11] Rarely, other ictal neurologic symptoms or signs—besides weakness or speech disturbances—may mimic strokes. For example, facial apraxia can be seen with frontal opercular seizures—clues to the diagnosis include concurrent facial clonic activity and profuse salivation.[7]

Postictus

Finally, the most common stage in which seizures mimic strokes is the postictal phase. Postictally, hemibody weakness has been called "Todd's paralysis." Its incidence ranges from 0.64-32%.[13] Tone may be flaccid, normal, or spastic. Reflexes can be diminished, normal, or increased. Occasionally, there is

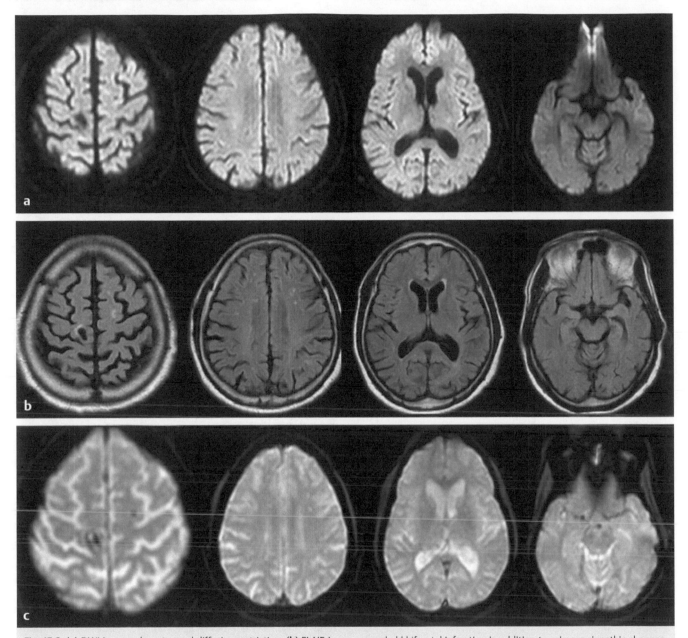

Fig. 47.2 (a) DWI images do not reveal diffusion restriction. (b) FLAIR images reveal old bifrontal infarction in addition to microangiopathic changes. (c) GRE images demonstrate foci of susceptibility corresponding to the old bifrontal infarcts.

associated aphasia or gaze palsy, and usually, no other associated major neurologic deficit. Postictal paresis typically lasts around 15 hours, but can be as short as 30 minutes or as long as 36 hours.[14] The duration of weakness does not appear to be related to the duration of the seizure itself. It occurs with every seizure in some patients, and sporadically in others. The patho-mechanism of negative neurologic signs postictally is up for debate—some theories include hypoxia from neuronal exhaustion, neurotransmitter depletion, hyperperfusion with AV shunting, or an increase in inhibitory discharges.[12,14,15]

In summary, seizures may be broken down into four phases: (1) prodrome, which does not usually mimic stroke; (2) aura, which occurs at the start of the ictus but has no observable signs and only infrequently mimics stroke; (3) observable ictus, which occasionally mimics stroke; and (4) postictus, which is

the most common stroke mimic. Seizures most commonly produce positive neurologic signs (gain of function), but it is when they cause negative (loss of function) signs—weakness, numbness, speech disturbances, or visual loss—that they can resemble cerebral ischemia.

Stroke and Seizure May Coexist

Strokes are the most common underlying cause of seizures among the elderly population.[7] When seizures begin in older individuals without a known history of strokes, occult cerebrovascular disease should be considered.[16] Among all age groups, seizures may occur poststroke in about 10% of patients.[17] They can occur "early"—defined as within 7 to 14 days of the stroke—or they can occur "late." There is minimal data on the frequency

Table 47.1 Pertinent questions on history when the differential diagnosis includes seizure and cerebral ischemia

Question	Purpose
Was there a prodrome or aura (e.g., rising epigastric sensation)?	May suggests seizure
Did all of the deficits start at once or was there a progression?	Acute onset of deficits simultaneously suggests stroke Progression over seconds to minutes suggests seizure
Urinary incontinence? Tongue bite?	May suggest seizure
Sustained eye or head deviation? Did the deviation switch sides at any point?	Activation of FEF in seizure causes contraversion, followed by ipsiversion postictally Loss of function of FEF in stroke causes ipsiversion
Any facial twitching or rhythmic jerking of the extremities?	Rhythmic jerking suggests seizure. However, must distinguish from tremor or other movement disorders
Was the patient confused after the episode?	May suggest postictal state. However, must distinguish from receptive aphasia
Does the patient remember the entire episode?	Amnesia or altered awareness may suggest seizure
Past history to suggest seizure (e.g., waking up with unexplained tongue bite or soreness). Past history of a risk factor for the development of epilepsy: intracranial infection, mass, injury. Previously identical stereotyped events.	May suggest seizure

Abbreviation: FEF, frontal eye field.

of seizures at the very onset of strokes. When defined as "immediate" or within 24 hours, a study by Szaflarski et al of over 6,000 patients found that about 3% of stroke patients experienced seizures.[17] Seizures are more common after hemorrhagic strokes (intracerebral hemorrhage/subarachnoid hemorrhage [SAH]; 8.4%) than ischemic (2.4%). Among those with ischemic strokes, seizures appear to be more common when the etiology is embolic.[17,18]

The mechanism of early versus late poststroke seizure likely differs: early poststroke seizure may result from hypoxia and biochemical dysfunction from the excitatory neurotransmitter cascade, while late poststroke seizure is more likely due to structural changes or gliosis, eventually leading to the process of epileptogenesis.[18,19] Indeed, late-onset seizures are linked to a greater risk of subsequent epilepsy compared with early poststroke seizures.[18] Although early-onset seizures may be less likely to evolve into epilepsy, they may increase the burden of ischemia by amplifying metabolic demand.[20]

Other common underlying diseases or mechanisms may cause the same patient to have both seizures and strokes. For details, see further reading section.[16,19]

47.2.2 Workup and Diagnosis

History

To determine whether a patient has had a stroke, seizure, both, or neither, collateral historians are usually necessary. The clinician should obtain a history from the patient, as well as the closest witness of the episode, avoiding as much as possible second- or third-hand information that is prone to error. The most proximal witnesses may be strangers, colleagues, friends, or family members.

As of yet, no single symptom, sign, or epidemiologic factor ably predicts whether the patient is presenting with a stroke or a mimic.[21] The physician should obtain a complete description of the event itself, as well as what preceded and followed it.

▶ Table 47.1 suggests some important questions to consider asking of the patient and/or witnesses.

Examination

The first step in the examination is assessment of stability including vitals. Autonomic dysfunction, including alterations in blood pressure and heart rate, may be seen in either strokes or seizures and may need to be urgently addressed.

The clinician would then ordinarily perform a rapid, standardized screening examination for stroke, the NIHSS. Strokes are not excluded by the presence of seizures on examination, since both can present simultaneously.

Assessment of possible seizures starts like any other neurologic examination with mental status. Impaired awareness is seen with generalized seizures, and occasionally with those of focal onset.[4] It may instead indicate an underlying neurologic or systemic cause for the patients' presentation. Altered mental status does not preclude a thorough neurologic examination: Even with altered mental status, the clinician should be diligent, as one may uncover subtle, ongoing seizure activity, postictal features, or an underlying explanatory lesion.

Besides mental status, key elements to an examination for seizure include sustained gaze or head deviation, spontaneous unidirectional or bidirectional nystagmus, and any abnormal movements including twitching of the facial muscles, tonic posturing or rhythmic (clonic) jerking, tone, and reflex testing. The clinician should note how these signs evolve over time, as one may note the "gain of function" of the ictus followed by postictal "loss of function," for example, sustained gaze deviation that switches sides. The clinician should observe whether there are associated automatisms such as picking at clothing, chewing, or rapid blinking.

Bedside funduscopic examination may reveal papilledema, suggesting a mass lesion. Nuchal rigidity may implicate meningitis. Examination of the skin may show signs of infection or an underlying neurocutaneous disorder. Dysmorphisms should be noted. Examination of the tongue may reveal a tongue bite, which is seen in about 22% of epileptic seizures.[22] The patient should be assessed for musculoskeletal injuries.

Investigations

Laboratory

When presented with possible seizures, laboratory investigations may serve three purposes:
1. Supporting the diagnosis of seizures versus the differential diagnosis.
2. Identifying an underlying cause for seizures.
3. Assessing complications of seizures.

1. Supporting the Diagnosis of Seizures

Four laboratory tests have been found to be helpful in supporting a clinical diagnosis of generalized tonic-clonic seizures when elevated: prolactin, ammonia, lactate, and creatine kinase. None so far have been able to rule out seizures or strokes as the alternative. Each biomarker rises and peaks at different time points, so the clinician must consider this, if one is to ably interpret the test. Sensitivities are low, and multiple variables can affect their levels. Overall, there is a paucity of high-quality evidence to support the routine use of biomarkers in order to confirm a seizure diagnosis.[13,22,23,24,25,26]

2. Identifying an Underlying Cause for Seizures

Seizures may be provoked by metabolic, infectious, endocrine, toxic, autoimmune, and other causes that may be supported by laboratory investigations. The following tests can be considered in the workup for unprovoked seizure: cell counts, glucose, thyroid studies, electrolytes and extended electrolytes, hepatic and renal function, serum and urine toxicologies, and alcohol and drug levels. Lumbar puncture should be considered when intracranial infection or SAH are suspected; otherwise, it is not usually indicated.[22,23,24]

3. Assessing Complications of Seizures

Laboratory investigations may help in identifying complications of seizures, including rhabdomyolysis, arrhythmia, and renal injury. Leukocytosis can be moderate after seizures but should resolve within 24 hours. Infection must be considered if there is fever or other suggestive clinical features.[23]

Electroencephalography

The utility of EEG in acutely differentiating seizures from strokes is limited, due to its low specificity. In particular, focal slowing may be seen in either process. Epileptiform activity also does not rule out strokes.[20,27] Conversely, the absence of epileptiform activity does not rule out seizures. Sensitivity is highest when done promptly.[24] The usefulness of EEG mainly lies in identifying subclinical seizure activity, and spotting an epileptogenic focus to help stratify recurrence risk. Patients who do not return to baseline within 30 to 60 minutes after seizures should be referred for (ideally continuous) EEG to rule out nonconvulsive status epilepticus.[22,23] Otherwise, EEG can be considered as an outpatient investigation.[24]

Imaging

CT: If both noncontrast CT and CTA are normal, then a stroke mimic such as seizure or migraine should be considered.[20]

CT perfusion: CT perfusion is emerging as a potential radiographic tool to distinguish stroke from seizure or postictal state. In seizures, hyperperfusion (increased CBF and CBV, decreased MTT) is expected ictally, and this may persist into the early postictal phase. Hyperperfusion is then usually, but not always, followed by hypoperfusion postictally.[27,28,29,30] In stroke, hypoperfusion is expected, and then if there is recanalization, hyperperfusion or "luxury perfusion" can be seen.[31] Changes to perfusion in a nonvascular distribution may suggest seizure.[28,32] Variations in vascular supply, such as the presence of a fetal posterior cerebral artery (PCA), should be considered as an alternative explanation and can be verified by CTA.

MRI: In centers that have emergent access to MRI, diffusion-weighted imaging (DWI)/apparent diffusion coefficient (ADC) may be used to rule out acute stroke which usually manifests as diffusion restriction corresponding to vascular territory. However, MRI can show peri-ictal changes, especially on DWI, fluid-attenuated inversion recovery (FLAIR) and T2-weighted images. Two patterns have been described: cytotoxic edema pattern which manifests as diffusion restriction with hyperintensity on DWI images with correspondingly reduced ADC values, and a vasogenic edema pattern which manifests as facilitated diffusion with high-signal intensity on DWI, ADC, FLAIR, and T2. The geographic distribution of these findings would involve regions of highest seizure activity such as the neocortex or mesolimbic structures and the peri-sylvan region, in addition to remote areas such as the homolateral pulvinar nucleus of the thalamus, contralateral cerebellum, basal ganglia, claustrum, and splenium of the corpus callosum. These findings are usually transient and normalize with no residual encephalomalacia, but partial normalization has been reported as well as emerging new findings such as cortical laminar necrosis, mesial temporal sclerosis, and focal brain atrophy, indicative of tissue damage.

MRI is often warranted after first presentation seizure, particularly if an intracranial cause is suspected. An outpatient study may be appropriate.

47.2.3 Decision-Making Process

The physician's ability to distinguish between strokes and seizures as a cause of acute neurologic deficit relies heavily on skilled history-taking and careful examination.[22] There is a short list of investigations that are useful in this context, mainly CT and CTA, which when normal raises the possibility of stroke mimic.[20] MRI-DWI/ADC can help exclude cerebral ischemia but is not available emergently in many centers.[33] CT perfusion may help in distinguishing seizure from stroke, and more studies are needed before this can be routinely adopted. A few laboratory studies may be used to help support a diagnosis of recent generalized tonic-clonic seizures; knowledge of the expected timing of the rise of each of these biomarkers is paramount[22,23]. Laboratory investigations cannot be used to exclude generalized tonic-clonic seizures or rule in mimics, due to poor sensitivities.[23] At this time, laboratory investigations are not routinely recommended. EEG is not helpful in distinguishing strokes from seizures, as it only rules in epileptic activity, which, however, does not exclude concomitant strokes.[20,27]

When the above strategies are insufficient and the clinician remains uncertain about the possibility of ongoing seizures, then benzodiazepines can be considered as a diagnostic and therapeutic trial. Ideally, this should be undertaken with continuous EEG monitoring, where the end point is clinical and electrographic resolution.

47.2.4 Management

Early treatment of strokes is paramount to increasing the probability of success with therapeutic interventions, namely, IV-tPA or interventional embolectomy. Equally important is early recognition and treatment of seizures. The longer the delay in seizure treatment, the less likely antiepileptic medications will be effective.[34,35] As seizures can be precipitated by acute strokes, treatments for both processes may need to be given concurrently.

For acute seizures that do not terminate spontaneously, benzodiazepines are first line. Lorazepam 2 to 4 mg (0.1 mg/kg) IV is a good starting point, with option to redose in 5 to 10 minutes. For thorough discussions on the treatment of status epileptics, selection of long-term antiepileptic therapy, and management of first presentation seizures, see the corresponding reviews outlined in the "Further Readings" section of this chapter.[35,36,37]

Many jurisdictions mandate reporting seizures to the corresponding transportation authority. Counseling should be provided to the patient—and his/her family, as appropriate—regarding the dangers of driving. Additional safety counseling should be offered for new seizure patients regarding the following: avoidance of heights, operating heavy machinery, bathing/swimming alone, and women's health issues.

47.2.5 Literature Synopsis

Distinguishing strokes from seizures relies heavily on clinical skills. Importantly, a diagnosis of seizures does not preclude concomitant strokes.[20] Clues to seizures include positive neurologic symptoms or signs, such as paresthesias, twitching, rhythmic jerking, nystagmoid eye movements, and sustained gaze deviation in the direction of the affected extremities. Postictally, drowsiness, reversal of the gaze deviation, and weakness are all possible. An underlying cause for seizures should be sought, as it can help to stratify risk of recurrent seizures.

A few investigations may support one's clinical suspicion for seizures or strokes. In the case of seizures, CT/CTA is expected to be normal.[20] CT perfusion can show various changes, especially hyperperfusion ictally and hypoperfusion postictally. A nonvascular distribution of these changes suggests seizures[28,32]; variations in vascular supply such a as fetal PCA can be verified by CTA. More studies are needed to validate the use of CT perfusion in this context. EEG may confirm seizures but does not rule out strokes. Laboratory investigations, when appropriately timed, may support a clinical diagnosis of recent generalized tonic-clonic seizures but cannot rule out this diagnosis or rule in alternatives such as stroke.[23]

Both strokes and seizures require prompt recognition and treatment to optimize outcomes. In the case of suspected seizures, benzodiazepines are first line. Longer-term treatment can be initiated concurrently, if appropriate. The clinician must be aware of local requirements for reporting to the transportation authorities. Safety counseling should always be undertaken in the case of new seizures.

47.2.6 Pearls and Pitfalls

- A diagnosis of seizures does not rule out concurrent strokes.
- When seizures mimic strokes, it is usually postictally, as in Todd's paresis; however, occasionally ictal paresis can occur.
- Laboratory investigations such as prolactin may support a clinical diagnosis of seizures when used properly and with correct timing. Due to low sensitivity, such laboratory investigations cannot be used to exclude seizures or suggest an alternate diagnosis such as strokes.
- CT perfusion is emerging as a potential tool to distinguish strokes from seizures and postictal paresis. More data are needed before it can be routinely adopted.
- If a patient does not return to baseline promptly after seizures, an EEG should be undertaken to rule out status epilepticus, and consideration should be given to empiric antiepileptic therapy.
- The clinician must follow local requirements for reporting seizures to the corresponding transportation authorities. Safety counseling should always be undertaken in the case of new seizures.

References

[1] Huff JS. Stroke differential diagnosis—mimics and chameleons. Foundation for Education and Research in Neurological Emergencies. Available at: www.uic.edu/com/ferne/pdf2. Accessed September 19, 2019

[2] Zinkstok SM, Engelter ST, Gensicke H, et al. Safety of thrombolysis in stroke mimics: results from a multicenter cohort study. Stroke. 2013; 44(4):1080–1084

[3] Geisler F, Ali EF, Ebinger M, et al. Evaluation of a score for the prehospital distinction between cerebrovascular disease and stroke mimic patients. Int J Stroke. 2019; 14(4):400–408

[4] Fischer RS, Acevedo C, Arzimanoglou A, et al. A practical clinical definition of epilepsy. ILAE official report. Epilepsia. 2014; 55(4):475–482

[5] Besag FMC, Vasey MJ. Prodrome in epilepsy. Epilepsy Behav. 2018; 83:219–233

[6] Liu Y, Guo XM, Wu X, Li P, Wang WW. Clinical analysis of partial epilepsy. Chin Med J (Engl). 2017; 130(3):318–322

[7] Daroff RB, Bradley WG. Bradley's Neurology in Clinical Practice. Philadelphia, PA: Elsevier/Saunders; 2012

[8] Perven G, So NK. Epileptic auras: phenomenology and neurophysiology. Epileptic Disord. 2015; 17(4):349–362

[9] Abou-Khalil B, Fakhoury T, Jennings M, Moots P, Warner J, Kessler RM. Inhibitory motor seizures: correlation with centroparietal structural and functional abnormalities. Acta Neurol Scand. 1995; 91(2):103–108

[10] Chowdhury FA, Connor S, Ferner R, Leschziner G. Focal inhibitory seizures: a cause of recurrent transient weakness. Pract Neurol. 2015; 15(6):460–462

[11] Foldvary-Schaefer N, Unnwongse K. Localizing and lateralizing features of auras and seizures. Epilepsy Behav. 2011; 20(2):160–166

[12] Villani F, D'Amico D, Pincherle A, Tullo V, Chiapparini L, Bussone G. Prolonged focal negative motor seizures: a video-EEG study. Epilepsia. 2006; 47(11):1949–1952

[13] Sato K, Arai N, Omori A, Hida A, Kimura A, Takeuchi S. Hyperammonaemia and associated factors in unprovoked convulsive seizures: a cross-sectional study. Seizure. 2016; 43:6–12

[14] Rolak LA, Rutecki P, Ashizawa T, Harati Y. Clinical features of Todd's post-epileptic paralysis. J Neurol Neurosurg Psychiatry. 1992; 55(1):63–64

[15] Binder DK. A history of Todd and his paralysis. Neurosurgery. 2004; 54(2):480–486, discussion 486–487

[16] Gibson LM, Hanby MF, Al-Bachari SM, Parkes LM, Allan SM, Emsley HC. Late-onset epilepsy and occult cerebrovascular disease. J Cereb Blood Flow Metab. 2014; 34(4):564–570

[17] Szaflarski JP, Rackley AY, Kleindorfer DO, et al. Incidence of seizures in the acute phase of stroke: a population-based study. Epilepsia. 2008; 49(6):974–981

[18] Bladin CF, Alexandrov AV, Bellavance A, et al. Seizures after stroke: a prospective multicenter study. Arch Neurol. 2000; 57(11):1617–1622

[19] Pohlmann-Eden B, Cochius JI, Hoch DB, Hennerici MG. Stroke and epilepsy: critical review of the literature. Cerebrovasc Dis. 1997; 7:2–9

[20] Sylaja PN, Dzialowski I, Krol A, Roy J, Federico P, Demchuk AM, Calgary Stroke Program. Role of CT angiography in thrombolysis decision-making for patients with presumed seizure at stroke onset. Stroke. 2006; 37(3):915–917

[21] Nguyen PL, Chang JJ. Stroke mimics and acute stroke evaluation: clinical differentiation and complications after intravenous tissue plasminogen activator. J Emerg Med. 2015; 49(2):244–252

[22] Gavvala JR, Schuele SU. New onset seizure in adults and adolescents: a review. JAMA. 2016; 316(24):2657–2668

[23] Nass RD, Sassen R, Elger CE, Surges R. The role of postictal laboratory blood analyses in the diagnosis and prognosis of seizures. Seizure. 2017; 47:51–65

[24] Beghi E, De Maria G, Gobbi G, Veneselli E. Diagnosis and treatment of the first epileptic seizure: guidelines of the Italian league against epilepsy. Epilepsia. 2006; 47 Suppl 5:2–8

[25] Albadareen R, Gronseth G, Landazuri P, He J, Hammond N, Uysal U. Postictal ammonia as a biomarker for electrographic convulsive seizures: a prospective study. Epilepsia. 2016; 57(8):1221–1227

[26] Matz O, Heckelmann J, Zechbauer S, et al. Early postictal serum lactate concentrations are superior to serum creatine kinase concentrations in distinguishing generalized tonic-clonic seizures from syncopes. Intern Emerg Med. 2018; 13(5):749–755

[27] Kubiak-Balcerewicz K, Fiszer U, Nagańska E, et al. Differentiating stroke and seizure in acute setting—perfusion computed tomography. J Stroke Cerebrovasc Dis. 2017; 26(6):1321–1327

[28] Gelfand JM, Wintermark M, Josephson SA. Cerebral perfusion-CT patterns following seizure. Eur J Neurol. 2010; 17(4):594–601

[29] Van Cauwenberge MGA, Dekeyzer S, Nikoubashman O, Dafotakis M, Wiesmann M. Can perfusion CT unmask postictal stroke mimics? A case-control study of 133 patients. Neurology. 2018; 91(20):e1918–e1927

[30] Shelly S, Maggio N, Boxer M, Blatt I, Tanne D, Orion D. Computed tomography perfusion maps reveal dynamics in postictal patients: a novel diagnostic tool. Isr Med Assoc J. 2017; 19(9):553–556

[31] Sotoudeh H, Shafaat O, Singhal A, Bag A. Luxury perfusion: a paradoxical finding and pitfall of CT perfusion in subacute infarction of brain. Radiol Case Rep. 2018; 14(1):6–9

[32] Dekeyzer S, Vanden Bossche S, Keereman V, Hemelsoet D, Van Driessche V. Stroke versus seizure–perfusion computed tomography in a patient with aphasia. J Belg Soc Radiol. 2015; 99(2):85–89

[33] Sanghvi D, Goyal C, Mani J. Stroke mimic: perfusion magnetic resonance imaging of a patient with ictal paralysis. J Postgrad Med. 2016; 62(4):264–266

[34] Zaccara G, Giannasi G, Oggioni R, Rosati E, Tramacere L, Palumbo P, et al. Challenges in the treatment of convulsive status epilepticus. Seizure. 2017; 47:17–24

[35] Hocker SE. Status epilepticus. Continuum (Minneap Minn). 2015; 21 5 Neurocritical Care:1362–1383

[36] Abou-Khalil BW. Antiepileptic drugs. Continuum (Minneap Minn). 2016; 22 (1 Epilepsy):132–156

[37] Bergey GK. Management of a first seizure. Continuum (Minneap Minn). 2016; 22(1 Epilepsy):38–50

48 Cerebral Amyloid Angiopathy

48.1 Case Description

48.1.1 Case 1: Patient with Seizures and Cognitive Impairment

Clinical Presentation

A 75-year-old man presented to the emergency department for assessment of loss of consciousness. While sitting on the edge of the bed and staring, he suddenly developed a generalized tonic clonic seizure that lasted 10 minutes. His past medical history was negative except for well-controlled hypertension and dyslipidemia. He did not have prior cerebrovascular events or cognitive deficits. His family history was negative for dementia. He lived with his family and was fully independent at baseline. On examination, he was confused, and not oriented to place or time. He had a right gaze preference and head deviation to the right, with continuous right-sided clonic movements. Given his complex presentation, he was promptly intubated for airway protection and received a loading dose of phenytoin.

48.1.2 Investigations and Imaging

- Noncontrast CT (NCCT) of the head at the time of presentation (► Fig. 48.1a) showed multifocal left occipital hyperattenuation, consistent with intraparenchymal hemorrhage (ICH). CT angiography (CTA) did not show any underlying vascular malformation and dural venous sinuses were patent.

- An MRI of the brain was performed 2 days later (► Fig. 48.1b–d), showing acute left occipital hemorrhage with associated vasogenic edema. There was no definite evidence of an underlying lesion. Scattered microhemorrhages with a posterior predilection at the cortical/subcortical junctions were suggestive of cerebral amyloid angiopathy (CAA).
- Electroencephalography (EEG) revealed intermittent frequent focal polymorphic delta theta waves involving the left anterior and mid temporal regions, reflective of underlying subcortical white matter dysfunction.

48.1.3 Treatment and Outcome

The patient remained intubated for 2 days; after extubation, he was delirious for 3 days without any signs of infection or electrolyte disturbance, but once subtherapeutic phenytoin levels were corrected his delirium resolved. He required two antiepileptic medications for breakthrough complex partial seizures: on levetiracetam 1,500 mg orally twice daily and phenytoin 300 mg orally once daily, the patient did not have any further seizure recurrence. Through his hospital stay, his blood pressure was well controlled with an average of less than 140/90 while on three antihypertensive agents. On cognitive assessment, his Mini Mental State Examination (MMSE) score was 17/30, with recall and attention domains mostly affected. At discharge, the patient could sit without assistance, but he needed assistance for mobility, bathing, grooming, and dressing. He was discharged home after 2 weeks with community care support and a modified Rankin scale (mRS) functional status of 3.

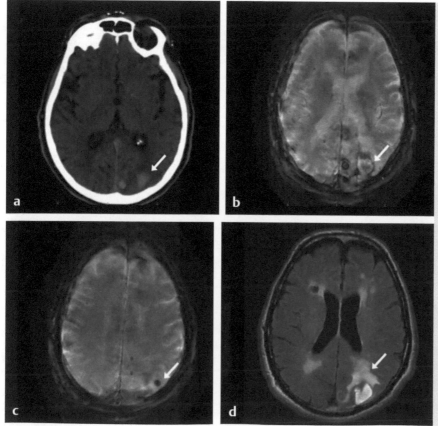

Fig. 48.1 (a) Noncontrast CT scan performed at the time of admission shows intraparenchymal hemorrhage within the left occipital lobe. (b). Gradient echo MRI sequence shows susceptibility effect from hemosiderin deposition in the left occipital hematoma cavity, and (c) previous subcortical microhemorrhage in the left parietooccipital region. (d) FLAIR MRI sequence shows vasogenic edema around the hematoma cavity, with evidence of previous white matter infarcts and chronic microangiopathy.

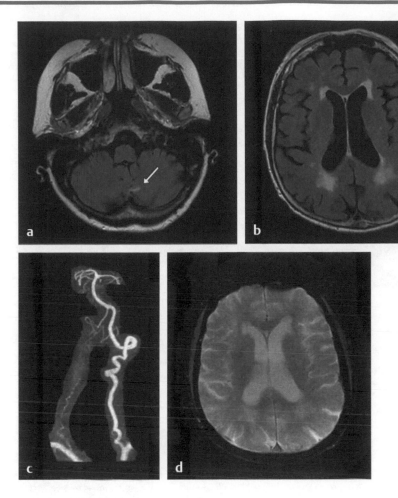

Fig. 48.2 (a) FLAIR MRI sequence shows ence-phalomalacia compatible with a small established infarct in the cerebellum, with (b) moderate periventricular FLAIR hyperintensity indicating chronic microangiopathy. (c) MR angiography shows a chronically occluded right vertebral artery. (d) At the time of this MRI, gradient echo sequences show no evidence of prior microhemorrhage.

48.1.4 Final Diagnosis

CAA presenting with intraparenchymal hemorrhage and multiple cerebral microbleeds.

48.2 Case 2: Patient with Rapidly Progressive Cognitive Decline

48.2.1 Clinical Presentation

An 82-year-old woman, with a history of polymyalgia rheumatica on low-dose prednisone, was originally referred to the stroke prevention clinic after the incidental discovery of a chronic cerebellar infarct on an MRI of the brain performed as part of a workup for gait instability and headache. The MRI showed a small area of encephalomalacia from remote infarct in the inferior cerebellar vermis and moderate white matter microangiopathy, but no evidence of prior hemorrhage (▶ Fig. 48.2). The right vertebral artery was chronically occluded on MR angiography. The patient had no known vascular risk factors such as hypertension, dyslipidemia, diabetes, or tobacco use, although she had taken hormone replacement therapy after menopause. Echocardiogram showed no cardiac source of embolus, so the patient was advised to take daily 81 mg aspirin and was discharged from the stroke clinic.

Sixteen months after being assessed at the stroke clinic, the patient presented to the emergency room. Her husband reported that the patient was cognitively intact until two months before, when he noticed that she had forgotten to pay bills. In the last month, she had become increasingly disoriented, her gait instability had worsened, and she had developed speech difficulties. Her husband brought her to the emergency room once she no longer recognized him.

48.2.2 Investigations and Imaging

- NCCT scan performed at the time of admission showed small volume subarachnoid hemorrhage (SAH) in the left cingulate sulcus (▶ Fig. 48.3a, b), with a background of white matter low attenuation and generalized brain parenchymal volume loss.
- C-reactive protein (CRP) was elevated at 42 mg/L, and erythrocyte sedimentation rate (ESR) was elevated at 39 mm/hour. The white blood cell count was at the upper limits of normal, 7.4×10^9/L. Rheumatologic investigations including antineutrophil cytoplasmic antibodies (ANCA), antinuclear antibodies (ANA), rheumatoid factor (RF), and anti-dsDNA antibodies were negative.
- Cerebrospinal fluid (CSF) analysis showed no evidence of infection with viruses, fungi, mycoplasma, tuberculosis, syphilis, or other bacteria. CSF cell count and differential were normal. Cytology showed no evidence of malignant cells. CSF glucose was low at 2.1 mmol/L, and CSF protein was high at 1.61 g/L.

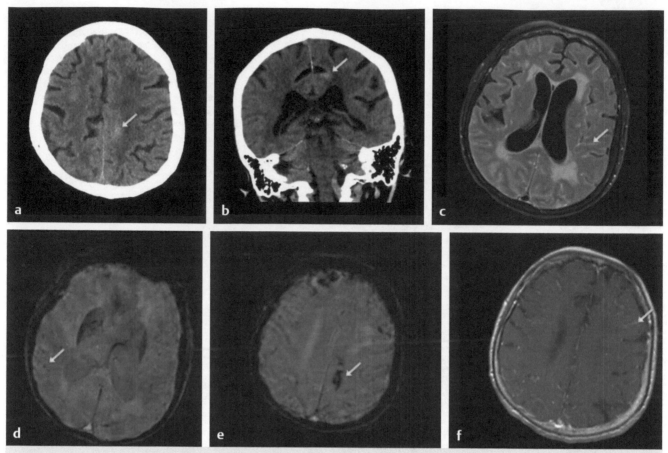

Fig. 48.3 (a) Noncontrast CT scan performed at the time of admission shows small volume hemorrhage in the left parasagittal frontoparietal region, localizing to the cingulate sulcus on the coronal reformat (b). (c) FLAIR sequence shows diffuse high signal in the cerebral sulci, and extensive white matter hyperintensity. (d) Susceptibility-weighted sequences show interval development of cortical/subcortical microhemorrhages, and (e) blood products in the left cingulate sulcus. (f) Postcontrast T1 sequence shows several areas of leptomeningeal enhancement.

- Contrast-enhanced MRI (▶ Fig. 48.3c–f) showed diffuse high fluid-attenuated inversion recovery (FLAIR) signal in the cerebral sulci, and extensive white matter hyperintensity, with multifocal leptomeningeal enhancement and interval development of cerebral subcortical microhemorrhages.
- A brain biopsy in the region of leptomeningeal enhancement in the right frontal lobe showed vasculocentric granulomatous inflammation. Immunohistochemistry for beta–amyloid showed abundant reactivity in leptomeningeal and cortical blood vessels, suggesting amyloid angiitis. Frequent neuritic and diffuse amyloid plaques were seen in the cortex.

48.2.3 Treatment and Outcome

At the time of admission, the patient was treated with high-dose intravenous (IV) methylprednisolone for five days, which resulted in mild cognitive improvement. The methylprednisolone was continued for a further five days with the addition of cyclophosphamide, and the patient was then switched to 50 mg of oral prednisone daily. Tapering of the prednisone resulted in deterioration, so MMF 500 mg PO BID was added.

Follow-up MRI (▶ Fig. 48.4) showed moderate reduction, but not resolution, in the leptomeningeal enhancement. After three months in hospital, the patient was discharged to a long-term care facility, as she required assistance with her activities of daily living (mRS score of 4).

48.2.4 Final Diagnosis

Amyloid-beta–related angiitis (ABRA), causing vasculocentric granulomatous inflammation and resulting SAH.

48.3 Discussion

CAA is a brain condition characterized by amyloid protein deposition within the media and adventitia of the leptomeningeal and cortical arterioles and small arteries of the brain cerebrum and cerebellum. CAA is classified based on the type of the amyloid protein involved in the process. The sporadic amyloid β-protein (Aβ)-type CAA is most commonly found in older individuals and in patients with Alzheimer disease (AD). So far, the following seven amyloid proteins have been reported in CAA: Aβ, cystatin C, prion protein, ABri/ADan, transthyretin, gelsolin, and immunoglobulin light chain amyloid.

Whereas the senile plaques of Alzheimer disease deposited within the neuropil are mostly composed of the longer 42–43 amino acid cleavage peptide Aβ42, the aggregates seen in CAA are typically composed of the shorter 40 amino acid peptide

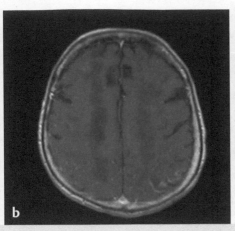
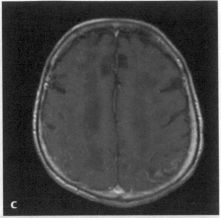

Fig. 48.4 MRI performed after 2 months of immunosuppression shows (**a**) progression of white matter FLAIR hyperintensity, and persistent high FLAIR signal in the cortical sulci. (**b**) Postcontrast leptomeningeal enhancement has decreased but not completely resolved. (**c**) Subcortical microhemorrhages have increased in number.

Aβ40. The Aβ42 peptide aggregates more readily than Aβ40 and therefore forms amyloid near its site of production from neurons within the brain parenchyma, while Aβ40 is transported by interstitial fluid flow to blood vessels, where it aggregates on vascular basement membranes.

48.3.1 Clinical Presentations of CAA

The accumulation of the amyloid causes CAA-associated vasculopathy and fragility of the arterioles and small arteries, leading to clinical or subclinical hemorrhagic lesions: lobar intracerebral macrohemorrhage, cortical microhemorrhage, and focal convexity SAH. The occipital lobe is preferentially affected, while CAA is uncommon in the basal ganglia, thalamus, and brainstem; spontaneous hemorrhages in these regions are more commonly hypertensive in etiology.

CAA-related lobar ICH is often multiple and recurrent. Clinical manifestations depend on the function of the brain region at the site of hemorrhage and include motor paresis, disturbance of consciousness, aphasia, and visual loss. Patients often present with headache at the acute stage, and dementia and seizures during chronic stages. Headache with meningeal signs is likely caused by SAH accompanying lobar ICH.

CAA is a frequent cause of cortical superficial siderosis/focal convexity SAH, a subtype of nonaneurysmal SAH, in patients older than 60 years and in those with AD. Notably, cortical superficial siderosis is closely associated with microhemorrhages in lobar locations in the general population; it is highly prevalent in CAA and is found in 60.5% of pathologically confirmed cases.

CAA-related cerebral hypoperfusion or occlusive small-vessel disease may cause progressive white matter lesions and cortical microinfarcts. Patients with CAA-related ICH exhibit occipital dominant white matter hyperintensities on MRI, compatible with the predilection of CAA pathology for posterior brain regions.

Dementia was noted in 74% of individuals with severe CAA at autopsy. Moderate-to-very severe CAA is associated with impaired performance in specific cognitive domains, most notably perceptual speed, which is separate from the effect of AD pathology.

48.3.2 Diagnostic Criteria for CAA

Definite confirmation of a CAA diagnosis is only possible on post-mortem histopathological examination of the brain. The modified Boston criteria (▶ Table 48.1) establish categories of definite, probable, and possible CAA which can help guide clinical diagnosis and management at the time of patient presentation. In general, the diagnosis of probable and possible CAA require imaging demonstration of lobar, cortical, or cortical/subcortical hemorrhage, and/or superficial siderosis, in patients older than 55 years. Alterative causes for intracerebral hemorrhage must be excluded.

48.3.3 Inflammatory Variants of CAA

CAA is commonly associated with activation of cells in the monocyte/macrophage lineage. CAA can therefore be accompanied by inflammation, presenting with subacute leukoencephalopathy that is responsive to immunosuppressive therapies. The clinical symptoms include subacute cognitive impairment or seizure, which are different from those of hemorrhagic stroke in noninflammatory CAA.

The inflammatory variants of CAA are closely related and include CAA-related inflammation (CAA-RI) and ABRA. In CAA-RI, the inflammation is primarily perivascular, whereas in ABRA it is centered within the media and adventitia of small arteries and arterioles. Imaging features of CAA-RI and ABRA are overlapping: in addition to the superficial siderosis and intraparenchymal hemorrhage present in noninflammatory inflammatory, CAA is also characterized by T2 and FLAIR white matter hyperintensity in the region of inflammation, often with leptomeningeal enhancement. The degree of white matter hyperintensity and leptomeningeal enhancement can be monitored on serial MRI as a marker of response to immunosuppression. Case 1 describes a noninflammatory presentation of CAA, while case 2 shows an inflammatory variant, shown on biopsy to be ABRA.

Table 48.1 Modified Boston criteria for diagnosis of CAA-related hemorrhage

Diagnostic category	Criteria
Definite CAA	Postmortem examination demonstrating: • Lobar, cortical, or cortical/subcortical hemorrhage • Severe CAA with vasculopathy • Absence of other diagnostic lesions
Probable CAA with supporting pathology	Clinical data and pathologic tissue (evacuated hematoma or cortical biopsy) demonstrating: • Lobar, cortical, or cortical/subcortical hemorrhage • Some degree of CAA in the specimen • Absence of other diagnostic lesions
Probable CAA	Clinical data and MRI or CT demonstrating: • Multiple hemorrhages restricted to lobar, cortical, or cortical/subcortical regions (cerebellar hemorrhage is allowed) • Alternatively, a single hemorrhage in one of these regions and focal[a] or disseminated[b] superficial siderosis • Age > 55 y • Absence of other causes of hemorrhage or superficial siderosis[c]
Possible CAA	Clinical data and MRI or CT demonstrating: • Single lobar, cortical, or cortical/subcortical hemorrhage • Alternatively, focal[a] or disseminated[b] superficial siderosis • Age > 55 y • Absence of other causes of hemorrhage or superficial siderosis[c]

Abbreviations: CAA, cerebral amyloid angiopathy; INR, international normalized ratio.
[a]Affecting three or fewer sulci.
[b]Affecting four or more sulci.
[c]Other causes of intracerebral hemorrhage include excessive warfarin with (INR) > 3, antecedent head trauma or ischemic stroke, tumor, vascular malformation, vasculitis, blood dyscrasia, or coagulopathy. INR > 3 and other nonspecific laboratory abnormalities are permitted for the diagnosis of CAA.

48.3.4 Imaging Investigations for CAA

Patients with CAA who present emergently with acute subarachnoid or intraparenchymal hemorrhage frequently have a NCCT performed as an initial study. Head CT is sensitive for the detection of intracerebral hematoma, and SAH within 6 hours of occurrence. Identification of these findings will prompt hospital admission and further investigation into the cause of hemorrhage. CTA may not only be useful to detect a spot sign indicating active extravasation but also help identify an underlying vascular malformation.

Contrast-enhanced MRI is the preferred modality for detection of imaging findings supportive of a diagnosis of possible or probable CAA. Gradient echo or susceptibility weighted sequences are useful for detection of cerebral microhemorrhages or superficial siderosis. Although acute or subacute cortical or subcortical infarctions can be recognized in CAA on diffusion-weighted images, cortical microinfarcts are often undetected on MRI because of their limited size. Higher magnetic field strengths may improve sensitivity for detection of microhemorrhages and microinfarcts.

As noted in Table 48.1, the diagnosis of possible or probable CAA requires exclusion of other etiologies for intracerebral hemorrhage, such as mass lesions or vascular malformations. In the setting of an acute intraparenchymal hematoma, mass effect from the hematoma may obscure an underlying lesion, so it is advisable to repeat the MRI after resolution of mass effect from the hematoma to more confidently exclude an underlying abnormality.

Multifocal cerebral microhemorrhages are occasionally encountered as an incidental finding on MRI scans of outpatients. In the clinical context of cognitive decline, this provides supportive evidence for the possible diagnosis of CAA. In the asymptomatic patient, other causes of microhemorrhage should be considered, including hypertension and diffuse axonal injury from prior trauma. The distribution of microhemorrhages may be helpful to distinguish the cause: as described above, CAA typically has a cortical/subcortical distribution in the cerebral hemispheres, while hypertension affects the basal ganglia, thalamus, and brainstem (perforator vascular territories). Diffuse axonal injury is typically seen in long white matter tracts including the corpus callosum and may be accompanied by other evidence of trauma such as healed fractures or encephalomalacia involving the inferior frontal lobes and anterior temporal lobes. Other diagnoses to consider include multiple hemorrhagic metastases in a patient with malignancy, or mycotic aneurysms in a patient with sepsis, endocarditis, or a right to left heart shunt.

Positron emission tomography (PET) with an amyloid avid ligand such as Pittsburgh Compound B (PiB) may show greater occipital uptake in CAA-related intracerebral hemorrhage. High PiB uptake in healthy elderly individuals may reflect incipient AD. PiB PET has low specificity for CAA, but a negative PiB scan rules out CAA with excellent sensitivity.

48.3.5 Biochemical Markers of CAA

A significant decrease in cerebrospinal fluid (CSF) levels of Aβ40 as well as Aβ42 was reported in patients with probable CAA, which suggests trapping of Aβ40 and Aβ42 in the cerebral vasculature. Furthermore, CSF levels of total tau and phosphorylated tau are higher in patients with probable CAA than in controls, but lower than in AD. CAA-related inflammation is associated with an increase in anti-Aβ antibodies in the CSF.

48.3.6 Treatment and Prognosis

Currently, no disease-modifying therapies are available for CAA. Subacute leukoencephalopathy associated with CAA-related inflammation or angiitis often responds to immunosuppressive treatment, but as demonstrated in Case 2 resolution of inflammation is often incomplete and requires ongoing immunosuppression.

The humanized monoclonal antibody ponezumab, which binds the C terminal residues 33–40 of the Aβ40 peptide, was the first medication tested in clinical trials for CAA. The specificity of the antibody for Aβ40, the predominant Aβ subtype in vascular deposits, made it a promising candidate therapy. Previous trials of ponezumab for AD had demonstrated an acceptable safety profile. A trial in 36 patients receiving three infusions on days 1, 30, and 60 of the trial unfortunately failed to meet its primary outcome target of improvement in cerebrovascular reactivity as measured by functional MRI.

Blood pressure control has been shown to be beneficial in patients with CAA: a subgroup analysis of the PROGRESS (Perindopril Protection Against Recurrent Stroke Study) trial showed that those with probable CAA (although with limited diagnostic evaluation) had a 77% reduction in ICH with blood pressure lowering. There is still no guidance on specific blood pressure targets or how aggressively this should be managed in patients without macrohemorrhage. In addition to preventing recurrent ICH, blood pressure control has a potential role in slowing the progression of CAA, as has been observed in age-related deep-perforating arteriopathy, but further evidence from clinical trials is needed.

Patients with CAA who require anticoagulation for other medical indications face a difficult balance of risk and benefit, since CAA confers an increased probability of ICH. With an average ICH recurrence rate in CAA of about 9% per year, antithrombotic strategies that increase the relative risk of ICH by more than about 50% are likely to outweigh the benefits from reduced risk of thrombosis.

48.4 Summary

CAA is a disease characterized by amyloid deposition in the small arteries of the brain, leading to an increased risk of lobar, cortical/subcortical, and subarachnoid hemorrhage. The most commonly deposited protein is the 40-amino acid form of the Aβ peptide, implying a complex and incompletely understood overlap with Alzheimer's disease. Clinical presentation may be acute, related to intracranial macrohemorrhage or seizure, or chronic with progressive cognitive decline. Gradient echo (GRE) or susceptibility-weighted MRI sequences are helpful in establishing the clinical diagnosis of possible or probable CAA through demonstration of intraparenchymal blood products and superficial siderosis, while excluding other etiologies. Inflammatory variants of CAA exist with a macrophage/monocyte infiltrate, leading to T2/FLAIR white matter hyperintensities and leptomeningeal enhancement. The inflammatory variants of CAA often respond to immunosuppression, but to date there is no other disease modifying therapy available for CAA.

Suggested Readings

Banerjee G, Carare R, Cordonnier C, et al. The increasing impact of cerebral amyloid angiopathy: essential new insights for clinical practice. J Neurol Neurosurg Psychiatry. 2017; 88(11):982–994

Yamada M. Cerebral amyloid angiopathy: emerging concepts. J Stroke. 2015; 17 (1):17–30

Yates PA, Sirisriro R, Villemagne VL, Farquharson S, Masters CL, Rowe CC, AIBL Research Group. Cerebral microhemorrhage and brain β-amyloid in aging and Alzheimer disease. Neurology. 2011; 77(1):48–54

Charidimou A, Peeters AP, Jäger R, et al. Cortical superficial siderosis and intracerebral hemorrhage risk in cerebral amyloid angiopathy. Neurology. 2013; 81(19):1666–1673

Shoamanesh A, Martinez-Ramirez S, Oliveira-Filho J, et al. Interrelationship of superficial siderosis and microbleeds in cerebral amyloid angiopathy. Neurology. 2014; 83(20):1838–1843

Renard D, Castelnovo G, Wacongne A, et al. Interest of CSF biomarker analysis in possible cerebral amyloid angiopathy cases defined by the modified Boston criteria. J Neurol. 2012; 259(11):2429–2433

Arima H, Tzourio C, Anderson C, et al. Chalmers. J Stroke. 2010; 41:394–396

Maxwell SS, Jackson CA, Paternoster L, et al. Genetic associations with brain microbleeds: Systematic review and meta-analyses. Neurology. 2011; 77(2):158–167

Baron JC, Farid K, Dolan E, et al. Diagnostic utility of amyloid PET in cerebral amyloid angiopathy-related symptomatic intracerebral hemorrhage. J Cereb Blood Flow Metab. 2014; 34(5):753–758

Nandigam RN, Viswanathan A, Delgado P, et al. MR imaging detection of cerebral microbleeds: effect of susceptibility-weighted imaging, section thickness, and field strength. AJNR Am J Neuroradiol. 2009; 30(2):338–343

Martucci M, Sarria S, Toledo M, et al. Cerebral amyloid angiopathy related inflammation: imaging findings and clinical outcome. Neuroradiology. 2014; 56 (4):283–289

Sakaguchi H, Ueda A, Kosaka T, et al. Cerebral amyloid angiopathy-related inflammation presenting with steroid-responsive higher brain dysfunction: case report and review of the literature. J Neuroinflammation. 2011; 8:116

49 Contrast Staining Masquerading as Hemorrhage

49.1 Case

Utility of dual-energy CT after endovascular stroke treatment.

49.2 Case Description

49.2.1 Clinical Presentation

A 52-year-old male presented at 23:15 on Sunday night, 60 minutes after being discovered with an altered conscious state. Past medical history was significant for ischemic heart disease with cardiac stents and automatic implantable cardioverter-defibrillator. Examination in the emergency department reveals a Glasgow coma scale (GCS) score of 12 with some motion in all limbs.

49.2.2 Imaging Workup and Investigations

- Initial noncontrast CT (NCCT) at 100 minutes post–stroke onset reveals no established ischemic changes with Alberta Stroke Program Early CT (ASPECTS) score of 10.
- CTA reveals occlusion of the extracranial and intracranial left internal carotid artery (ICA) and middle cerebral artery (MCA; ▶ Fig. 49.1).
- No CTP was performed at the time due to excessive motion artefact.
- Delayed code stroke was activated as the emergency staffs were attempting to stabilize the patients' agitated state, and CTP was performed.
- CTP at 5 hours post–onset reveals perfusion abnormality in the left MCA territory, with elevated mean transit time and normal cerebral blood volume maps, suggesting the presence of a small core and large penumbra.
- Examination by the stroke team revealed a National Institutes of Health Stroke Scale (NIHSS) score of 28. The patient was now outside the intravenous tissue plasminogen activator (IV-tPA) treatment timeframe. Endovascular treatment was contemplated.

49.2.3 Diagnosis

Left ICA and MCA occlusion with a small core infarct size based on CT findings.

49.2.4 Treatment

- Endovascular team was contacted, and repeat CT of the brain was performed at 6.5 hours (05:00) post–symptom onset with minimal core evident—ASPECTS score of 7 (▶ Fig. 49.2).
- Endovascular team in the hospital at 05:50 was unable to proceed with conscious sedation due to concerns regarding airway protection. Patient was intubated and moved onto the neuroangiography table at 06:50. Groin puncture occurred at 07:00.

Endovascular Treatment

- Initial digital subtraction angiography (DSA) revealed extensive thrombus burden, extending from cavernous ICA to the terminus and into both A1 and M1 MCA segments.
- Multiple passes with Penumbra 054 for thromboaspiration, and Treveo stentriever.
- Recanalization of the ICA, anterior cerebral artery (ACA), and MCA was achieved, with final thrombolysis in cerebral infarction (TICI) 2a reperfusion after 120 minutes of procedure time.

Posttreatment Imaging

- Postprocedural dual-energy CT imaging at 12 hours post–onset reveals hyperattenuation in the left basal ganglia, left temporal lobe, and in the left sylvian fissure.
- Since this could be due to post procedural hemorrhage, CT images with iodine subtraction are reconstructed (▶ Fig. 49.3).
- This confirmed that the hyperattenuation was due to contrast staining and not intracranial hemorrhage.

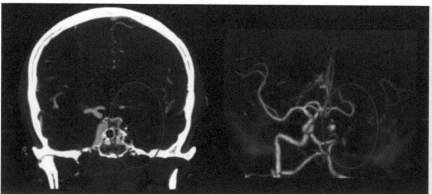

Fig. 49.1 CTA coronal maximum intensity projection and 3D reconstruction demonstrate occlusion of the left internal carotid artery, extending to the carotid terminus, proximal left anterior cerebral artery, and into the left middle cerebral artery.

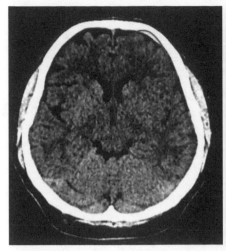

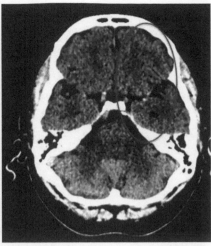

Fig. 49.2 NCCT in a 52-year-old male, performed 6.5 hours after onset. There is loss of gray-white differentiation in the left insular cortex and left lentiform nucleus. Additional left inferior temporal change (not shown) with ASPECTS score of 7.

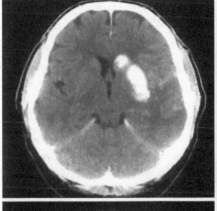

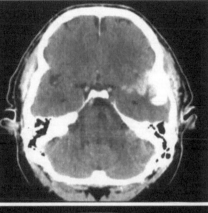

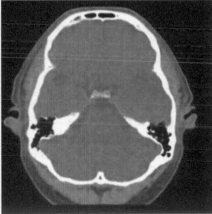

Fig. 49.3 Normal CT (top row) and water (bottom row) maps from dual-energy CT. On the normal CT, there is increased attenuation in the left caudate, lentiform nucleus and temporal lobe, as well as increased attenuation within the sylvian fissure and frontotemporal sulci. No increased attenuation is evident on the water maps (also known as "virtual non contrast"), indicating that the increased attenuation is attributable to contrast staining rather than hemorrhage. Note that these were the corresponding areas of ischemic change evident on the pretreatment CT, since these areas have disruption of the blood–brain barrier.

Outcome

- Repeat CT the following day revealed some contrast washout, and delayed CT at 8 weeks revealed final infarct volume similar to initial CT scans (▶ Fig. 49.4).
- After 4 months, the patient was able to function independently with slight dysphasia and residual hemiparesis, with a mRS score of 2.

49.3 Discussion

Dual-energy CT has ever increasing clinical application throughout the various imaging disciplines, including neuroradiology. The principle of dual-energy CT is the acquisition of two datasets for the same anatomical location with different kVp, allowing decomposition of the imaged object based on the different attenuation coefficients obtained at each kVp. There are three main techniques to facilitate dual-energy acquisition. First, two X-ray tubes may be positioned at right angles within the CT gantry, allowing simultaneous acquisition via two separate detector arrays, each X-ray tube operating at a different kVp. This technique enables the high-temporal resolution required for some clinical applications, but can limit the field of view. Second, a single tube may be utilized with a dual-layer detector array, with each layer optimized to absorb photons at higher or lower energy levels, and each subsequently

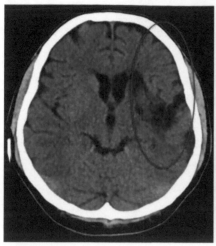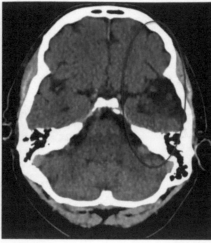

Fig. 49.4 NCCT at 8 weeks revealed final infarct volume similar to initial CT scans. Note that the encephalomalacia is limited to the areas with contrast staining from infarction prior to endovascular treatment.

reconstructed independently. Finally, a single X-ray tube may rapidly switch between the two desired kVp levels, paired with a single detector array.

Neuroradiology applications of dual-energy CT include generating "virtual" noncontrast images from data obtained during a contrast enhanced study; automatic "bone removal" during post processing; reduced beam hardening artefact; improved detection of underlying enhancing mass lesions in the setting of parenchymal hematoma; postprocessing removal of calcified carotid artery plaque for CTA; and differentiating between iodinated contrast media and parenchymal blood.[1,2,3,4,5,6,7,8] The last two applications are of particular interest to neurovascular and interventional neuroradiologists.

When referenced against DSA, dual-energy CTA with automated post processing "plaque removal" has good quantification of stenoses and superior accuracy for detection of relevant stenosis compared to standard CTA reconstructions. The "plaque removal" technique does have the potential to overestimate high-grade stenosis as occlusion, and is thus complementary to standard reconstructions rather than a replacement.[2,6]

Use of dual-energy CT to differentiate between blood and iodinated contrast media may be useful in different clinical settings. Dual-energy CT allows differentiating between iodine and blood based on the differences in attenuation of each that occur at the two selected kVP levels. Postprocessed virtual noncontrast map (water map) and iodine maps may be viewed as standalone images, or fused onto source images.[9,10,11,12]

Parenchymal hyperattenuation is frequently observed following intra-arterial therapy for acute ischemic stroke, representing blood, contrast staining, or a combination of both.[13,14,15,16,17] Early studies reported that the presence of parenchymal hyperattenuation after intra-arterial thrombolysis was a risk factor contributing to secondary hemorrhage and a poor prognostic factor.[14,15] More recently, the significance of parenchymal hyperattenuation after mechanical clot extraction has been evaluated with varied findings. In a series of 48 patients, parenchymal and/or subarachnoid hyperattenuation carried no risk of symptomatic hemorrhage or negative prognosis.[17] In a larger series of 101 patients, parenchymal hyperattenuation was associated with a four-fold risk of hemorrhagic transformation, but had no negative prognostic implication.[16] In a study of

50 patients, the presence of "blood–brain barrier disruption" was associated with a poorer outcome.[18] "Blood–brain barrier disruption" was defined as "spontaneous deposition of iodinated contrast medium in the parenchyma of the ischemic core," but was "differentiated from contrast extravasation secondary to endovascular therapy complications." Detail with regard to distinguishing between hemorrhage and contrast staining is lacking in this study, and the significance of the findings is uncertain with regard to the prognostic implication of parenchymal hyperattenuation. Regardless of prognosis, identifying hemorrhage and distinguishing it from contrast staining may have treatment implications by influencing the decision to anticoagulate, and identifying patients who may need early or closer imaging surveillance.

Distinguishing between parenchymal hyperattenuation and hemorrhage may be achieved with serial CT imaging. Contrast staining typically "washes out" within 24 to 48 hours, with hemorrhage persisting as increased parenchymal attenuation. Alternatively, MRI with blood sensitive sequences may be utilized. In the acute setting, if there is dense contrast staining, the attenuation of the contrast may exceed that of blood, allowing the presence of contrast staining to be established on conventional CT; however, an associated hemorrhage cannot be excluded. Less dense or heterogeneous contrast staining may appear identical to blood, and thus be indistinguishable on conventional CT. Dual-energy CT is emerging as a valuable tool to acutely distinguish between blood and contrast staining in the setting of intra-arterial therapy for acute stroke. Generating iodine and water maps allows contrast staining to be distinguished from hemorrhage, with each appearing as high attenuation on their relative maps, as well as in the assessment of relative amounts of each if they coexist.[4,5] A major advantage of dual-energy CT is that there is no need to delay or repeat imaging to determine if hemorrhage is present, and thus treatment decisions, particularly with regards to anticoagulation, can be instituted immediately. In addition, there is no increase in radiation dose over conventional CT. One pitfall with this technique is calcification, as this appears as increased attenuation on both water and iodine maps. In the current case, the iodine and water maps revealed that the increased parenchymal attenuation was due solely to contrast staining, with no hemorrhage present at the time of the posttreatment CT examination.

49.4 Pearls and Pitfalls

- Increased parenchymal and subarachnoid attenuation after endovascular stroke therapy may reflect blood, contrast staining, or both.
- Contrast staining typically "washes out" within 24 to 48 hours.
- Calcification appears as high attenuation on both iodine and water maps with dual-energy CT, and is a potential pitfall when distinguishing between hemorrhage and contrast staining.

References

[1] Ferda J, Novák M, Mírka H, et al. The assessment of intracranial bleeding with virtual unenhanced imaging by means of dual-energy CT angiography. Eur Radiol. 2009; 19(10):2518–2522

[2] Thomas C, Korn A, Ketelsen D, et al. Automatic lumen segmentation in calcified plaques: dual-energy CT versus standard reconstructions in comparison with digital subtraction angiography. AJR Am J Roentgenol. 2010; 194(6):1590–1595

[3] Thomas C, Korn A, Krauss B, et al. Automatic bone and plaque removal using dual energy CT for head and neck angiography: feasibility and initial performance evaluation. Eur J Radiol. 2010; 76(1):61–67

[4] Phan CM, Yoo AJ, Hirsch JA, Nogueira RG, Gupta R. Differentiation of hemorrhage from iodinated contrast in different intracranial compartments using dual-energy head CT. AJNR Am J Neuroradiol. 2012; 33(6):1088–1094

[5] Gupta R, Phan CM, Leidecker C, et al. Evaluation of dual-energy CT for differentiating intracerebral hemorrhage from iodinated contrast material staining. Radiology. 2010; 257(1):205–211

[6] Uotani K, Watanabe Y, Higashi M, et al. Dual-energy CT head bone and hard plaque removal for quantification of calcified carotid stenosis: utility and comparison with digital subtraction angiography. Eur Radiol. 2009; 19 (8):2060–2065

[7] Kim SJ, Lim HK, Lee HY, et al. Dual-energy CT in the evaluation of intracerebral hemorrhage of unknown origin: differentiation between tumor bleeding and pure hemorrhage. AJNR Am J Neuroradiol. 2012; 33(5):865–872

[8] Watanabe Y, Tsukabe A, Kunitomi Y, et al. Dual-energy CT for detection of contrast enhancement or leakage within high-density haematomas in patients with intracranial haemorrhage. Neuroradiology. 2014; 56(4):291–295

[9] Ederies A, Demchuk A, Chia T, et al. Postcontrast CT extravasation is associated with hematoma expansion in CTA spot negative patients. Stroke. 2009; 40(5):1672–1676

[10] Demchuk AM, Dowlatshahi D, Rodriguez-Luna D, et al. PREDICT/Sunnybrook ICH CTA study group. Prediction of haematoma growth and outcome in patients with intracerebral haemorrhage using the CT-angiography spot sign (PREDICT): a prospective observational study. Lancet Neurol. 2012; 11 (4):307–314

[11] Romero JM, Kelly HR, Delgado Almandoz JE, et al. Contrast extravasation on CT angiography predicts hematoma expansion and mortality in acute traumatic subdural hemorrhage. AJNR Am J Neuroradiol. 2013; 34(8):1528–1534

[12] Letourneau-Guillon L, Huynh T, Jakobovic R, Milwid R, Symons SP, Aviv RI. Traumatic intracranial hematomas: prognostic value of contrast extravasation. AJNR Am J Neuroradiol. 2013; 34(4):773–779

[13] Wildenhain SL, Jungreis CA, Barr J, Mathis J, Wechsler L, Horton JA. CT after intracranial intraarterial thrombolysis for acute stroke. AJNR Am J Neuroradiol. 1994; 15(3):487–492

[14] Nakano S, Iseda T, Kawano H, Yoneyama T, Ikeda T, Wakisaka S. Parenchymal hyperdensity on computed tomography after intra-arterial reperfusion therapy for acute middle cerebral artery occlusion: incidence and clinical significance. Stroke. 2001; 32(9):2042–2048

[15] Yoon W, Seo JJ, Kim JK, Cho KH, Park JG, Kang HK. Contrast enhancement and contrast extravasation on computed tomography after intra-arterial thrombolysis in patients with acute ischemic stroke. Stroke. 2004; 35 (4):876–881

[16] Lummel N, Schulte-Altedorneburg G, Bernau C, et al. Hyperattenuated intracerebral lesions after mechanical recanalization in acute stroke. AJNR Am J Neuroradiol. 2014; 35(2):345–351

[17] Parrilla G, García-Villalba B, Espinosa de Rueda M, et al. Hemorrhage/contrast staining areas after mechanical intra-arterial thrombectomy in acute ischemic stroke: imaging findings and clinical significance. AJNR Am J Neuroradiol. 2012; 33(9):1791–1796

[18] Costalat V, Lobotesis K, Machi P, et al. Prognostic factors related to clinical outcome following thrombectomy in ischemic stroke (RECOST study). 50 patients prospective study. Eur J Radiol. 2012; 81(12):4075–4082

50 HaNDL

50.1 Case Description

50.1.1 Clinical Presentation

A 21-year-old male presented with confusion, nausea, vomiting and severe headache, as well as abdominal pain and mild right-sided weakness. The onset of symptoms was not witnessed, as he was found at home by his parents, and was last seen well earlier the same day. In the emergency room, his presentation activated the acute stroke protocol. Examination revealed a left hemispheric syndrome with expressive and receptive language deficits, mild hemiparesis, and inattention. He was unable to answer questions but could follow simple commands. He also had dysconjugate gaze with double vision to rightward gaze.

Collateral history from his family revealed that he had been admitted to another hospital 3 weeks previously with a similar presentation. At that time, he had developed gradual onset of confusion, with right-sided paresthesia, followed by headache and abdominal pain. His clinical status had progressed to stupor with severe right-sided weakness, ongoing headache, nausea and vomiting. Over the course of 24 to 48 hours, he had gradually recovered to baseline. MRI of the brain at that time, according to his family, had not shown significant abnormality. Subsequent records from the previous admission were obtained which showed he had undergone lumbar puncture. Cerebrospinal fluid (CSF) analysis revealed a raised white cell count (WBC; 173/µL), mildly elevated protein (71 mg/dL), and normal glucose level.

The patient had also experienced recent onset of headaches with nausea, vomiting, photophobia and phonophobia, and abdominal pain, with three episodes over the preceding 3 months. He also had a history of depression. Otherwise, he was healthy, with no comorbidities, no cardiovascular risk factors, and no relevant family history. The only regular preadmission medication was escitalopram 10 mg daily.

50.1.2 Imaging Workup and Investigations

Noncontrast CT (NCCT), CTA, MRI, MRA, MR perfusion (MRP), and digital subtraction angiography were all performed on the day of admission.

NCCT of the brain was performed initially and appeared normal, with no evidence of infarction, hyperdense vessel sign, or hemorrhage (▶ Fig. 50.1a). No intracranial proximal large artery occlusion was seen on intracranial CTA (▶ Fig. 50.1b). Note was however made of generalized paucity of distal arterial branches over the left hemisphere compared to the contralateral right side (▶ Fig. 50.1c–e).

MRI demonstrated generalized hyperintensity throughout the left hemispheric cortex on T2 FLAIR and diffusion-weighted imaging, with subtle reduced apparent diffusion coefficient (ADC) value in the cortex of the left parietal region (▶ Fig. 50.2a–c). MRP demonstrated reduced cerebral blood flow (CBF) throughout the left cerebral hemisphere compared to the contralateral side (▶ Fig. 50.2d). Contrast-enhanced MRA

of the extracranial arterial system showed no upstream arterial lesion to explain this, with normal appearance of the extracranial arteries (▶ Fig. 50.2e). There was no evidence of leptomeningeal enhancement or abnormal enhancement elsewhere on postgadolinium imaging of the brain (not shown).

Catheter angiography was performed, demonstrating a wedge-shaped area of mildly delayed arteriovenous contrast transit time involving the posterior left middle cerebral artery (MCA) territory (▶ Fig. 50.3a, b). There was no evidence of arterial irregularity or areas of stenosis to suggest a vasculitis or other vascular abnormality. The remainder of the examination was unremarkable. The site of abnormality correlated to the site of maximum abnormality on the patients' previous CTA and MRI examinations.

EEG showed some slowing in the left frontotemporal region but no epileptiform discharges. This was deemed mildly abnormal.

Lumbar puncture was performed. CSF analysis again revealed elevated white cell count (WBC 35/µL (95% lymphocytes), raised protein (47 mg/dL), and normal glucose. CSF culture was negative and viral culture was negative for Herpes Simplex Virus 1 and 2 as well as negative for varicella zoster and EBV. CSF cytology was negative for malignancy, although it did demonstrate chronic inflammation that included small T lymphocytes. There was no evidence of a lymphoproliferative disorder.

Porphyria screen was negative. Liver enzymes were normal. Testing for hypercoagulable state revealed no abnormalities. A molecular screen was performed for any genetic abnormality, with no significant abnormality revealed.

50.1.3 Diagnosis

HaNDL—Syndrome of transient *H*eadache and *N*eurological *D*eficits with cerebrospinal fluid *L*ymphocytosis.

50.1.4 Treatment and Follow-up

The symptoms and signs gradually started to resolve within the first 6 hours of hospitalization, with just subtle parietal symptoms and mild language difficulties remaining by day 2 of admission. He subsequently made a complete recovery. He was commenced on verapamil, prior to discharge, as a prophylactic agent to prevent future headaches. Antiplatelet medication was not administered. Follow-up MRI 1 month following presentation was normal (▶ Fig. 50.4). At 1-year clinic follow-up, he remained asymptomatic with no further episodes and no further headaches.

50.2 Companion Case

50.2.1 Clinical Presentation

An 18-year-old female presented to the emergency room with a moderate to severe throbbing headache, of onset over hours, in a frontal distribution with radiation to the left ear. This was associated with nausea and vomiting as well as photophobia and phonophobia. There was no history of fever, rash or neck

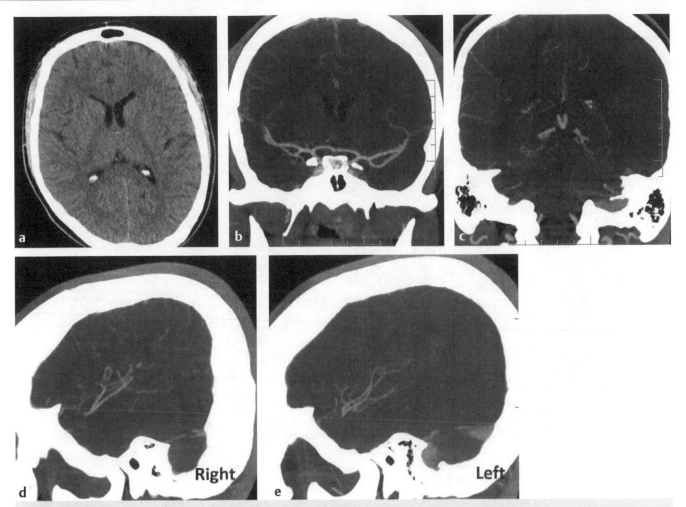

Fig. 50.1 Non-contrast enhanced CT of the brain was performed initially and appeared normal, with no evidence of infarction, no hyperdense vessel sign, and no hemorrhage (**a**). No intracranial proximal large artery occlusion was seen on intracranial CTA (**b**). Note was however made of generalized paucity of distal arterial branches over the left hemisphere compared to the contralateral right side (**c–e**).

stiffness. There was no recent travel. Her vaccinations were up to date. She was discharged from the emergency room with a diagnosis of migraine.

Following discharge, her headaches remained intermittently present; 2 days later, she developed a fever, prompting her to again visit the hospital. A lumbar puncture showed 500×10^6 leukocytes/mL, with 96% lymphocytes. Cultures and viral studies were negative. She was treated for presumed aseptic meningitis with intravenous Acyclovir. She improved markedly during admission and was discharged on oral Acyclovir.

She continued to improve, with only a mild, intermittent residual headache. However, 2 weeks later, she had a relapse, with severe headache, nausea, vomiting, and fatigue. Her father noted her speech to be incoherent. She also had two episodes of arm numbness, one on the right and one bilateral. She was again taken to the emergency department and examination was notable for lethargy, drowsiness, and fluent aphasia.

50.2.2 Imaging Workup and Investigations

A lumbar puncture was again performed, revealing 513×10^6 leukocytes/mL with 99% lymphocytes, 1% monocytes, and no visualized Mollaret cells. Protein was 1.06 g/L and glucose was 3.6 mmol/L. Cytology showed reactive lymphocytes. Viral polymerase chain reaction including herpes simplex virus and varicella zoster virus were negative. Bacterial and fungal cultures and cultures for acid fast bacilli were also all negative. HIV testing was also negative, as were screening autoimmune studies. Finally, a contrast-enhanced MRI and MRA were all found to be normal.

50.2.3 Diagnosis

Transient HaNDL.

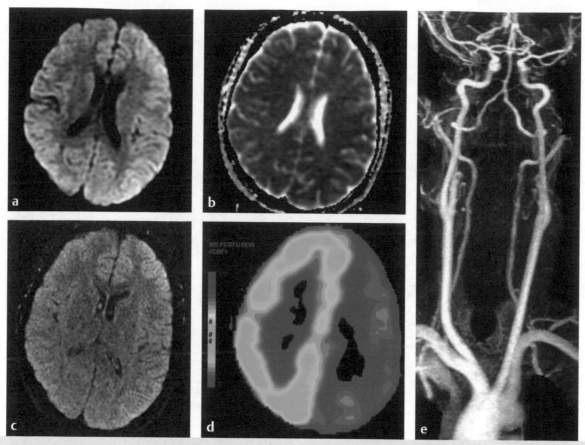

Fig. 50.2 MRI demonstrated generalized hyperintensity throughout the left hemispheric cortex on T2 FLAIR and diffusion-weighted imaging, with subtle reduced ADC value in the cortex of the left parietal region (**a, b, c**). MR perfusion demonstrated reduced CBF throughout the left cerebral hemisphere compared to the contralateral side (**d**). Contrast-enhanced MRA of the extracranial arterial system showed no upstream arterial lesion to explain this, with normal appearance of the extracranial arteries (**e**).

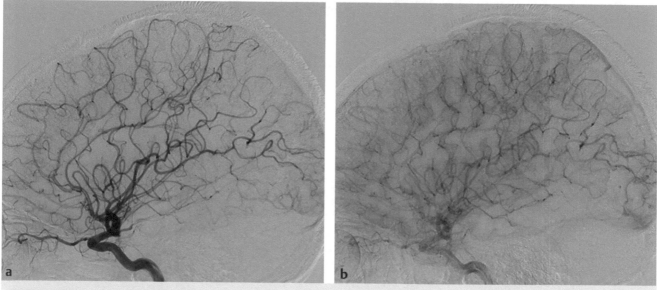

Fig. 50.3 Catheter angiography was performed and demonstrated a wedge-shaped area of mildly delayed arteriovenous contrast transit time involving the posterior left MCA territory (**a,b**).

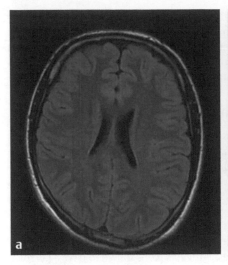
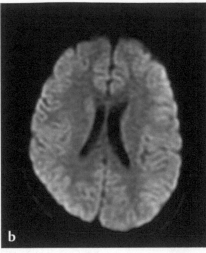

Fig. 50.4 Follow up MRI one month following presentation was normal, with resolution of previously seen abnormality on FLAIR and diffusion weighted imaging.

50.2.4 Treatment

The patient was treated supportively, with analgesia as required. Her symptoms rapidly improved over the course of the day and by the following day, she was back to her baseline with no further need for analgesia.

50.3 Discussion

50.3.1 Background

HaNDL was first described in 1981 in a case series of seven patients with headaches accompanied by neurologic deficits, occurring over 1 to 12 weeks.[1] In the decades since, several case reports and case series have described the phenomenon as well as its imaging correlates. The typical descriptions consist of migraine-like headache episodes (typically 1–12) accompanied by neurological deficits, most commonly including hemiparesthesia, hemiparesis, or aphasia. CSF studies demonstrate lymphocytic pleocytosis and symptoms resolve within a period of 3 months.[2]

The etiology of the syndrome has not been well elucidated. However, studies have demonstrated alterations in CBF using various modalities including single photon emission tomography (PET)[2] and CTP.[4] Similarly, occipital lobe perfusion deficits have been noted in migraine with aura. A study of MCA transcranial doppler flow[4] has also shown fluctuations in flow velocity and pulsatility, suggesting alterations in arteriolar tone which have also been implicated in migraine. Such findings as well as the clinical similarities underlie the hypothesis that the pathophysiology of HaNDL resembles that of migraine. Given the commonly reported prodromal viral-like illness and inflammatory findings on lumbar puncture, a viral trigger has also been hypothesized.

50.3.2 Workup and Diagnosis

Patient History

Historical features in HaNDL are variable and may closely resemble other considerably more common disorders such as acute ischemic stroke or meningitis.

The International Classification of Headache Disorders, 3rd edition (ICHD-3)[5] has developed the following diagnostic criteria:

a) Episodes of migraine-like headache fulfilling criteria B and C.
b) Both of the following:
1. Accompanied or shortly preceded by the onset of at least one of the following transient neurological deficits lasting > 4 hours: (a) hemiparesthesia, (b) dysphasia, and (c) hemiparesis.
2. Associated with CSF lymphocytic pleocytosis (> 15 white cells per mL), with negative etiological studies.
c) Evidence of causation demonstrated by either or both of the following:
1. Headache and transient neurological deficits have developed or significantly worsened in temporal relation to the CSF lymphocytic pleocytosis, or led to its discovery.
2. Headache and transient neurological deficits have significantly improved in parallel with improvement in CSF lymphocytic pleocytosis.
d) Not better accounted for by another ICHD-3 diagnosis.

Onset of neurologic deficits has been described as abrupt in some cases, or more progressive in others. For example, numbness can begin in one hand and progress through the arm and finally affect the face and tongue. The duration of deficits has been reported as long as three days.[3]

Examination and Investigations

Physical examination in HaNDL will typically correspond to the neurologic deficits described by the patient or those providing collateral history. On mental status examination, acute confusional states have sometimes been observed.[6] Papilledema is not common but has also been described. Language examination is crucial, with motor aphasia the most commonly observed language deficit.[2] Sensory examination can reveal primary or cortical sensory deficits, and motor examination may reveal pyramidal pattern weakness or pronator drift.

CSF studies are an important adjunctive test, and diagnosis requires a pleocytosis with a lymphocytic predominance. Up to 760 cells/mL have been observed on CSF analyses.[5] Total protein level and CSF pressure are often elevated as well. Antibodies against the CACNA1A calcium channel have been uniformly negative in those cases tested. However, antibodies to CACNA1 H, a T-type calcium channel, have been described.[7] Regions of electrographic slowing may be observed on EEG.[8]

Imaging Findings

Routine imaging, including CT and MRI of the brain, are often normal in HaNDL. However, there have been case reports of sulcal enhancement on contrast-enhanced MRI. On perfusion imaging modalities, including CTP scans or single photon emission computed tomography (SPECT) scans, relative hypoperfusion of the affected hemisphere or vascular territory has also been observed during the ictal phase. Imaging modalities which assess cerebral perfusion are sometimes employed in the setting of acute stroke, and may show such perfusion abnormalities in HaNDL, without evidence of an intracranial arterial occlusion and without abnormalities of the arteries in the neck.

50.3.3 Decision-Making Process

The diagnosis of HaNDL relies on the exclusion of various more common and potentially treatable conditions which may be suspected according to a given patient's clinical presentation. If there is an infectious prodrome or fever, the exclusion of intracranial infections including Lyme, syphilis, or granulomatous meningitis is necessary with an urgent lumbar puncture. If the onset of neurologic deficits is acute, this would usually be in keeping with a vascular insult, and the exclusion of an acute vascular event such as ischemic stroke would be crucial. Neuroimaging, including arterial and potentially also venous imaging, will often clarify this possibility. A brain MRI to rule out a stroke or other structural lesion is also often essential.

Depending on the clinical context, other important differential diagnoses to consider include parainfectious and inflammatory causes of meningitis or encephalitis, including Mollaret's meningitis, which also presents with a relapsing course and meningeal signs. CSF studies are usually helpful in this regard. Neoplastic causes such as leptomeningeal carcinomatosis or paraneoplastic causes are also important to consider, but may be ruled out depending on the clinical context and imaging findings.

In summary, in the setting of a headache, completely resolving neurologic deficits, CSF lymphocytic pleocytosis, with the exclusion of stroke, CNS infection, intracranial malignancy, and in the absence of a family history of hemiplegic migraine, the diagnosis of HaNDL can be entertained. Another consistent feature would be the recurrence of similar symptomatology one or more times within a period of 3 months. The clinician must be vigilant for other potential underlying etiologies, and the risk factors contributing to vascular disease, infection or malignancy that would render an alternative diagnosis far more likely in a particular patient.

50.3.4 Management

Because it is a self-limited, episodic condition, the management of HaNDL is largely supportive. Some success has been noted with short courses of therapy such as nonsteroidal anti-inflammatory drugs, beta-blockers, ergotamine, and steroids.[9] However, given the tendency for the episodes to be relatively short and the characteristic resolution of the syndrome as a whole within 3 months, no long-term prophylactic therapy is generally instituted to manage HaNDL.

50.3.5 Literature Synopsis

HaNDL is a syndrome which is becoming increasingly recognized among clinicians. Nevertheless, there have only been two large case series published thus far,[2,10] and the precise epidemiology remains unclear.

The headache in HaNDL is typically throbbing in quality. Photophobia, phonophobia, and nausea have been reported, although not in all cases. Even though the character of the headache does resemble that of migraine, only 24 to 26% of patients in large case aggregates were shown to have a personal history and 42% a family history of migraine. Approximately one quarter to one half of patients have a viral prodrome or fever in conjunction with the episodes. There does not appear to be a clear gender bias, with one series suggesting females are more commonly affected and the other showing the reverse.

In the pediatric population, a review of the literature revealed 13 published cases, where the mean age of onset was 14, 71% were female and 11 out of 13 patients experienced at least one recurrent attack.[9]

Clinical and imaging correlates remain variable. In the majority of cases, standard imaging is normal but SPECT and other perfusion imaging techniques during the ictal phase have in some published cases demonstrated hemispheric perfusion abnormalities.

50.3.6 Pearls and Pitfalls

- Although there have been reports of territorial hypoperfusion in the context of HaNDL, much of the affected territory may not be hypoperfused to the extent that it results in ischemic symptoms.
- In the setting of possible ischemic stroke, the degree of discordance between perfusion imaging and symptoms, as well as the absence of an acute vessel occlusion, may provide sufficient contravening evidence to prevent the use of intravenous thrombolytics. This is particularly relevant if a history consistent with HaNDL is available to the clinician in the acute setting.
- HaNDL may be mistaken for ischemic stroke, aseptic meningitis, or classic migraine, depending on the clinical presentation, which is highly variable. It is important to be cognizant of these possibilities when making the diagnosis.

References

[1] Bartleson JD, Swanson JW, Whisnant JP. A migrainous syndrome with cerebrospinal fluid pleocytosis. Neurology. 1981; 31(10):1257–1262

[2] Gómez-Aranda F, Cañadillas F, Martí-Massó JF, et al. Pseudomigraine with temporary neurological symptoms and lymphocytic pleocytosis. A report of 50 cases. Brain. 1997; 120(Pt 7):1105–1113

[3] Pettersen JA, Aviv RI, Black SE, Fox AJ, Lim A, Murray BJ. Global hemispheric CT hypoperfusion may differentiate headache with associated neurological deficits and lymphocytosis from acute stroke. Stroke. 2008; 39(2):492–493

[4] Kappler J, Mohr S, Steinmetz H. Cerebral vasomotor changes in the transient syndrome of headache with neurologic deficits and CSF lymphocytosis (HaNDL). Headache. 1997; 37(8):516–518

[5] et al. The international classification of headache disorders, 3rd edition (beta version). Cephalgia. 2013; 33(9):629–808

[6] Parissis D, Ioannidis P, Balamoutsos G, Karacostas D. Confusional state in the syndrome of HaNDL. Headache. 2011; 51(8):1285–1288

[7] Kürtüncü M, Kaya D, Zuliani L, et al. CACNA1 H antibodies associated with headache with neurological deficits and cerebrospinal fluid lymphocytosis (HaNDL). Cephalalgia. 2013; 33(2):123–129

[8] Barón J, Mulero P, Pedraza MI, et al. HaNDL syndrome: correlation between focal deficits topography and EEG or SPECT abnormalities in a series of 5 new cases. Neurologia. 2015; 31(5):305–10

[9] Filina T, Feja KN, Tolan RW, Jr. An adolescent with pseudomigraine, transient headache, neurological deficits, and lymphocytic pleocytosis (HaNDL Syndrome): case report and review of the literature. Clin Pediatr (Phila). 2013; 52(6):496–502

[10] Berg MJ, Williams LS. The transient syndrome of headache with neurologic deficits and CSF lymphocytosis. Neurology. 1995; 45(9):1648–1654

51 Appendix: Essential Terms, Trials, and Tools

51.1 Introduction

Throughout this text, reference is made to various clinical, radiological terms and interventional devices which are further contextualized by major trials of the modern era. The following is an explanation and elaboration of the current state of the art for the endovascular management of stroke.

51.2 Recanalization and Reperfusion Scoring

Several radiographic classifications have been published in the past decades for evaluating the effect of the endovascular treatment after an acute ischemic stroke (AIS). The success of the treatment can be evaluated by the assessment of either the recanalization of the affected vessel and/or the reperfusion of the brain tissue.

Despite often interchanged, recanalization and reperfusion represent two interconnected, but different, aspects of revascularization, and the two terms cannot be considered interchangeable. Distinguishing between these parameters is clinically important. For example, an artery may be completely recanalized, but distal clot embolization may limit distal reperfusion. This may significantly limit the neurologic recovery, potentially increasing the risk of hemorrhage as a result of hyperperfusion of ischemic tissue. On the other hand, distal reperfusion may be achieved, but the artery may have incomplete recanalization predisposing to a higher rate of reocclusion with subsequent clinical deterioration.[1] Of the two parameters, reperfusion is more strongly associated with tissue and clinical outcomes because of its measurement of tissue-level effects.[2,3] Therefore, reperfusion is the best marker of effective revascularization, whereas recanalization is an important metric of the treatment effect on the target lesion. Because of their intimate relationship, both measures have been shown to predict improved clinical outcomes after intra-arterial treatment.[2,3,4,5,6,7,8,9,10,11] Drugs, devices, or combinations may differ in their ability to achieve and maintain recanalization and reperfusion.

51.2.1 Reperfusion Scales

Perfusion is usually evidenced by a capillary blush on digital subtraction angiography (DSA). After intra-arterial treatment, reperfusion is defined as the antegrade restoration of a capillary blush, thus not from collateral pial supplies. As such, reperfusion scales account for distal emboli and would identify treatment modalities that achieve revascularization without clot fragmentation and distal embolization. The two most common reperfusion scales are the thrombolysis in myocardial infarction (TIMI) and thrombolysis in cerebral infarction (TICI) systems.

The Thrombolysis in Myocardial Infarction Scoring System

TIMI is a scoring system initially devised for the assessment of reperfusion in acute myocardial infarction.[12,13] This simple angiographic score is now accepted worldwide and used with AIS to assess recanalization, angiographic reperfusion, or both.[14] TIMI score is graded from 0 to 3, according to angiographic demonstration of blood flow (▶ Table 51.1).

The main advantage of this scoring system is represented by its simplicity, being widely accepted and known among neurologist and neurointerventionalists. However, variability of the subjective perception of the grading definition represents the main disadvantage of its use across clinical trials.

The Thrombolysis in Cerebral Infarction Grading System

The TICI is a grading system first described by Higashida et al[15] in 2003. It assesses the extent of tissue reperfusion, as represented by the capillary blush on DSA and was conceived to standardize the angiographic outcome after endovascular treatment of ischemic stroke.

This scale identifies three different grades, from "0—no perfusion" to "3—complete perfusion" and represents a modified version of the TIMI scale (▶ Table 51.2).

Interestingly, it provides a subcategorization of the grade 2, partial perfusion, describing those cases in which contrast passes through the obstruction but with rates of entry and washout slower than normal (2a and 2b). Despite being criticized because of some internal inconsistencies,[16] TICI scale is still widely used in literature.

In 2013, a modified treatment in cerebral infarction (mTICI) score[17] was proposed by a consensus group. The name of the scale was changed to better reflect the increased use of

Table 51.1 The thrombolysis in myocardial infarction grading system

Grade	Angiographic appearances
0	No perfusion
1	Perfusion past the initial occlusion, but no distal branch filling
2	Perfusion with incomplete or slow distal branch filling
3	Full perfusion with filling of all distal branches, including M3, 4

Table 51.2 The thrombolysis in cerebral infarction scale

Grade	Angiographic appearances
0	No perfusion
1	Penetration with minimal perfusion
2a	Only partial filling (less than two-thirds) of the entire vascular territory is visualized
2b	Complete filling of all of the expected vascular territory is visualized but the filling is slower than normal
3	Complete perfusion

Table 51.3 Modified treatment in cerebral infarction (mTICI) score

Grade	Angiographic appearances
0	No perfusion
1	Antegrade reperfusion past the initial occlusion, but limited distal branch filling with little or slow distal reperfusion
2a	Antegrade reperfusion of less than half of the previously occluded target artery previously ischemic territory
2b	Antegrade reperfusion of more than half of the previously occluded target artery ischemic territory
3	Complete antegrade reperfusion of the previously occluded target artery ischemic territory, with absence of visualized occlusion in all distal branches

Table 51.4 The anterior occlusive lesion (AOL) scale

Grade	Angiographic appearances
0	No recanalization of the primary occlusive lesion
1	Incomplete or partial recanalization of the primary occlusive lesion with no distal flow
2	Incomplete or partial recanalization of the primary occlusive lesion with any distal flow
3	Complete recanalization of the primary occlusion with any distal flow

endovascular therapies, and a simplification of the TICI 2 component was added. In the new scale, the score 2 was subdivided as "mTICI 2a—reperfusion of less than half of the occluded target" and "mTICI 2b—reperfusion of more than half of the occluded target" (▶ Table 51.3).

mTICI has proven to be superior to TIMI for predicting functional outcome and mortality after intra-arterial therapy,[9,10,18] supporting its use as the standard reperfusion grading scale. Furthermore, mTICI 2b to 3 is the optimal threshold for predicting 90-day independence and should be used as the target angiographic end point for technical success, instead of the traditional end point[9] of TIMI 2 to 3.

A further modification was proposed in 2014,[19] with the introduction of the "grade 2c—near-complete perfusion except for slow flow or distal emboli in a few distal cortical vessels." To date, this has not yet reached consensus approval, with some proposing an expanded treatment in cerebral infarction (eTICI) score after investigators found a significant difference in outcomes for patients with partial recanalization between those with reperfusion of 50 to 66%, 67 to 89%, and 90 to 90% in addition to those previously defined by mTICI.

51.2.2 Recanalization Scale: The Arterial Occlusive Lesion Scoring System

The arterial occlusive lesion (AOL) is a grading scale devised to assess the degree of recanalization at the target arterial lesion (TAL). It was introduced in the IMS I pilot trial to evaluate recanalization directly.[14] The AOL scoring system describes arterial patency at the site of occlusion based on the degree of luminal opening, simply assigning a score from 0 to 3, which represents the range from no recanalization to complete recanalization with any distal flow (▶ Table 51.4).

This method was compared with TIMI reperfusion scoring in the IMS I trial to determine the relationship between recanalization and reperfusion; there was no statistical difference between the two methods of prediction of clinical outcome ($p = 0.11$), although numerically TIMI reperfusion had a higher association.[14] This analysis confirmed that recanalization is related to reperfusion, and both may be important in overall clinical outcomes.

51.3 The National Institute of Health Stroke Scale

The National Institute of Health Stroke Scale or NIHSS is a diagnostic tool used to determine the severity of a stroke, providing a quantitative measure of stroke-related neurologic deficits. This scale has three major purposes:
1. To evaluate the severity of the stroke.
2. To help determine the appropriate treatment.
3. To predict patient outcome.

Eleven different elements are assessed to evaluate specific abilities (▶ Table 51.5):
1. Level of consciousness (LOC).
2. Best gaze.
3. Visual field testing.
4. Facial paresis.
5. Arm motor function.
6. Leg motor function.
7. Limb ataxia.
8. Sensory.
9. Best language.
10. Dysarthria.
11. Extinction and inattention.

The score for each ability is a number between 0 and 4, 0 being normal functioning and 4 being completely impaired. The patient's NIHSS score is calculated by adding the number for each element of the scale; 42 is the highest score possible. In the NIHSS, the higher the score, the more impaired a stroke patient is. As a general rule, a score over 16 predicts a strong probability of patient death, while a score of 6 or lower indicates a strong possibility for a good recovery. Each 1-point increase on the scale lowers the possibility of a positive outcome for the patient by 17%.

The NIHSS score is important for patients because it determines the course of action and treatment following a stroke. First, healthcare staff apply the NIHSS score as soon as possible after the onset of symptoms, which would typically be in the ambulance or emergency department of a hospital. It will also be applied at regular intervals, and/or whenever the patient's condition changes significantly. It is important to keep a good history of stroke patients' NIHSS score because it allows healthcare professionals to monitor their progress, tailor their treatment, and quantify their improvement or decline over time.

Table 51.5 The National Institute of Health Stroke Scale

Category	Score/Description		
1a. Level of consciousness	0—Alert 1—Drowsy 2—Stuporous 3—Coma		
1b. LOC questions (month, age)	0—Answer both correctly 1—Answer one correctly 2—Incorrect		
1c. LOC commands (open/close eyes, make fist/let go)	0—Obeys both correctly 1—Obeys one correctly 2—Incorrect		
2. Best gaze (eyes open—patient follows examiner's finger or face)	0—Normal 1—Partial gaze palsy 2—Forced deviation		
3. Visual fields (introduce visual stimulus/threat to patient's visual field quadrants)	0—No visual loss 1—Partial hemianopia 2—Complete hemianopia 3—Bilateral hemianopia		
4. Facial paresis (show teeth, raise eyebrows, and squeeze eyes shut)	0—Normal 1—Minor 2—Partial 3—Complete		
5a. Motor arm—Left 5b. Motor arm—Right (elevate arm to 90 degrees if patient is sitting, 45 degrees if supine)	0—No drift 1—Drift 2—Can't resist gravity 3—No effort against gravity 4—No movements x—Untestable (joint fusion or limb amputation)	Left Right	
6a. Motor leg—Left 6b. Motor leg—Right (elevate leg to 30 degrees with patient supine)	0—No drift 1—Drift 2—Can't resist gravity 3—No effort against gravity 4—No movements x—Untestable (joint fusion or limb amputation)	Left Right	
7. Limb ataxia (finger-nose, heel down shin)	0—No ataxia 1—Present in one limb 2—Present in two limbs		
8. Sensory (pin prick to face, arm, trunk, and leg)	0—Normal 1—Partial loss 2—Severe loss		
9. Best language (name item, describe a picture and read sentences)	0—No aphasia 1—Mild to moderate aphasia 2—Severe aphasia 3—Mute		
10. Dysarthria (evaluate speech clarity by patient repeating listed words)	0—Normal articulation 1—Mild to moderate slurring of words 2—Near to unintelligible or worse X—intubated or other physical barriers		
11. Extinction and inattention (use information prior to testing to identify neglect or double simultaneous stimuli testing)	0—No neglect 1—Partial neglect 2—Complete neglect		

51.4 The Alberta Stroke Program Early CT Score

The Alberta Stroke Program Early CT Score (ASPECTS) is a 10-point quantitative score used to assess early ischemic changes on noncontrast head CT scan in patients suspected of having acute large vessel anterior circulation occlusion. It is a simple and reliable tool, recognized worldwide as part of the assessment for eligibility in receiving interventional mechanical thrombectomy treatment. Initially conceived exclusively for anterior circulation stroke,[20] it has been adapted for posterior circulation[21] as well.

ASPECTS is based on assessment of two standardized regions of the middle cerebral artery (MCA) territory: the basal ganglia level, where thalamus, caudate, and basal ganglia, are visible, and the supraganglionic level, which includes the corona radiata and centrum semiovale. Early ischemic changes should be visible on at least two consecutive cuts to ensure that it is truly abnormal rather than a volume averaging effect.

ASPECTS is calculated subtracting 1 point from 10 for any evidence of early ischemic change for each of the following regions:
- C: Caudate.
- I: Insular ribbon.
- IC: Internal capsule.
- L: Lentiform nucleus.
- M1: Anterior MCA cortex.
- M2: MCA cortex lateral to the insular ribbon.
- M3: Posterior MCA cortex.
- M4: Anterior MCA territory immediately superior to M1.
- M5: Lateral MCA territory immediately superior to M2.
- M6: Posterior MCA territory immediately superior to M3.

A normal CT scan receives ASPECTS of 10 points, while a score of 0 indicates diffuse involvement throughout the MCA territory. An ASPECTS score less than or equal to 7 predicts a worse functional outcome at 3 months.

The ASPECTS scoring system has been also adapted for use in the posterior circulation and referred to as pc-ASPECTS.[5] The same approach is used for the pc-ASPECTS, with different areas of interest. From 10 points, 1 point each is subtracted for early ischemic changes detected on the left or right thalamus, cerebellar hemisphere, or posterior cerebral artery territory, respectively, and 2 points each for involvement of any part of the midbrain or pons.

51.5 Common CT/CTA Protocols

51.5.1 Noncontrast Head Computed Tomographic Scan

Noncontrast computed tomography (CT) remains the primary imaging modality for the initial assessment of a patient who comes to the emergency department with suspected stroke.[22,23] It is able to easily identify early signs of stroke but is mainly used to rule out the most common intracranial pathologies that can mimic an AIS, such as tumor or intracerebral hemorrhage.

51.5.2 CT Angiography

CT angiography (CTA) usually represents the next step in the radiological assessment of a patient with suspected AIS. Usually, thin-section helical CT images are obtained in the arterial phase after injection of intravenous contrast. Software allows those thin-section axial CT images to be reformatted in any plane enabling a more complete evaluation of vessels with a three-dimensional reproduction of the intracranial vasculature. Imaging of the entire intra- and extracranial circulation beginning at the aortic arch and continuing through the circle of Willis can frequently be performed within 60 seconds.[24,25,26]

51.5.3 CT Perfusion

CT perfusion represents a crucial point in the radiological assessment of a stroke patient. It is more widely available than magnetic resonance imaging (MRI) and can be performed quickly on any standard helical CT scanner right after unenhanced CT. It is based on a rapid intravenous infusion of contrast followed by several imaging of brain sections. This modality is able to assess and quantify the total amount and the speed of the blood flow through the different parts of the brain, thus identifying a stroke and potential areas of reversible and salvageable brain tissue in the ischemic penumbra.[26]

By definition, the cerebral blood flow (CBF) is equal to the cerebral blood volume (CBV) divided by the mean transit time (MTT). The MTT is the time difference between the arterial inflow and venous outflow,[26,27,28] and represents the most sensitive measure used to evaluate for flow abnormalities.

The area of the brain undergoing hypoperfusion has both decreased CBF and CBV. Decreased total CBV is the most specific indicator for an area actually undergoing irreversible ischemia or infarct and is nonsalvageable. Areas of the brain that are at risk for injury known as the ischemic penumbra show decreased CBF with normal to increased CBV. CT perfusion imaging can identify the penumbra, helping with selection of those patients who may still benefit by intravenous, intra-arterial or mechanical reperfusion.

CT perfusion does have some limitations. First of all, it requires multidetector CT and a special software which needs to be set up by trained technologist. The software package that is used for CT perfusion analyzes the images obtained, and color-coded maps representing many levels of the brain are produced to help differentiate the potential cause of the flow abnormalities.

51.6 European Cooperative Acute Stroke Study II Trial Hemorrhage Classification

The European Cooperative Acute Stroke Study II Trial (ECASS II) was designed to evaluate the safety and efficacy of intravenous thrombolysis with alteplase (0.9 mg/kg) within 6 hours of stroke onset.[29] A new classification system was proposed for assessment of postthrombolytic hemorrhagic transformations (▶ Table 51.6).

Table 51.6 European Cooperative Acute Stroke Study II Trial (ECASS II) Hemorrhage Classification

Type	Radiographic appearances
Hemorrhagic infarction 1 (HI1)	Small petechiae along the margins of the infarct
Hemorrhagic infarction 2 (HI2)	Confluent petechiae within the infarcted area but no space-occupying effect
Parenchymal hemorrhage 1 (PH1)	Blood clots in 30% or less of the infarcted area with some slight space-occupying effect
Parenchymal hemorrhage 2 (PH2)	Blood clots in more than 30% of the infarcted area with substantial space-occupying effect

Table 51.8 Collateral circulation score on CT angiography

Grade	CT angiographic appearances
1	Absent
2	Less the contralateral unaffected site
3	Equal to the contralateral unaffected site
4	More than the contralateral unaffected site
5	Exuberant

Table 51.7 Collateral circulation on digital subtraction angiography

Grade	Angiographic appearances
0	No collaterals visible to the ischemic site
1	Slow collaterals to the periphery of the ischemic site with persistence of some of the defect
2	Rapid collaterals to the periphery of ischemic site with persistence of some of the defect and to only a portion of the ischemic territory
3	Collaterals with slow but complete angiographic blood flow of the ischemic bed by the late venous phase
4	Complete and rapid collateral blood flow to the vascular bed in the entire ischemic territory by retrograde perfusion

Table 51.9 Collateral circulation score on CT angiography

Grade	CT angiographic appearances
1	Absent
2	Less than the contralateral unaffected site
3	Equal to the contralateral unaffected site
4	More than the contralateral unaffected site
5	Exuberant

Table 51.10 Contrast injection rates and imaging framing rates for common selective catheterizations

	Contrast injection rate, (mL/s)/ total mL	Framing rate, frames/s
Cervical arch	20/40	3
Extracranial ICA with catheter in the CCA	4–5/7–8	2
Cerebral angiography with catheter in the CCA	7–8/11–12	2–3
ECA with the catheter in the ECA	4–5/6–7	2
Posterior cerebral angiography with catheter in the vertebral artery	6–7/9–10	2

Abbreviations: ICA, internal carotid artery; CCA, common carotid artery; ECA, external carotid artery.

51.7 Collateral Circulation Score

Collateral flow plays a crucial role in maintaining tissue viability in case of AIS due to proximal large vessel occlusion (LVO). The preservation of flow through leptomeningeal collaterals is known to reduce ischemic brain damage, especially after a proximal arterial occlusion. More recently, the collateral circulation was shown to play an important role in infarct core volume,[30] and a good collateral grade was mandatory in selecting patients for intra-arterial intervention.[31] Collaterals may sustain the penumbra prior to recanalization, but the influence of baseline collateral flow on the final infarct size following endovascular or reperfusion therapies remains unknown.

The first trial with a specific estimation of collateral flow was the PROACT-II trial.[32] Collateral flow is usually assessed either with DSA, which still represents the "gold standard" (▶ Table 51.7), or CTA (▶ Table 51.8). Lima et al[33] in 2010 described a new CTA-based grading system. Briefly, the extent of vascularity was graded at two heights: around the Sylvian fissure and at the cerebral convexity as follows: 0 = absent, 1 = less than the contralateral unaffected side, 2 = equal to the contralateral unaffected side, 3 = more than the contralateral unaffected side, and 4 = exuberant (▶ Table 51.9). The sum of these scores is considered to be the total collateral grade ranging from 0 to 8.

51.8 Thrombectomy Devices

Several thrombectomy devices have been approved and used in the last decade for the treatment of AIS (▶ Table 51.10, ▶ Table 51.11, ▶ Table 51.12, ▶ Table 51.13). They are based on different mechanisms, and can be used alternatively, being the treatment usually tailored according to clinical and radiological findings. Two main systems are in use: stent retrievers and aspiration devices.

51.8.1 Stent Retrievers

Stent retrievers are devices that use a simple mechanism: a microcatheter is inserted up to the clot and then withdrawn together with the clot inside a proximal, larger, catheter.

Solitaire FR

The Solitaire FR is a device available in four sizes: 4 × 15 mm, 4 × 20 mm, 6 × 20 mm, and 6 × 30 mm. It can be fully deployed, fully resheathed, and recovered. Its stent-like design with closed-

Table 51.11 Summary of key features of aspiration catheters

Device (company)	Aspiration method	Available models	Distal inner diameter in inches	Working length in cm
ARC ARC Mini (Medtronic)	Manual	ARCA-132 ARCA-160	0.061 0.035	132 160
Navien (Medtronic)	Manual	RFXA058 RFXA072	0.058 0.072	125 or 130
Sofia (MicroVention)	Manual	DA5115ST DA5125ST DA6115ST	0.055 0.070	115 125 115
Sofia Plus (MicroVention)	Manual	DA6125ST DA6131ST	0.070	125 131
ACE reperfusion catheter (Penumbra)	External pump	ACE60 ACE64 ACE68	0.060 0.064 0.068	132
MAX reperfusion catheter (Penumbra)	External pump	3 MAX 4 MAX 5 MAX	0.035 0.041 0.054	153 139 132
AXS catalyst distal access catheter (Stryker)	Manual	AXS Catalyst 5 AXS Catalyst 5 AXS Catalyst 6	0.058 0.058 0.060	115 132 132

cell structure provides optimal clot interaction, which allows immediate blood flow restoration and clot retrieval. If revascularization is not achieved with one pass, the process can be repeated with the same device three to five times using the same steps.

Trevo

The Trevo device is designed for removal of acute occlusive thrombus in vessels ranging from 1.5 to 3.5 mm in diameter. The device consists of a 180-cm proximal 0.018-in core wire with a 75-cm tapered transition region and a closed-cell, stent-like section at the distal end. The overall length of the device is 44 mm, with an unconstrained diameter of 4 mm. The distal end has a soft radiopaque tip designed to allow safe and accurate deployment with fluoroscopic visualization. The distal end of the device is tapered to provide higher radial force, with the ability to be deployed into distal, smaller vessels. The proximal end of the device is also tapered for easy resheathing. The Trevo device has a hydrophilic coating to reduce friction during use.

Impressive recanalization results and safety were recently reported for the Solitaire FR device in the Solitaire FR with the Intention for Thrombectomy (SWIFT)[34] and the Trevo retriever in the Thrombectomy REvascularization of large Vessel Occlusions[35] (TREVO 2) randomized trials versus the MERCI retriever, as well as by comparison with the results of the Mechanical Embolus Removal in Cerebral Ischemia (MERCI) trial.[36]

They promote immediate reperfusion in 80 to 90% of cases, reestablishing oxygen supply to the ischemic brain region and enhance the efficacy of thrombolytic drugs in the circulation. The advantage of stent retrievers compared to regular stents is that stent retrievers require no anticoagulation or antiplatelet therapy, as the stent is not permanently implanted. Also, stent retrievers can be resheathed and used repeatedly, even in small peripheral vessel branches. The MERCI Clot retriever was one of the first introduced and evaluated in a trial.[36] New systems have been recently introduced, showing higher recanalization rate.

51.8.2 Aspiration Devices

Penumbra

The Penumbra system (Penumbra Inc., Alameda, CA) is the most diffused aspiration device. It is specifically designed for treatment of patients with AIS secondary to occlusive disease in large intracranial vessels, including the internal carotid artery (ICA), M1 and M2 segments of the MCA, and basilar and vertebral arteries. With a combination of aspiration through a specially designed catheter and clot fragmentation with a clot separator, the Penumbra device is able to successfully remove thrombus and perform revascularization in a minimally invasive fashion. The Penumbra system is composed of five fundamental devices: a reperfusion catheter, a separator, an aspiration pump, the pump and canister tubing, and the aspiration tubing.

In general, the aspiration catheter is advanced up to, or sometimes past, the site of occlusion, and then the separator device is introduced through the aspiration catheter. An electric pump provides negative pressure, while the separator device is moved in and out of the aspiration catheter, progressively dislodging clot fragments that are then aspirated into the catheter. The designed result is revascularization of the affected vessel while minimizing the risk of distal clot emboli.

In case of residual thrombus after revascularization with aspiration, the thrombus removal ring is used to directly engage and remove the thrombus. An alternative technique to the proximal aspiration method described earlier is to take the reperfusion catheter beyond the clot on the initial placement and then unsheathe the separator into the distal vasculature. While on aspiration, leave the separator in position and move the reperfusion catheter back and forth across the clot, effectively "coring" the clot with the catheter.

Occasionally, a thrombus may not be amenable to aspiration using the Penumbra device secondary to a very firm

Table 51.12 Summary of key features of included stent retrievers

Device (company)	Available models	Stent diameter and length in mm	Delivery catheter: minimum inner diameter in inches
Aperio (Acandis; UK Supplier: Neurologic)	01–000700 01–000701 01–000702 01–000703	3.5 × 28 4.5 × 30 4.5 × 40 6 × 40	0.0165–0.021 0.0165–0.021 0.021–0.027 0.021–0.027
Catch + (Balt; UK Supplier Sela Medical)	Catch + Mini Catch + Catch + Maxi	3 × 15 4 × 20 6 × 30	0.017 0.021 0.024
EmboTrap II (Cerenovus Johnson and Johnson)	ET-007–521 ET-007–533	5 × 21 5 × 33	0.021 0.021
ReVive SE (Cerenovus Johnson and Johnson)	ReVive SE	4.5 × 30	0.021–0.027
Solitaire 2 (Medtronic)	SFR2–4-15 SFR2–4-20 SFR2–4-40 SFR2–6-20 SFR2–6-30	4 × 15 4 × 20 4 × 40 6 × 20 6 × 30	0.021 0.021 0.021 0.027 0.027
Solitaire Platinum (Medtronic)	SRD3–4-20–05 SRD3–4-20–10 SRD3–4-40–10 SRD3–6-20–10 SRD3–6-24–06 SRD3–6-40–10	4 × 20 4 × 20 4 × 40 6 × 20 6 × 24 6 × 40	0.021 0.021 0.021 0.027 0.027 0.027
ERIC (MicroVention)	ERIC 3 ERIC 3 ERIC 4 ERIC 4 ERIC 6	3 × 15 3 × 20 4 × 24 4 × 30 6 × 44	0.017 0.017 0.021 0.021 0.027
pREset (Phenox)	PRE-4–20 PRE-6–30	4 × 20 6 × 30	0.021 0.021
pREset LITE (Phenox)	PRE-LT-3–20 PRE-LT-4–20	3 × 20 4 × 20	0.0165 0.0165
Tigertriever (Rapid Medical; UK supplier: Neurologic)	TRPP3166 TRPP3155	3 × 23 6 × 32	0.017 0.021
Trevo ProVue (Stryker)	90184	4 × 20	0.021
Trevo XP ProVue (Stryker)	90182 90183 90185 90186	4 × 20 3 × 20 4 × 30 6 × 25	0.021 0.017 0.021 0.027

consistency that prevents fragmentation. In these instances, an additional alternative thrombectomy method may be used. Kang et al[37] in 2011 described a novel technique called "forced suction thrombectomy," based on the use of the reperfusion catheter as a vacuum device to suction the thrombus directly. In this modified technique, the Penumbra separator and removal ring are not used.

5 MAX ACE

The 5 MAX ACE device is a further advance in the use of aspiration to effect successful clot retrieval. Its emergence has temporally corresponded with the increased adoption of the ADAPT technique. This technique involves placing a 5 MAX ACE

aspiration device at the clot, aspirating, and then withdrawing the clot while continuously aspirating. A recent study of 57 prospectively captured patients found that the ADAPT technique was successful in 28 of 37 (75%) patients.[38] On average, patients improved from NIHSS score of 16.3 to 4.2. While caution must be exercised as this is a new technique and catheter, it appears that aspiration-based stroke thrombectomy has been significantly improved with the ACE catheter, achieving higher rates of recanalization in a more rapid timeframe.

51.8.3 Permanent Stents

Despite the high recanalization rates achieved with the MERCI retriever (Concentric Medical Inc., Mountain View, CA),

Table 51.13 Summary of key features of included balloon guide catheters

Device (company)	Size (F)	Length (cm)	Internal diameter (inch)
Concentric balloon guide catheter (Stryker)	6	95	0.059
FlowGate 2 balloon guide catheter (Stryker)	8	85 95	0.084
MERCI balloon guide catheter (Stryker)	8 9	80, 95 80, 95	0.078 0.085
Cello balloon guide catheter (Medtronic)	7 8 8 9	110 108 102 98	0.051 0.067 0.075 0.085

mechanical thrombectomy, and the Penumbra thromboaspiration device in the setting of AIS, good clinical outcomes were relatively limited with both devices (36% with the MERCI and 25% with the Penumbra). This led to the adoption of the concept of intracranial stenting for AIS, with the goals of reducing the procedure time and more rapidly restoring flow to the affected area.

Self-expanding stents are preferred to balloon-mounted stents for this application. In theory, self-expanding stents reduce the risk of vessel dissection and rupture by reducing barotrauma on the blood vessel wall. These stents provide easier navigation to the target vessel and adaptation to the anatomy of the affected vessel. Most recently, stent retrievers have been successfully used for large-vessel revascularization with better effectiveness and improved outcomes as compared to the MERCI device. Their use also avoids permanent implantation of intracranial stents and attendant complications.

Although a recanalization rate as high as 100% can be achieved with permanent implantation of a self-expanding stent, the dual-antiplatelet therapy required to prevent in-stent thrombosis in such cases represents a major disadvantage that can lead to an increased risk of hemorrhagic complications. Furthermore, most acute intracranial artery occlusions are embolic in nature with a normal underlying blood vessel that would not benefit from placing a permanent stent versus thrombus retrieval. Most occlusions involve one or more major branches, and deployment of currently available stents is associated with obligatory jailing of these branch points, with attendant ischemia of the affected territory. Similarly, jailing of perforator territories can be associated with perforator ischemia.

Stent retrievers are still considered a step forward because they provide similar immediate recanalization, but because they are used to retrieve a clot, there is no permanent jailing of large branches or small perforators. However, instead of stents that jail the entire thrombus in place immediately upon deployment, the stent retrieval necessarily induces clot fragmentation, which raises concern for recurrent occlusion or distal or uninvolved territory embolization as the clot is retrieved.

51.9 Tool Terminology Glossary

51.9.1 Flexibility

An indication of the bending stiffness of the material. The flexural modulus is a coefficient of elasticity which represents the ratio of stress to strain as a material is deformed under dynamic load.

51.9.2 Internal Diameter (ID)

Internal diameter of a catheter. Generally measured in inch for a catheter and in French size for a sheath. Note: "Sheath sizes are labeled based on ID."

51.9.3 Kink Resistance

Refers to the ability of a tube to withstand bending and coiling without deforming or "kinking." Kinking weakens the structural strength of the tube and can block or slow down the transference of media or devices. Kink resistance is to a large extent a function of wall thickness and shore hardness.

51.9.4 Lubricity (Coefficient of Friction)

Measures the frictional properties or tackiness of material. A low coefficient of friction is usually desired in medical applications to minimize bodily trauma and tissue irritation.

51.9.5 Outer Diameter (OD)

Outer diameter of a catheter. Generally measured in French size, although microcatheters are often measured in millimeters. Note: "Catheter sizes are labeled based on OD."

51.9.6 Shore Hardness

The relative resistance of a material's surface to indentation by an indenter of specified dimensions under specified load. Shore hardness refers to the general stiffness of a material. Hardness is measured according to the durometer and Rockwell scales.

51.9.7 Tensile Strength

Tensile properties are a measure of the force required to stretch a plastic and the percent of stretching the plastic can withstand before breaking. Ultimate tensile strength is the maximum stress a material withstands at the point of rupture. A good tensile strength allows for design of thinner wall thicknesses, which result in smaller diameters. A high tensile strength also aids in ease of catheter insertion. Related to this is ultimate elongation, which is the total elongation by percentage of a sample at the point of rupture.

51.9.8 Torque

A measure of force related to the rotational stability of the tube. If rotated at one end, a tube with a high degree of torque will rotate at nearly the same ratio at the other (untouched) end. A

Table 51.14 Common neurodiagnostic catheters by region

Region	Catheters
Cervical arch	Multiside holed
CCA	Angled (Berenstein), Reverse curve (Simmons)
ECA	Angled (Berenstein)
Intracranial ICA	Microcatheter

Abbreviations: CCA, common carotid artery; ECA, external carotid artery; ICA, internal carotid artery.

high degree of torque can be desirable in invasive applications. Braiding of tubes is a method used to increase torque.

51.10 Curves of Catheters and Selective Catheters Types

Angiography can be performed from the femoral or radial arteries. The radial artery could be a safe alternative for interventions involving the right vertebral and carotid arteries where radial artery access is often easier to accomplish. Selective carotid angiography is usually performed after obtaining an aortic arch aortogram in the left anterior oblique view, which allows the operator to visualize the origin of the brachiocephalic trunk and left common carotid artery (▶ Table 51.14).

Using the same left anterior oblique angle, the brachiocephalic trunk is engaged with a diagnostic catheter. Once the origin of the common carotid artery has been engaged with a guidewire, the catheter is advanced into the common carotid artery over the wire. Care must be taken to clear the catheters and manifold of air and debris before injecting into the carotid artery. Carotid angiograms are obtained in the anterior, posterior, oblique, and lateral views.

Because of the dense bony structure of the skull, it is preferable to use digital subtraction techniques for diagnostic images of the intracranial vascular anatomy. A 12-in or larger image intensifier is optimal for intracranial angiography. It is important to emphasize using DSA for the intracranial portion of the ICA and its branches in the anterior posterior and lateral views. This enables assessment of the circle of Willis and demonstrates the presence of any collateral circulation.

51.11 Modern Inclusion/Eligibility Criteria

Updated guidelines from the American Heart Association (AHA) and the American Stroke Association (ASA) extend the time limit on mechanical clot removal from 6 up to 24 hours in select patients,[39] recommending thrombectomy in eligible patients 6 to 16 hours after a stroke.[40,41] They also broaden the eligibility criteria by allowing patients who are ineligible for intravenous tissue plasminogen activator to undergo mechanical thrombectomy within 6 hours.

The following are six recommendations of the new guidelines reported with class of recommendation (COR) and level of evidence (LOE) assigned.

1. Patients should receive mechanical thrombectomy with a stent retriever if they meet all the following criteria:
   - Prestroke modified Ranking scale (mRS) score of 0 to 1.
   - Causative occlusion of the ICA or MCA segment 1 (M1).
   - Age ≥ 18 years.
   - NIHSS score of ≥ 6.
   - ASPECTS of ≥ 6.
   - Treatment can be initiated (groin puncture) within 6 hours of symptom onset.
   COR: I
   LOE: A
2. Although the benefits are uncertain, the use of mechanical thrombectomy with stent retrievers may be reasonable for carefully selected patients with AIS in whom treatment can be initiated (groin puncture) within 6 hours of symptom onset and who have causative occlusion of the MCA segment 2 (M2) or MCA segment 3 (M3) portion of the MCAs.
   COR: IIb
   LOE: B-R
3. Although the benefits are uncertain, the use of mechanical thrombectomy with stent retrievers may be reasonable for carefully selected patients with AIS in whom treatment can be initiated (groin puncture) within 6 hours of symptom onset and who have causative occlusion of the anterior cerebral arteries, vertebral arteries, basilar artery, or posterior cerebral arteries.
   COR: IIb
   LOE: C-EO
4. Although its benefits are uncertain, the use of mechanical thrombectomy with stent retrievers may be reasonable for patients with AIS in whom treatment can be initiated (groin puncture) within 6 hours of symptom onset and who have prestroke mRS score > 1, ASPECTS < 6, or NIHSS score < 6, and causative occlusion of the ICA or proximal MCA (M1). Additional randomized trial data are needed.
   COR: IIb
   LOE: B-R
5. In selected patients with AIS within 6 to 16 hours of last known normal who have LVO in the anterior circulation and meet other DAWN or DEFUSE 3 eligibility criteria, mechanical thrombectomy is recommended.
   COR: I
   LOE: A
6. In selected patients with AIS within 16 to 24 hours of last known normal who have LVO in the anterior circulation and meet other DAWN eligibility criteria, mechanical thrombectomy is reasonable.
   COR: IIa
   LOE: B-R

51.12 Main Trials

The following is a list of the major trials for stroke. See ▶ Table 51.15, ▶ Table 51.16, ▶ Table 51.17, and ▶ Table 51.18.

Table 51.15 Designs of the major trials by era

Trial name	Arms	Size	Era	Centers	Age range	Clinical criteria	Vessel occlusion	Time window (onset to groin puncture)	CT criteria	Advanced imaging criteria
MR RESCUE	Rescue EVT vs. standard	118	2004–2011	North America—22 centers	18–85 y	NIHSS 6–29	CTA/MRA showing persistent occlusion post IVT—ICA, M1 or M2	<8 h	None	Penumbra assessment with multimodal CT or MRI for stratification but not for trial eligibility
IMS III	Bridging vs. IVT	656	Aug 2006–Apr 2012	58 centers (US, Canada, Australia, Europe)	18–82 y	NIHSS ≥10 or NIHSS 8–9 with proven vessel occlusion (ICA, M1, BA)	Not required at randomization	<5 h	None	None
SYNTHESIS	EVT vs. IVT	362 (181 vs. 181)	Feb 2008–Apr 2012	Italy—24 centers	18–80 y	NIHSS >25 excluded	Not required at randomization	<4.5 h	None	None
PISTE	Bridging vs. IVT	65 (33 vs. 32)	Apr 2013–Apr 2015	10 centers (UK)	≥18 y	NIHSS ≥6	I-ICA, M1, M2 Extracranial ICA excluded	<5.5 h	Evidence of extensive established infarction excluded	None
THERAPY	Bridging vs. IVT	108 (55 vs. 53)	Mar 2012–Oct 2014	36 centers (US and Germany)	18–85 y	NIHSS ≥8	I-ICA, M1	eligible for tPA (<4.5 h)	Any acute ischemic changes >1/3 MCA excluded	Clot length ≥8 mm
MR CLEAN	EVT vs. standard	500 (233 vs. 267)	Dec 2010 – Mar 2014	Netherlands – 16 centers	≥18 yr	NIHSS ≥2	I-ICA, M1, M2, A1, A2 Additional extra-cranial ICA or dissection at discretion of treating physician	<6 hr	None	None
ESCAPE	EVT vs. standard	315 (165 vs. 150)	Feb 2013–Oct 2014	22 centers (Canada, US, Ireland, South Korea, UK)	≥18 y	NIHSS >5	I-ICA, M1, 2-M2s, A1 Additional extracranial ICA or dissection at discretion of treating physician	<12 h	ASPECTS >5	CTA filling >50% of MCA pial collaterals, CTP = vlCBF/CBV ASPECTS >5
EXTEND_IA	Bridging vs. IVT (Solitaire only)	75 (35 vs. 35)	Aug 2012–Oct 2014	10 centers (9 Aus, 1 NZ)	≥18 y	No NIHSS cut-off	ICA, M1 or M2 dissection excluded	<6 h	None	Target mismatch: mismatch >1.2, rCBF core < 70 mL, 6 s Tmax penumbra >10 mL
SWIFT PRIME	Bridging vs. IVT (Solitaire only)	196 (98 vs. 98)	Dec 2012–Nov 2014	39 centers (US and Europe)	18–80	NIHSS 8–29	I-ICA, M1 Extracranial ICA excluded (including dissection)	<6 h	Revised small core (ASPECTS >5)	Initially target mismatch (core <50 mL, 10 s Tmax lesion <100 mL, penumbra > 15 mL and mismatch ≥ 1.8)

(Continued)

Table 51.15 (Continued) Designs of the major trials by era

Trial name	Arms	Size	Era	Centers	Age range	Clinical criteria	Vessel occlusion	Time window (onset to groin puncture)	CT criteria	Advanced imaging criteria
REVASCAT	EVT vs. standard (Solitaire only)	206 (103 vs. 103)	Nov 2012–Dec 2014	4 centers Spain (Catalonia)	18–80	NIHSS > 5	I-ICA, M1	< 8 h	ASPECTS > 6 (> 5 on DWI)	No recanalization on CTA/MRA after ≥ 30 min from start of tPA infusion If CTA/MRA performed > 4.5 h from onset then CBV ASPECTS, CTA-SI ASPECTS. or DWI-MR ASPECTS must be performed
THRACE	Bridging vs. IVT	412 (208 vs. 204)	June 2010–Feb 2015	26 centers France (mothership only model)	18–80	NIHSS 10–25 I	I-ICA, M1, upper 1/3 basilar artery *Ipsilateral E-ICA, stenosis/ occlusion excluded*	< 5 h	None	None
DEFUSE 3	Outcome in patient undergoing ETV with good collaterals vs. poor collaterals on CTA	130 (97 vs. 33)	April 2016–August 2017	38 centers in the United States	18–90	NIHSS ≥ 6	ICA or MCA-M1 occlusion	6–16 h	None	ICA or MCA-M1 occlusion (carotid occlusions can be cervical or intracranial; with or without tandem MCA lesions) by MRA or CTA *and* Target mismatch profile on CT perfusion or MRI (ischemic core volume is < 70 mL, mismatch ratio is ≥ 1.8 and mismatch volume is ≥ 15 mL)
DAWN	Outcome in thrombectomy + standard medical care vs. standard medical care alone	206 (107 vs. 99)	Sep 2014–Feb 2017	26 centers in US, Canada, Europe, and Australia	≥ 18 y	Patients had to have a mismatch between the severity of the clinical deficit and the infarct volume: those in Group A were 80 y of age or older, had a NIHSS score of 10 or higher and had an infarct volume of < 21 mL; those in Group B were younger than 80 y, had a score of 10 or higher on the NIHSS, and had an infarct volume of < 31 mL; and those in Group C were younger than 80 y, had a score of 20 or higher on the NIHSS, and had an infarct volume of 31 to < 51 mL	ICA or MCA-M1 occlusion	6–24 h	None	No evidence of intracranial hemorrhage on CT or MRI, and no evidence of an infarct involving more than one-third of the territory of the MCA on CT or MRI at baseline

Abbreviations: CTA, computed tomography angiography; CTP, CT perfusion; EVT, endovascular thrombectomy; I-ICA, intracranial internal carotid artery; IVT, intravitreal injection; MCA, middle cerebral artery; M1, first portion of the middle cerebral artery, from the origin to the bifurcation/trifurcation; M2, second portion of the middle cerebral artery; NIHSS, National Institutes of Health Stroke Scale; ASPECTS, Alberta Stroke Program Early CT Score; vlCBF, very low cerebral blood volume.

Table 51.16 Major trial baseline characteristics

Trial name	Age (median)	Male (%)	NIHSS (median)	Vessel occlusion	Tandem lesion (extracranial ICA occlusion)	ASPECTS (median)	IVT (%)	Retrievable stent (%)
MR RESCUE[a]	66	50	16	71% ICA or M1	nr	predicted core 36 mL	47	0
IMS III	69	50	17	18% of EVT group had no occlusion	nr	nr	100	4
SYNTHESIS	66	59	13	2% no occlusion	nr	nr	0	41
PISTE	67	39	18	90% carotid T/L or M1	3%	9	100	68
THERAPY	67	62	17	89% I-ICA or M1	Excluded	7.5	100	13% (majority used aspiration thrombectomy)
MR CLEAN	66	58	17	92% I-ICA, carotid T or M1	32%	9	87 (44% drip and ship)	82
ESCAPE	71	48 (87% white)	16	96% carotid T/L or M1	13%	9	73	73
EXTEND_IA	69	49	17	88% I-ICA or M1	n/r	nr (median core 12 mL)	100	100
SWIFT PRIME	65	55 (89% white)	17	86% carotid T/L or M1	Excluded	9	100 (44% drip and ship)	100
REVASCAT	65	55	17	90% carotid T/L or M1		7	70	70
THRACE	66	57	18	98% ICA or M1	Excluded	nr	100 (100% mothership)	77
DEFUSE 3	70.5 (59–80)	49.5% (86.8% white)	16	82% MCA	nr	8	100%	nr
DAWN	69.4 vs. 70.7	42 vs. 51	17	83 vs. 77% M1	nr	nr	51	100

Abbreviations: EVT, endovascular thrombectomy; I-ICA, intracranial internal carotid artery; IVT, intravitreal injection; MCA, middle cerebral artery; M1, first portion of the middle cerebral artery, from the origin to the bifurcation/trifurcation; NIHSS, National Institutes of Health Stroke Scale; ASPECTS, Alberta Stroke Program Early CT Score; nr, not reported.
[a]MR RESCUE values reported for penumbral group receiving embolectomy.

Table 51.17 Individual process times

Trial name	Onset to IVT (median, min)	Onset to randomization (median, min)	Onset to groin puncture (median, min)	Onset to first reperfusion (median, min)	Groin puncture to reperfusion (median, min)	IVT to groin puncture (median, min)	CT to groin puncture (median, min)	CT to reperfusion (median, min)
MR RESCUE	nr	nr	381	nr	nr	nr	124	nr
IMS III	122	nr	208	nr	nr	nr	nr	nr
SYNTHESIS	165	148	225	nr	nr	nr	nr	nr
PISTE	120	150	209	259	49[a]	82	58[b]	nr
THERAPY	108	181	227	nr	nr	nr	123	nr
MR CLEAN	85	204	260	332	nr	nr	nr	nr
ESCAPE	110	169	208	241	30	51	51	84
EXTEND_IA	127	256	210	248	43	74	93	nr
SWIFT PRIME	111	191	244	252	nr	nr	58	87
REVASCAT	118	223	269	355	59	nr	67	nr
THRACE	150	168	250	nr	nr	nr	nr	nr
DEFUSE 3	nr	10:15 h (10:16 vs. 9:46)	11:35 h (11:28 vs. 11:48)	12:34 h (12:23 vs. 12:39)	nr	nr	nr	nr
DAWN	nr	4.8 vs. 5.6	nr	nr	nr	nr	nr	Nr

Abbreviations: IVT, intravitreal injection; nr, not recorded.
[a]Groin puncture to device removal.
[b]Randomization to groin puncture.

Table 51.18 Major trial outcomes by era

Trial name	Recanalization (%, EVT vs. control)	Reperfusion (mTICI 2b/3, %)	Primary outcome	mRS at day 90	mRS 0–2 at day 90	Final infarct volume (mL)	sICH (PH-2, %)	Death at day 90 (%)	New AIS in a different territory (%)	SAE (%)
MR RESCUE	69	27	mRS 3.8 vs. 3.4	3.8 vs. 3.4	21 vs. 26	32 vs. 32	9 vs. 6	18 vs. 21	1.4	62
IMS III	81 ICA; 86 M1; 88 M2	38 ICA; 44 M1; 44 M2	mRS 0–2: 41 vs. 39%	nr	41 vs. 39	nr	6 vs. 6	19 vs. 21	nr	nr
SYNTHESIS	nr	nr	mRS 0–1: 30 vs. 35%	nr	42 vs. 46	nr	6 vs. 6	8 vs. 6	nr	nr
PISTE	69	87	OR 2.12 mRS 0–2; p=0.2	nr	51 to 40 vo NNT=9	nr	0 vs. 0	7 vs. 4	nr	45 vs. 34
THERAPY	nr	70	mRS 0–2: 38 vs. 30%; p=0.44	nr	38 vs. 30 ns	nr	9.3 vs. 9.7	12 vs. 24	nr	42 vs. 48
MR CLEAN	75 vs. 33	59	mRS 3 vs. 4 day 90	3 vs. 4	33 vs. 19 NNT=7	49 vs. 79	6 vs. 5	21 vs. 22	5.6	47 vs. 42
ESCAPE	nr vs. 31 (mAOL 2–3)	72	cOR 2.6	2 vs. 4	53 vs. 29 NNT=4	nr	4 vs. 3	10 vs. 19 (significant)	nr	21 vs. 18
EXTEND_IA	94 vs. 43 (TIMI 2–3)	86	24 h reperfusion: 100 vs. 37% Early neurological recovery: 82 vs. 37%	1 vs. 3	71 vs. 40 NNT=3	23 vs. 53	0 vs. 6	9 vs. 20 (p=0.18)	5.7	nr
SWIFT PRIME	nr	88	Shift analysis. p=0.0002	2 vs. 3	60 vs. 36 NNT=4	nr	1 vs. 3	9 vs. 12 (p=0.5)	nr	36 vs. 31
REVASCAT	nr	66	cOR 1.7	nr	44 vs. 28 NNT=6	16 vs. 39	5 vs. 2	18 vs. 16	5	30 vs. 25
THRACE	78	69	mRS 0–2 at day 90: 53 vs. 42%	nr	53 vs. 42 NNT=9	nr	2 vs. 2	12 vs. 13	6	8 vs. 7
DEFUSE 3	42 vs. 12	38 vs. 9	mRS 0–2 at day 90: 29 vs. 13%	nr	29 vs. 13	At 24 h 32.9 mL vs. 65.7 mL	6 vs. 2	18 vs. 8	nr	nr
DAWN	82 vs. 39	nr	mRS at day 90: 5.5 ± 3.8 vs. 3.4 ± 3.1	5.5 ± 3.8 vs. 3.4 ± 3.1	nr	At 24 h 8 vs. 22 mL (median)	6 vs. 3	20 vs. 18	nr	7 procedure-related complications

Abbreviations: cOR, common Odd Ratio; EVT, endovascular thrombectomy; tPA tissue plasminogen activator; nr, not recorded; mAOL, modified arterial occlusion lesion score; TIMI, thrombolysis in myocardial infarction score; mTICI, modified thrombolysis in cerebral infarction score; mRS, modified Ranking scale; sICH, symptomatic intracranial hemorrhage; PH-2, parenchymal hematoma 2, i.e., > 30% of the infarcted area with significant space-occupying effect, or clot remote from infarcted area; AIS, acute ischemic stroke; SAE, serious adverse events.

References

[1] Alexandrov AV, Grotta JC. Arterial reocclusion in stroke patients treated with intravenous tissue plasminogen activator. Neurology. 2002; 59(6):862–867

[2] Soares BP, Tong E, Hom J, et al. Reperfusion is a more accurate predictor of follow-up infarct volume than recanalization: a proof of concept using CT in acute ischemic stroke patients. Stroke. 2010; 41(1):e34–e40

[3] Tomsick T, Broderick J, Carrozzella J, et al. Interventional Management of Stroke II Investigators. Revascularization results in the interventional management of stroke II trial. AJNR Am J Neuroradiol. 2008; 29(3):582–587

[4] Zaidat OO, Suarez JI, Sunshine JL, et al. Thrombolytic therapy of acute ischemic stroke: correlation of angiographic recanalization with clinical outcome. AJNR Am J Neuroradiol. 2005; 26(4):880–884

[5] Fields JD, Lutsep HL, Smith WS, MERCI Multi MERCI Investigators. Higher degrees of recanalization after mechanical thrombectomy for acute stroke are associated with improved outcome and decreased mortality: pooled analysis of the MERCI and Multi MERCI trials. AJNR Am J Neuroradiol. 2011; 32(11):2170–2174

[6] von Kummer R, Holle R, Rosin L, Forsting M, Hacke W. Does arterial recanalization improve outcome in carotid territory stroke? Stroke. 1995; 26 (4):581–587

[7] Arnold M, Nedeltchev K, Remonda L, et al. Recanalisation of middle cerebral artery occlusion after intra-arterial thrombolysis: different recanalisation grading systems and clinical functional outcome. J Neurol Neurosurg Psychiatry. 2005; 76(10):1373–1376

[8] Nam HS, Lee KY, Kim YD, et al. Failure of complete recanalization is associated with poor outcome after cardioembolic stroke. Eur J Neurol. 2011; 18(9):1171–1178

[9] Yoo AJ, Simonsen CZ, Prabhakaran S, et al. Cerebral Angiographic Revascularization Grading Collaborators. Refining angiographic biomarkers of revascularization: improving outcome prediction after intra-arterial therapy. Stroke. 2013; 44(9):2509–2512

[10] Suh SH, Cloft HJ, Fugate JE, Rabinstein AA, Liebeskind DS, Kallmes DF. Clarifying differences among thrombolysis in cerebral infarction scale variants: is the artery half open or half closed? Stroke. 2013; 44(4):1166–1168

[11] Rha JH, Saver JL. The impact of recanalization on ischemic stroke outcome: a meta-analysis. Stroke. 2007; 38(3):967–973

[12] Chesebro JH, Knatterud G, Roberts R, et al. Thrombolysis in Myocardial Infarction (TIMI) Trial, Phase I: A comparison between intravenous tissue plasminogen activator and intravenous streptokinase. Clinical findings through hospital discharge. Circulation. 1987; 76(1):142–154

[13] Braunwald E, Knatterud GL, Terrin ML, et al. The Thrombolysis in Myocardial Infarction (TIMI) Trial. Phase I findings. N Engl J Med. 1985; 312(14):932–936

[14] Khatri P, Neff J, Broderick JP, Khoury JC, Carrozzella J, Tomsick T, IMS-I Investigators. Revascularization end points in stroke interventional trials: recanalization versus reperfusion in IMS-I. Stroke. 2005; 36(11):2400–2403

[15] Higashida RT, Furlan AJ, Roberts H, et al. Technology Assessment Committee of the American Society of Interventional and Therapeutic Neuroradiology, Technology Assessment Committee of the Society of Interventional Radiology. Trial design and reporting standards for intra-arterial cerebral thrombolysis for acute ischemic stroke. Stroke. 2003; 34(8):e109–e137

[16] Kallmes DF. TICI: if you are not confused, then you are not paying attention. AJNR Am J Neuroradiol. 2012; 33(5):975–976

[17] Zaidat OO, Yoo AJ, Khatri P, et al. Cerebral Angiographic Revascularization Grading (CARG) Collaborators, STIR Revascularization working group, STIR Thrombolysis in Cerebral Infarction (TICI) Task Force. Recommendations on angiographic revascularization grading standards for acute ischemic stroke: a consensus statement. Stroke. 2013; 44(9):2650–2663

[18] Sugg R, Holloway W, Martin C, Akhtar N, Rymer M. Recanalization vs reperfusion as vascular end points in acute ischemic stroke endovascular intervention. J Neurointerv Surg. 2011

[19] Almekhlafi MA, Mishra S, Desai JA, et al. Not all "successful" angiographic reperfusion patients are an equal validation of a modified TICI scoring system. Interv Neuroradiol. 2014; 20(1):21–27

[20] Barber PA, Demchuk AM, Zhang J, Buchan AM. Validity and reliability of a quantitative computed tomography score in predicting outcome of hyperacute stroke before thrombolytic therapy. ASPECTS Study Group. Alberta Stroke Programme Early CT Score. Lancet. 2000; 355(9216):1670–1674

[21] Puetz V, Sylaja PN, Coutts SB, et al. Extent of hypoattenuation on CT angiography source images predicts functional outcome in patients with basilar artery occlusion. Stroke. 2008; 39(9):2485–2490

[22] Douglas AC, Wippold FJ, II, Broderick DF, et al. ACR appropriateness criteria headache. J Am Coll Radiol. 2014; 11(7):657–667

[23] Salmela MB, Mortazavi S, Jagadeesan BD, et al. Expert Panel on Neurologic Imaging. ACR Appropriateness Criteria® cerebrovascular disease. J Am Coll Radiol. 2017; 14 5S:S34–S61

[24] Torres-Mozqueda F, He J, Yeh IB, et al. An acute ischemic stroke classification instrument that includes CT or MR angiography: the Boston Acute Stroke Imaging Scale. AJNR Am J Neuroradiol. 2008; 29(6):1111–1117

[25] Wintermark M, Ko NU, Smith WS, Liu S, Higashida RT, Dillon WP. Vasospasm after subarachnoid hemorrhage: utility of perfusion CT and CT angiography on diagnosis and management. AJNR Am J Neuroradiol. 2006; 27(1):26–34

[26] Srinivasan A, Goyal M, Al Azri F, Lum C. State-of-the-art imaging of acute stroke. Radiographics. 2007; 26(Suppl 1):S75–S95

[27] Lin K, Rapalino O, Law M, Babb JS, Siller KA, Pramanik BK. Accuracy of the Alberta Stroke Program Early CT score during the first 3 hours of middle cerebral artery stroke: comparison of noncontrast CT, CT angiography source images, and CT perfusion. AJNR Am J Neuroradiol. 2008; 29(5):931–936

[28] Konstas AA, Goldmakher GV, Lee TY, Lev MH. Theoretic basis and technical implementations of CT perfusion in acute ischemic stroke, part 2: technical implementations. AJNR Am J Neuroradiol. 2009; 30(5):885–892

[29] Hacke W, Kaste M, Fieschi C, et al. Second European-Australasian Acute Stroke Study Investigators. Randomised double-blind placebo-controlled trial of thrombolytic therapy with intravenous alteplase in acute ischaemic stroke (ECASS II). Lancet. 1998; 352(9136):1245–1251

[30] Cheng-Ching E, Frontera JA, Man S, et al. Degree of collaterals and not time is the determining factor of core infarct volume within 6 hours of stroke onset. AJNR Am J Neuroradiol. 2015; 36(7):1272–1276

[31] Goyal M, Demchuk AM, Menon BK, et al. ESCAPE Trial Investigators. Randomized assessment of rapid endovascular treatment of ischemic stroke. N Engl J Med. 2015; 372(11):1019–1030

[32] Roberts HC, Dillon WP, Furlan AJ, et al. Angiographic collaterals in acute stroke—relationship to clinical presentation and outcome: The PROACT II trial. Stroke. 2001; 32(1):336–336

[33] Lima FO, Furie KL, Silva GS, et al. The pattern of leptomeningeal collaterals on CT angiography is a strong predictor of long-term functional outcome in stroke patients with large vessel intracranial occlusion. Stroke. 2010; 41 (10):2316–2322

[34] Saver JL, Goyal M, Bonafe A, et al. SWIFT PRIME Investigators. Solitaire™ with the Intention for Thrombectomy as Primary Endovascular Treatment for Acute Ischemic Stroke (SWIFT PRIME) trial: protocol for a randomized, controlled, multicenter study comparing the Solitaire revascularization device with IV tPA with IV tPA alone in acute ischemic stroke. Int J Stroke. 2015; 10(3):439–448

[35] Asadi H, Dowling R, Yan B, Wong S, Mitchell P. Advances in endovascular treatment of acute ischaemic stroke. Intern Med J. 2015; 45(8):798–805

[36] Smith WS, Sung G, Starkman S, et al. MERCI Trial Investigators. Safety and efficacy of mechanical embolectomy in acute ischemic stroke: results of the MERCI trial. Stroke. 2005; 36(7):1432–1438

[37] Kang D-H, Kim Y-S, Park J, Hwang Y-H. Rescue forced suction thrombectomy using the reperfusion catheter of the Penumbra System for thromboembolism during coil embolization of ruptured cerebral aneurysms. Neurosurgery. 2012; 70

[38] Turk AS, Spiotta A, Frei D, et al. Initial clinical experience with the ADAPT technique: a direct aspiration first pass technique for stroke thrombectomy. J Neurointerv Surg. 2018; 10 Suppl 1:i20–i25

[39] Powers WJ, Rabinstein AA, Ackerson T, et al. American Heart Association Stroke Council. 2018 Guidelines for the early management of patients with acute ischemic stroke: a guideline for healthcare professionals from the American Heart Association/American Stroke Association. Stroke. 2018; 49 (3):e46–e110

[40] Albers GW, Marks MP, Kemp S, et al. DEFUSE 3 Investigators. Thrombectomy for stroke at 6 to 16 hours with selection by perfusion imaging. N Engl J Med. 2018; 378(8):708–718

[41] Nogueira RG, Jadhav AP, Haussen DC, et al. DAWN Trial Investigators. Thrombectomy 6 to 24 hours after stroke with a mismatch between deficit and infarct. N Engl J Med. 2018; 378(1):11–21

Index